Magnesium
in the
Central Nervous System

This book is available as a free fully-searchable PDF
from

www.adelaide.edu.au/press

Black and white images in this print edition
are in colour

You can read the print and PDF in tandem

Magnesium in the Central Nervous System

EDITED BY

ROBERT VINK

Discipline of Anatomy and Pathology & Adelaide Centre for Neuroscience Research, School of Medical Sciences, The University of Adelaide, Adelaide, South Australia, Australia

MIHAI NECHIFOR

Department of Pharmacology, "Gr. T. Popa" University of Medicine and Pharmacy, Iasi, Romania

UNIVERSITY OF ADELAIDE PRESS

THE UNIVERSITY of ADELAIDE

SUB CRUCE LUMEN

Published in Adelaide by

University of Adelaide Press
Barr Smith Library
The University of Adelaide
South Australia
5005
press@adelaide.edu.au
www.adelaide.edu.au/press

The University of Adelaide Press publishes externally refereed scholarly books by staff of the University of Adelaide. It aims to maximise the accessibility to its best research by publishing works through the internet as free downloads and as high quality printed volumes on demand.

Electronic Index: this book is available from the website as a down-loadable PDF with fully searchable text. Please use the electronic version to serve as the index.

For the full Cataloguing-in-Publication data please contact National Library of Australia

Magnesium in the central nervous system / edited by Robert Vink and Mihai Nechifor.

I Vink, Robert.
II Nechifor, Mihai.

1 Magnesium—Physiological effect.
2 Magnesium in the body.
3 Central nervous system.

ISBN (electronic) 978-0-9870730-5-1
ISBN (paperback) 978-0-9870730-6-8

Book design: Robert Vink
Cover design: Emma Spoehr. Photograph with permission, istockphoto.com

List of Contributors

Bulent Ahishali

Istanbul University, Istanbul Faculty of Medicine, Department of Physiology & Department of Histology and Embryology, Capa 34093 Istanbul, Turkey

Jean-Pierre Bali

Université Montpellier I, 34000 Montpellier, France

Jean-Marie Billard

Université Paris Descartes, Faculté de Médecine René Descartes, Centre de Psychiatrie et Neurosciences, UMR 894, Paris, 75014, France

Kym Campbell

Centre for Neuromuscular and Neurological Disorders, University of Western Australia & Australian Neuromuscular Research Institute, Department of Neurosurgery, Sir Charles Gairdner Hospital, Nedlands, Western Australia, Australia

Yves Cazals

UMR6231, Université Paul Cézanne, Marseille, France

Zheng Chen

Department of Psychiatry & Institute for Geriatric Clinic and Rehabilitation, Beijing Geriatric Hospital, Beijing 100095, China

Dehua Chui

Neuroscience Research Institute & Department of Neurobiology, Key Laboratory for Neuroscience, Ministry of Education & Ministry of Public Health, Health Science Center, Peking University, Beijing 100191, China

Naomi L. Cook

Discipline of Anatomy and Pathology, School of Medical Sciences & Adelaide Centre for Neuroscience Research, The University of Adelaide, Adelaide, South Australia, Australia

Frances Corrigan

Discipline of Anatomy and Pathology, School of Medical Sciences & Adelaide Centre for Neuroscience Research, The University of Adelaide, Adelaide, South Australia, Australia

Magdalena D. Cuciureanu

Department of Pharmacology, "Gr. T. Popa" University of Medicine and Pharmacy 16, Iasi, Romania

Sang-Hwan Do

Department of Anesthesiology and Pain medicine, Seoul National University Bundang Hospital, Seongnam, South Korea

George A. Eby III

George Eby Research Institute, 14909-C Fitzhugh Road, Austin, Texas, USA

Karen L. Eby

George Eby Research Institute, 14909-C Fitzhugh Road, Austin, Texas, USA

Mounir N. Ghabriel

Discipline of Anatomy and Pathology, School of Medical Sciences & Adelaide Centre for Neuroscience Research, The University of Adelaide, Adelaide, South Australia, Australia

Tomoyo Hashimoto

Department of Internal Medicine (Neurology and Rheumatology), Shinshu University School of Medicine, Nagano, Japan

Michael R. Hoane

Restorative Neuroscience Laboratory, Brain and Cognitive Science Program, Department of Psychology Southern Illinois University, Carbondale, Illinois, USA

Xavier Holy

Institut de Recherche Biomédicale des Armées, Antenne de Brétigny, Brétigny-sur-Orge, France

Stefano Iotti

Dipartimento di Medicina Interna, dell'Invecchiamento e Malattie Nefrologiche, Università di Bologna, Italy and Istituto Nazionale di Biostrutture e Biosistemi, Roma, Italy

Mehmet Kaya

Istanbul University, Istanbul Faculty of Medicine, Department of Physiology & Department of Histology and Embryology, Capa 34093 Istanbul, Turkey

Neville W. Knuckey

Centre for Neuromuscular and Neurological Disorders, University of Western Australia, & Australian Neuromuscular Research Institute, Department of Neurosurgery, Sir Charles Gairdner Hospital, Nedlands, Western Australia, Australia

Marzia Leidi

Università di Milano, Dipartimento di Scienze Cliniche Luigi Sacco, Via G.B. Grassi 74, 20157 Milano, Italy

Yi Liu

Neuroscience Research Institute & Department of Neurobiology, Key Laboratory for Neuroscience, Ministry of Education & Ministry of Public Health, Health Science Center, Peking University, Beijing 100191, China

Jeanette A.M. Maier

Università di Milano, Dipartimento di Scienze Cliniche Luigi Sacco, Via G.B. Grassi 74, 20157 Milano, Italy

Emil Malucelli

Dipartimento di Medicina Interna, dell'Invecchiamento e Malattie Nefrologiche' Università di Bologna, Italy

Lucia Mastrototaro

Istituto di Patologia Generale e Centro di Ricerche Oncologiche Giovanni XXIII, Università Cattolica del Sacro Cuore, Rome, Italy

Alexander Mauskop

The New York Headache Center, 30 East 76th Street, New York, NY, USA

Bruno P. Meloni

Centre for Neuromuscular and Neurological Disorders, University of Western Australia, & Australian Neuromuscular Research Institute, Department of Neurosurgery, Sir Charles Gairdner Hospital, Nedlands, Western Australia, Australia

Marianne Mousain-Bosc

Ecole de l'ADN, Museum d'Histoire Naturelle de Nîmes, 19, Grand'rue, 30000 Nimes, France

Harald Murck

Clinic of Psychiatry and Psychotherapy, University of Marburg, Marburg, Germany

Hyo-Seok Na

Department of Anesthesiology and Pain medicine, Seoul National University Bundang Hospital, Seongnam, South Korea

Mihai Nechifor

Department of Pharmacology, "Gr. T. Popa" University of Medicine and Pharmacy, Iasi, Romania

Kiyomitsu Oyanagi

Department of Brain Disease Research, Shinshu University School of Medicine, Nagano Japan

Victoria Papadopol

Regional Centre of Public Health Iaşi, Romania

Florent Raffin

Institut de Recherche Biomédicale des Armées, Antenne de la Tronche, La Tronche, France

Andrea M.P. Romani

Department of Physiology and Biophysics, School of Medicine, Case Western Reserve University, Cleveland, Ohio USA

Harry Rubin

Department of Molecular and Cell Biology, Life Sciences Addition, University of California, Berkeley, CA, USA

Jung-Hee Ryu

Department of Anesthesiology and Pain medicine, Seoul National University Bundang Hospital, Seongnam, South Korea

Jeffrey L. Saver

UCLA Stroke Center, Geffen School of Medicine of the University of California, Los Angeles, CA, USA

Isabelle Sendowski

Institut de Recherche Biomédicale des Armées, Antenne de la Tronche, La Tronche, France

Christian Siatka

Ecole de l'ADN, Museum d'Histoire Naturelle de Nîmes, 19, grand'rue, 30000 Nimes, France

Yuetao Song

Department of Psychiatry & Institute for Geriatric Clinic and Rehabilitation, Beijing Geriatric Hospital, Beijing 100095, China

Sidney Starkman

UCLA Stroke Center, Geffen School of Medicine of the University of California, Los Angeles, CA, USA

Valentina Trapani

Istituto di Patologia Generale e Centro di Ricerche Oncologiche Giovanni XXIII, Università Cattolica del Sacro Cuore, Rome, Italy

Walter M. van den Bergh

Department of Intensive Care, Academic Medical Center, 1100 DD Amsterdam, The Netherlands

Corinna van den Heuvel

Discipline of Anatomy and Pathology, School of Medical Sciences & Adelaide Centre for Neuroscience Research, The University of Adelaide, Adelaide, South Australia, Australia

Robert Vink

Discipline of Anatomy and Pathology, School of Medical Sciences & Adelaide Centre for Neuroscience Research, The University of Adelaide, Adelaide, South Australia, Australia

Weishan Wang

Department of Psychiatry & Institute for Geriatric Clinic and Rehabilitation, Beijing Geriatric Hospital, Beijing 100095, China

Federica I. Wolf

Istituto di Patologia Generale e Centro di Ricerche Oncologiche Giovanni XXIII, Università Cattolica del Sacro Cuore, Rome, Italy

Lisa A. Yablon

The New York Headache Center, 30 East 76th Street, New York, NY, USA

Huan Yang

Neuroscience Research Institute & Department of Neurobiology, Key Laboratory for Neuroscience, Ministry of Education & Ministry of Public Health, Health Science Center, Peking University, Beijing 100191, China

Jia Yu

Department of Psychiatry & Institute for Geriatric Clinic and Rehabilitation, Beijing Geriatric Hospital, Beijing 100095, China

Honglin Zhang

Department of Psychiatry & Institute for Geriatric Clinic and Rehabilitation, Beijing Geriatric Hospital, Beijing 100095, China

Preface

The brain is the most complex organ in our body. Indeed, it is perhaps the most complex structure we have ever encountered in nature. Both structurally and functionally, there are many peculiarities that differentiate the brain from all other organs. The brain is our connection to the world around us and by governing nervous system and higher function, any disturbance induces severe neurological and psychiatric disorders that can have a devastating effect on quality of life.

Our understanding of the physiology and biochemistry of the brain has improved dramatically in the last two decades. In particular, the critical role of cations, including magnesium, has become evident, even if incompletely understood at a mechanistic level. The exact role and regulation of magnesium, in particular, remains elusive, largely because intracellular levels are so difficult to routinely quantify. Nonetheless, the importance of magnesium to normal central nervous system activity is self-evident given the complicated homeostatic mechanisms that maintain the concentration of this cation within strict limits essential for normal physiology and metabolism. There is also considerable accumulating evidence to suggest alterations to some brain functions in both normal and pathological conditions may be linked to alterations in local magnesium concentration.

This book, containing chapters written by some of the foremost experts in the field of magnesium research, brings together the latest in experimental and clinical magnesium research as it relates to the central nervous system. It offers a complete and updated view of magnesium's involvement in central nervous system function and in so doing, brings together two main pillars of contemporary neuroscience research, namely providing an explanation for the molecular mechanisms involved in brain function, and emphasizing the connections between the molecular changes and behavior.

It is the untiring efforts of those magnesium researchers who have dedicated their lives to unraveling the mysteries of magnesium's role in biological systems that has inspired the collation of this volume of work.

Robert Vink
Mihai Nechifor

List of Contributors v

Preface viii

Section 1: Magnesium in Normal Brain

Chapter 1 **Free magnesium concentration in human brain** 3
Stefano Iotti and Emil Malucelli

Chapter 2 **Intracellular magnesium homeostasis** 13
Andrea M.P. Romani

Chapter 3 **Magnesium transport across the blood-brain barriers** 59
Mounir N. Ghabriel and Robert Vink

Chapter 4 **Intracellular free Mg^{2+} and $MgATP^{2-}$ in coordinate control of protein synthesis and cell proliferation** 75
Harry Rubin

Chapter 5 **Magnesium and the Yin-Yang interplay in apoptosis** 85
Valentina Trapani, Lucia Mastrototaro and Federica I. Wolf

Chapter 6 **Brain magnesium homeostasis as a target for reducing cognitive ageing** 99
Jean-Marie Billard

Section 2: Magnesium in Neurological Diseases

Chapter 7 **The role of magnesium therapy in learning and memory** 115
Michael R. Hoane

Chapter 8 **The role of magnesium in headache and migraine** 125
Lisa A. Yablon and Alexander Mauskop

Chapter 9 **Magnesium in edema and blood-brain barrier disruption** 135
Mehmet Kaya and Bulent Ahishali

Chapter 10 **Magnesium and hearing loss** 145
Isabelle Sendowski, Xavier Holy, Florent Raffin and Yves Cazals

Chapter 11 **The role of magnesium in pain** 157
Hyo-Seok Na, Jung-Hee Ryu and Sang-Hwan Do

Chapter 12 **The role of magnesium in traumatic CNS injury** 167
Naomi L. Cook, Frances Corrigan and Corinna van den Heuvel

Chapter 13 **The use of magnesium in experimental cerebral ischaemia** 181
Bruno P. Meloni, Kym Campbell and Neville W. Knuckey

Chapter 14 **Magnesium in subarachnoid hemorrhage** 193
Walter M. van den Bergh

Chapter 15 **Magnesium in clinical stroke** 205
Jeffrey L. Saver and Sidney Starkman

Chapter 16 **Magnesium in cancer: more questions than answers** 217
Marzia Leidi, Federica I. Wolf and Jeanette A.M. Maier

Chapter 17 **Magnesium in Parkinson's disease: an update in clinical and basic aspects** 229
Kiyomitsu Oyanagi and Tomoyo Hashimoto

Section 3: Involvement of Magnesium in Psychiatric Diseases

Chapter 18	**Magnesium and Alzheimer's disease** *Dehua Chui, Zheng Chen, Jia Yu, Honglin Zhang, Weishan Wang Yuetao Song, Huan Yang and Yi Liu*	**239**
Chapter 19	**Magnesium and stress** *Magdalena D. Cuciureanu and Robert Vink*	**251**
Chapter 20	**Magnesium in neuroses** *Victoria Papadopol and Mihai Nechifor*	**269**
Chapter 21	**Magnesium, hyperactivity and autism in children** *Marianne Mousain-Bosc, Christian Siatka and Jean-Pierre Bali*	**283**
Chapter 22	**Magnesium in psychoses (schizophrenia, bipolar disorder)** *Mihai Nechifor*	**303**
Chapter 23	**Magnesium and major depression** *George A. Eby III, Karen L. Eby and Harald Murck*	**313**
Chapter 24	**Magnesium in drug abuse and addiction** *Mihai Nechifor*	**333**

Electronic Index: this book is available from the website adelaide.edu.au/press as a free downloadable PDF with fully searchable text. Please use the electronic version to serve as the index.

Section 1

Magnesium in Normal Brain

Free magnesium concentration in human brain

Stefano Iotti [1,2,✉] *and Emil Malucelli* [1]

[1] Dipartimento di Medicina Interna, dell'Invecchiamento e Malattie Nefrologiche, Università di Bologna, Italy.
[2] Istituto Nazionale di Biostrutture e Biosistemi, Roma, Italy.
✉ stefano.iotti@unibo.it

Abstract

The cytosolic free magnesium concentration can be assessed *in vivo* in human brain by phosphorus magnetic resonance spectroscopy. This technique has been employed in human brain providing new hints on the Mg^{2+} homeostasis and on its involvement on the cellular bioenergetics. The free cytosolic [Mg^{2+}] measured in the human brain is about half of that assessed in the human skeletal muscle. This result is likely related to the lower ATP concentration of brain tissue. The possibility to assess the cytosolic [Mg^{2+}] in human brain opened the chance to study the involvement of Mg^{2+} in different neurological pathologies, and particularly in those where the defective mitochondrial energy production represents the primary causative factor in pathogenesis. The results obtained, studying patients affected by different types of mitochondrial cytopathies, helped to clarify the functional relationship between the energy metabolism and free [Mg^{2+}], providing evidences that the cytosolic [Mg^{2+}] is a function of the energy charge of brain cells and a defective mitochondrial respiration causes a derangement of cytosolic [Mg^{2+}] homeostasis. A reduced cytosolic [Mg^{2+}] has been also found in the occipital lobes of patients with different types of migraine and cluster headache, showing among migraine patients, a trend in keeping with the severity of clinical phenotype. In addition, the assessment by phosphorus magnetic resonance spectroscopy of brain [Mg^{2+}] can help in the differential diagnosis of Multiple System Atrophy and Parkinson's disease, offering a new diagnostic tool that may help to differentiate neurodegenerative diseases sharing common clinical features.

Introduction

Inorganic phosphate (Pi), phosphocreatine (PCr), and ATP are the principal Mg^{+2} ligands among the phosphorylated molecules present in the cell cytosol detectable by phosphorus magnetic resonance spectroscopy (^{31}P-MRS) (Figure 1). Nevertheless, in the cytosol matrix magnesium is primarily bound to ATP. As a consequence, in the living organism, ATP is present mainly in the form $MgATP^{2-}$ (Iotti *et al*, 1996) (Figure 2) that is the active species in enzyme binding (Kuby and Noltman, 1959), as well as the energy producing form in active transport (Skou, 1982; Repke, 1982) and muscular contraction (Ramirez, Marecek 1980; Wells *et al*, 1980).

The amount of magnesium bound to ATP shifts the resonance frequencies measured by ^{31}P-MRS of signals coming from the three phosphoric groups α, β, γ of the molecule (chemical shift). Due to the chemical equilibrium between the Mg bound to ATP and free Mg^{2+}, the chemical shift of ATP signals is function of free Mg^{2+} concentration (Figure 3). The *in vivo* assessment of cytosolic Mg^{2+} concentration ([Mg^{2+}]) in human brain needs a specific calibration curve that should satisfy precise criteria. In particular, the calibration curve should take into account: i) other ions present in the cell cytosol competing with Mg^{2+} in binding ATP such as: H^+, Na^+, K^+ and ii) other ligands such as ADP, PCr and Pi competing with ATP in binding Mg^{2+} (Iotti *et al*, 1996).

Operatively, [Mg^{2+}] is assessed by ^{31}P-MRS from the chemical shift of β-ATP being measured from the signal of either α-ATP (Gupta *et al*, 1984; Williams and Smith, 1995) or PCr (Taylor *et al*, 1991; Halvorson *et al*, 1992). The reliability of the *in vivo* measurements depends on the availability of an appropriate *in vitro* calibration method to determine the limits of chemical shifts of unbound ATP and Mg-ATP complexes. As a result, the calibration method has to take into account the two issues mentioned above together with other variables such as the ionic strength, temperature and pH of the medium. Besides, to have a precise measurement of β-ATP chemical

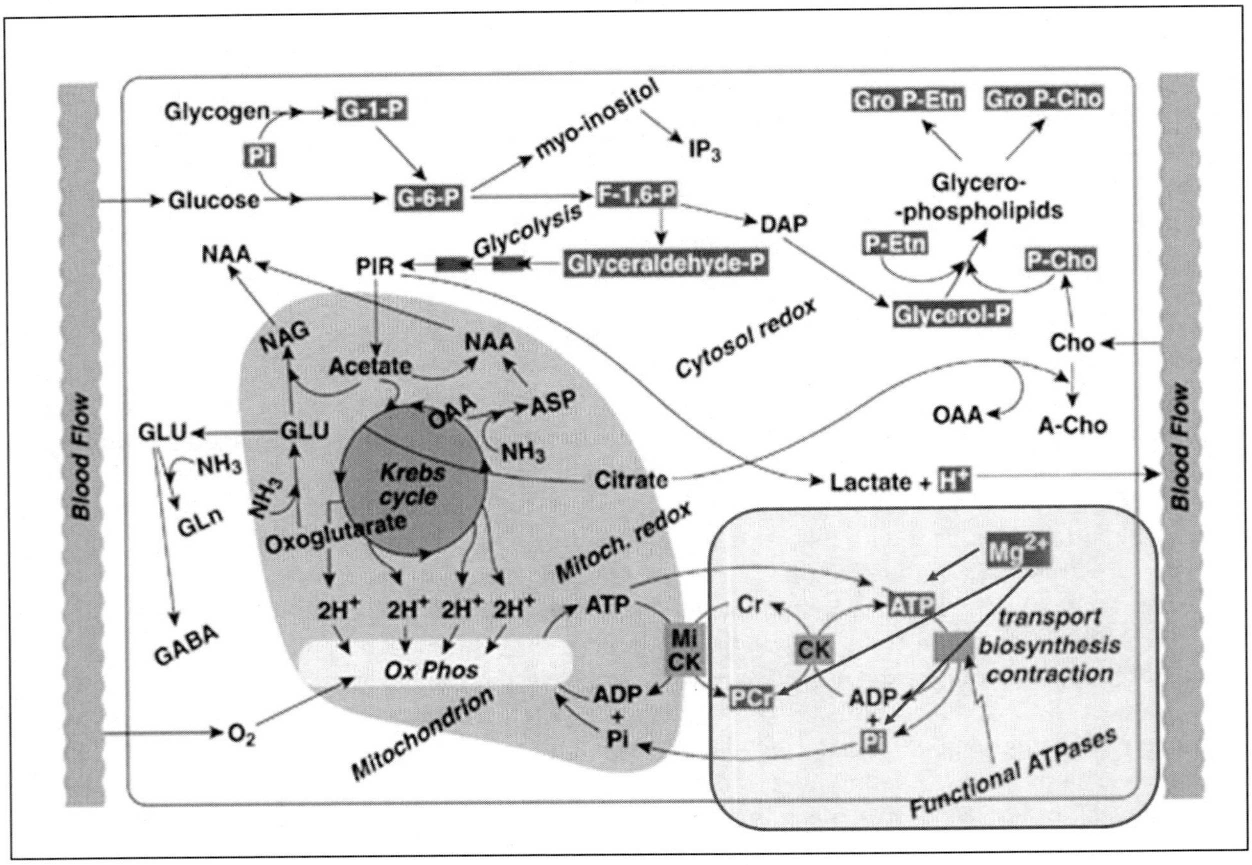

Figure 1. Scheme of the main phosphorylated molecules present in the brain cell cytosol detectable by phosphorus magnetic resonance spectroscopy. Inorganic phosphate (Pi), phosphocreatine (PCr), and ATP are the principal magnesium ligands.

shift it must be taken into account that the shifts of both α-ATP and PCr change as a function of [Mg^{2+}] (Iotti *et al*, 1996). The earlier works of Gupta (Gupta *et al*, 1978; Gupta *et al*, 1983; Gupta *et al*, 1984) were based on the assumption of the presence of only one ATP-Mg complex. In the 90s several studies were published proposing more accurate calibration methods taking into account equilibria involving few different chemical species (Mosher *et al*, 1992; Halvorson *et al*, 1992; Golding and Golding, 1995). Nevertheless, the influence of the ionic strength (I) of the medium on the equilibrium constants of the species present in the calibration solutions must be taken into account as discussed in one report published in those years (Mottet *et al*, 1994).

In the next paragraph the methodological approach used to build the calibration curve for the [Mg^{2+}] determination in human brain by ^{31}P-MRS is analytically presented.

Building a calibration curve for the [Mg^{2+}] determination in human brain by ^{31}P MRS

The accuracy and reliability of *in vivo* assessment of [Mg^{2+}] mainly depend on the availability of calibration curves based on precise *in vitro* NMR measurements performed on appropriate solutions that mimic, as far as possible, the *in vivo* conditions of the tissue to be studied. As a consequence these solutions will contain molecules involved in multiple equilibria in which several ligands (Lewis base) interact with metal ions (Lewis acid), and among them Mg^{2+} and H^+. Typically, to build a calibration curve, a titration of the species of interest must be performed, linking its concentration to the experimental NMR measurement. [Mg^{2+}] can be assessed by ^{31}P MRS from the chemical shift of β-ATP signal, which in turn depends on the fraction of total ATP bound to Mg^{2+}. Quite problematic is the use of a Mg electrode to measure [Mg^{2+}] in a complex

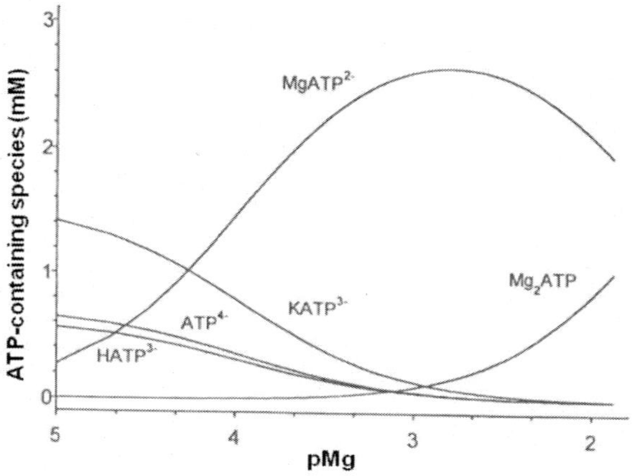

Figure 2. Concentration of the major ATP-containing species present in solutions mimicking the cell brain cytosol plotted *versus* pMg. Solutions composition were: ATP = 3 mM, phosphocreatine = 4.5 mM, K_2HPO_4 = 1.0 mM, and variable amounts of $MgCl_2$ at pH = 7.00, 37 °C and ionic strength 0.25 M. Adapted from Iotti *et al*, 1996.

mixture, having to deal with interferences and lack of accuracy.

A convenient approach to measure the $[Mg^{2+}]$ in a multi-equilibrium system is using appropriate algorithms and software, which are currently available, allowing a quantitative chemical speciation of any component present in solution, given a set of stability and acidic dissociation constants. In this approach, a pivotal step is the definition of the chemical model better describing the multi-equilibrium system present in solution. After the characterization of ligands and Lewis acids as the basic species, the next step is the delineation of all the possible equilibria between them.

In the calibration curve specifically developed for the *in vivo* assessment of $[Mg^{2+}]$ in human brain (Iotti *et al*, 1996) the chemical model was defined by choosing four ligands: ATP^{4-}, PO_4^{3-}, Cl^- and PCr^{2-} and four Lewis acids: Na^+, K^+, Mg^{2+} and H^+ as basic species, giving raise to the multi-equilibrium system shown in Figure 4.

An obligatory prerequisite for the analysis of spectra recorded *in vitro* is a reliable and homogeneous set of equilibrium constants to be used in the quantitative speciation of the experimental solutions. Therefore, if the equilibrium

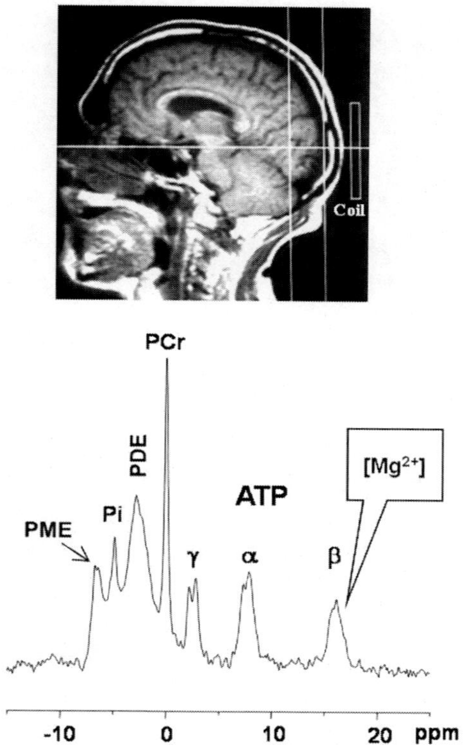

Figure 3. Top: Sagittal slice image of human brain acquired by magnetic resonance imaging. The brain volume within vertical axes defines the region of occipital lobes. Bottom: ^{31}P-MRS spectra acquired from occipital lobes placing the surface coil directly on the skull. Abbreviations: Pi, inorganic phosphate; PCr, phosphocreatine; α, β, γ, ATP phosphoric groups; PME, phosphomonoesters; PDE, phosphodiesters. Brain cytosolic $[Mg^{2+}]$ is assessed from the chemical shift of β-ATP.

constants reported in the literature do not conform to the conditions of temperature and ionic strength used in the experiments, suitable corrections, using Van't Hoff and/or Davies equations , have to be applied to account for the different conditions of NMR experiments (Iotti *et al*, 1996).

Furthermore, the literature is rich with data pertaining to interactions between metal ions and ligands in solution, but the reported values are often characterized by extremely variable levels of precision and accuracy. Williams and colleagues (Duffield *et al*, 1991) discussed the problems related to the determination of the magnitude of quantities of biological/environ-

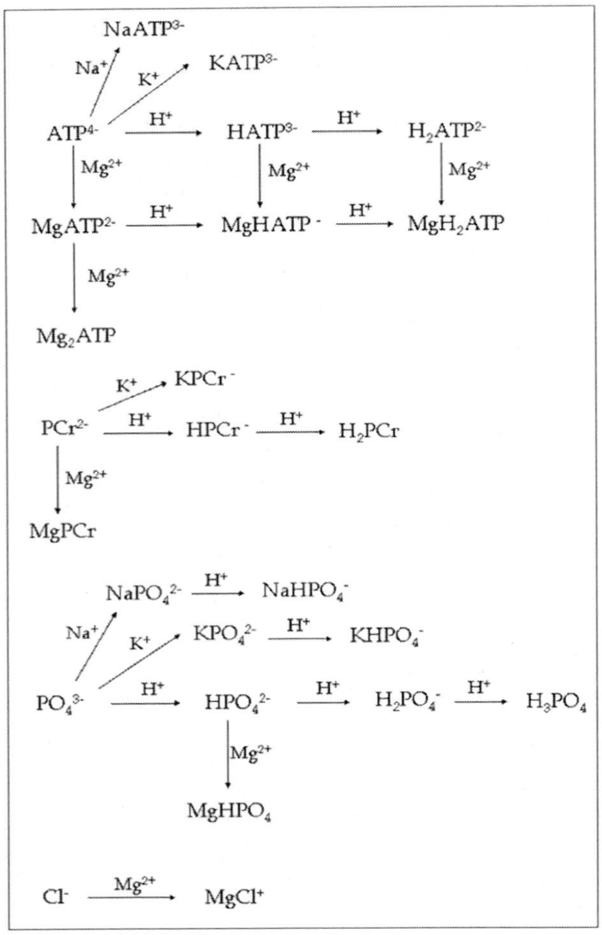

Figure 4. Scheme of the chemical model used to build the calibration curve for the assessment of brain cytosolic [Mg^{2+}] by ^{31}P-MRS. Four ligands (ATP^{4-}, PO_4^{3-}, Cl^-, and PCr^{2-}) and four Lewis acids (Na^+, K^+, Mg^{2+}, and H^+) were chosen as basic species.

mental interest and to its associated error. When these quantities are used for the chemical speciation of natural systems, the results bear an uncertainty directly related to the errors which affect the original quantities. Hence, a careful examination of the published values of equilibrium constants for the reactions involved in the chemical model chosen, must be performed.

Another consideration to bear in mind is when using protonation constants that have been determined with the so-called "incomplete convention" (Halvorson *et al*, 1992), in which hydrogen ion activity is used instead of hydrogen ion concentration in the expression used to define the equilibrium constants. This can generate confusion when such constants are used together with others that are expressed solely in terms of concentration. Therefore a coherent and internally consistent set of equilibrium constants has to be collected, which are valid at 37 °C and at I = 0.25 M, the conditions of solutions that mimic the *in vivo* environment.

To handle the relevant number of different equilibria taken into consideration, an algorithm was developed that allowed a quantitative chemical speciation of the Mg^{2+}-binding molecules with the goal of building a semi-empirical equation that correlates the chemical shift of the β-ATP signal measured by *in vitro* NMR measurements in the calibration solutions to [Mg^{2+}] calculated, taking into account the amount of Mg^{2+} bound to all constituents in solution. As a result, the concentrations of all species present under a given set of conditions (i.e. total concentrations of all reagents) were determined by the program HYSS (Alderighi *et al*, 1999), a specific software program, utilized for chemical speciation. Using this software it was possible to derive the concentration of free magnesium in any condition. HYSS requires two sets of data: a chemical model and the experimental conditions. The model was the one reported in Figure 4, by specifying values for the equilibrium constants $\beta_{abc....}$ and the corresponding stoichiometric coefficients *a, b, c,* ...., considering that the general reaction between reagents A, B, C ... to give a chemical species of formula AaBbCc...:

$$aA+bB+cC+\ldots \rightleftharpoons AaBbCc$$

is associated with an equilibrium constant $\beta_{abc...}$:

$$\beta_{abc} = \frac{[AaBbCc\ldots]}{[A]^a[B]^b[C]^c}$$

Electric charges have been omitted for the sake of simplicity. By using this approach and different calibration solutions prepared to mimic the *in vivo* metabolic conditions of brain, it has been possible to obtain, following an heuristic procedure, the following equation:

$$pMg = x_1 - \log_{10} [(d - x_2)^{x_3}/(x_4 - d)^{x_5}]$$

where x_1, x_2, x_3, x_4, x_5 are the calculated parameters, δ is the measured chemical shift, and pMg = $-\log_{10}$ [Mg^{2+}]. This equation can be seen as a more general expression of the typical titration curve in which x_1 is the pK of the equilibrium involved and with x_3, x_5 = 1. More precisely, two different equations were obtained, where pMg is expressed as a function of the chemical shifts of β-ATP from PCr (δ_β) or from α-ATP ($\delta_{\alpha\beta}$) (Iotti *et al*, 1996). However, the calibration curve obtained using δ_β as experimental variable showed to be more accurate than that obtained using $\delta_{\alpha\beta}$ (Iotti *et al*, 1996). This is because the measurements of $\delta_{\alpha\beta}$ in spectra obtained *in vivo* are usually less accurate than those of δ_β, due to the unresolved resonances of α-ADP, NAD, NADH underlying up-field the α-ATP peak. Furthermore, PCr resonates alone and is symmetric, allowing a more accurate identification of the centroid of the peak. Therefore, δ_β should be preferable to $\delta_{\alpha\beta}$ as experimental variable for the *in vivo* measurements of brain cytosolic free [Mg^{2+}]. According to this, the equation to be used is:

$$pMg = 4.24 - \log_{10}[(\delta_\beta - 18.58)^{0.42} / (15.74 - \delta_\beta)^{0.84}]$$

The specific software package MAGIC-BC based on the equation reported above has been made available at http://www.cermiv.unibo.it. It is worth underlying that, in principle, by this approach it is possible to assess the concentration of any species independently of the degree of complexity of the system under investigation, with the restriction of only two requisites: i) a precise definition of the chemical model and ii) the knowledge of the equilibrium constants of the chemical reactions involved.

Cytosolic [Mg^{2+}] in human brain

The cytosolic [Mg^{2+}] assessed by ^{31}P-MRS in the occipital lobes of human brain of 36 control subjects (22 men and 14 women) of mean age 36.4 ± 17.1 (SD) (16 - 67 years) was 0.182 mM (Iotti *et al*, 1996). Brain studies were performed on occipital lobes by placing the surface coil directly on the skull in the occipital region and precisely positioned by imaging the brain as shown in Figure 3. The free cytosolic [Mg^{2+}] measured in the human brain is about half of that assessed in the human calf muscle (Iotti *et al*, 2000, Iotti and Malucelli, 2008). This result is likely related to the lower ATP concentration of brain tissue (3 mM) compared to that of skeletal muscle (8 mM), ATP being the major binding site present in the cellular milieu. Nevertheless, the value found of 0.182 mM is lower than that obtained by others (Taylor *et al*, 1991; Halvorson *et al*, 1992). This is not a surprising result as the model considered in building this calibration curve contains more species that bind Mg^{2+} than in all other approaches published. As a consequence a lower value of cytosolic free [Mg^{2+}] has to be expected. If the model described previously, upon which the cytosolic [Mg^{2+}] assessment is based, had taken into account more species binding Mg^{2+}, the resulting value of brain [Mg^{2+}] would be even lower. Therefore, we believe that the present brain [Mg^{2+}] value is a good estimate of the cytosolic free ion concentration, which however could still be slightly overestimated.

In the cohort of subjects studied there was no significant difference in cytosolic [Mg^{2+}] as a function of age and sex. This shows that the sum of anions binding Mg^{2+} *in vivo* does not change in the brain cortex during the life span studied and/or that regulatory mechanisms exist to maintain the cytosolic free [Mg^{2+}] constant. The possibility to assess the free cytosolic [Mg^{2+}] in the human brain opened the chance to study the involvement of Mg in different neurological pathologies. Particularly interesting are mitochondrial cytopathies and migraines in which the defective mitochondrial energy production is respectively the primary causative or putative pathogenetic factor.

Brain [Mg^{2+}] in mitochondrial cytopathies

^{31}P-MRS was used to assess the free [Mg^{2+}] in the occipital lobes of patients affected by different types of mitochondrial cytopathies due to known enzyme and/or mitochondrial DNA defects to clarify the functional relationship between the energy metabolism and the concentration of cytosolic free magnesium (Barbiroli *et al*, 1999a). In particular, 19 subjects (9 women and 10 men) of mean age 43 ± 19 (SD) (13-75 years) with mitochondrial cytopathies were studied (see Table 1). Treatment with oral CoQ10 (150 mg/day) was given for six months to 9 patients. All patients displayed significantly low cytosolic [Mg^{2+}], well below the 95% confidence interval of control values (Figure 5). Since the mtDNA mutations and enzyme defects found in these patients (Table 1) are known to be primarily responsible for brain defective mitochondrial respiration, this outcome strongly suggest that

Table 1. Patients with mitochondrial cytopathies due to known enzyme/mtDNA defect/s. COX = cytochrome oxidase. Patients 1-4, 10, 12-14 and 16 were treated with CoQ10 (150 mg/day for six months). Adapted from Barbiroli *et al*, 1999a.

Patients numbers	Sex/age (years)	Diagnosis	Enzyme defect or mtDNA bp mutation/deletion
1*	F/61	CPEO	COX
2*	M/75	CPEO	COX
3*	F/69	CPEO	mtDNA deletion
4*	M/66	CPEO	COX
5	F/21	LHON	3460
6	M/26	LHON	11778
7	M/33	LHON	11778
8	F/61	LHON	11778
9	F/54	LHON	11778
10*	M/33	LHON	3460
11	M/51	LHON	11778 + 4216 + 13708
12*	M/56	LHON	11778
13*	M/36	LHON	11778
14*	M/25	LHON	11778
15	F/41	NARP	8993
16*	F/13	NARP	8993
17	F/16	MERFF	8344
18	M/49	MELAS	3243
19	F/38	MEM	mtDNA deletion

Abbreviations: * treated with CoQ10; CPEO, chronic progressive external ophthalmoplegia; LHON, Leber's hereditary optic neuropathy; NARP, neuropathy ataxia and retinitis pigmentosa; MEM, mitochondrial encephalomyopathy; MERF, myoclonic epilepsy with ragged red fibres; MELAS, mitochondrial myopathy encephalopathy, lactic acidosis, and stroke.

the low cytosolic [Mg^{2+}] found in these patients was secondary to failure of the respiratory chain.

Nine of the 19 patients investigated were treated with CoQ, which improved the efficiency of the respiratory chain (Barbiroli *et al*, 1999a). Administration of CoQ also increased cytosolic [Mg^{2+}] in all treated patients (Figure 5). The increased efficiency of oxidative phosphorylation following treatment with CoQ accompanied by an increased cytosolic free [Mg^{2+}] gives further support to the hypothesis that changes in brain cytosolic [Mg^{2+}] were secondary to the improved efficiency of mitochondrial energy production. According to this view, the cytosolic [Mg^{2+}] is a function of the energy charge of brain cells and a defective mitochondrial respiration causes a derangement of cytosolic [Mg^{2+}] homeostasis. This interpretation is consistent with the observations of several reports that indicate mitochondria as the primary pool for the increase and decrease in cellular magnesium content, suggesting that mitochondria might act as magnesium stores (Kubota *et al*, 2005; Farruggia *et al*, 2006) and play a key role in regulating magnesium homeostasis (Fatholahi *et al*, 2000; Murphy, 2000).

Brain [Mg^{2+}] in different types of migraine and cluster headache

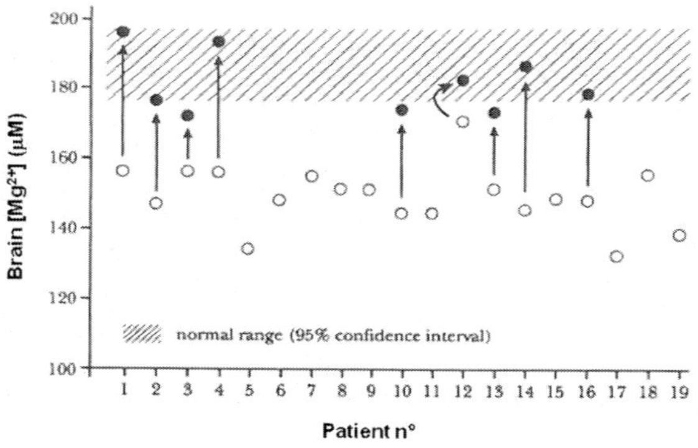

Figure 5. Brain cytosolic [Mg^{2+}] assessed in the occipital lobes of patients with mitochondrial cytopathies (open symbols). The values from nine of these patients after treatment with CoQ are shown by closed symbols. Dashed areas represent the 95% confidence intervals of 36 healthy control subjects. Adapted from Barbiroli *et al*, 1999a.

Low cytosolic free magnesium has been found in the brains of patients with migraine with and without aura during attacks (Ramadan *et al*, 1989) and interictally in young patients with migraine with aura (Lodi *et al*, 1997). It has been suggested that low free magnesium may contribute to the bioenergetic deficit in headache patients as magnesium is essential for mitochondrial membrane stability and coupling of oxidative phosphorylation (Welch and Ramadan, 1995). Migraine headache is a common feature in patients with mitochondrial encephalomyopathies where deficient brain mitochondrial oxidation is due to mutations of mitochondrial DNA. In fact, several studies contributed to disclose an altered energy metabolism in the brain of patients with different types of migraine and cluster headache (Barbiroli *et al*, 1992; Montagna *et al*, 1994; Montagna *et al*, 1997), although the molecular mechanisms leading to oxidative deficit in migraine and cluster headache are unknown. On the other hand, as shown in the previous section, the reduction in cytosolic [Mg^{2+}] seems to be secondary to the bioenergetics deficit in the brains of patients with different mitochondrial encephalomyopathies. These outcomes provided the rationale to perform an extensive study to assess the brain Mg^{2+} by ^{31}P-MRS in different form of migraines and in cluster headache (Lodi *et al*, 2001). The study was performed in 78 patients with different forms of migraine in attack-free periods (7 with migraine stroke, 13 with migraine with prolonged aura, 37 with migraine with typical aura or basilar migraine, 21 with migraine without aura), and 13 patients with cluster headache. In the occipital lobes of all subgroups of migraine and in cluster headache patients cytosolic [Mg^{2+}] was significantly reduced. Among migraine patients the level of cytosolic free [Mg^{2+}] correlated with the severity of clinical phenotype, showing the lowest values in patients with migraine stroke and the highest in patients with migraine without aura, as shown in Figure 6 (Lodi *et al*, 2001). Again, the results of this study sustain the hypothesis that the reduction of cytosolic [Mg^{2+}] in tissues with defective mitochondrial functionality is secondary to the bioenergetics deficit, hence the reduction of brain cytosolic free [Mg^{2+}] is unlikely to be a direct consequence of hypomagnesemia.

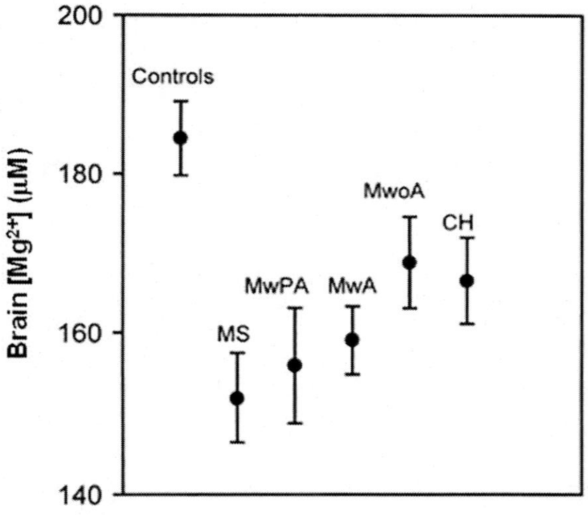

Figure 6. Concentration of cytosolic [Mg^{2+}] in the occipital lobes of patients with migraine and cluster headache compared with healthy control subjects. Abbreviations: MS, migraine stroke; MwPA, migraine with prolonged aura; MwA, migraine with typical aura or basilar migraine; MwoA, migraine without aura; CH, cluster headache. All values are reported as mean ± SE. Adapted from Lodi *et al*, 2001.

Brain [Mg^{2+}] in the differential diagnosis of multiple system atrophy and idiopathic Parkinson's disease

An *in vivo* study by ^{31}P-MRS showed that the combined measurement of [PCr], and free [Mg^{2+}], could help to differentiate patients with Multiple System Atrophy (MSA) from those with Parkinson's disease (PD) (Barbiroli *et al*, 1999b). MSA is a group of multisystem degenerative diseases that have several clinical features of Parkinson's disease. Furthermore, not all the signs in MSA become evident at the same time, rendering difficult the differentiation from PD. Therefore, differentiating MSA from PD can be complicated and the diagnosis of MSA represents a clinical challenge. The study was carried out on the occipital lobes of 15 patients MSA, 13 patients with idiopathic PD.

In the occipital lobes of MSA patients we found a ^{31}P-MRS spectroscopy pattern suggestive of defective brain mitochondrial respiration with low [PCr] and high [Pi]. However, the brain cytosolic [Mg^{2+}] of MSA patients did not differ significantly from control values, displaying a peculiar pattern compared to mitochondrial cytopathies . On the other hand, PD patients did not exhibit in their occipital lobes the metabolic pattern typical of mitochondrial malfunction, showing an increased [Pi], decreased cytosolic [Mg^{2+}] and unchanged [PCr] and pH. Although there is a highly significant difference in both [PCr] and [Mg^{2+}] between MSA and PD patients when compared as groups, there is a small overlap of [PCr] and [Mg^{2+}] values between the two groups when considering single individuals (Barbiroli *et al*, 1999b). However, taking into consideration both variables at the same time, the individual patients with MSA can be separated from the individual patients with PD

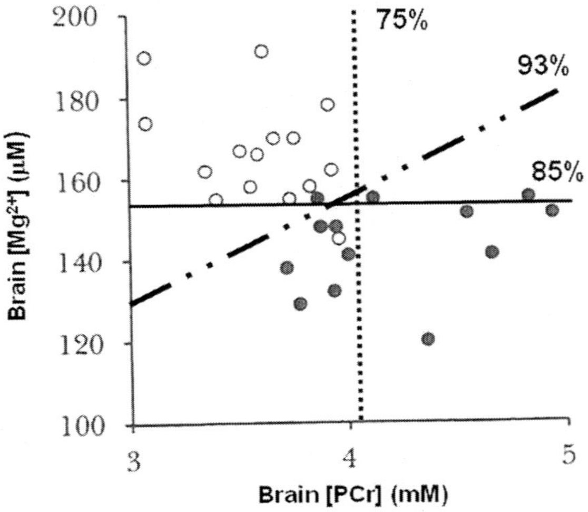

Figure 7. Plot of the distribution patterns of 13 patients with Idiopathic Parkinson's Disease (closed symbols) and 15 patients with Multiple System Atrophy (open symbols) as a function of brain [PCr] and free [Mg^{2+}] assessed by ^{31}P-MRS. [PCr] and [Mg^{2+}] alone were able to classify respectively 75% and 85% of the patients. Discriminant analysis using contemporarily these two independent parameters correctly classified 93% of cases. Adapted from Barbiroli et al, 1999b.

with a probability of 93%, the degree of uncertainty being due to two cases (one case in each group, Figure 7). The results of the study revealed an abnormal bioenergetics in MSA and a decreased cytosolic [Mg^{2+}] content in PD, offering a new diagnostic tool that may help to differentiate MSA from PD.

Acknowledgments

This work was supported by an RFO grants from the University of Bologna and PRIN 2007ZT39FN from MIUR to Stefano Iotti.

References

Alderighi L, Gans P, Ienco A, Peters D, Sabatini A, Vacca A (1999) Hyperquad simulation and speciation (HySS): a utility program for the investigation of equilibria involving soluble and partially soluble species. *Coord Chem Rev* 184:311-318.

Barbiroli B, Montagna P, Funicello R, Iotti S, Monari L, Pierangeli G, Zaniol P, Lugaresi E (1992) Abnormal brain and muscle energy metabolism shown by ^{31}P magnetic resonance spectroscopy in patients affected by migraine with aura. *Neurology* 42:1209-1214.

Barbiroli B, Iotti S, Cortelli P, Martinelli P, Lodi R, Carelli V, Montagna P (1999a) Low brain intracellular free magnesium in mitochondrial cytopathies. *J Cereb Blood Flow Metab* 19:528-532.

Barbiroli B, Martinelli P, Patuelli A, Lodi R, Iotti S, Cortelli P, Montagna P (1999b) Phosphorus magnetic resonance spectroscopy in multiple system atrophy and Parkinson's disease. *Mov Disord* 14:430-435.

Duffield JR, Marsicano F, Williams D R (1991) Chemical speciation modelling and thermodynamic database compilation–I. Data uncertainties. *Polyhedron* 10:1105-1111.

Farruggia G, Iotti S, Prodi L, Montalti M, Zaccheroni N, Savage PB, Trapani V, Sale P, Wolf FI (2006) 8-Hydroxyquinoline derivatives as fluorescent sensors for magnesium in living cells. *J Am Chem Soc* 128:344-350.

Fatholahi M, LaNoue K, Romani A, Scarpa A (2000) Relationship between total and free cellular Mg($^{2+}$) during metabolic stimulation of rat cardiac myocytes and perfused hearts. *Arch Biochem Biophys* 374:395-401.

Golding EM, Golding RM (1995) Interpretation of ^{31}P MRS spectra in determining intracellular free magnesium and potassium ion concentration. *Magn Reson Med.* 33:467-474.

Gupta RK, Benovic JL, Rose Z B (1978) The determination of the free magnesium level in the human red blood cell by ^{31}P NMR. *J Biol Chem* 252:6172-6176.

Gupta RK, Gupta P, Yushok WD, Rose ZB (1983) Measurements of the dissociation constant of MgATP at physiological nucleotide levels by a combination of ^{31}P NMR and optical absorbance spectroscopy. *Biochem Biophys Res Commun* 117:210-216.

Gupta RK, Gupta P, Moore RD (1984) NMR studies of intracellular metal ions in intact cells and tissues. *Ann Rev Biophys Bioeng* 13:221-246.

Halvorson HR, Vande Linde AMQ, Helpern JA, Welch KMA (1992) Assessment of magnesium concentration by ^{31}P NMR *in vivo*. *NMR Biomed* 5:53-58.

Iotti S, Frassineti C, Alderighi L, Sabatini A, Vacca A, Barbiroli B (1996) In vivo assessment of free magnesium concentration in human brain by ^{31}P-MRS. A new calibration curve based on a mathematical algorithm. *NMR Biomed* 9:24-32.

Iotti S, Frassineti C, Alderighi L, Sabatini A, Vacca A, Barbiroli B (2000) *In vivo* ^{31}P-MRS assessment of cytosolic [Mg($^{2+}$)] in the human skeletal muscle in different metabolic conditions. *Magn Reson Imag* 18:607-614.

Iotti S, Malucelli E (2008) In vivo assessment of Mg^{2+} in human brain and skeletal muscle by ^{31}P-MRS. *Magnesium Research* 21:157-162.

Kubota T, Shindo Y, Tokuno K, Komatsu H, Ogawa H, Kudo S, Kitamura Y, Suzuki K, Oka K (2005) Mitochondria are intracellular magnesium stores: investigation by simultaneous fluorescent imagings in PC12 cells. *Biochim Biophys Acta* 1744(1):19-28.

Kuby SA, Noltman EA (1959) ATP-Creatine Transphosphorylase, in: P.D. In: *The Enzymes*, (Boyer Ed), 2nd ed, New York, PA: Academic Press, 515–603.

Lodi R, Montagna P, Soriani S, Iotti S, Arnaldi C, Cortelli P et al. (1997) Deficit of brain and skeletal muscle bioenergetics and low brain magnesium in juvenile migraine: an in vivo ^{31}P magnetic resonance spectroscopy interictal study. *Pediatr Res* 42:866-71.

Lodi R, Iotti S, Cortelli P, Pierangeli G, Cevoli S, Clementi V, Soriani S, Montagna P, Barbiroli B (2001) Deficient energy metabolism is associated with low free magnesium in the brains of patients with migraine and cluster headache. *Brain Res Bull* 54:437-441.

Montagna P, Cortelli P, Monari L, Pierangeli G, Parchi P, Lodi R, Iotti S, Frassineti C, Zaniol P, Lugaresi E (1994) ^{31}P-magnetic resonance spectroscopy in migraine without aura. *Neurology* 44:666-669.

Montagna P, Lodi R, Cortelli P, Pierangeli G, Iotti S, Cevoli S, Zaniol P, Barbiroli B (1997) Phosphorus magnetic resonance spectroscopy in cluster headache. *Neurology* 48:113-118.

Mosher TJ, Williams GD, Doumen C, LaNoue KF, Smith MB (1992) Errors in the calibration of MgATP chemical shift limit: effects on the determination of free magnesium by ^{31}P NMR spectroscopy. *Magn Reson Med* 24:163-169.

Mottet I, Demeure R, Gallez B, Grandin C, Van Beers BE, Pringot J (1994) Experimental ^{31}P NMR study of the influence of ionic strength on the apparent dissociation constant of MgATP. *Magma* 2:101-107.

Murphy E, (2000) Mysteries of Magnesium Homeostasis. *Circ Res* 86:245-248.

Ramadan NM, Halvorson H, Vande-Linde A, Levine SR, Helpern JA, Welch KMA (1989) Low brain magnesium in migraine. *Headache* 29:590-593.

Ramirez F, Marecek JF (1980) Coordination of magnesium with adenosine 5'-diphosphate and triphosphate. *Biochim. Biophys Acta* 589:21-29.

Repke KRH (1982) On the mechanism of energy release, transfer, and utilization in sodium-potassium ATPase transport work: old ideas and new findings. *Ann N Y Acad Sci* 402:272-286.

Skou C (1982) The sodium-potassium ATPase: coupling of the reaction with ATP to the reaction with sodium ion and potassium ion. *Ann N Y Acad Sci* 402:169-184.

Taylor JS, Vigneron DB, Murphy-Boesch J, Nelson SJ, Kessler HB, Coia L, Curran W., Brown TR (1991) Free magnesium levels in normal human brain and brain tumors: ^{31}P chemical-shift imaging measurements at 1.5 T. *Proc Natl Acad Sci USA* 88:6810-6814.

Welch KMA, Ramadan NM (1995) Mitochondria, magnesium and migraine. *J Neurol Sci* 134:9-14.

Wells JA, Knoeber C, Sheldon MC, Werber MM, Yount RG (1980) Cross-linking of myosin subfragment 1. Nucleotide-enhanced modification by a variety of bifunctional reagents. *J Biol Chem* 255:11135-11140.

Williams GD, Smith MB (1995) Application of the accurate assessment of intracellular magnesium and pH from the ^{31}P shift of ATP to cerebral hypoxia-ischemia in neonatal rat. *Magn Reson Med* 33:853-857.

Intracellular magnesium homeostasis

Andrea M.P. Romani ✉

Department of Physiology and Biophysics, School of Medicine, Case Western Reserve University, Cleveland, Ohio, USA.
✉ amr5@po.cwru.edu

Abstract

Magnesium (Mg^{2+}) is the fourth most abundant cation in the whole body and the second most abundant cation within the cell. Numerous cellular functions and enzymes, including ion channels, metabolic cycles, and signaling pathways are regulated by Mg^{2+}. Our understanding of how cells regulate Mg^{2+} homeostasis and transport has registered significant progress in recent time. Yet, several aspects of Mg^{2+} homeostasis within cellular organelles, and the nature of the Mg^{2+} extrusion mechanisms at the cell membrane are still undefined. The present work attempts to provide a comprehensive and updated review of the mechanisms regulating cellular Mg^{2+} homeostasis in eukaryotic cells under physiological conditions and the modifications these mechanisms undergo in various human and animal pathologies.

Introduction

Mammalian cells contain high concentrations of total and free magnesium ion (Mg^{2+}). These concentrations are essential to regulate numerous cellular functions and enzymes, including ion channels, metabolic cycles, and signaling pathways. While the increasing number of observations supports a key regulatory role for Mg^{2+} within the cell, our understanding of how Mg^{2+} homeostasis is regulated at the cellular and subcellular level remains sketchy and incomplete. There are both conceptual and methodological reasons for this limitation. The relative slow turn-over of Mg^{2+} across the plasma membrane or other biological membranes in the absence of metabolic and hormonal stimuli, the absolute abundance of total and free Mg^{2+} within the cell, and the limited occurrence of significant changes in free [Mg^{2+}] have all contributed for a long time to the assumption that cellular Mg^{2+} concentration does not change significantly, and is consistently at a level adequate for its role as a co-factor for various cellular enzymes and proteins. Consequently, this conceptual assumption has limited the interest to develop techniques and methodologies able to rapidly and accurately quantify changes in cellular Mg^{2+} content. In the last two decades, however, an increasing number of experimental and clinical observations have challenged this assumption. More than 1000 entries in the literature highlight the regulatory role of Mg^{2+} on various cellular functions and cycles, and indicate the occurrence of major fluxes of Mg^{2+} in either directly across the plasma membrane of various mammalian cells under a variety of metabolic or hormonal stimuli. In turn, these fluxes have resulted in appreciable changes in cytosolic free [Mg^{2+}] and total Mg^{2+} content within the cell and cellular organelles. Furthermore, genetic and electrophysiological approaches in bacteria, yeast and mammalian cells have identified several Mg^{2+} entry mechanisms that operate either at the cell membrane level or in the membrane of cellular organelles such as mitochondria and Golgi. At the same time, the increased interest in biological functions regulated by Mg^{2+} has stimulated the development of methodological approaches aimed at better detecting and quantifying variations in cellular Mg^{2+} level, and renewed interest in relating alterations in Mg^{2+} homeostasis with the onset of specific pathologies and complications in human patients. All these different aspects will be elucidated in the present review to provide a framework as comprehensive as possible to correlate changes in cellular Mg^{2+} homeostasis and content with variations in the function of specific enzymes, which ultimately affect the *modus operandi* of different cellular organelles and cell types.

Cellular Mg^{2+} distribution

Direct and indirect measurement of total cellular Mg^{2+} content by various techniques consistently indicates that total Mg^{2+} concentration ranges between 17 to 20mM in the majority of mammalian cell types examined (Romani and Scarpa, 1992; Wolf *et al*, 2003). Determinations of total and free Mg^{2+} concentrations by electron probe X-rays microanalysis (EPXMA), ^{31}P-NMR, selective Mg^{2+}-electrode, ^{13}C-NMR citrate/isocitrate ratio or fluorescent indicators (Table I in Romani and Scarpa, 1992, and in Wolf and Cittadini, 2003) localize major amounts of Mg^{2+} within mitochondria, nucleus, and endo-(sarco)-plasmic reticulum, with total concentrations ranging between 15 to 18 mM in each of these organelles. Binding of Mg^{2+} by phospholipids, proteins, nucleic acids, chromatin and nucleotides has been invoked to explain the persistence of such a high Mg^{2+} concentration within these organelles. Although the specific modality and nature of these bindings have not been fully investigated, experimental evidence indicates that only a small fraction of such a large Mg^{2+} content is actually free in the lumen of these structures. Concentrations of 0.8 and 1.2 mM free [Mg^{2+}] have been measured in the matrix of cardiac and liver mitochondria (Jung *et al*, 1990; Rutter *et al*, 1990). No determinations of free [Mg^{2+}] are available for the nucleus and the endo-(sarco)-plasmic reticulum. The porous structure of the nuclear envelope makes it reasonable to envision that the intranuclear free [Mg^{2+}] is similar to the concentration measured in the cytoplasm. The free [Mg^{2+}] within the endo-(sarco)-plasmic reticulum lumen cannot be reliably determined due to the elevated millimolar concentration of Ca^{2+} inside the organelle (Somlyo *et al.* 1985), and the high affinity of the fluorescent dyes Mag-Fura or Mag-Indo for Ca^{2+} (50mM) as compared to Mg^{2+} (1.5 mM) (Hofer and Machen, 1993). A third considerable pool of Mg^{2+} (~4-5mM) is present in the cytoplasm in the form of a complex with ATP, and other phosphonucleotides and phosphometabolites (Scarpa and Brinley, 1981). Because of its abundance (~ 5mM) and Mg^{2+} binding affinity (K_d ~78μM), ATP constitutes the largest metabolic pool able to bind Mg^{2+} within the cytoplasm and the mitochondria matrix as well (Luthi *et al*, 1999). The binding/buffering capacity of ATP, phosphonucleotides and phosphometabolites, and possibly proteins, maintains cytosolic *free* [Mg^{2+}] between 0.5-1mM, or less than 5% of total cellular Mg^{2+} content in almost all the cells and tissues examined (Table I in Romani and Scarpa, 1992). Similar values have been obtained using fluorescent dyes, ^{31}P-NMR and citrate/isocitrate ratio (Romani and Scarpa, 1992). Overall, these results support the presence of a very limited chemical Mg^{2+} gradient across the cell membrane, and across the membrane of cellular organelles. In erythrocytes, which lack cellular Mg^{2+} compartmentation, Flatman and Lew (Flatman and Lew, 1981) have observed three kinetically distinct binding pools for Mg^{2+}: a low capacity, high affinity pool represented by cell proteins, and two pools that correspond reasonably well to ATP and 2,3-diphosphoglycerate (2,3-DPG), respectively (Gunther *et al*, 1995). This model has been further refined by Raftos et al (Raftos *et al*, 1999) to take into account Mg^{2+} binding by hemoglobin under oxygenated and not oxygenated conditions.

Limited information is available about the ability of proteins to bind Mg^{2+} within the cell and cellular organelles. Aside from calmodulin (Oki *et al*, 1997), troponin C (Wang *et al*, 1998), parvalbumin (Allouche *et al*, 1999), and S100 protein (Ogoma *et al*, 1992), there is no indication as to whether other cytosolic or intra-organelle proteins can bind substantial amounts of Mg^{2+} and contribute to the elevated concentrations of total Mg^{2+} measured within the mitochondria or discrete regions of the endo-(sarco)-plasmic reticulum. An early report by Bogucka and Wojitczak (Bogucka and Wojitczak, 1971) has suggested the presence of two proteins able to bind Mg^{2+} with high affinity/low capacity and high capacity/low affinity, respectively, in the intermembraneous space of the mitochondrion. However, no subsequent study has confirmed their presence or identified the proteins. The presence of Mg^{2+} binding sites has been indicated for several other cellular proteins, but no clear information is available as to whether these proteins do bind Mg^{2+} under basal conditions and whether binding changes to a significant extent following hormonal or metabolic stimuli, or under pathological conditions. Moreover, the potential physiological relevance of Mg^{2+} binding by any of the mentioned proteins has been called into question by the observation that parvalbumin *null* mice do not exhibit hypomagnesaemia or significant changes in tissue Mg^{2+} handling and homeostasis (Belge *et al*, 2007).

Taking into account the cellular distribution and assuming a Mg^{2+} concentration in plasma and extracellular fluid of 1.2-1.4 mM, one-third of which is binding extracellular proteins (e.g. albumin) or other biochemical moieties (Geigy, 1984), it appears that most mammalian cells are at or near *zero trans* condition as far it concerns the chemical free [Mg^{2+}] concentration across the cell membrane or the biomembrane of cellular organelles (e.g. mitochondria). Because the electrochemical equilibrium potential for cellular free [Mg^{2+}] is approximately 50mM in most mammalian cells under resting conditions (Flatman, 1984), it is evident that mechanisms must operate in the cell membrane to maintain cytosolic *free* Mg^{2+} and total cellular Mg^{2+} content within the measured levels.

Mg^{2+} transport mechanisms

Eukaryotes retain their cellular Mg^{2+} content virtually unaltered under resting conditions even when exposed to a significant gradient across the cell membrane (e.g. culturing in virtually *zero* extracellular Mg^{2+} content) (Wolf *et al*, 2003; Romani, 2007). Atomic absorbance spectrophotometry determinations and radioisotopic equilibrium indicate Mg^{2+} turnover rates ranging from 1 hour (adipocytes) to several days (lymphocytes) as a result of structural and functional specificity of different tissues and cells (Romani, 2007). Within the same cell types discrepancies can be observed based upon the experimental conditions or the modality of isolation, e.g. cells *in situ* versus freshly isolated cells versus cells in culture. For example, cardiac ventricular myocytes attain ^{28}Mg equilibrium within 3 hours in the whole animal but require 72-80 hours, as dispersed cells incubated at 37°C, or even a longer period of times when exposed to 20°C (Polimeni and Page, 1974; Rogers *et al*, 1960; Rogers, 1961). Lymphocytes also present differences in amplitude (or operation) of Mg^{2+} transport depending on whether they are freshly isolated (Wolf *et al*, 1997) or cultured (Maguire and Erdos, 1978) cells.

For a long time, the slow Mg^{2+} turnover observed in various tissues or cells has contributed to the erroneous idea that Mg^{2+} content in mammalian cells does not change, or changes at such a slow pace that it lacks physiological significance. In the last twenty years, this notion has been completely reverted by a large body of experimental evidence, which indicates that large fluxes of Mg^{2+} can cross the plasma membrane of eukaryotic cells within minutes from the application of metabolic or hormonal stimuli, with relatively small changes in free Mg^{2+} level (Romani, 2007; Grubbs and Maguire, 1987; Romani and Scarpa, 2000; Romani and Maguire, 2002). Lymphocytes (Gunther and Vormann, 1990; Wolf *et al*, 1997), erythrocytes (Matsuura, 1993), cardiac myocytes (Vormann and Gunther, 1987; Romani and Scarpa, 1990a) and liver cells (Jakob *et al*, 1989; Romani and Scarpa, 1990b; Gunther *et al*, 1991) are just a few examples of the mammalian cells that have been reported to extrude 10% to 20% of their total cellular Mg^{2+} content in less than 10min from the application of adrenergic or metabolic stimuli. The amplitude and rapidity of these fluxes presuppose the presence and operation of powerful transport mechanisms able to move large amounts of Mg^{2+} in and out of mammalian cells following various stimuli (for a list of experimental models and conditions see Romani and Scarpa, 2000). In addition, the operation of Mg^{2+} entry mechanisms appears to be tightly coupled with the ability of the cell to rapidly and efficiently buffering the magnesium ions accumulated, as suggested by the limited changes in cytosolic free [Mg^{2+}]i in the large majority of conditions tested (Fatholahi *et al*, 2000; Kubota *et al*, 2005).

The Mg^{2+} transport mechanisms operating at the level of the cell membrane or in the membrane of cellular organelles are represented by channels and exchangers. While channels are predominantly involved in Mg^{2+} accumulation, exchangers mediate essentially Mg^{2+} extrusion. The majority of recently identified Mg^{2+} entry mechanisms operate in the cell membrane but two of them have been located in the mitochondrial membrane and the Golgi system, respectively. For the most part, these entry mechanisms present a modest selectivity for Mg^{2+}, and do not appear to be involved in Mg^{2+} extrusion. No information is currently available about the mechanisms that contribute to maintain an elevated Mg^{2+} concentration within the lumen of the endoplasmic (sarcoplasmic) reticulum.

What it follows is a general description of our current knowledge about the channels and exchangers involved in Mg^{2+} transport across biological membranes (summarized in Table 1).

Channels

Magnesium ions enter the cell via channels or channel-like mechanisms. Channels able to transport Mg^{2+} into the cell have been originally described in prokaryotes (Kehres *et al*, 1998; Moncrief and Maguire, 1999), including protozoans (Preston, 1990), but recently several Mg^{2+} entry mechanisms with channels or channels-like features have been identified in eukaryotic cells. Some of these mechanisms exhibit a relatively high specificity for Mg^{2+} but they can permeate other divalent cations as well. Whereas the majority of these channels are located in the cell membrane or perhaps translocate between early endosomal vesicles and the cell membrane, other are specifically located in the mitochondrial membrane or in the Golgi cysternae. Because the identification and characterization of these eukaryotic Mg^{2+} transporting channels is far from being complete, information relative to their regulation is still largely fragmentary. The abundance of mechanisms favoring Mg^{2+} entry into the cell also raises the question as to what extent the different mechanisms cooperate to modulate Mg^{2+} entry or exert an absolute (or relative predominance) in specific cells under well defined conditions.

TRPM Channels

TRPM7 (Nadler *et al*, 2001) and TRPM6 (Schlingmann *et al*, 2002) were the first channels identified as being able to transport Mg^{2+} into mammalian cells. While Fleig and her group (Nadler *et al*, 2001) reported a preferential Mg^{2+} permeation through the LTRPC7 channel (i.e. TRPM7 based on the current nomenclature), genetic analysis (Schlingmann *et al*, 2002) indicated, more or less at the same time, that TRPM6, another member of the melastatin subfamily of TRP channels, exhibits a selective Mg^{2+} permeation. At variance of the ubiquitous nature of TRPM7, TRMP6 is specifically localized in the colon and the distal convolute tubule of the nephron, a distribution that strongly emphases the role of TRPM6 in controlling whole body Mg^{2+} homeostasis via intestinal absorption and renal resorption. In contrast, it would appear that TRPM7 is more in control of Mg^{2+} homeostasis in individual cells.

The original observations have led to a flurry of studies aimed at better understanding the role, regulation and interaction of these channels with other cellular components involved to a varying degree in Mg^{2+} homeostasis, and presently more than 190 publications relative to TRPM7 and 110 publications relative to TRPM6 can be found in the literature. Although sharing several similarities in terms of structure and operation, these two channels differ in various aspects ranging from location to hormonal modulation.

• *TRPM7*

The key role of TRPM7 in transporting Mg^{2+} into cells and modulating cell growth was first evidenced by Nadler et al (2001). At the time, the channel was identified as LTRPC7 or long TRP channel 7 owing to the presence of a particularly long extension outside the channel segment (Yamaguchi *et al*, 2001). Due to the presence of an alpha-kinase domain at the C-terminus (Ryazanova *et al*, 2001) and its functional homology to eEF2-kinase (Ryazanov, 2002), this protein was already known as CHAK1 (channel kinase 1) (Ryazanova *et al*, 2001). Shortly after the observation of Nadler et al (2001), Runnels et al (2001) evidenced the peculiar structure of TRPM7, combining a channel structure with an alpha-kinase domain at the C-terminus. Although originally investigated for a possible role in Ca^{2+} signaling in lymphocyte, it became rapidly apparent that the channel would preferentially carry Mg^{2+} and Ca^{2+} (Nadler *et al*, 2001) but also trace amounts of divalent cations such as Ni^{2+} and Zn^{2+} (Bessac and Fleig, 2007; Monteilh-Zoller *et al*, 2003).

Located on the human chromosome 15 at the locus 15q21, the protein is formed by 1865 amino acids arranged to possibly form 10 transmembrane domains, with both the C- and N-termini internalized. The protein is ubiquitously expressed albeit to a varying extent in all mammalian cells tested so far. The functional structure is supposed to be a tetramer but disagreement exists as to whether it is formed by 4 identical monomers or by a combination of TRPM7 and TRPM6 (see following section) arranged with a varying stoichiometry in different portion of the cell membrane or in different cell types. Voets and colleagues reported the functional expression of TRPM6 channels in HEK-

Table 1. Mg^{2+} transporters in eukaryotes

	Family	Members	Apparent K_m	Type of Transporter	Reference
<u>**Entry Mechanisms**</u>					
Cell Membrane	TRPM	TRPM6	~0.7 mM	Channel	Schlingmann *et al.*, 2002
		TRPM7	~0.7 mM	Channel	Nadler *et al.*, 2001
	Claudins	Claudin 16 (PCLN-1)	~0.7mM	Channel	Simon *et al.*, 1999
		Claudin-19	~0.7mM	Channel	Hou *et al.*, 2009
	MagT1	MagT1	0.2 mM	Channel	Goytain and Quamme, 2005a
					Zou and Clapham, 2009
	SLC41	SLC41A1	0.7 - 3 mM	Carrier	Goytain and Quamme, 2005b
		SLC41A2	0.7 - 3 mM	Carrier	Goytain and Quamme, 2005c
					Sahni *et al.*, 2007
	ACDP	ACDP1	~0.7 mM	Carrier	Goytain and Quamme, 2005d
		ACDP2	~0.5 mM	Carrier	Goytain and Quamme, 2005d
	NIPA	NIPA1 (SPG6)	0.7 mM	Carrier	Goytain *et al.*, 2007
		NIPA2	0.7 mM	Carrier	Goytain *et al.*, 2008a
	Huntingtin	Huntingtin1 (HIP14)	0.87 mM	Carrier	Goytain *et al.*, 2008b
		HIP14L	0.74 mM	Carrier	Goytain *et al.*, 2008b
Mitochondria	Mrs2	Mrs2/AtMrs2, Lpe10	~1.5 mM	Channel	Koliske *et al.*, 2003
Golgi	MMgt	MMgT1	1.5 mM	Channel	Goytain and Quamme, 2008
		MMgT2	0.6 mM	Channel	Goytain and Quamme, 2008

	Family	Members	Apparent Km	Type of Transporter	Reference
Exit Mechanisms					
Cell Membrane	Na^+/Mg^{2+} Exchanger	ND	15-20 mM	Antiport	Gunther and Vormann, 1984 Tashiro and Konishi, 1997 Cefaratti *et al*, 1998
	Na^+-Independent	ND (choline?)	~20mM	Exchanger(?)	Ebel *et al*, 2002
	SLC41	SLC41A1	~0.7 mM	Carrier	Kolisek *et al*, 2008
	H^+/Mg^{2+} exchanger	AtMHX#	~15mM	exchanger	Shaul *et al*, 1999

Identified only in plants and yeast and not in mammalian/human cells.

293 cells with electrophysiological properties similar to those of TRPM7 (Voets *et al*, 2004). In contrast, Chubanov et al (2004) reported the absence of functional currents through TRPM6 when the channel is expressed by itself in either HEK-293 cells or *X. Laevis* oocytes, and suggested that TRPM7 co-expression was required for TRPM6 to incorporate into channel complexes at the plasma membrane level. Schmitz *et al.* (Schmitz *et al*, 2005) subsequently confirmed the association of TRPM6 and TRPM7 channel proteins to obtain a functional structure. Yet, a detailed functional characterization of the TRPM6/7 chimeric channel remained undefined (Chubanov *et al*, 2005) until Yue and collaborators addressed the issue in two elegant electrophysiology studies (Li *et al*, 2006; Li *et al*, 2007). In these studies, the authors demonstrate that TRPM6 and TRPM7 can indeed form a chimeric heterotetramer, and that TRPM6, TRPM7, and TRPM6/7 constitute three distinct ion channels with different divalent cation permeability, pH sensitivity, and unique single channel conductance. In addition, these authors reported that 2-APB can differentially regulate the channel activities of TRPM6, TRPM7, and TRPM6/7, markedly increasing Mg^{2+} and Ca^{2+} entry through TRPM6 (Li *et al*, 2006). Based on these results, it would then appear that TRPM6 can form either functional homotetrameric channels or heterotetrameric TRPM6/7 channels (Gwanyanya *et al*, 2004). A corollary of this observation would be that TRPM6, TRPM7, and TRPM6/7 channels may play different roles under various physiological or pathological conditions in different tissues. A detailed mapping of the distribution of homomeric TRPM7 *versus* heteromeric TRPM6/7 channels in various tissues, however, is still lacking, leaving their relative role largely undefined.

More recently, some light has been shed on the modality of TRPM7 regulation. At the direct channel level, TRPM7 inward current is markedly enhanced by protons, which compete with Ca^{2+} and Mg^{2+} for binding sites, most likely at the level of the channel pore, thereby releasing the blockade of divalent cations on inward monovalent currents (Bessac and Fleig, 2007; Monteilh-Zoller *et al*, 2003). Not only extracellular protons significantly increased monovalent cation permeability, but higher proton concentrations are required to induce 50% of maximal increase in TRPM7 currents under conditions in which extracellular Ca^{2+} and Mg^{2+} concentrations are increased. Following the increase in extracellular H^+ concentration, in fact, the apparent affinity for Ca^{2+} and Mg^{2+} is significantly diminished. This set of observation suggests that at physiological pH, Ca^{2+} and Mg^{2+} bind to TRPM7 and inhibit the monovalent cation currents. At higher H^+ concentrations, instead, the affinity of TRPM7 for Ca^{2+} and Mg^{2+} is decreased, thus allowing monovalent cations to permeate the channel (Jiang *et al*, 2005). Another level of regulation appears to be provided by PIP2, as initially reported by Clapham and his collaborators (Runnels *et al*, 2002). This observation was not confirmed by Fleig's group, which instead reported a regulatory role by cAMP (Takezawa *et al*. 2004). More recently, however, Langeslag *et al*. (Langeslag *et al*, 2007) have observed that the depletion in PIP2 level resulting from PLC-activation counteracts TRPM7 activation. It would therefore appear that either PLC-activation accelerates TRPM7 'rundown' via PIP2 depletion or PIP2 depletion plays a feedback regulatory role on the channel activation by PLC (Langeslag *et al*, 2007). Additional evidence for a regulatory role by PIP2 on TRPM7 has been provided by Mubagwa's group (Gwanyanya *et al*, 2006; Macianskiene *et al*, 2008). This group, in fact, has reported that inhibition of phospholipase C or addition of exogenous PIP2 decreases the run-down of the channel whereas the extracellular addition of phenylephrine accelerates it (Macianskiene *et al*, 2008). In addition, this group has observed that both ATP (Gwanyanya *et al*, 2006) and non-hydrolysable GTP analogs modulate the channel activity, most likely by forming MgATP and by accelerating the channel run-down via phospholipase-C activation, respectively (Macianskiene *et al*, 2008). The regulatory role of PIP2 on TRPM7 is further emphasized by the experimental evidence that agonists like bradykinin or angiotensin-II, which activate phospholipase-C coupled receptors via Gq signaling (Touyz *et al*, 2006; Langeslag *et al*, 2007) can modulate the channel activity via PIP2 metabolism. Interestingly, TRPM7 activation only takes place in the presence of a physiological cellular $[Mg^{2+}]_i$, whereas reducing this concentration below its physiological level with EDTA-AM results in a PLC-mediated inactivation of TRPM7 activity, most likely via PIP2 depletion (Langeslag *et al*, 2007).

The interaction between TRPM7 and phosphatidyl-inositol metabolites is further supported by the observation that TRPM7 is required for a sustained phosphoinositide-3-kinase signaling in lymphocytes (Sahni and Scharenberg, 2008). In the presence of a physiological concentration of extracellular Mg^{2+}, TRPM7-deficient cells rapidly down-regulate their rate of growth as a result of a signaling deactivation downstream PI3-Kinase (Sahni and Scharenberg, 2008), the phenotype being rescued by supplementing the culture medium with Mg^{2+} (Sahni and Scharenberg, 2008).

A structural peculiarity of TRPM7 is the presence of an alpha-kinase at the C-terminus, which specifically phosphorylates serine and threonines located in an alpha-helix (Middelbeek *et al*, 2010). Initial experimental evidence (Runnels *et al*, 2002) invoked an essential role of this kinase domain in modulating channel activation and gating. Subsequent studies, however, failed to fully support this initial claim, as they indicated that TRPM7 channels lacking the kinase domain could still be activated by internal Mg^{2+} depletion (Schmitz *et al*, 2003). One consequence of lacking the kinase domain, however, is the inability of properly phosphorylating and consequently activating downstream cellular components. Yet, little is know about the molecular mechanisms activating the kinase domain. A recent study by Clark et al (2006) strongly suggests that autophosphorylation plays a significant role in target recognition by the TRMP7 kinase domain. Phosphomapping by mass spectrometry has confirmed the massing autophosphorylation of TRPM7 kinase domain, which – in turn – increases the rate of substrate phosphorylation. The phosphomapping has also identified the majority (37 out of 46) of the autophosphorylation sites in a Ser/Thr rich region immediately preceding the kinase catalytic domain (Clark *et al*, 2008). Deletion of this region does not affect the intrinsic catalytic activity of the kinase but prevents substrate phosphorylation, confirming the role of this region in substrate recognition (Clark *et al*, 2008). Although this Ser/Thr region is poorly conserved at the amino acid sequence in TRPM6, the kinase domain of this channel appears to require a similar massive autophosphorylation of its Sr/Thr residues for proper substrate recognition and efficient target phosphorylation (Clark *et al*, 2008).

So far, only annexin I (Dorovkov and Ryazanov, 2004), myosin IIA heavy chain (Clark *et al*, 2008a; Clark *et al*, 2008b), and calpain (Su *et al*, 2006) have been clearly identified as substrates phosphorylated by TRPM7 kinase domain. Although the number of targets is rather restricted, it appears that TRPM7 is playing a double role within cells by regulating Mg^{2+} homeostasis on the one hand, and cellular functions centered on cell adhesion, contractility and (anti)-inflammatory processes on the other hand. This double role of TRPM7 within cells, in particular smooth muscle cells, is emphasized by a recent observation by Touyz and colleagues (Paravicini *et al*, 2009). In this study, the authors report that aortic segments of mice exhibiting low intracellular Mg^{2+} levels present increased medial cross-section and increased TRPM7 expression but decreased levels of annexin-I expression. As annexin-I has a major anti-inflammatory role (Parente and Solito, 2004), the results of this study suggest a potential regulatory role of TRPM7 in regulating vascular structure and integrity, as well as inflammation.

As our understanding of TRPM7 expression and regulation has improved, evidence of a major functional role of the channel in neuronal function and survival under hypoxia or ischemic-reperfusion conditions has increased. Owing to its ability to transport either Ca^{2+} or Mg^{2+}, TRPM7 exhibits an ambivalent role based upon the permeating cation. Following activation by reactive oxygen/nitrogen species and prolonged oxygen and glucose deprivation, TRPM7 favors Ca^{2+} fluxes that result in a toxic event for neurons (Aarts *et al*, 2003). In contrast, Mg^{2+} permeation of the channel enhances anti-apoptotic and cell-survival mechanisms, preventing the anoxic death of neurons (Clark *et al*, 2006). The essential role of TRPM7 in detecting extracellular divalent cations is supported by a recent study by Wei et al (2007), which indicates that activation of the channel by low extracellular divalent cations is lethal to the cell. At the same time, Jiang *et al.* (Jiang *et al*, 2008) have reported that occlusion of the middle cerebral artery for 1 hour enhances TRPM7 expression in ipsilateral hippocampus, with deleterious consequences for the neurons. The increased expression of TRPM7 and its consequences are largely counteracted by pre-treatment with nerve growth factor via activation of TrkA pathway (Jiang *et al*, 2008). More recently, application of 5-lipoxygenase inhibitors can block TRPM7 current without affecting protein expression and cell membrane concentration, *de facto* preventing cell death (Chen *et al*, 2010).

The involvement of TRPM7 is not restricted to the sympathetic nervous system but extends to the parasympathetic system as well, in which the channel facilitates the fusion of cholinergic vesicles with the plasma membrane without affecting large dense core vesicle secretion (Brauchi *et al*, 2008).

Despite the data accumulated since its identification as a preferential Mg^{2+} channel, a recent report by Clapham's group has cast some concern about the effective role of TRPM7 in regulating Mg^{2+} homeostasis (Jin *et al*, 2008). In their report, the authors indicate that TRPM7 null mouse present an altered embryonic development, and that tissue specific deletion of the channel in T cell lineage disrupts thymopoiesis, leading to the progressive depletion of thymic medullary cells. Deletion of TRPM7, however, did not affect acute accumulation of Mg^{2+} nor impacted total cellular Mg^{2+} content in T cells. The synthesis of several growth factors, however, was significantly dysregulated, resulting in an altered differentiation of thymic epithelial cells (Jin *et al*, 2008). TRPM7, therefore, appears to be the first TRP channel with a non-redundant and actually essential role in embryogenesis and thymopoiesis. Whether these defects are the result on an altered Ca^{2+} rather than Mg^{2+} homeostasis it is presently undefined. It is also unclear how the removal of this protein results in an altered cellular differentiation process.

• *TRPM6*

The unique localization of TRPM6 channels in the colon and the renal distal convolute tubule, two epithelia otherwise highly impermeable to salt re-absorption, highlights the specific role of this channel in controlling intestinal Mg^{2+} absorption and renal Mg^{2+} resorption, and consequently contributing to whole-body Mg^{2+} homeostasis.

The *TRPM6* gene was originally identified as the site of various mutations responsible for Hypomagnesaemia with Secondary Hypocalcaemia (HSH), a rare autosomal recessive disease characterized by Mg^{2+} and Ca^{2+} wasting, whose symptoms could be ameliorated by massive intravenous Mg^{2+} administration followed by oral Mg^{2+} supplementation (Schlingmann *et al*, 2002). Surprisingly, while hypocalcaemia is completely alleviated by this treatment, the patients continue to present serum Mg^{2+} level around 0.5-0.6 mmol/L, i.e. about half the physiological level (Schlingmann *et al*, 2002). Because the primary defect in these patients is at the level of the TRPM6 expressed in the intestine (Schlingmann *et al*, 2002), the excess Mg^{2+} supplementation is rapidly filtered at the glomerular level and increases passive renal absorption via paracellin-1 (see next section). Trans-cellular absorption via renal TRPM6, however, remains depressed and unable to restore physiological serum Mg^{2+} level (Schlingmann *et al*, 2002).

At the functional level, experimental evidence suggests that the channel forms a tetramer within the plasma membrane. As indicated in the previous Section, questions remain as to whether the channel forms a homo-tetramer, or a hetero-tetramer with TRPM7, with a varying stoichiometry. Irrespective of the possibilities, several TRPM6 mutations have been identified (Walder *et al*, 2002). The majority of these mutations result in the expression of a truncated and non-functional channel (Walder *et al*, 2002). The missense mutation $S^{141}L$, on the other hand, occurs at the N-terminus of the channel and prevents its proper assembly as a homo-tetramer, or a hetero-tetramer with TRPM7 (Walder *et al*, 2002). Another missense identified in humans is the $P^{1017}R$ mutation (Walder *et al*, 2002), which appears to occur in a region putatively identified as the pore region of the channel. Yet, this mutation affects negatively and more significantly TRPM7 function when this protein is co-expressed with TRPM6 (Walder *et al*, 2002). More recently, TRPM6 null mice have been developed by Sheffield and his collaborators (Walder *et al*, 2009). The heterozygous *Trpm6*$^{+/-}$ have for the most part normal electrolyte levels aside for a modest low plasma Mg^{2+} level (~0.67 vs. 0.75, (Walder *et al*, 2009). The majority of the homozygous *Trpm6*$^{-/-}$ animals die by embryonic day 12.5. Most of the few animals that survive to term present significant neural tube defects, consisting primarily of both exencephaly and spina bifida occulta. Administration of high Mg diet to dams improves offspring survival to weaning (Walder *et al*, 2009).

A peculiarity TRPM6 shares with TRPM7 is the presence of an alpha-kinase domain at the C-terminus. Originally, TRPM6 was known as CHAK2 (channel kinase 2) (Ryazanov, 2002) due to the presence of this kinase domain, which presents a functional homology to eEF2-kinase (Ryazanov, 2002). At variance of other kinases, this domain phosphorylates serine and threonine residues located within an alpha-helix instead of a beta-sheet (Ryazanova *et al*, 2001; Ryazanov, 2002; Middelbeek *et al*, 2010). Owing to their dual function as a channel and a kinase, TRPM6 and TRPM7 are currently referred to as *chanzymes*. As in the case of TRPM7, removal of the kinase domain does not abolish entirely the channel activity but modulates the extent to which the channel is regulated by intra-cellular free Mg^{2+} or MgATP complex (Chubanov *et al*, 2004; Schmitz *et al*, 2005; Chubanov *et al*, 2005; Li *et al*, 2005; Thebault *et al*, 2008). Hence, the targets phosphorylated by the kinase must be located downstream the protein. At variance of what reported for the kinase domain of TRPM7 (see previous Section) no phosphorylation substrate for the TRPM6 kinase has been clearly identified up-to-date, with the exception of TRPM7 itself. Data from the Ryazanov's group clearly indicate that the TRPM6 kinase domain can phosphorylate TRPM7 channel within a heterotetramer structure while the opposite does not occur (Schmitz *et al*, 2005). Due to the limited information available, it is largely undefined as to whether the kinase domain of TRPM7 and TRMP6 phosphorylate similar or different substrates in the tissues in which these chanzymes are specifically expressed.

How exactly the expression and/or activity of TRPM6 channel are modulated *in vivo* is slowly being elucidated. Estrogens (17ß-estradiol) markedly upregulate TRPM6 mRNA in both colon and kidney while having no effect on TRPM7 mRNA (Groenestege *et al*, 2006; Cao *et al*, 2009). In the absence of estrogen, the repressor of estrogen receptor activity (REA) binds to the 6th, 7th and 8th beta-sheets of TRPM6 kinase domain in a phosphorylation-dependent manner and inhibits TRPM6 activity (Cao *et al*, 2009). Short-term estrogen administration dissociates the binding between REA and TRPM6, resulting in an increased channel activity (Cao *et al*, 2009). Dietary Mg^{2+} restriction also upregulates TRPM6 mRNA in both colon and kidney but does not affect TRPM7 mRNA (Groenestege *et al*, 2006; Rondon *et al*, 2008). In contrast, an Mg^{2+} enriched diet upregulates TRPM6 mRNA only in the colon, in keeping with an increased intestinal absorption (Groenestege *et al*, 2006). Mice selected for the their low erythrocyte and plasma Mg^{2+} status exhibit hypomagnesaemia and hypomagnesuria, and increased TRPM6 expression in kidney and intestine when fed a severely Mg^{2+}-deficient diet (Rondon *et al*, 2008). Feeding the mice an Mg^{2+} adequate diet resulted, instead, in hypomagnesaemia and hypermagnesuria, and lower intestinal and renal TRPM6 expression (Rondon *et al*, 2008). These changes in TRPM6 expression and Mg^{2+} level in blood and urine were not observed in mice exhibiting normal or high erythrocyte and plasma Mg^{2+} level (Rondon *et al*, 2008). It is becoming progressively apparent, therefore, that genetic factors control TRPM6 expression and activity, and that dietary Mg^{2+} restriction increases Mg^{2+} resorption, the process correlating well with an increased TRPM6 expression in both intestine and kidney Groenestege *et al*, 2006; Rondon *et al*, 2008).

As already observed for TRPM7, intracellular ATP specifically decreased TRPM6 current (Chubanov *et al*, 2004; Schmitz *et al*, 2005; Chubanov *et al*, 2005; Li *et al*, 2005; Thebault *et al*, 2008). The inhibitory site resides in the conserved ATP-binding motif GXG(A)XXG within the alpha-kinase domain (Thebault *et al*, 2008). Either the full deletion of the kinase domain or point mutations within the ATP-binding motif ($G^{1955}D$) completely prevents the inhibitory effect of intracellular ATP. The effect of ATP, however, is independent of alpha-kinase autophosphorylation activity (Thebault *et al*, 2008).

The activity of TRPM6 channels can also be modulated by cellular signaling molecules. Bindels and collaborators (Cao *et al*, 2008) have reported that over-expression of RACK1 (receptor for activated protein kinase C) results in a direct binding of this protein to the alpha-kinase domain of TRPM6, and possibly TRPM7 due to the high homology (>84%) between the two kinase domains. The TRPM6 site binding RACK1 is restricted to the region between amino acids 1857 and 1885 (6th, 7th and 8th b sheets). Interestingly, these are the same sheets involved in REA regulation Cao *et al*, 2009). The interplay between REA and RACK1 in modulating the channel activity, however, still remains undefined. Accessibility analysis of the RACK1 binding site suggests that 18 of the 28 amino acids of this site are localized at the surface of the TRPM6 alpha-kinase domain (Cao *et al*, 2008). As a result of this interaction, the channel activity of TRPM6 and TRPM7 are inhibited. As it could be anticipated, co-expression of RACK1with a alpha-kinase deleted TRPM6 mutant fails to suppress channel activity. The inhibitory effect of RACK1 fully depends on the autophosphorylation of threonine 1851 (T^{1851}) within the kinase domain. This residue is localized at the end of the 4th alpha-helix adjacent to the RACK1 binding site. Mutation of T^{1851} to alanine (T^{1851}A) or to aspartate (T^{1851}D) significantly decreases TRPM6 autophosphorylation while leaving unaltered RACK1 binding. The inhibitory effect of RACK1 on the channel activity, however, is completely abolished only in the case of T^{1851}A mutation while it persists in the case of T^{1851}D mutation (Cao *et al*, 2008). Interestingly, T^{1851}D autophosphorylation strongly depends on Mg^{2+} concentration, steadily increasing for concentrations between 0.1 to 1mM. In contrast, T^{1851}A mutant is less sensitive to intracellular Mg^{2+} concentrations as compared to the wild type (IC_{50} ~0.7 vs. 0.5mM, respectively). Under conditions in which protein kinase C is activated (e.g. pre-incubation with PMA), the inhibitory effect of RACK1 on TRPM6 channel activity is completely prevented (Cao *et al*, 2008). The inhibition, however, can be restored by pre-treatment with the PKC inhibitor chelerythrine (Cao *et al*, 2008), suggesting a competing effect of PKC for RACK1.

A recent study of Groenestege et al (2007) has evidenced the role of EGF as an autocrine/ paracrine magnesiotropic hormone. By engaging its receptor in the basolateral domain of the distal convolute tubule, EGF is able to activate TRPM6 at the apical domain of the cell and induce cellular Mg^{2+} accumulation. Point mutation in the pro-EGF (P^{1070}L) retains EGF secretion to the apical membrane and disrupts this cascade of events, ultimately resulting in the Mg^{2+} wasting typical of isolated recessive renal hypo-magnesemia (IRH). An alteration of the axis EGF/TRPM6/Mg^{2+} reabsorption/renal Mg^{2+} wasting is also observed in cancer patients undergoing treatment with antibodies anti-EGFR (Cunningham *et al*, 2004; Dimke *et al*, 2010), as the antibody antagonizes the stimulation of TRPM6 activity via EGF. The modality by which EGF modulates TRPM6 activity and/or expression appears to involve ERK1/2 signaling. A report by Ikari et al (2008) indicates that the stimulation of NRK-52E cells by EGF results in an increased phosphorylation of ERK1/2 and an increased expression of TRPM6 in a time-dependent manner (Ikari *et al*, 2008) via modulation by adaptin protein-1 (AP-1) (Ikari *et al*, 2010). The process is prevented by the use of antagonists for integrin a_vb3 or for MEK1/MEK2 activity, or by the use of siRNA for TRPM6 (Ikari *et al*, 2008). How exactly EGF, integrin, and ERK1/2 interact to enhance TRPM6 expression needs further elucidation. It is in fact unclear whether the activation of this signaling axis is connected to the release of RACK1-mediated inhibition of TRPM6 activity mentioned previously (Cao *et al*, 2008). The modality by which apically accumulated Mg^{2+} is transported across the cell to be delivered to basolateral domain of the cell to be extruded into the blood stream also needs further elucidation. One hypothesis is that parvalbumin and calbindin-D_{28k}, two proteins abundantly present within cells of the distal convolute tubule of the nephron, can operate the transcellular transport of Mg^{2+} accumulated at the apical domain, or at least accelerate the rate of delivery at the basolateral domain. However, as mentioned previously, parvalbumin *null* mice do not show detectable defects in Mg^{2+} excretion or homeostasis (Belge *et al*, 2007), *de facto* questioning whether parvalbumin does play a role in the process or other proteins can compensate for its absence in the *null* model.

Claudins

Paracellin 1 (claudin 16) was the first Mg^{2+} transporting protein to be identified in mammals (Simon *et al*, 1999). The identification was rendered possible by the genetic analysis of patients affected by Familial Hypomagnesaemia with Hypercalciuria and Nephrocalcinosis (FHHNC), a disease characterized by massive renal Mg^{2+} and Ca^{2+} wasting that leads rapidly and irreversibly to renal failure (Simon *et al*, 1999). At variance of what described for patients with TRPM6 mutations (Section 3.1.3.2), the symptoms and the progressive renal deterioration in FHHNC patients are not ameliorated by Mg^{2+} supplementation (Simon *et al*, 1999). The gene responsible for this disease was identified by Lifton and collaborators in 1999 and named *Paracellin-1* (*PCLN-1*) (Simon *et al*, 1999). More than 20 mutations affecting paracellin-1 trafficking or permeability have been identified up-to-date (Kausalya *et al*, 2006). *PCLN-1* encodes for paracellin-1 (PCLN-1), also termed claudin-16. This protein is a member of the claudin family ((Lal-Nag and Morin, 2009), which comprehends a group of tight junction proteins that present 4 transmembrane spans coordinated by 2 extracellular loops, and both C- and N-termini on the cytoplasm side.

Claudin-16 mediates paracellular Ca^{2+} and Mg^{2+} fluxes throughout the nephron. Yet, discrepancy exists about the modality by which these fluxes are generated. Data obtained in LLC-PK1 (a porcine renal cell line) suggest that claudin-16 mediates paracellular Na^{+}-permeation which, in turn, generates a positive potential within the lumen that acts as the driving force for Mg^{2+} and Ca^{2+} resorption (Hou *et al*, 2005). In contrast, data in MDCK cells indicate a decrease in Na^{+}-permeability and an increase in Mg^{2+} permeability (Ikari *et al*, 2006). It is unclear whether these discrepancies reflect a different *modus operandi* in cell lines of differing origin, or depend on the experimental conditions utilized in the two studies. It is evident, however, that *PCLN-1* expression is modulated based upon the magnesium concentration present in the extracellular medium (Efrati *et al*, 2005).

At the functional level, claudin-16 has to be delivered correctly to the tight junction where it interacts with the scaffolding protein ZO-1 (Muller *et al*, 2003). The association and dissociation of claudin-16 and ZO-1 appear to be regulated via PKA-mediated phosphorylation of Ser^{217} in claudin-16 (Muller *et al*, 2003). The dephosphorylation of this residue, as it occurs upon activation of the Calcium Sensing Receptor (CaSR) (Khan and Conigrave, 2010) results in the dissociation of claudin-16 from ZO-1 and its accumulation in the lysosomal compartment (Ikari *et al*, 2006). Mutations of Ser 217 can therefore accelerate claudin-16 turn-over and modulate its function. Mutation of Threo233 (T233R) also impairs the interaction between claudin-16 and ZO-1, and favors the accumulation of claudin-166 into lysosomes (Muller *et al*, 2003; Ikari *et al*, 2006). More recently, evidence has emerged indicating the involvement of another claudin isoform, claudin-19, in mediating Mg^{2+} and Ca^{2+} resorption (Hou *et al*, 2009) by forming a head-to-head cation-selective complex with claudin-16 at the level of the tight junction. While the channel function of claudin-16 may not depend on its association with claudin-19, claudin-19 plays an indispensable role in recruiting claudin-16 to form a co-polymer at the level of the tight junction and in switching the channel from anion to cation selective (Hou *et al*, 2009). The heteromeric association between claudin-16 and claudin-19 is dramatically affected by point mutations in claudin-16 ($L^{145}P$, $L^{151}F$, $G^{191}R$, $A^{209}T$, and $F^{232}C$) and claudin-19 ($L^{90}P$ and $G^{123}R$), which abolish the physiological synergism between the two proteins and result in the development of FHHNC.

MagT1

This protein was identified by Goytain and Quamme (2005a) in human epithelial cells that upregulate the encoding gene following exposure to low-Mg^{2+} concentrations in the culture medium. The protein encoded by this gene has an estimated molecular weight of 38 KDa and 5 transmembrane domains. The mature MagT1 protein, however, would contain 4 transmembrane spans owing to the cleavage of the first transmembrane segment located near the C-terminus. At variance of SLC41 (Section 3.3.1) and Mrs2 (discussed in the next Section), MagT1 does not exhibit any significant degree of homology to prokaryotic Mg^{2+} transporters, but has some similarities with the oligosaccharide transferase complex OST3/OST6 that regulates protein glycosylation in the endoplasmic reticulum in yeast (Shibatani *et al*, 2005). The murine orthologue of MagT1 is highly expressed in liver, heart, kidney and colon, with detectable levels in lung, brain and spleen (Goytain and Quamme, 2005a). For the most part, MagT1 levels in these tissues are consistent with the mRNA levels, the only exception being the liver in which a low protein level is detected (Goytain and Quamme, 2005a). At variance of the other transporters described in this section, MagT1 appears to possess high specificity for Mg^{2+} (K_m = 0.23mM). The Mg^{2+}-elicited currents are not inhibited by Ca^{2+} but can be inhibited by Ni^{2+}, Zn^{2+} and Mn^{2+}, although the required concentrations (>0.2mM) far exceed the physiological concentrations of these cations in extracellular fluids. Interestingly, nitrendipine at ~10mM can inhibit the Mg^{2+} current whereas the more common nifedipine does not, even at much higher concentrations (Goytain and Quamme, 2005a). Virtually no information is available about N33, a second member of the MagT family. Although able to transport Mg^{2+}, this protein does not show the same high specificity presented by MagT1 for the cation, and can also mediate the transport of Fe^{2+}, Mn^{2+} and Cu^{2+} (Goytain and Quamme, 2005a).

Based upon these observations MagT1 appears to possess channel-like characteristics and a high selectivity for Mg^{2+}. The latter evidence strongly suggests that this transporter can play an essential role in regulating Mg^{2+} homeostasis in mammalian cells. Support to this hypothesis is provided by the report of Zhou and Clapham (Zhou and Clapham, 2009) that knock-out of MagT1, and its human homolog TUSC3, in HEK-293 cells results in a major reduction of cellular Mg^{2+} content. These authors also provide evidence that either protein can complement the yeast Mg^{2+} transporter ALR1 (Zhou and Clapham, 2009). Interestingly, the mRNA levels of MagT1 but not those of TUSC3 increase markedly following exposure of expressing cells to low extracellular Mg^{2+} concentrations for 1 day and 2 days. Incubation of the cells in high extracellular Mg^{2+} concentration has no effect on the expression of either protein (Zhou and Clapham, 2009).

Mrs2

This protein was identified during a screening aimed at isolating nuclear genes suppressing RNA splicing defects in yeast mitochondrial introns (Wiesenberger *et al*, 1992). The three main characteristics observed in yeasts deficient in Mrs2 are: 1) a splicing phenotype, 2) a significant reduction in cytochromes, and 3) a deficit in mitochondria respiration to the point that the yeasts become unable to grow on non-fermentable substrates.

Structurally, Mrs2 shows short regions of homology to the bacterial transporter CorA (Bui *et al*, 1999), and shares a similar membrane topology with 2 transmembrane domains. Mutants lacking Mrs2 can be rescued by CorA fused to the mitochondrial N-terminus leader sequence of Mrs2, which guarantees proper insertion in the mitochondrial membrane. These mutants also present a decrease in mitochondrial Mg^{2+} content, which strongly supports a key role of Mrs2 in regulating mitochondrial Mg^{2+} homeostasis. Studies carried out with the fluorescent indicator Mag-Fura indicate a marked decrease in mitochondrial matrix Mg^{2+} level in yeast lacking Mrs2 protein whereas the over-expression of the protein results in a rapid and marked increase in matrix free Mg^{2+} (Kolisek *et al*, 2003). Mrs2 apparently functions as a channel, and its function is modulated by mitochondrial Dy as well as by inhibitors of F0-F1-ATPase or ANT, which substantially decrease Mg^{2+} influx. Highly conserved motifs in the middle region of the protein, corresponding to the coiled-coil portion of the channel, appear to be essential to form functional channels, or to gate the channel. More recently, Schweyen and his collaborators (Piskacek *et al*, 2009) have confirmed in HEK293 cells some of the mitochondrial modifications observed in yeasts. These authors, in fact, have reported that HEK 293 cells deprived of Mrs2 (Piskacek *et al*, 2009) lack complex I expression in mitochondria and present reduced level of mitochondrial Mg^{2+}. Furthermore, the cells show a change in configuration as well as an increased incidence in apoptosis, which within 2 weeks results in a complete loss of cell viability (Piskacek *et al*, 2009). It still remains to be elucidated whether the decrease in mitochondrial Mg^{2+} simply depends on the absence of Mrs2, or is related to some extent to the absence of complex I, which affects mitochondrial Dy and consequently Mg^{2+} retention within the organelle (Akerman, 1981).

Mammalian cells express a single orthologue of Mrs2, which can rescue Mg^{2+} deficient yeast strain (Zsurka *et al*, 2001). Hence, it appears that the mammalian/human Mrs2 homologue functions in a manner similar to the yeast homologue in mediating Mg^{2+} entry in mitochondria. Under conditions in which Mrs2p is absent, the operation of an alternative but much slower mitochondrial Mg^{2+} entry mechanism is observed. Although this pathway restores Mg^{2+} homeostasis only partially, it does rescue the phenotype of Mrs2 deficient yeast, ensuring their survival. No information is presently available about the identity, abundance, and regulation of this alternative transporter in mitochondria. Taken together, the data on Mrs2 suggest that Mg^{2+} is dynamically regulated within the mitochondrion, in which it plays a significant role in modulating mitochondrial dehydrogenases and oxygen consumption (Panov and Scarpa, 1996a; Panov and Scarpa, 1996b).

MMgTs

This gene family comprehends two proteins termed MMgT1 and MMgT2 (for membrane Mg^{2+} transporter 1 and 2) by Goytain and Quamme, who identified them by microarray analysis screening (Goytain and Quamme, 2008). The chromosomal location of these proteins in the mouse is XA5 for MMgT1 and 11B2 for MMgT2. In the rat, the respective locations are Xq36 for MMgT1 and 10q23 for MMgT2. Human MMgT1 is instead located on Xq26.3 (Goytain and Quamme, 2008). Immunohistochemistry assessment indicates that MMgT1 and MMgT2 are essentially located in the Golgi complex and post-Golgi vesicles, where they may contribute to the regulation of Mg^{2+} dependent enzymes involved in protein assembly and glycosylation (Goytain and Quamme, 2008). This localization, however, does not exclude that these proteins may play a role in modulating Mg^{2+} homeostasis at sites downstream the Golgi network. Widely distributed in tissues, these proteins are formed by 131 (MMgT1) and 123 (MMgT2) amino acids assembled into two predicted transmembrane domains. This suggests that these proteins can form homo-oligomeric and possibly hetero-oligomeric channels to favor Mg^{2+} permeation. MMgT-mediated Mg^{2+} uptake is saturable with a Km ~1.5mM for MMgT1 and ~0.6mM for MMgT2, and these values do not vary significantly with voltage. However, MMgT1 and MMgT2 are not specific for Mg^{2+} but they can transport other cations as well. Some slight differences in cation permeation exist between the two isoforms. Whereas MMgT1 mediates Sr^{2+}, Fe^{2+}, Co^{2+} and Cu^{2+} transport in addition to Mg^{2+}, MMgT2 favors Sr^{2+}, Co^{2+}, Cu^{2+}, Ba^{2+} and Mn^{2+} transport [**112**]. Electrophysiological experiments indicate that Mg^{2+}-generated current in MMgT1 are inhibited by 0.2mM Mn^{2+} but not by Gd^{3+} or Ni^{2+}. Consistent with what reported for other Mg^{2+} transport mechanisms, MMgT1 mRNA increases ~2.5 fold in the kidney cortex of mice on low-Mg^{2+} diet and ~3.5 fold in MDCT epithelial cells culture in low Mg^{2+} medium. Under similar experimental conditions MMgT2 mRNA increases ~1.5 fold in kidney cortex and ~3 fold in MDCT cells (Goytain and Quamme, 2008).

We refer the interested audience to reviews by Schmidt *et al.* (Schmitz *et al*, 2007), Bindels' group (Alexander *et al*, 2008), and Quamme (Quamme, 2010) for a more in-depth elucidation of the specifics of TRPM6/7 channels and other Mg^{2+} entry mechanisms summarily described in this Section.

Exchangers

While Mg^{2+} entry appears to be mediated by channels or channels-like mechanisms, Mg^{2+} extrusion is mediated by two mechanisms operating as exchangers. Based upon the electrochemical requirements favoring Mg^{2+} extrusion, these mechanisms are referred to as Na^+-dependent and Na^+-independent Mg^{2+} exchanger, respectively (Table 1). Because neither of these two mechanisms has been cloned, information about their operation, abundance and tissue specificity remains mostly circumstantial or indirect based upon experimental conditions or pharmacological inhibition.

Na-dependent (Na^+/Mg^{2+} Exchanger)

The first evidence of the operation of a Mg^{2+} transport mechanism in mammalian cells was provided by Gunther and Vormann in 1984 (Gunther *et al*, 1984). In this and a subsequent publication (Gunther and Vormann, 1985), these authors detailed the presence and operation of an amiloride-inhibited, Na^+-dependent, Mg^{2+} extrusion mechanism in chicken red blood cells. This initial observation has been subsequently confirmed by other groups in mammalian red blood cells (Feray and Garay, 1986; Flatman and Smith, 1990; Xu and Willis, 1994) including human erythrocytes (Ludi and Schatzmannm 1987; Vormann *et al*, 1984; Raftos *et al*, 1999), and in a variety of mammalian cell types (see Romani and Scarpa, 2000 for a list). In addition, observation from Vormann and Gunther (Vormann and Gunther, 1987; Gunther and Vormann, 1992a), Wolf and collaborators (Wolf *et al*, 1996; Wolf *et al*, 1997), and our laboratory (Romani and Scarpa, 1990a; Romani and Scarpa 1990b; Romani *et al*, 1993a; Romani *et al*, 1993b; Fagan and Romani, 2000; Fagan and Romani, 2001; Cefaratti and Ruse, 2007; Cefaratti and Romani, 2007) has provided compelling evidence that this Na^+-dependent, amiloride-inhibited Mg^{2+} extrusion mechanisms is specifically coupled to cAMP-production within the cells. From the experimental stand-point it is irrelevant whether cellular cAMP increases via stimulation of b-adrenergic, glucagon, or PGE2 receptors, or via administration of forskolin or cell-permeant cyclic-AMP analogs. All these conditions, in fact, result in the activation of the Na^+-dependent Mg^{2+} extrusion mechanism via phosphorylation. Conversely, pre-treatment of cells with inhibitors of adenylyl cyclase (e.g. Rp-cAMP) completely blocks Mg^{2+} mobilization irrespective of the modality utilized to enhance cAMP level (Wolf *et al*, 1997).

Because the Mg^{2+} extrusion mediated by this exchanger strictly depends on the presence of a physiological concentration of Na^+ in the extracellular milieu (Romani *et al*, 1993a; Fagan and Romani, 2000), it is generally accepted that the Na^+-dependent Mg^{2+} extrusion mechanisms is a Na^+/Mg^{2+} exchanger. As this Mg^{2+} extrusion mechanism has not been functionally cloned, we lack detailed information about its membrane abundance, structure, proximity to other cellular transporters with whom it may possibly interact, and stoichiometry. Early reports by Gunther and Vormann (1984, 1985) suggest the operation of electroneutral bases ($2Na^+_{in}$:1 Mg^{2+}_{out}) at least in chicken or turkey erythrocytes. This notion has not been confirmed in mammalian erythrocytes including human red blood cells, in which the exchanger appears to operate electrogenically on a $1Na^+_{in}$:1 Mg^{2+}_{out} ratio (Ludi and Schatzmann, 1987; Flatman, 1990; Xu and Willis, 1994). The discrepancy between these reports is not apparent although it may depend on the experimental model (i.e. cell isolation vs. cultured cells), composition of incubation medium, or modality of cellular Mg^{2+} loading. Irrespective of the stoichiometry of exchange and the experimental model, however, all the obtained results consistently indicate a K_m for Na^+ between 15 to 20 mM (Gunther, 1996; Tashiro and Konishi, 1997; Cefaratti *et al*, 1998). Pharmacological inhibition has done little to enhance our understanding of the modality of operation of the putative Na^+/Mg^{2+} exchanger. Amiloride, imipramine and quinidine represent the three most widely utilized inhibitors of Na^+-dependent Mg^{2+} extrusion (Gunther and Vormann, 1984; Feray and Garay, 1988; Gunther and Vormann, 1992a). However, because of their limited specificity, it is unclear as to whether they inhibit the Na^+/Mg^{2+}-exchanger directly, or indirectly by operating on other transport mechanisms including Na^+ and K^+ channel, ultimately altering the cell membrane potential and the driving force for Mg^{2+} transport across the plasma membrane.

Despite intense research, the Na^+/Mg^{2+} exchanger is not cloned as yet. Work by Schweigel, Martens and colleagues (Schweigel *et al*, 2000) in mammalian rumen support the operation of a Na^+/Mg^{2+} exchanger with kinetic parameters and characteristics similar to those described by other groups in a various mammalian cell types. Furthermore, by using a hybridoma screening procedure, this group has generated monoclonal antibodies against the Na^+/Mg^{2+} exchanger present in porcine red blood cells. Incubation of sheep rumen epithelial cells in the presence of these antibodies has resulted in a significant inhibition of Mg^{2+} extrusion *via* this exchanger (Schweigel *et al*, 2000). Western blot analysis utilizing these antibodies has evidenced a protein band of ~70 KDa mr, which could tentatively correspond to the Na^+/Mg^{2+} exchanger (Schweigel *et al*, 2000). This is the first time that information about the molecular size of the elusive Na^+/Mg^{2+} exchanger is obtained, and the utilization of these antibodies could represent an ideal tool to identify and recognize this transporter in mammalian tissue.

Na^+-independent

Under conditions in which no extracellular Na^+ is available to exchange for intracellular Mg^{2+}, an alternative Na^+-independent Mg^{2+} extrusion mechanism becomes evident. The specificity of this transporter, however, is far from being characterized. Different cations including Ca^{2+} or Mn^{2+} as well as anions (e.g. HCO_3^-, Cl^-, or choline) (Gunther, 1993; Ebel *et al*, 2002) have been reported to be utilized by this mechanism to extrude Mg^{2+} from the cell. Hence, it remains unclear whether we are in the presence of distinct transport mechanisms, or in the presence of a transporter that can operate as an antiporter for cations or a synporter for cations and anions based upon the experimental conditions. Also, it is unclear whether the Na^+-independent pathway is activated by hormonal stimulation. Results obtained in liver cells (Keenan *et al*, 1996; Fagan and Romani, 2000; Fagan and Romani, 2001) indicate that the stimulation by mix adrenergic agonists (e.g. epinephrine) elicit a Mg^{2+} extrusion that is equivalent to the sum of the amounts of Mg^{2+} mobilized by the separate stimulation of a_1-

and b-adrenergic receptors. More specifically, the selective stimulation of a_1-adrenergic receptors by phenylephrine requires the presence of physiological concentrations of both Na^+ and Ca^{2+} in the extracellular medium to elicit Mg^{2+} extrusion from liver cells (Fagan and Romani, 2000; Fagan and Romani, 2001). As phenylephrine stimulation appears to operate via Ca^{2+}-CaM to induce Mg^{2+} extrusion, it is undefined whether this signaling pathway represents an alternative modality of activation of the Na^+/Mg^{2+} exchanger, or it activates instead a different Mg^{2+} extrusion mechanism that can be reconciled at least in part with the afore mentioned Na^+-independent mechanism. Adding to the uncertainty, Ebel and collaborators (Ebel *et al*, 2002) have suggested that in red blood cells and hepatocytes the Na^+-independent Mg^{2+} extrusion occurs via the choline transporter, which can be inhibited rather specifically by cinchona alkaloids.

One controversial issue is whether the Na^+-dependent and Na^+-independent mechanisms operate as ATPases or require ATP for their operation. Reports by Gunther and collaborators (Gunther *et al*, 1990; Ebel *et al*, 2004) indicate a certain dependence of Na^+-dependent Mg^{2+} extrusion on the presence of a physiological concentration of cellular ATP, the absence or decrease in cellular ATP content resulting in a reduced Mg^{2+} efflux from the cell (Gunther *et al*, 1990; Ebel *et al*, 2004). In the particular case of red blood cells, ATP and 2,3 bisphosphoglycerate both contribute to Mg^{2+} homeostasis and transport (Gunther *et al*, 1995). A regulatory effect of ATP on Mg^{2+} extrusion is not observed in purified liver plasma membrane vesicles (Cefaratti *et al*, 1998). It is true that no Mg^{2+} extrusion is observed in alkaline phosphatase-treated basolateral liver plasma membrane vesicles in the absence of ATP (Cefaratti and Romani, 2007), but this observation can reasonably be explained by the requirement of ATP to phosphorylate and activate the Na^+/Mg^{2+} exchanger in the presence of PKA catalytic subunit (Cefaratti and Romani, 2007).

Mg^{2+}/H^+

This exchange mechanism, originally identified in *A. thaliana* and termed AtMHX, appears to be present in all plants (Shaul *et al*, 1999). This transporter presents 11 putative transmembrane domains, is exclusively localized in the vacuolar membrane of the plant, and electrogenically exchanges protons with Mg^{2+} or Zn^{2+}. Interestingly, the ectopic overexpression of the transporter in tobacco plants sensitizes the plant to grow in the presence of elevated concentrations of Mg^{2+} (or Zn^{2+}) (Shaul *et al*, 1999). Presently, no corresponding gene and transporter have been identified in mammalian cells, although evidence for a direct or indirect exchange of Mg^{2+} for H^+ under certain conditions has been provided by Gunther (Gunther and Vormann, 1990a). An enhanced extrusion of cellular Mg^{2+} has been observed in cells incubated in an acidic extracellular environment, in which an inwardly oriented H^+ gradient is imposed, provided that extracellular Na^+ is present (Gunther and Vormann, 1990a; Dalal and Romani, 2010). Amiloride derivates that inhibit with high affinity the Na^+/H^+ exchanger are ineffective at blocking Mg^{2+} extrusion under these experimental conditions (Gunzel and Schlue, 1996), thus excluding that Mg^{2+} extrusion depends on the operation in reverse of the Na^+/H^+ exchanger in parallel with the forward operation of the Na^+/Mg^{2+} exchanger.

Carriers

This section groups several novel Mg^{2+} transport mechanisms of murine or human origin identified as a result of diet restriction (i.e. Mg^{2+}-deficient diet) or medium restriction (i.e. low extracellular Mg^{2+} content). Due to the limited information available and controversies in their *modus operandi*, these transport mechanisms are non-descriptively classified as carriers.

SLC41

This family of Mg^{2+} transport mechanisms includes three members (A1, A2, and A3) that are distantly related to the prokaryotic MgtE channel identified by Maguire (Smith *et al*, 1995). We will discuss predominantly SLC41A1 and A2 isoforms since no study has addressed function and structure of the SLC41A3 isoform.

SLC41A1 was the first member of this family to be identified (Wabakken *et al*, 2003). Based on the hydrophobic profile, this protein of ~56 kDa Mr was predicted to possess 10 transmembrane domains, two of which presented a discrete level of homology with MgtE (Wabakken *et al*, 2003). Northern blot analysis indicates a wide distribution of the *SLC41A1* gene, but its abundance varies markedly among tissues, the highest expression being in heart and testis and the lowest being in hematopoietic tissues and cells (Wabakken *et al*, 2003). While modest under basal conditions, the expression of this gene is markedly up-regulated in the renal cortex of mice fed low Mg^{2+} diet for several days (Goytain and Quamme, 2005b). Functional expression of mouse SLC41A1 in *X. oocyte* indicates that this protein can transport Mg^{2+} but also Fe^{2+}, Cu^{2+}, Zn^{2+} and Cd^{2+} while Ca^{2+} is not transported nor inhibits Mg^{2+} transport (Goytain and Qaumme, 2005b). The original characterization of Mg^{2+} generated current, which would be tentatively consistent with SLC41A1 operating as a channel (Goytain and Qaumme, 2005b) or an electrogenic exchanger similar to the Na/Ca exchanger (Quednau *et al*, 2004), contrasts with a recent report by Kolisek et al (2008). In this study the authors strongly advocate for SLC41A1 operating as a carrier and predominantly favoring Mg^{2+} efflux rather than influx. Following overexpression of SLC41A1 in HEK293 cells 1) no detectable Mg^{2+} currents is observed; 2) incubation of cells in Mg^{2+}-free media results in a significant reduction of total Mg^{2+} content and $[Mg^{2+}]_i$; 3) the amplitude of Mg^{2+} loss depends on the number of SLC41A1 molecules expressed in the membrane and the induction time, and 4) the changes in $[Mg^{2+}]i$ are temperature sensitive but insensitive to the Mg^{2+} channel blocker CoHexamine (Kolisek *et al*, 2008. Furthermore, Kolisek and collaborators suggest that SLC41A1 forms high molecular weight complexes within the cell membrane with masses ranging from 1236 KDa to ~360 kDa, in stark contrast to the 56 KDa Mr of the monomer (Kolisek *et al*, 2008). Whether this observation indicates that the SLC41A1 monomer forms large multimeric complexes and/or interacts with auxiliary proteins is presently undefined. The reason for the absence of Mg^{2+}-generated currents in this study as compared to the original observation by Goytain and Quamme (2005b) is not apparent. One possibility is that the murine (Goytain and Qaumme, 2005b) and human orthologs (Kolisek *et al*, 2008) operate differently. Based upon their high degree (>90%) of homology the mouse and human SLC41A1 are expected to operate in a similar manner. Yet, the possibility that point mutations can dramatically alter SLC41A1 ion specificity and modality of function cannot be completely dismissed. In this respect, it has to be noted that Goytain and Quamme (2005b) did not report a dependency of SLC41A1 operation on Na^+ or other cations or anions following expression in *X. oocytes* whereas Kolisek and collaborators (Kolisek *et al*, 2008) observed a marked Cl^- conductance following expression in HEK293 cells, which was abolished by DIDS. Whether this reflects the operation of additional transport mechanisms or the presence of structural differences in the cell membrane of HEK293 cells as compared to *X. oocyte* are possibilities that need further investigation.

Two additional SLC41 isoforms were identified in both humans and mice. SLC41A2 also transport Mg^{2+} as well as other divalent cations albeit with a different selectivity and inhibition profile than SLC41A1 (Goytain and Qaumme, 2005c). Aside from Mg^{2+}, SLC41A2 can carry Ba^{2+}, Ni^{2+}, Co^{2+}, Fe^{2+} and Mn^{2+} but not Ca^{2+}, Cu^{2+} or Zn^{2+}. At variance of SLC41A1, Mg^{2+} transport via SLC41A2 is inhibited by Ca^{2+} (Goytain and Qaumme, 2005c). Both SLC41A1 and A2 generate Mg^{2+} currents in *X. oocyte*, and the ionic uptake is voltage dependent with an apparent affinity of 0.75 mM and 0.31 mM, respectively (Goytain and Qaumme, 2005b; Goytain and Qaumme, 2005c). Also SLC41A2 is widely expressed in mammalian tissues, but the expression is not affected by low Mg^{2+} diet (Goytain and Qaumme, 2005c). At the structural level, SLC41A2 shares >70% homology with SLC41A1, and is supposed to have also 10 transmembrane domains, although this hypothesis is not supported by a recent study (Sahni *et al*, 2007) that suggests instead a structural arrangement in 2 five trans-membrane spans linked together by a supplementary span motif. Hydrophobicity analysis indicates that the C- and N- termini are located on different sites of the cell membrane (Sahni *et al*, 2007), a configuration that will be consistent with a total of 11 trans-membrane segments.

ACDP2

The human ACDP gene family was identified by Wang and collaborators (Wang *et al*, 2003a) as a possible candidate of the urofacial syndrome. Mapped to 10q23-10q24 chromosome, this gene family comprises 4 isoforms differentially located in human tissues. ACDP1 is essentially restricted to brain. ACDP2 is more widely expressed, but still retains the highest expression in brain while being absent in skeletal muscle. Both ACDP3 and ACDP4 are ubiquitous, but have the highest expression in heart (Wang *et al*, 2003b). The murine distribution of ACDP isoforms is very similar to that observed in humans (Wang *et al*, 2004). Termed ancient conserved domain protein because all isoforms have one domain in common that appears to be phylogenetically conserved from bacteria to man (Wang *et al*, 2003a), these proteins share >50% homology to the CorC transporter, which together with CorB and CorD plays a role in Mg^{2+} efflux in prokaryotes. Over-expression of ACDP2 in *X. oocytes* indicates that this protein can transport a broad range of divalent cations including Mg^{2+}, Co^{2+}, Mn^{2+}, Sr^{2+}, Ba^{2+}, Cu^{2+}, and Fe^{2+} while Zn^{2+} can inhibit its activity (Goytain and Quamme, 2005d). Mg^{2+} transport via ACDP2 is voltage dependent and occurs with a Km of ~0.5mM. The transport, however, operates independently of Na^{+} or Cl^{-} ions (Goytain and Quamme, 2005d). As in the case of SLC41A1, the *ACDP2* gene becomes over-expressed following a Mg^{2+} deficient diet (Goytain and Qaumme, 2005).

NIPA

Located in the SPG6 locus of chromosome 15q11-q13, the *NIPA1* gene is so called for 'non-imprinted in Prader-Willi/Angelman syndrome, a disease characterized by a complex developmental and multisystem disorder (Butler, 1990). Located among about 30 genes linked to this disease (Butler, 1990), *NIPA1* has also been implicated in autosomal dominant hereditary spastic paraplegia (HSP). The human and mouse genome contain four members of the NIPA family, termed NIPA1 trough NIPA4, with an overall similarity of ~40%. Homology between human and mice proteins is high at around 98%. Studies conducted by Goytain and Quamme indicate that both NIPA1 and NIPA2 (Goytain *et al*, 2007; Goytain *et al*, 2008a) can operate as Mg^{2+} transporter. Characterized by a sequence of 323 (NIPA1) and 359 amino acids (NIPA2) arranged to form 9 and 8 transmembrane spans, respectively, these two proteins can be distinguished based on their K_m and specificity for Mg^{2+}. While both proteins transport Mg^{2+} in a saturable fashion, NIPA1 has a K_m for Mg^{2+} of ~0.66mM (Goytain *et al*, 2007) as compared to 0.31mM for NIPA2 (Goytain *et al*, 2008a). In addition, NIPA2 is highly specific for Mg^{2+} while NIPA1 can also transport Sr^{2+}, Fe^{2+} or Co^{2+}, albeit to a lesser extent (Goytain *et al*, 2007). NIPA3, instead, transports Sr^{2+}, Ba^{2+}, Fe^{2+} and Cu^{2+} whereas NIPA4 transport Sr^{2+} and Ba^{2+}. Interestingly, point mutations in NIPA1 (i.e. $G^{100}R$ or $T^{45}R$) represent the basis for the insurgence of autosomal dominant HSP (Rainier *et al*, 2003). Both the glycine and threonine residues are conserved among ortholog NIPA1 channels in different species. There are no similar consensus sites in the paralogs NIPA2, NIPA3 and NIPA4, implying that the folding of these proteins might be different. Although NIPA2 appears to be normal in HSP patients, it cannot functionally replace NIPA1 to ameliorate HSP symptoms, nor can NIPA3 or NIPA4 substitute for the defective NIPA1. This is somewhat surprising for NIPA2 as the gene encoding for this proteins is part of the 30 gene clusters associated with the Prade-Willi syndrome together with *NIPA1*. Presently, there is no information available as to whether the Prade-Willi syndrome presents alterations in Mg^{2+} homeostasis.

Huntingtin

The use of oligonucleotide microarray analysis to screen for Mg^{2+}-regulated transcripts in epithelial cells indicates Huntingtin-interacting protein 14 (HIP14) and its related protein HIP14-like (HIP14L) as significantly (~ 3fold) upregulated by low-extracellular Mg^{2+} (Goytain *et al*, 2008b). Formed by approximately 532 amino acids organized in 6 transmembrane spans, HIP14 presents a strong sequence similarity to the ankyrin repeat protein Akr1p (Li and Li, 2004), and a 69% homology to HIP14L. In addition, HIP14 possesses a cytoplasmic DHHC cysteine-rich domain. Defined by the Asp-His-His-Cys sequence motif, this domain confers palmitoyl-acyltransferase activity to the protein and gives it the ability to palmitoylate membrane components and modulate their structure. Mg^{2+} accumulation via HIP14 and HIP14L appears to be electrogenic, voltage-dependent, and saturable with K_m of ~0.87 and ~0.74mM, respectively (Goytain *et al*, 2008b). Inhibition of palmitoylation activity by 2-Br-palmitate or deletion of the DHHC domain decreases HIP14 mediated Mg^{2+} accumulation by ~50%, suggesting that palmitoylation is not required for basal Mg^{2+} transport. The widespread tissue distribution and intracellular localization of HIP14 (nuclear and perinuclear regions, Golgi complex, mitochondria, microtubules, endosomes, clathrin-coated and noncoated vesicles, and plasma membrane (Yanai *et al*, 2006) has implicated this protein in numerous cellular processes including transcriptional regulation, mitochondrial bioenergetics, structural scaffolding, vesicle trafficking, endocytosis, and dendrite formation (Yanai *et al*, 2006). Its primary location however, appears to be in the Golgi and post-Golgi vesicles (Yanai *et al*, 2006; Goytain *et al*, 2008b). Hence, it can be hypothesized that the ability of this protein to favor Mg^{2+} accumulation is linked to some extent to the role HIP14 plays in the physiological functioning of the compartments in which the protein is located. At the pathological level, the neuropathology of Huntington disease and the occurrence of progressive neurodegenerative disorders, cognitive deficits and choreic movements typical of this disease are linked to the abnormal expansion of glutamine residues from <34 to >37 at the 18th amino acid position (Li and Li, 2004). Presently, the mechanism responsible for the insurgence of these defects is unknown (Li and Li, 2004). Similarly unknown is whether the poly-glutamine expansion alters Mg^{2+} transport, and whether perturbation of Mg^{2+} homeostasis plays any role in the uprising of the neuronal defects typical of Huntington disease.

Mg^{2+} transport in purified plasma membrane vesicles

Because of the lack of functional cloning, several laboratories including ours have resorted to the use of plasma membrane vesicles to better characterize how different Mg^{2+} extrusion mechanisms operate in particular cell types. The plasma membrane model presents several advantages including: 1) the possibility to provide a well defined ionic extra- and intra-vesicular milieu composition to determine the modality of operation of the various Mg^{2+} transporters; and 2) the ability to investigate the operation of the different Mg^{2+} extrusion mechanisms in the absence of Mg^{2+} buffering by ATP, proteins or other cytosolic components, and partitioning within intracellular organelles. By purifying total liver plasma membrane or cardiac sarcolemmal vesicles as well as specific hepatic subpopulations enriched in basolateral or apical domains, our laboratory has been able to provide a better understanding of the selective location and specificity of the Na^+- dependent and Na^+-independent Mg^{2+} extrusion mechanisms in liver cells and cardiac myocytes.

The Na^+-dependent extrusion mechanism located in the basolateral domain of the hepatocyte is selectively activated by Na^+ (Cefaratti *et al*, 1998; Cefaratti *et al*, 2000), and specifically inhibited by imipramine (Cefaratti *et al*, 2000), but not amiloride and amiloride derivates (Cefaratti *et al*, 2000). Furthermore, the operation of the exchanger is completely inhibited by pre-treatment of basolateral vesicles with alkaline phosphatase, and restored by loading the vesicles with ATP and PKA catalytic subunit (Cefaratti and Ruse, 2007; Cefaratti and Romani, 2007), leaning further support to the notion that this exchange mechanism becomes operative upon phosphorylation by cAMP. The Na^+/Mg^{2+} exchanger continues to operate in the presence of *zero trans* Mg^{2+} across the plasma membrane (*i.e.*, 20 mM Mg^{2+} inside and outside the vesicles), an indication that Mg^{2+} extrusion does not depend on the trans-membrane gradient for Mg^{2+} but rather on that of Na^+, with a K_m lower than 20mM (Cefaratti *et al*, 1998), in good agreement with kinetic data obtained in isolated hepatocytes (Romani *et al*, 1993b) and other cell types (Tashiro and Konishi, 1997). Experiments based on TPP^+ distribution have confirmed the electrogenicity of this exchange mechanism in plasma membrane vesicles, and suggested a $1Na^+_{in}$ for $1Mg^{2+}_{out}$ exchange ratio under the majority of experimental conditions tested (Cefaratti *et al*, 1998; Cefaratti *et al*, 2000; Cefaratti and Ruse, 2007). Interestingly, removal of intravesicular Cl-switches the stoichiometric ratio of the exchanger from electrogenic to electroneutral (i.e. $2Na^+_{in}$ for $1Mg^{2+}_{out}$) (Cefaratti and Romani, 2011). Moreover, in the presence of intra-vesicular Cl^- an extrusion of ~35nmol Cl^-/mg protein is observed within 1min from the addition of external Na^+, in concomitance with the extrusion of Mg^{2+} and the accumulation of external Na^+ into the vesicles (Cefaratti and Romani, 2011). Chloride ion extrusion is not inhibited by anion transport inhibitors like DNDS, DIDS, or niflumic acid, nor is blocked by NKCC1 inhibitors like bumetanide or furosemide (Cefaratti and Romani, 2011), thus excluding that it occurs via one of these mechanisms. The only agent able to block the Cl^- extrusion is imipramine (Cefaratti and Romani, 2011), which specifically blocks the Na^+/Mg^{2+} exchanger operating in the basolateral domain of the hepatocyte (Cefaratti *et al*, 2000). Hence, it would appear that Cl^- can be extruded either via the Na^+/Mg^{2+} exchanger or via Cl^- channels for partial charge compensation (Cefaratti and Romani, 2011). The possibility of a Cl^- extrusion via the Na^+/Mg^{2+} exchanger has been suggested by Rasgado-Flores *et al.* (Rasgado-Flores *et al*, 1994) in dialyzed squid axons, and it would also be in good agreement with the observation by Gunther and collaborators that intracellular Cl- has a stimulatory role on the activity of the Na^+/Mg^{2+} antiport in red blood cells (Ebel and Gunther, 2003).

The basolateral domain of the hepatocyte is not the only site in which the operation of a Mg^{2+} extrusion mechanism has been observed. Experiments carried out in liver plasma membrane vesicles enriched in apical domain indicate the presence of two apparently distinct, unidirectional Mg^{2+} transport mechanisms, which extrude intravesicular Mg^{2+} for extravesicular Na^+ and Ca^{2+}, respectively (Cefaratti *et al*, 2000).

This apical Na^+-dependent Mg^{2+} transporter presents a K_m for Na^+ comparable to the basolateral transporter, and selectively uses Na^+ over other monovalent cations in a manner similar to the basolateral exchanger. Like the basolateral antiport, this exchanger transports electrogenically $1Na^+_{in}{:}1Mg^{2+}_{out}$ (Cefaratti *et al*, 2000). From the pharmacological stand-point the apical and basolateral exchanger can be distinguished based on the specific inhibition of the apical exchanger by amiloride (Cefaratti *et al*, 2000), although it retains a significant level of sensitivity to imipramine inhibition, whereas only imipramine can block the basolateral antiport (Cefaratti *et al*, 2000). The apical exchanger can also be distinguished from the basolateral antiport based on its inability to operate in reverse mode (Cefaratti *et al*, 2000).

The Ca^{2+}-dependent Mg^{2+} extrusion mechanism is specifically located in the apical domain of the hepatocytes, is activated by micromolar Ca^{2+} concentration ($K_m \leq 50\mu M$), and is insensitive to alkaline phosphatase pre-treatment (Cefaratti and Ruse, 2007; Cefaratti and Romani, 2007). The Mg^{2+} extrusion elicited by this antiport occurs on electro-neutral basis (i.e. $1Ca^{2+}_{in}{:}1Mg^{2+}_{out}$) (Cefaratti and Ruse, 2007). The exchanger, however, is not Ca^{2+} specific, as Mg^{2+} extrusion is observed following the extravesicular addition of micromolar concentrations of other divalent cations ($Ca^{2+}>>Co^{2+}=Mn^{2+}>Sr^{2+}>>Ba^{2+}>Cu^{2+}>>Cd^{2+}$) (Cefaratti *et al*, 2000). Similarly to the apical Na^+/Mg^{2+} antiport, the Ca^{2+}-dependent mechanism is inhibited by amiloride or imipramine (Cefaratti *et al*, 2000). This observation raises the question as to whether we are in the presence of two distinct apical mechanisms, modulated by Na^+ and cations, respectively. Several lines of evidence, however, do not fully support this possibility. First, the co-addition of Na^+ and Ca^{2+} in purified apical plasma membrane vesicles subpopulations does not appear to significantly enlarge Mg^{2+} extrusion (Romani, personal observation). Second, amiloride inhibits both exchangers to a comparable extent at a similar concentration (Cefaratti *et al*, 2000). Third, alkaline phosphatase treatment does not affect the Mg^{2+} extrusion elicited by either exchanger in apical liver plasma membrane vesicles (Cefaratti and Ruse, 2007; Cefaratti and Romani, 2007). Fourth, neither of these exchangers can operate in reverse at variance of the basolateral Na^+/Mg^{2+} antiport. Taken together, these observations suggest the operation of a non-selective exchange mechanism able to utilize monovalent or divalent cations to promote Mg^{2+} extrusion. At the present time, the physiological implication for the operation of such an exchanger in the apical domain of the hepatocyte is not fully clear. Circumstantial evidence, however, might support a possible role of Mg^{2+} in limiting Ca^{2+} sedimentation in the bile with consequent formation of bile stones (Moore, 1990).

The operation of functionally similar Na^+- and Ca^{2+}-dependent Mg^{2+} extrusion mechanisms has also been observed in cardiac sarcolemma vesicles (Cefaratti and Romani, 2007). As in the case of liver plasma membrane vesicles, cardiac sarcolemma vesicles do not require intravesicular ATP for the operation of Mg^{2+} transporters (Cefaratti and Romani, 2007), and pretreatment of the vesicles with alkaline phosphatase specifically inhibits the Na^+-dependent Mg^{2+} extrusion mechanism (Cefaratti and Romani, 2007). For technical reasons, it is presently unknown whether the Ca^{2+}/Mg^{2+} exchanger in sarcolemmal vesicles can also utilize Na^+ to promote Mg^{2+} extrusion.

The operation of specific Mg^{2+} accumulation mechanisms has also been observed in plasma membrane vesicles from brush border cells of rabbit ileum (Juttner and Ebel, 1998) and from the duodenum and jejunum of rat (Baillien and Cogneau, 1995). By using membrane vesicles from rabbit ileum and cell permeant and non-permeant Mag-Fura, Juttner and Ebel have observed the operation of a saturable Mg^{2+} uptake mechanism when the intracellular Na^{+} concentration is higher than the extracellular one (Baillien and Cogneau, 1995). This process becomes inoperative when the Na^{+} gradient is reversed (*i.e.*, $[Na^{+}]_i<[Na^{+}]_o$), the vesicles are in *zero trans* condition for Na^{+}, or external Na^{+} is removed. At variance with the transporter observed in liver plasma membrane, the pathway in ileum vesicles is not reversible and appears to be electroneutral. Yet, it possesses a K_m for Na^{+} of 16mM, a value similar to the K_m calculated in liver plasma membranes (Cefaratti *et al*, 1998), in smooth muscle cells from guinea pig tenia caecum (Tashiro and Konishi, 1997), and in chicken erythrocytes (Schatzmann, 1993). Another similarity with the transporter operating in basolateral liver plasma membranes is the lack of inhibition by amiloride analogs. In good agreement with reports from Gunther and collaborators (Ebel and Gunther, 2003), this transporter is modulated by intravesicular anions, especially Cl^{-} and SCN^{-}, and markedly stimulated by antagonists of anion transport (*e.g.*, H_2-DIDS) (Juttner and Ebel, 1998).

The main difference between plasma membrane vesicles from duodenum and jejunum (Baillien and Cogneau, 1995) is that a single Mg^{2+} uptake mechanism operates in the duodenum with a K_m of 0.8mM, whereas two transporters operate in the jejunum with K_m values of 0.15 and 2.4mM, respectively. In both these experimental models, Mg^{2+} but not Ca^{2+} accumulation is reduced in the presence of alkaline phosphatase inhibitors (Baillien *et al*, 2005), suggesting that Ca^{2+} and Mg^{2+} are transported via distinct pathways. This hypothesis is further supported by the observation that Mg^{2+} accumulation is inhibited by amiloride but not by Ca^{2+} channel antagonists. Consistent with the report by Juttner and Ebel (Juttner and Ebel, 1998), Mg^{2+} accumulation is stimulated by an intravesicular electronegative potential or an alkaline pH_o (Baillien and Cogneau, 1995). The effect of external pH, however, is lost when $[Mg^{2+}]_o$>1mM (Baillien and Cogneau, 1995). Under the latter condition, Mg^{2+} accumulation is enhanced by the presence of Na^{+} or K^{+} in the extravesicular space but is inhibited by the presence of divalent cations ($Co^{2+}>Mn^{2+}>Ca^{2+}>Ni^{2+}>Ba^{2+}>Sr^{2+}$) (Baillien and Cogneau, 1995).

Regulation of Mg^{2+} transport and homeostasis

While mammalian cells retains their basal Mg^{2+} content virtually unchanged under resting conditions, compelling evidence supports the ability of different hormones to induce the movement of large amount of Mg^{2+} in either direction across the eukaryotes cell membrane. As a result of these movements, changes in serum, total and to a lesser extent free Mg^{2+} content have been observed. Further, these changes have resulted in detectable variations in Mg^{2+} level within organelles, especially mitochondria, with major repercussions on cellular bioenergetics. A full understanding of the physiological relevance of these changes in cellular Mg^{2+} content is far from complete. Yet, a picture is slowly emerging, which relates changes in total Mg^{2+} content to the utilization of metabolites (e.g. glucose) or to meaningful changes in Mg^{2+} content within discrete portions of the cell or cellular organelles, whereby variations in total Mg^{2+} content translate into changes in concentrations able to modulate the activity of specific enzymes located within these compartments.

Mg^{2+} extrusion

Several classes of hormones induce Mg^{2+} extrusion from various cell types or perfused tissues. For the most part, these hormones are catecholamine or hormones that increase cellular cAMP level by activating different GPCR receptors at the cell membrane level. The extrusion elicited by these agents affects to a varying extent the Mg^{2+} pools present within cytoplasm as well as within cellular compartments. The extrusion across the cell membrane primarily occurs via the Na^{+}/Mg^{2+} exchanger previously described although a (partial) contribution of the Na^{+}-independent pathway cannot be excluded. Magnesium extrusion can also be observed following metabolic treatments that decrease cellular ATP content, the main Mg^{2+} buffering component. Interestingly, several of the hormones that induce Mg^{2+} extrusion also elicit a glucose output from hepatocytes. Hence, it would appear that at least in this organ Mg^{2+}

extrusion is functionally associated with glucose transport and utilization.

Cyclic-AMP Dependent Extrusion

Elliot and Rizack were the first to report an accumulation of Mg^{2+} in adipocytes stimulated by adreno-corticotrophic hormone in 1974, although they did not elucidate the modality of transport (Elliot and Rizack, 1974). The first extensive characterization of an hormonal effect on Mg^{2+} transport was provided by Maguire and colleagues in S49 lymphoma cells and primary lymphocytes stimulated by beta-adrenergic agonist or PGE1 (Bird and Maguire, 1978; Erdos and Maguire, 1980; Erdos and Maguire, 1983; Grubbs *et al*, 1984)). Maguire and Erdos (Maguire and Erdos, 1978) also provided the first observation that stimulation of protein kinase C enhanced Mg^{2+} influx in S49 cells whereas beta-adrenergic stimulation inhibited the process. Observation carried out in S49 cells lacking protein kinase A or adenylyl cyclase, however, indicated that cAMP was not mediating the inhibitory effect of beta-adrenergic agonists (Maguire and Erdos, 1978; Maguire and Erdos, 1980). At variance of what observed in primary lymphocytes (Wolf *et al*, 1997), Mg^{2+} transport in S49 cells appears to be independent of extra- cellular Na^{+} concentration or membrane potential (Grubbs R.D. and Maguire M.E., unpublished observation). Further, Mg^{2+} turnover in S49 required more than 40 hours as compared to the much faster Ca^{2+} turn-over, which was accomplished in less than 3 hours (Grubbs *et al*, 1985).

These initial observations were followed by a long series of report supporting the notion that b-adrenergic agonists and other hormones control Mg^{2+} homeostasis in mammalian cells. In the majority of eukaryotic cells, hormones or agents that increase cellular cAMP level elicit a significant extrusion of Mg^{2+} into the extracellular space or the circulation (Vormann and Gunther, 1987; Romani and Scarpa, 1990a; Romani and Scarpa, 1990b). This effect has been observed in cardiac ventricular myocytes (Vormann and Gunther, 1987; Romani and Scarpa, 1990a; Romani *et al*, 1993a; Howarth *et al*, 1994), liver cells (Romani and Scarpa, 1990b; Gunther *et al*, 1991; Romani *et al*, 1993b; Fagan and Romani, 2000; Fagan and Romani, 2001), red blood cells (Matsuura *et al*, 1993), thymocytes (Gunther and Vormann, 1990b), and Erhlich ascites cells (Wolf *et al*, 1994) among other cells (see Romani and Scarpa, 2000 for a more comprehensive list), as well as in whole anesthetized animals (Gunther and Vormann, 1992; Keenan *et al*, 1995). In all cellular models, Mg^{2+} extrusion is a fast process that reaches the maximum within 8min from the application of the stimulus irrespective of the hormone (catecholamine, isoproterenol, glucagon, PGE1, or arachidonic acid) (Vormann and Gunther, 1987; Gunther and Vormann, 1990a; Romani and Scarpa, 1990a; Romani and Scarpa 1990b; Matsuura *et al*, 1993; Howarth *et al*, 1994; Wolf *et al*, 1994) or agent (i.e. forskolin or cell permeant cyclic AMP analogs) (Vormann and Gunther, 1987; Gunther and Vormann, 1990a; Romani and Scarpa, 1990a; Romani and Scarpa, 1990b; Matsuura *et al*, 1993; Romani *et al*, 1993b; Fagan and Romani 2000; Fagan and Romani, 2001) utilized to increase cellular cAMP level. The key role of cAMP in modulating Mg^{2+} extrusion is further emphasized by the observation that pretreatment with hormones or agents that either decrease cAMP production (e.g. carbachol (Romani and Scarpa, 1990a; Romani and Scarpa, 1990b; Romani *et al*, 1993b), insulin (Romani *et al*, 2000) or prevent PKA activation (e.g. Rp-cAMP (Wolf *et al*, 1997) inhibits cellular Mg^{2+} mobilization. In an open perfusion system, the amount of Mg^{2+} extruded from the organ returns towards baseline level within 8min from the application of the agonist irrespective of its dose or persistence in the perfusate (Romani and Scarpa, 1990a; Romani and Scarpa, 1990b), suggesting a rapid mobilization of Mg^{2+} from a well defined cellular pool that is rapidly depleted of its content. This notion is further supported by the evidence that submaximal doses of agonist sequentially infused within a few minutes from each other elicit Mg^{2+} extrusions of progressively decreasing amplitudes (Gunther and Vormann, 1990a). Under all these conditions, limited changes in cytosolic free $[Mg^{2+}]_i$ are observed (Fatholahi *et al*, 2000; Amano *et al*, 2000), suggesting that Mg^{2+} is rapidly released from its binding and buffering sites, or form cellular organelle(s) and extruded across the cell membrane. Independent of the hormone utilized the cAMP-mediated Mg^{2+} extrusion occurs via the putative Na^{+}/Mg^{2+} exchanger described previously. In fact, either the removal of extracellular Na^{+} (Gunther, 1996) or the presence of agents like amiloride (Vormann and Gunther, 1987; Gunther, 1996), which inhibits Na^{+} transport albeit in a non-specific manner, abolishes to a large extent the Mg^{2+} extrusion. Under either of these conditions, the amplitude of Mg^{2+} extrusion across the cell membrane is hampered and a more sustained rise in cytosolic free $[Mg^{2+}]_i$ is observed (Fatholahi *et al*, 2000; Amano *et al*, 2000), supporting the notion that blocking Na^+ transport prevents Mg^{2+} from being extruded across the cell membrane but not its released from binding/buffering sites and/or cellular pool(s) into the cytoplasm.

Cyclic-AMP Independent Extrusion

In 1989, Jakob and collaborators reported the first observation that phenylephrine can also elicit Mg^{2+} extrusion from liver cells via alpha$_1$-adrenergic stimulation (Jakob *et al*, 1989). Subsequently, our laboratory (Keenan *et al*, 1996; Fagan and Romani, 2000) confirmed this observation and provided the first evidence that the stimulation of α_1- and β-adrenergic receptor are not alternative but rather additive and complementary processes in eliciting Mg^{2+} extrusion from liver cells, especially when the two classes of receptors are stimulated by mix adrenergic agonists such as epinephrine or norepinephrine (Keenan *et al*, 1996; Fagan and Romani, 2000). Pre-treatment with insulin only abolishes β-adrenergic receptor mediated Mg^{2+} extrusion but leaves unaffected the Mg^{2+} mobilization mediated via α_1-adrenergic receptors (Keenan *et al*, 1996). The inhibitory effect of insulin persists even in cells treated with cell-permeant cAMP analogs (Keenan *et al*, 1996). A similar inhibitory effect of insulin on b-adrenergic receptor mediated, cAMP-modulated Mg^{2+} extrusion has been observed in cardiac myocytes (Romani *et al*, 2000). This inhibition has been largely interpreted as the consequence of an inhibitory effect of insulin on the b-adrenergic receptor (Karoor *et al*, 1995) or a positive effect of the hormone on the cytosolic phosphodiesterase degrading cAMP (Smoake *et al*, 1995). A more recent report by Romero and collaborators (Ferreira *et al*, 2004), however, suggests that insulin can also modulate directly the Na^+/Mg^{2+} exchanger, at least in red blood cells.

Fagan and Romani (Fagan and Romani, 2000; Fagan and Romani, 2001) further investigated the modality of Mg^{2+} extrusion following α_1-adrenergic receptor stimulation in liver cells. Their observation indicates that phenylephrine-induced Mg^{2+} extrusion strictly depends on the activation of capacitative Ca^{2+} entry (Fagan and Romani, 2001). Inhibition of IP_3-induced Ca^{2+} release from the endoplasmic reticulum, chelation of cytosolic Ca^{2+}, or inhibition of Ca^{2+} entry at the plasma membrane level all result in the complete inhibition of Mg^{2+} extrusion from the hepatocyte (Fagan and Romani, 2001). The scant information available about possible binding of Mg^{2+} by cellular proteins prevented the authors from ascertaining whether the extruded Mg^{2+} was mobilized from the ER or displaced from cytosolic binding sites following the massive entry of Ca^{2+} across the hepatocyte cell membrane (Fagan and Romani, 2001, and refs. therein). Extracellular Na^+ and Ca^{2+} are both required for the phenylephrine-induced Mg^{2+} extrusion to occur (Fagan and Romani, 2001). The absence of extracellular Ca^{2+}, in fact, decreases the amplitude of Mg^{2+} extrusion by ~15% to 20% whereas extracellular Na^+ is responsible for the remaining 80% to 85% of the extrusion. It is presently unclear whether Mg^{2+} extrusion occurs via the Ca^{2+}-activated Na^+-dependent mechanism observed in the apical domain of the hepatocyte, or whether Na^+ is required to maintain membrane potential and facilitate Ca^{2+} entry across the hepatocyte cell membrane. It has to be noted, however, that in the absence of receptor activation, thapsigargin administration can mimic phenylephrine stimulation and elicit Mg^{2+} extrusion from the hepatocyte, even in the absence of extracellular Ca^{2+} (Fagan and Romani, 2001), although to a lesser extent. Hence, it would appear that an optimal level of cytosolic Ca^{2+} has to be attained in order for Mg^{2+} extrusion to occur via displacement from cellular binding sites or via a Ca^{2+}-calmodulin-activated mechanism (Fagan and Romani, 2001).

Mg^{2+} homeostasis and glucose

The presence of redundant Mg^{2+} extrusion mechanisms or modalities of activation of a common Mg^{2+} extrusion pathway raises the question of the physiological significance of Mg^{2+} mobilization in mammalian cells. In the case of cardiac myocytes, an increase in extracellular Mg^{2+} level has been associated with a modulatory effect on the open probability of the L-type Ca^{2+}-channels (Wang and Berlin, 2006) and a temporary decrease in SA node action potential (Howarth *et al*, 1994). In the case of liver cells, instead, Mg^{2+} transport has been associated with a regulatory role on glucose transport and utilization. Under conditions in which hormones like catecholamine (Keenan *et al*, 1996; Fagan and Romani, 2000), glucagon (Fagan and Romani, 2000), or phenylephrine (Keenan *et al*, 1996; Fagan and Romani, 2000) elicit Mg^{2+} extrusion from liver cells, a concomitant release of hepatic glucose, mostly via glycogenolysis, has been observed (Fagan and Romani, 2000). Interestingly, inhibition of Mg^{2+} extrusion by amiloride or imipramine also results in a marked inhibition of hepatic glucose output (Fagan and Romani, 2000). The converse is also true. Inhibition of glucose transport activity by phlorethin results in a qualitatively similar inhibition of Mg^{2+} extrusion from liver cells (Fagan and Romani, 2000). The presence of a close functional 'link' between glucose and Mg^{2+} homeostasis is further emphasizes by the observation that overnight starvation results in the complete depletion of hepatic glycogen and glucose as well as in a marked decrease (minus 15%) of total Mg^{2+} content as a consequence of the activation of the pro-glycemic hormones catecholamine and glucagon (Torres *et al*, 2005). Noteworthy, this decrease in hepatic Mg^{2+} content is equivalent to that elicited via *in vitro* stimulation of perfused livers by the same hormones (Torres *et al*, 2005), or that observed in the liver of type-I diabetic animals (Fagan *et al*, 2004), which are markedly decreased in cellular glycogen. The functional link between glucose and Mg^{2+} homeostasis is also observed under conditions in which glucose accumulation is stimulated by insulin or similar hormones in cardiac ventricular myocytes (Romani *et al*, 2000) or pancreatic beta cells (Henquin *et al*, 1983). In both experimental models, the amount of Mg^{2+} accumulated within the cells is directly proportional to the amplitude of glucose accumulation. Conversely, decreasing extracellular Mg^{2+} concentration directly reduces the amount of glucose accumulated within the cells (Fagan and Romani, 2000; Romani *et al*, 2000).

Although indirect, a clear proof of the glucose/Mg^{2+} relationship is provided by diabetic conditions. Work by Altura's group (Resnick *et al*, 1993) and more recently by Resnick (Resnick, 1993) and Barbagallo (Barbagallo and Dominguez, 2007) indicate that cellular Mg^{2+} content is markedly decreased under type-I and type-II diabetes. Originally observed in red blood cells (Resnick *et al*, 1993; Resnick, 1993; Barbagallo and Dominguez, 2007), the decrease has also been reported in various other tissues including muscles, liver (Fagan *et al*, 2004), and cardiac myocytes (Reed *et al*, 2008). Interestingly, Mg^{2+} extrusion via β-adrenergic signaling remains operative and is actually up-regulated in liver cells from diabetic animals (Fagan *et al*, 2004) while it is markedly inhibited in cardiac myocytes from the same animals (Reed *et al*, 2008). Whether this reflects a differential operation and modulation of β_2-adrenergic receptors in liver cells *vs.* β_1-adrenergic receptors in cardiac cells is not completely clear. Both cell models show a marked inhibition of the Mg^{2+} entry mechanism(s), which persists also in liver plasma membrane vesicles (Fagan *et al*, 2004; Cefaratti *et al*, 2004). Addition of glucose or glycogen to plasma membrane vesicles from diabetic animals renormalizes the amplitude of Mg^{2+} extrusion, but is ineffective at restoring Mg^{2+} accumulation in vesicles (Cefaratti *et al*, 2004). The defect in total cellular Mg^{2+} content appears to be strongly associated with the decrease in protein synthesis and ATP production detected in the cells (Reed *et al*, 2008). Supplementation of exogenous insulin restores both these parameters as well as Mg^{2+} homeostasis and extrusion provided that insulin is administered for at least two weeks (reed *et al*, 2008). As indicated previously, it appears that the role of insulin in modulating Mg^{2+} homeostasis is not restricted to controlling glucose homeostasis and accumulation or the release of pro-glycemic hormones like glucagon, but extends to a direct modulation of the Na^{+}/Mg^{2+} exchanger (Ferreira *et al*, 2004). The latter effect would not only directly increase cellular Mg^{2+} content but it could also reverberate on the insulin receptor itself. Data obtained in animals maintained on low Mg^{2+} diet indicate that a decrease in cellular Mg^{2+} content affects the ability of the insulin receptor to properly phosphorylate the downstream insulin receptor substrate (IRS) and propagate the signaling within muscle cells (Suarez *et al*, 1995). This result might be of relevance in explaining the decrease in glucose accumulation observed in skeletal muscles under diabetic conditions (Suarez *et al*, 1995).

Mg^{2+} homeostasis and ATP

Hormonal stimuli represent the most dynamic modality by which a cell can rapidly extruded 10%

to 15% of its total cellular Mg^{2+} content within a few minutes from the application of the agonist. Mg^{2+}, however, can also be extruded following the treatment with various agents that impact cellular ATP content and production. Cyanide (Harman *et al*, 1990; Dalal and Romani, 2010), mitochondrial uncouplers (Akerman, 1981; Kubota *et al*, 2005), fructose (Gaussin *et al*, 1997), ethanol (Tessman and Romani, 1998), or hypoxia (Gasbarrini *et al*, 1992) are just some of the agents whose addition impact cellular Mg^{2+} homeostasis. All these agents, in fact, have in common that they decrease cellular ATP content by either preventing the mitochondrial electron chain from generating ATP at various levels (cyanide or uncouplers), or by acting as an ATP trap (fructose), or by altering the redox state of pyridine nucleotide within the mitochondrion or the cell (ethanol). As ATP represents the major buffering component for Mg^{2+} within the cell (Scarpa and Brinley, 1981; Luthi *et al*, 1999), a decrease in this phosphonucleotide moiety results in an increase in cytosolic free $[Mg^{2+}]i$, and ultimately in a detectable extrusion from the cell (Harman *et al*, 1990; Gasbarrini *et al*, 1992; Gaussin *et al*, 1997; Tessman and Romani, 1998; Dalal and Romani, 2010). The Mg^{2+} extrusion can be observed to a larger extent in erythrocytes, which possess limited cellular buffering capacity and no compartmentation (Hwa *et al*, 1993), but it can also be observed in cells that present additional buffering by proteins or cellular organelles in addition to phosphonucleotides (Harman *et al*, 1990; Gasbarrini *et al*, 1992; Gaussin *et al*, 1997; Tessman and Romani, 1998; Dalal and Romani, 2010). In the case of fructose, the changes in cytosolic Mg^{2+} have been associated with an activation of the glycogen phosphorylase, which ultimately results in glycogenolysis activation and glucose utilization to restore ATP levels (Gaussin *et al*, 1997). In the majority of these experimental conditions, the increase in cytosolic free $[Mg^{2+}]i$ is usually modest, and considerably lower than the increase expected to occur based upon the corresponding decrease in ATP level, which strongly supports the notion that Mg^{2+} is for the most part extruded from the cell. Furthermore, as ATP level decreases as a result of mitochondria poisoning or changes in pyridine nucleotide ratio, it would appear that not phosphorylation but the rise in cytosolic Mg^{2+} albeit modest is sufficient to activate the Mg^{2+} extrusion mechanism and limit the rise in cytosolic free Mg^{2+} concentration to approximately 100-200 mM at the most Harman *et al*, 1999).

Cellular ATP plays a key role in regulating Mg^{2+} extrusion. Evidence for this role has been provided in the giant squid axon (Di Polo and Beauge', 1988) as well as in mammalian hepatocytes (Gunther and Hollriegl, 1993) or erythrocytes (Gunther *et al*, 1995). In squid axon, the Na^+-dependent Mg^{2+} extrusion requires a physiological level of ATP. As the phospho-nucleotide level decreases, so does the amplitude of extrusion (Gunther and Hollriegl, 1993). In erythrocytes and hepatocytes, instead, ATP appears to regulate the Na^+-independent Mg^{2+} extrusion process (Gunther and Hollriegl, 1993; Gunther *et al*, 1995). The exact role of ATP in regulating the process, however, is unclear as it does not appear that the extrusion process is mediated by an ATPase mechanism. This notion is supported by the observation that a decrease in cellular ATP level (as it occurs for example under diabetic or alcoholic conditions) paradoxically results in an increased extrusion of Mg^{2+} via the Na^+-dependent mechanism in a manner directly proportional to the decrease in ATP level (Tessman and Romani, 1998; Fagan *et al*, 2004). Hence, it appears that the role of ATP is predominantly that of a ligand for Mg^{2+} both in the cytoplasm and the mitochondrial matrix (Scarpa and Brinley, 1981; Luthi *et al*, 1999), and that a decrease in ATP results in an increase in free Mg^{2+} and its consequent extrusion from the cell.

Mg^{2+} accumulation

The identification of several Mg^{2+} entry mechanisms strongly support the hypothesis that cellular Mg^{2+} is dynamically maintained through the operation of entry and exit mechanisms that are differentially regulated by hormones and metabolic conditions. A striking difference is there, however, between the Mg^{2+} exit and the Mg^{2+} entry mechanisms. In the case of Mg^{2+} extrusion mechanisms we have a good understanding of the signaling activating these mechanisms but we lack any structural information about the mechanisms themselves. In the case of Mg^{2+} entry mechanisms, instead, we do have structural information about several of these mechanisms but for the most part we lack detailed information about their individual activation by hormones or second messengers, and their possible cooperation under specific conditions.

Role of Protein Kinase C

Experimental evidence indicates that mammalian cells can accumulate large amounts of Mg^{2+} as a result of hormonal stimulation. Hormones like carbachol, vasopressin, angiotensin-II, or insulin have been indicated as able to either inhibit cAMP-mediated Mg^{2+} extrusion or reverse the extrusion into Mg^{2+} accumulation in various cell types (Romani and Scarpa, 1990a; Romani *et al*, 2000). The list of cells that respond to hormonal stimulation by accumulating Mg^{2+} is rather long [see Romani and Scarpa, 2000 for a list], and involve all kind of cells: cardiac myocytes (Romani and Scarpa, 1990a; Romani *et al*, 2000), smooth muscle cells (Touyz and Schiffrin, 1996), hepatocytes (Romani and Scarpa, 1990b; Romani *et al*, 1992), platelets (Hwang *et al*, 1993), lymphocytes (Grubbs and Maguire, 1986), fibroblasts (Ishijima and Tatibana, 1994), and pancreatic beta cells (Henquin *et al*, 1983), just to name a few. In addition to inhibiting cAMP production, several of the hormones indicated above can activate protein kinase C (PKC) as part of their cellular signaling. Evidence supporting a role of PKC in mediating Mg^{2+} accumulation has been provided by several laboratories. Maguire and collaborators have indicated that administration of phorbol-myristate acetate (PMA), which directly activates PKC, elicits a marked accumulation of Mg^{2+} in S49 lymphoma cells (Erdos and Maguire, 1983). A similar effect of PMA has been reported by Somogyi's group in thymocytes (Csermely *et al*, 1987), and by our laboratory in cardiac myocytes (Romani *et al*, 1992) and hepatocytes (Romani *et al*, 1992). Furthermore, our group has reported that down-regulation of PKC by exposure to a large dose of PMA for 3 hours completely abolishes the ability of cardiac and liver cells to accumulate Mg^{2+} while leaving unaffected the responsiveness of these cells to adrenergic agonists (Romani *et al*, 1992). An inhibitory effect has also been observed following administration of the PKC inhibitors calphostin (Touyz and Schiffrin, 1996) or staurosporine (Gunther and Vormann, 1995). Alteration in PKC distribution and activity and defective accumulation of Mg^{2+} has been observed in arterial smooth muscle cells (Yang *et al*, 2001), hepatocytes of animals exposed to alcohol (Torres *et al*, 2010), and in liver cells of diabetic animals (Tang *et al*, 1993).

Protein kinase C activation is only part of the integral response of hormones like angiotensin-II or vasopressin. The interaction of these hormones with their receptor, in fact, activates phospholipase C which, in turn hydrolyses PIP2 to generate diacylglycerol (DAG) and IP3. In turn, these two molecules activate protein kinase C and IP3 receptor in the ER, respectively. Activation of the latter receptor results in a marked but transient increase in cytosolic Ca^{2+}, and in a more sustained entry of Ca^{2+} through the capacitative Ca^{2+} entry mechanism. Hence, Ca^{2+} signaling is an integral component of the cellular response elicited by these hormones. Yet, the contribution of this second messenger in mediating Mg^{2+} accumulation is poorly defined. Liver cells loaded with Bapta-AM, which effectively chelates cytosolic Ca^{2+}, are unable to extrude and accumulate Mg^{2+} following stimulation by phenylephrine and PMA, respectively (Romani *et al*, 1993b). The artificial increase in cytosolic Ca^{2+} elicited by thapsigargin administration also prevents Mg^{2+} accumulation (Romani *et al*, 1993b) and actually induces a Mg^{2+} extrusion from the liver cell if applied for more than 3-5 min (Romani *et al*, 1993b; Fagan and Romani, 2001). Because of the different time-scale and amplitude of the changes in cellular Ca^{2+} and Mg^{2+} content (Romani *et al*, 1993b), it is difficult to properly correlate these experimental variations. Cytosolic free Ca^{2+} transiently increases several orders of magnitude while cytosolic free Mg^{2+}, which is already in the millimolar or submillimolar range, increases by ~10-15% (Fatholahi *et al*, 2000) at the most, although in absolute terms this amount is far larger than the overall change in cytosolic Ca^{2+} mass.

An unresolved point of inconsistency in the role of Ca^{2+} and PKC signaling in regulating Mg^{2+} accumulation is provided by the reports that the administration of phenylephrine, which activates PKC signaling in addition to the inositol 1,4,5 trisphosphate/Ca^{2+} pathway, does not elicit Mg^{2+} accumulation but induces a Mg^{2+} extrusion from liver cells (Fagan and Romani, 2001). This point raises the question as to what modulates the differential response of the cell to the administration of phenylephrine or vasopressin.

One possibility could be that different PKC isoforms are activated under one condition and not the other. For example, hepatocytes possess 3 classical and at least 2 novel PKC isoforms (Tang *et al*, 1993). Thus, it is reasonable to envisage that one isoform (or class of isoforms) is involved in mediating Mg^{2+} accumulation whereas another isoform (or class of isoforms) is involved in modulating Mg^{2+} extrusion. Consistent with this hypothesis, recent data from our laboratory suggests that PKCe is essential for Mg^{2+} accumulation to occur (Torres *et al*, 2010). Under conditions in which the expression of this isoform is inhibited by antisense or its translocation to the cell membrane is prevented - for example - by ethanol administration, no Mg^{2+} accumulation can be detected in liver cells (Torres *et al*, 2010). Interestingly, this PKC isoform has the highest affinity for Mg^{2+} among all PKC isoenzymes, with a K_m of ~1mM (Konno *et al*, 1989), close to the physiological free $[Mg^{2+}]_i$ measured in the cytoplasm of the hepatocyte (Corkey *et al*, 1986; Fatholahi *et al*, 2000) and other mammalian cells as well (Touyz and Schiffrin, 1996). Although the mechanism ultimately responsible for Mg^{2+} accumulation into the hepatocyte has not been identified, it is worth considering the recent observation by Bindels and collaborators that in the absence of PKC activation or following RACK1 over-expression, RACK1 can bind to TRPM6, and possibly TRPM7, at the level of the kinase domain and inhibit the channel activity (Cao *et al*, 2008).

Role of MAPKs

These results mentioned above, however, do not exclude the possibility that additional signaling pathways (e.g. MAPKS) are involved in determining the differing response of the hepatocyte under apparently similar stimulatory conditions. In agreement with previous report from Altura's group (Yang *et al*, 2000) and Touyz's laboratory (Touyz and Yao, 2003), our laboratory has evidenced that pharmacological inhibition of ERK1/2 and p38 MAPKs in liver cells abolishes PKC mediated Mg^{2+} accumulation (Torres *et al*, 2006). In this respect, it has to be noted that the inhibition of MAPKs hampers Mg^{2+} accumulation in vascular smooth muscle cells, and significantly affect cyclin activity (Touyz and Yao, 2003) and consequently the ability of the cells to progress in the cell cycle (Touyz and Yao, 2003). This effect may occur via changes in nuclear functions directly regulated by Mg^{2+}, as proposed by Rubin (Rubin, 2005) and/or via changes in nuclear functions of ERK2, which depends on Mg^{2+} level to properly dimerize, translocate and activate specific nuclear targets (Waas and Dalby, 2003). The role of ERK1/2 in Mg^{2+} regulation is further emphasized by the recent report that increased phosphorylation of ERK1/2 and increased expression of TRPM6 has been observed upon EGF administration to renal epithelial cells (Ikari *et al*, 2008; Ikari *et al*, 2010). The role of these MAPKs, however, is far from being elucidated as this kinase appears to be involved to some extent in also mediating Mg^{2+} extrusion (Kim *et al*, 2005; Torres *et al*, 2006).

Role of EGF

As mentioned, direct and indirect evidence suggests a key role of EGF in modulating Mg^{2+} accumulation, at least in kidney cells. The administration of EGF controls proper operation of TRPM6 in the apical domain of renal epithelial cells to promote Mg^{2+} accumulation (Ikari *et al*, 2008; Thebault *et al*, 2009; Ikari *et al*, 2010). Point mutations in EGF sequence result in limited function of TRPM6, and limited or no Mg^{2+} accumulation within the cells (van der Wjist *et al*, 2009). The modulation of TRPM6 appears to occur via MAPKs signaling, most likely ERK1/2 coupled to activator protein-1 (AP-1) (Ikari *et al*, 2010). Indirect evidence of EGF regulation is provided by the evidence that antibodies against EGF used in several form of colon cancer (Cunningham *et al*, 2004; Dimke *et al*, 2010) induce Mg^{2+} wasting and hypomagnesaemia.

Serum Mg^{2+} level and Mg^{2+} sensing mechanism

The experimental evidence that mammalian cells accumulate or extrude Mg^{2+} under a variety of experimental conditions suggests the presence of a *sensor* for the cytosolic Mg^{2+} concentration, whereby the cell would operate accordingly either extruding the excess cation or accumulating it to restore the 'set-point'. Compelling evidence for the presence of such a *sensor* mechanism is provided by the observation that prolonged exposure to 0mM $[Mg^{2+}]_o$ decreases cytosolic *free* Mg^{2+} concentration by approximately 50% in cardiac ventricular myocytes (Quamme and Rabkin, 1990), MDKC (Quamme and Dai, 1990), or MDCT cells (Dai *et al*, 1997). The new cytosolic Mg^{2+} level is maintained as long as the cells are incubated in the presence of 0 mM $[Mg^{2+}]_o$, but returns to the normal level as soon as $[Mg^{2+}]_o$ is increased (Quamme and Rabkin, 1990; Quamme and Dai, 1990; Dai *et al*, 1997), in a frame of time that is directly proportional to the extracellular Mg^{2+} concentration utilized (Quamme and Rabkin, 1990; Quamme and Dai, 1990; Dai *et al*, 1997). The process is prevented by the presence of the L-type Ca^{2+}-channel inhibitors verapamil or nifedipine, or La^{3+} in the extracellular milieu (Quamme and Rabkin, 1990). The absence of significant changes in cytosolic free Ca^{2+} concentration under these experimental conditions suggests a direct effect of these inhibitory agents on the Mg^{2+} entry mechanism (Quamme and Rabkin, 1990). This observation led the authors to propose the operation of a specific Mg^{2+} channel in these cells, anticipating the identification of TRPM6 (Schlingmann *et al*, 2002) and TRPM7 (Nadler *et al*, 2001) as specific Mg^{2+} channels.

Mg^{2+} accumulation is favored by ion re-distribution. In fact, renal epithelial cells accumulate Mg^{2+} as a result of phosphate (Dai *et al*, 1997) or potassium (Dai *et al*, 1991) redistribution across the cell membrane. The dependence of Mg^{2+} accumulation on K^+ redistribution across the plasma membrane suggests that Mg^{2+} transport is the result of changes in membrane potential, possibly for charge compensation (Schweigel *et al*, 1999; Tashiro *et al*, 2002; Schweigel and Martens, 2003). In this respect, it is interesting to note that pathological conditions characterized by a marked decrease in tissue Mg^{2+} content (*e.g.*, diabetes) (Fagan *et al*, 2004) are also characterized by an inability to properly transport potassium (Mondon *et al*, 1974; Taylor and Agius, 1988). Whether the effect on K^+ occurs through changes in membrane potential, or indirectly via a reduced operation of the Na^+/K^+-ATPase coupled to the operation in reverse of the Na^+/Mg^{2+} exchanger (Gunther and Vormann, 1995) is matter for future investigation.

Humans and many mammals present a circulating Mg^{2+} level of ~1.2-1.4 mEq/L (Geigy, 1984; Mudge, 1989). Clinical and experimental evidence indicates that serum Mg^{2+} level decreases in humans and animals in several chronic diseases (Fagan *et al*, 2004). Yet, there is a remarkable lack of information as to whether serum Mg^{2+} undergoes circadian fluctuations following hormonal or non-hormonal stimuli (*e.g.*, fasting or exercise). The infusion of catecholamine in conscious humans (Joborn *et al*, 1985; Bailly *et al*, 1990) or ovine (Rayssiguier, 1977), or the administration of isoproterenol (Guideri, 1992) or epinephrine in the presence of α_1-adrenoceptor blockade (Rayssiguier, 1977) have provided contrasting results. More recent results, however, would indicate that isoproterenol infusion elicits in a marked dose- and time-dependent increase in circulating Mg^{2+} content (Gunther and Vormann, 1992; Keenan *et al*, 1995). The increase is serum Mg^{2+} is maximal within 20min from the agent administration (Keenan *et al*, 1995), and remains unchanged up to 2 hours even following the removal of the agonist (Keenan *et al*, 1995). This time frame indicates that the increase in serum Mg^{2+} does not dependent on the increase in heart rate and the decrease in mean arterial pressure elicited by the β-adrenergic agonist (Keenan *et al*, 1995). In fact, the infusion of sodium nitroprusside, which mimics the decrease in mean arterial pressure induced by isoproterenol, has not effect on serum Mg^{2+} level (Keenan *et al*, 1995). The persistence of an elevated serum Mg^{2+} level for up to 2 hours also implies that operation of secondary and not fully elucidated mechanisms activated by the stimulation of β-adrenergic receptor. Consistent with the larger distribution of β_2 versus β_1 adrenergic receptors in the all body (Molinoff, 1984; Barnes, 1995), the increase in serum Mg^{2+} occurs *via* the specific activation of β_2-adrenergic receptor, as it is mimicked by the administration of the selective β_2-adrenergic agonist salbutamol, and it is inhibited by the specific β_2-blocker ICI-118551 (Keenan *et al*, 1995). Due to the amplitude of the increase in Mg^{2+} level into the bloodstream, it is reasonable to envisage that the adrenergic agonists are mobilizing Mg^{2+} from more than one tissue (Keenan *et al*, 1995). The involvement of bone has been proposed by Gunther and co-workers (Gunther and Vormann, 1992) based on the observation that the infusion of carbonic anhydrase inhibitor prevents isoproterenol-mediated Mg^{2+} mobilization into the blood of anesthetized rats. Based upon the pre-infusion level of serum Mg^{2+}, the glomerular filtration rate (1.62 mL/min), and the fractional excretion (17%) (Shafik and Quamme, 1989), changes in renal excretion do not appear to contribute significantly to the increase in serum Mg^{2+} level, at least during the first two hours following adrenergic agonist infusion. It is interesting to note, however, that hormones that increase plasma Mg^{2+} by mobilizing the cation from different organs or tissues usually increase Mg^{2+} resorption in the Henle's loop, *de facto* preventing any net loss of Mg^{2+}.

The inconsistency of changes in serum Mg^{2+} level observed in the literature, however, does not have a clear explanation. Several factors may contribute to this incongruity, including the proportion of b-adrenergic receptor subtypes in different experimental models, the ability of adrenergic agonists to stimulate with various potency different adrenergic receptors subtypes, and the modality, rate and duration of drug infusion. This inconsistency has also hampered our ability to assign a physiological significance to the eventual increase in serum Mg^{2+} level following catecholamine infusion. The observation that serum Mg^{2+} level increases under certain conditions may imply that specific organs or tissues have the ability to *sense* these changes and act accordingly. Presently, no specific Mg^{2+} sensing mechanism has been identified. However, the Ca^{2+} sensing receptor (Brown *et al*, 1993) can senses changes in circulating Mg^{2+} level in a range of concentrations far higher than those of Ca^{2+} (Nemeth and Scarpa, 1987) but consistent with the increase in serum Mg^{2+} level reported in the literature (Gunther and Vormann, 1992; Keenan *et al*, 1995). The observation that in distal convoluted tubule cells (MDCT) of the mouse the Ca^{2+}-sensing receptor can be activated with comparable sensitivity by both extracellular Ca^{2+} and Mg^{2+} (Bapty *et al*, 1998a) suggests interesting hypotheses in terms of whole body physiology. The activation of this sensor mechanism would inhibit glucagon- or vasopressin-mediated entry of Mg^{2+} into the cell (Bapty *et al*, 1998b) and favor the elimination of the cation with the urine. This would then explain the clinical and experimental evidence that hypermagnesemia and hypercalcemia inhibit hormone-stimulated cAMP-mediated resorption of Mg^{2+} and Ca^{2+} along the different segments of the nephron (Quamme and Dirks, 1980). Also, it would represent a distal regulatory mechanism to restore magnesemia to a physiological level following the increase observed in anesthetized animals infused with adrenergic agonists (Gunther and Vormann, 1992; Keenan *et al*, 1995). Whether this sensing mechanism and/or its associated modulatory components are altered under diabetic conditions in which an increased magnesuria is observed it remains to be elucidated.

At variance of an increase in calcemia, which is associated with muscle weakness and arrhythmia, an increase in serum Mg^{2+} level appears to be well tolerated *in vivo*. Rats infused with boluses of Mg^{2+} that increase serum Mg^{2+} level by 50% do not exhibit significant systemic hemodynamic changes but show a marked increase in coronary artery flow (Dipette *et al*, 1987). Baboons infused with pharmacological doses of Mg^{2+} sufficient to prevent epinephrine-induced cardiac arrhythmias show a significant attenuation of the epinephrine-induced increase in mean arterial pressure and systemic vascular resistance (Stanbury, 1948). It would appear, therefore, that an elevated level of $[Mg^{2+}]_o$ can regulate catecholamine release from peripheral and adrenal sources (James *et al*, 1988) and modulate cardiac contractility (Howarth *et al*, 1994). Taken together, these observations suggest that an increase in serum Mg^{2+} level following adrenergic stimulation can: 1) act as a feed-back mechanism to modulate catechol-amine release and activity; and 2) contribute to improved blood flow and O_2 delivery to the heart and possibly other tissues at a time when an increase in energy production is expected.

Physiological role of intracellular Mg^{2+}

The conclusions presented in the previous sections strongly suggest a key role for Mg^{2+} as an indispensable component for enzymes, phospho-metabolites, and channel activity (Grubbs and Maguire, 1987; Romani and Scarpa, 1992). Several glycolytic enzymes, including hexokinase, phosphofructokinase, phosphoglycerate mutase, phosphoglycerate kinase, enolase and pyruvate kinase, show activation at low and inhibition at high Mg^{2+} concentrations (Otto *et al*, 1974; Garfinkel and Garfinkel, 1988). The adenylate cyclase is another example of an enzyme directly regulated by Mg^{2+} (reviewed in Maguire, 1984). All these processes occur at Mg^{2+} concentrations between 0.5 to 1mM, which are well within the fluctuations in free $[Mg^{2+}]_i$ measured in the cytoplasm of various cells including hepatocyte

(Corkey *et al*, 1986). With the exception of the glycolytic enzymes, studies attempting to evidence a regulatory role of Mg^{2+} for cytosolic enzymes have been disappointing, mostly because of the underlying assumption that Mg^{2+} would operate as Ca^{2+} in modulating enzyme activity. At variance from Ca^{2+}, Mg^{2+} concentration in the cytoplasm and extracellular fluids is in the millimolar or submillimolar range. Consequently, an increase or decrease in cytosolic Mg^{2+} level equivalent to the changes observed for Ca^{2+} will go largely undetected by the common fluorescent or ^{31}P-NMR techniques. Heretofore, a role of Mg^{2+} as transient regulator of cytosolic enzymes appears to be unlikely. It has to be noted that even under conditions in which hormonal and non-hormonal stimuli elicit major fluxes of Mg^{2+} across the cell plasma membrane in either direction, massive translocations of Mg^{2+} that increase or decrease the total cellular Mg^{2+} content by 1 to 2mM (or 5-10% of total cell content) result in minor or no changes in cytosolic free $[Mg^{2+}]_i$ (Harman *et al*, 1990; Romani *et al*, 2000). This disconnect can be explained by assuming that the source or destination of transported Mg^{2+} is a cellular compartment or organelle, or a major binding site, or that Mg^{2+} is highly buffered. Hence, regulation of cellular functions by Mg^{2+} should not be necessarily expected to occur in the cytosol but within organelles, and in the plasma, where Mg^{2+} concentration can rapidly increase or decrease more than 20% (Gunther and Vormann, 1992; Keenan *et al*, 1995).

In the following pages we will highlight what is known about regulatory effects of extracellular or intracellular Mg^{2+} on the operation of cation channels in the plasma membrane, as well as on mitochondria respiration and volume following changes in Mg^{2+} concentration within the organelle.

Ca^{2+}- and K^+-channels

The first report of a regulatory effect of intracellular free Mg^{2+} on calcium channels was by White and Hartzell (1988). These authors reported that increasing intracellular free $[Mg^{2+}]_i$ from 0.3 to 3.0mM by internal perfusion had a dual effect in cardiac ventricular myocytes. It had a small effect on basal L-type Ca^{2+}-channels current (I_{Ca}) but decreased by more than 50% the amplitude of I_{Ca} elevated by cAMP-dependent phosphorylation. The effect of Mg^{2+} was not due to changes in cAMP concentration or in the velocity of phosphorylation but appeared to be a direct effect on the phosphorylated channel or on the channel dephosphorylation rate (White and Hartzell, 1988). Similar results were also reported by Agus and Morad (1991) in guinea pig cardiac myocytes. The block induced by Mg^{2+}on the Ca^{2+} current depended on a direct effect on the inactivation state of the channel as the block persisted in the presence and in the absence of cAMP and was not reversed by elevation of extracellular Ca^{2+} concentration or addition of catecholamine (Agus and Morad, 1991). The effect of Mg^{2+} on Ca^{2+}-channels is not restricted to cardiac cells or to an intra-cellular site of action. Bara and Guiet-Bara (2001) have shown that in vascular smooth muscle cells and endothelial cells in human placenta $MgCl_2$ (and to a lesser extent $MgSO_4$) regulates the influx of Ca^{2+} through voltage-gated Ca^{2+} channels by acting at an extracellular site on the channel, thus modulating the tonus of the vessels. Evidence for a similar block by extracellular Mg^{2+} on T-type Ca^{2+}-channels has been provided by Serrano *et al.* (2000). The modulatory effect of Mg^{2+} appears to take place at the EF-hand motif of the COOH-terminus of $Ca_v1.2$ channels as recently evidence by Catterall and his group (Brunet *et al*, 2006).

Extracellular Mg^{2+} also modulates the activity of store-operated Ca^{2+} channels. Studies in intact, pressurized rat mesenteric arteries with myogenic tone indicate that 10 mM extracellular Mg^{2+} can mimic nifedipine in preventing or reversing the vasoconstriction elicited by phenylephrine administration, but not that induced by K^+ depolarization (Zhang *et al*, 2002). Therefore, Mg^{2+} abolishes the vasoconstriction attributed to Ca^{2+} entry through store-operated channels, which are activated following phenylephrine administration, contributing to maintain both myogenic tone and α_1-adrenoceptor-induced tonic vasoconstriction. These data may have direct implication to explain some of the modifications that occur under hypertensive conditions, in which a decrease in plasma Mg^{2+} has often been reported.

Intracellular Mg^{2+} also affects he operation of store-operated calcium release-activated Ca^{2+} (CRAC) channels (Prakriya and Lewis, 2002). CRAC channels are highly Ca^{2+}-selective under physiological ionic conditions whereas removal of extracellular divalent cations makes them freely permeable to monovalent cations, in particular Na^+. Experimental evidence indicates that intracellular Mg^{2+} can modulate the activity and selectivity of these channels therefore affecting monovalent cation permeability. While an effect of intracellular Mg^{2+} on CRAC channels cannot be completely excluded, a report by Prakriya and Lewis (2002) suggests that the channels modulated by intracellular Mg^{2+} are not CRAC channels, but a different class of channels that open when Mg^{2+} is washed out of the cytosol. These channels have therefore been termed Mg^{2+}-inhibited cation (MIC) channels, as they present distinctive functional parameters in terms of inhibition, regulation, ion permeation and selectivity (Prakriya and Lewis, 2002).

Potassium channels are also targets for Mg^{2+}. Matsuda (1991) has reported that the presence of Mg^{2+} on the cytoplasmic side of the inwardly rectifying K^+ channel blocks the outward currents without affecting the inward currents. The Mg^{2+} block is achieved at a half-saturation concentration of 1.7μM. When the Mg^{2+} concentration is elevated to 2-10μM, the outward current fluctuated between two intermediate sublevels in addition to the fully open and closed configuration. However, these concentrations of Mg^{2+} are far from being physiological and it is difficult to envision the occurrence of a similar regulatory effect under normal conditions without invoking Mg^{2+} microcompartmentation. A regulatory role of intracellular Mg^{2+} on K_v channels in vascular smooth muscle cells has been observed by Tammaro *et al.* (2005). These authors have observed that an increase in intracellular Mg^{2+} in a range of concentrations consistent with its physiological variations can slow down the kinetic of activation of the K_v channel, cause inward rectification at positive membrane potentials, and shift the voltage-dependent inactivation (Tammaro *et al*, 2005). Overall, this represents a novel mechanism for the regulation of this channel in the vasculature. Intracellular Mg^{2+} also modulates large-conductance (BK type) Ca^{2+}-dependent K^+ channels by either blocking the pore of BK channels in a voltage-dependent manner, or by activating the channels independently of changes in Ca^{2+} and voltage by preferentially binding to the channel open conformation at a site different from Ca^{2+} sites. Interestingly, Mg^{2+} may also bind to Ca^{2+} sites and competitively inhibit Ca^{2+}-dependent activation (Shi *et al*, 2002).

The inhibitory effect of Mg^{2+} is not restricted to cell membrane channels. Experimental evidence by Bednarczyk et al (2005) indicates that Mg^{2+} in the mitochondrial matrix can modulate gating and conductance of mitochondrial K_{ATP} channels, which play a key role under ischemia/reperfusion conditions.

Mitochondrial dehydrogenases

Mitochondria represent one of the major cellular pools for Mg^{2+}, its concentration being 14 to 16 mM (Gunther, 1986). Evidence from this (Romani *et al*, 1991) and other laboratories (Zhang and Melvin, 1992; Zhang and Melvin, 1996; Kubota *et al*, 2005) suggests that Mg^{2+} can be mobilized from mitochondria under various conditions including hormone-mediated increase in cytosolic cAMP level through a mechanism(s) that has not been fully elucidated but it appears to involve the adenine nucleotide translocase (Romani *et al*, 1991). Several reviews have analyzed in detail how Mg^{2+} homeostasis is regulated in the organelle (Flatman, 1984; Gunther, 1986; Ogoma *et al*, 1992), and we refer to those reviews for further information. This section will focus on some recent evidence about a role of intra- and extra-mitochondrial Mg^{2+} on the activity of specific mitochondrial proteins.

It is commonly accepted that changes in matrix Ca^{2+} can affect the rate of mitochondrial dehydrogenases and therefore the rate of respiration (McCormack *et al*, 1990; Hansford, 1994). Yet, limited evidence supports a similar role for Mg^{2+} although the activity of several mitochondrial dehydrogenases has been observed to increase within minutes from the application of hormonal or metabolic stimuli despite the absence of a detectable increase in mitochondrial Ca^{2+} (Moravec and Bond, 1991; Moravec and Bond, 1992). The role of matrix Mg^{2+} as regulator of dehydrogenases and consequently mitochondrial respiration has been investigated by measuring the activity of several dehydrogenases in mitochondria under conditions in which matrix Ca^{2+} and/or Mg^{2+} concentration were varied. From those data, it appears that α-ketoglutarate dehydrogenase and pyruvate dehydrogenase are not regulated by changes in mitochondrial Mg^{2+}, whereas Mg^{2+} removal increases several fold the activity of succinate and glutamate dehydrogenases (Panov and Scarpa, 1996a; Panov and Scarpa, 1996b). This evidence would therefore indicate that changes in matrix Mg^{2+} content (in combination with or in alternative to changes in mitochondrial Ca^{2+}) can control mitochondria respiration, at least under well defined conditions. In this respect, mitochondrial Mg^{2+} content appears to change quite significantly during transition from state 3 to state 4 (Brierley *et al*, 1987), affecting at the same time the amplitude of mitochondria respiration. In addition, data from our laboratory (Romani *et al*, 1991), Zhang and Melvin (1996), and Kubota et al (2005) would suggest that mitochondrial Mg^{2+} can be mobilized by catecholamine stimulation via cAMP. Hence, the enhanced mitochondrial respiration elicited by catecholamine could depend, at least in part, on cAMP-mediated modulation of mitochondrial Mg^{2+}, which, in turn, will stimulate directly some dehydrogenases while rendering others more susceptible to the Ca^{2+} concentrations present in the mitochondrial matrix.

The regulatory effect of Mg^{2+} on mitochondrial function is not restricted to the dehydrogenases activity but affects also the anion channel present in the mitochondrial membrane (Beavis and Powers, 2004) as well as the opening of the permeability transition pore (Dolder *et al*, 2003). The mitochondrial inner membrane anion channel (IMAC) transports various anions, and is involved in regulating the organelle volume in conjunction with the K^+/H^+ antiporter. Although its fine regulation is not completely elucidated as yet, experimental evidence suggests that matrix Mg^{2+} and protons inhibit IMAC, maintaining the channel in its closed state (Beavis and Powers, 2004). Kinetic studies by Beavis and collaborators further support a main role of Mg^{2+} in maintaining the channel in a condition that would allow fine modulation by small changes in pH and proton distribution under physiological conditions (Beavis and Powers, 2004).

The permeability transition pore (PTP) is a proteinaceous pore that opens in the inner mitochondrial membrane following a marked decrease in membrane potential and results in the rapid equilibration and redistribution of matrix and extramitochondrial solutes down their concentrations gradient. While it is still debated exactly which proteins participate in the pore formation and how the pore opens, it is well established that an increase in mitochondrial Ca^{2+} content facilitates the opening whereas an increase in mitochondrial Mg^{2+} antagonizes it. This effect can be appreciated well in yeasts, which do not possess a canonical PTP (Bradshaw and Pfeiffer, 2006). According to one model of regulation, creatine kinase can regulate the opening of the permeability transition pore by tightly associating to the mitochondrial membrane and remaining in an active state (Dolder *et al*, 2003). Both these processes are Mg^{2+}-dependent, and Mg^{2+} removal from the extramitochondrial environment results in a decline in creatine kinas activity and in the opening of the permeability transition pore Dolder *et al*, 2003).

Considering the effect of Mg^{2+} on mitochondrial function and channels (see previous section), it appears that Mg^{2+} plays more than one role within this organelle regulating: 1) mitochondrial volume; 2) ion composition; 3) ATP production; and 4) metabolic interaction with the hosting cell.

Reticular G6Pase

The Endoplasmic Reticulum (ER) represents one of the major cellular Mg^{2+} pools, with a total concentration of 14 to 18mM (Romani and Scarpa, 1992). Yet, limited information is available about any major role of luminal Mg^{2+} on reticular functions other than protein synthesis (Rubin, 2005). It is also unknown whether Mg^{2+} is buffered or chelated by endoluminal proteins in the same way Ca^{2+} is complexed. Furthermore, we do not have any information about the transport mechanism(s) that allow(s) ER (and SR) to attain and maintain such a large luminal Mg^{2+} concentration.

Work by Volpe and collaborators (Volpe *et al.* 1990; Volpe and Vezu', 1993), Gusev and Niggli (Gusev and Niggli, 2008), and Laver and Honen (Laver and Honen, 2008) suggests that cytosolic and perhaps luminal Mg^{2+} concentration can have a major effect in limiting Ca^{2+} uptake into the ER/SR and its release from the organelle via IP_3 (Volpe *et al.* 1990) and ryanodine receptor (Laver and Honen, 2008). In the latter case, a direct effect of Mg^{2+} on the receptor has been observed (Gusev and Niggli, 2008; Laver and Honen, 2008).

Less clear is whether a similar effect takes also place at the level of the IP_3 receptor. More recently, our laboratory has reported that cytosolic Mg^{2+} can have a regulatory role on the activity of reticular glucose 6-phosphatase (G6Pase) in liver cells (Doleh and Romani, 2007). This effect is biphasic, with an optimal stimulatory effect at ~0.5mM $[Mg^{2+}]_i$ and an inhibitory effect at higher concentrations (Doleh and Romani, 2007). The effect of Mg^{2+} appears to take place at the level of the G6Pi transport component of the G6Pase enzymatic complex in that it can be inhibited by EDTA (as Mg^{2+} chelating agent) or taurocholic acid, which permeabilizes the ER membrane and allows G6Pi to bypass the transport mechanism and be delivered directly to the catalytic site of the G6Pase within the ER lumen (Doleh and Romani, 2007). Investigation is in progress to determine whether Mg^{2+} exerts a similar modulatory effect on other ER enzymes.

Cell pH and volume

As mentioned in Section 4.1.4, exposure of the cell to cyanide (Dalal and Romani, 2010), fructose (Gaussin *et al*, 1997), hypoxia, Harman *et al*, 1990; Gasbarrini *et al*, 1992), ethanol (Tessman and Romani, 1998), or choline chloride (Romani *et al*, 1993b) results in a marked cellular acidification associated with a decrease in cellular ATP content and a major Mg^{2+} extrusion. This extrusion is the consequence of a decrease in buffering capacity (ATP loss) as well as binding affinity. Now, a report by Yamaguchi and Ishikawa (2008) highlights a new and important regulatory role of intracellular Mg^{2+} on the operation of the electrogenic Na^+-HCO_3^- co-transporter NBCe1-B in a range of concentrations that are consistent with the variations in Mg^{2+} content measured within the cytoplasm of various cell types (Grubbs and Maguire, 1987). This regulatory effect is exerted by Mg^{2+} and not by MgATP, and requires a functional N-terminus on the NBCe1-B transporter (Yamaguchi and Ishikawa, 2008). It is still unclear whether Mg^{2+} binds the N-terminus of the transporter directly or exerts its effects via an intermediate, Mg^{2+}-modulated regulatory protein (Yamaguchi and Ishikawa, 2008). At a cytosolic $[Mg^{2+}]$ of ~1mM (a physiological Mg^{2+} concentration measured in the cytosol of various cells (Corkey *et al*, 1986; Grubbs and Maguire, 19897), the NBCe1-B current is inhibited by ~50%, and no detectable current can be measured for *free* Mg^{2+} concentrations of 3-5mM.

More or less at the same time, the group of Hirano and collaborators reported that increasing cellular Mg^{2+} content has a stimulatory role on the expression of aquaporin 3 in CaCo-3 cells (Okahira *et al*, 2008). This isoform of aquaporin is highly expressed in the gastro-intestinal tract, in which it absorbs water, glycerol and urea. The effect of Mg^{2+} on aquaporin mRNA expression appears to involve cAMP/PKA/CREB signaling, as well as we MEK1/2 and MSK1 (Okahira *et al*, 2008), suggesting short- and long-term regulation on the activity and expression of this protein. It is presently undefined whether Mg^{2+} exerts a similar regulatory role on other aquaporin isoforms. Moreover, as aquaporin 3 is also expressed in brain, erythrocytes, kidney, and skin, a modulatory role of Mg^{2+} on the protein expression in these tissues may have major relevance for various physiological and/or pathological conditions.

Taken together, these two sets of information suggest that Mg^{2+} can have a major regulatory role on cellular pH, cellular volume, and cellular cation concentration, especially Na^+. Also, as aquaporin 3 mediates glycerol and urea accumulation, possible repercussions on fatty acid metabolism and urea cycle must be taken into proper consideration.

Cell cycle

Cell cycle (Maguire, 1988; Sgambato *et al*, 1999; Touyz et Yao, 2003), cell proliferation (Wolf *et al*, 2009b) and cell differentiation (Covacci *et al*, 1998; Wolf *et al*, 1998; Di Francesco *et al*, 1998) have all been associated with the maintenance of an optimal cellular Mg^{2+} level. Under conditions in which cellular Mg^{2+} accessibility is restricted or reduced, cell proliferation and cell cycle progression are markedly impaired. A decrease in extracellular Mg^{2+} content also affects cell differentiation (Covacci *et al*, 1998; Wolf *et al*, 1998; Di Francesco *et al*, 1998). The mechanisms by which a decrease in cellular Mg^{2+} content affects these cellular processes have been attributed to defective MAPKs (Touyz and Yao, 2003) and p27 (Sgambato *et al*, 1999) signaling, increased oxidative stress level (Wolf *et al*, 2009b), and decreased MgATP levels (Di Francesco *et al*, 1998; Rubin, 2005). Because cellular MgATP level is at a level optimal for protein synthesis (Rubin, 2005), any alteration in this metabolic parameter will have major repercussion on the proper functioning of the cell. In addition, extracellular Mg^{2+} levels regulate integrins signaling, *de facto* modulating the interaction among cells and between cells and extracellular matrix (Trache *et al*, 2010). Hence, consistent with the long-term regulatory function of Mg^{2+} proposed by Grubbs and Maguire (1987) several years ago, all these observations underlie the important role of Mg^{2+} to guarantee cell cycle progression and retention of proper cell morphology and function, avoiding undesired progression towards cell death or neoplastic destiny (Wolf *et al*, 2009a).

Conclusions

In the last few years, our understanding of cellular and whole body Mg^{2+} homeostasis has significantly advanced. While it still lags behind as compared to the knowledge available for other ions such as Ca^{2+}, H^{+}, K^{+} or Na^{+}, yet the identification of putative Mg^{2+} channels and transport mechanisms in the membrane of the cell or mitochondria, as well as an improved understanding of the signaling pathways and conditions regulating Mg^{2+} transport is providing new tools to address essential questions about the physiological role Mg^{2+} plays inside the cell and in the whole body.

References

Aarts M, Iihara K, Wei WL, Xiong ZG, Arundine M, Cerwinski W, MacDonald JF, Tymianski M (2003) A key role for TRPM7 channels in anoxic neuronal death. *Cell* 115:863-877.

Agus ZS, Morad M (1991) Modulation of cardiac ion channels by magnesium. *Annu Rev Physiol* 53:299-307.

Akerman KE (1981) Inhibition and stimulation of respiration-linked Mg^{2+} efflux in rat heart mitochondria. *J Bioenerg Biomembr* 13:133-139.

Alexander RT, Hoenderop JG, Bindels RJ (2008) Molecular determinants of magnesium homeostasis: insight from human disease. *J Am Soc Nephrol* 19:1451-1458.

Allouche D, Parello J, Sanejouand YH (1999) Ca^{2+}/Mg^{2+} exchange in parvalbumin and other EF-hand proteins. A theoretical study. *J Mol Biol* 285:857-873.

Amano T, Matsubara T, Watanabe J, Nakayama S, Hotta N (2000) Insulin modulation of intracellular free magnesium in heart: involvement of protein kinase C. *Brit J Pharmacol* 130:731-738.

Baillien M, Cogneau M (1995) Characterization of two mechanisms of ^{28}Mg uptake in rat jejunal brush border membrane vesicles. *Magnesium* 8:331-339.

Baillien M, Wang H, Cogneau M (1995) Uptake of ^{28}Mg by duodenal and jejunal brush border membrane vesicle in the rat. *Magnesium* 8:315-329.

Bailly C, Imbert-Teboul M, Roinel N, Amiel C (1990) Isoproterenol increases Ca, Mg, and NaCl reabsorption in mouse thick ascending limb. *Am J Physiol* 258:F1224-F1231.

Bapty BW, Dai LJ, Ritchie G, Canaff L, Hendy GN, Quamme GA (1998) Mg^{2+}/Ca^{2+} sensing inhibits hormone-stimulated uptake in mouse distal convolute tubule cells. *Am J Physiol* 275:F353-F360.

Bapty BW, Dai LJ, Ritchie G, Jirik F, Canaff L, Hendy GN, Quamme GA (1998) Extracellular Mg^{2+}- and Ca^{2+}-sensing in mouse distal convoluted tubule cells. *Kidney Intern* 53:583-592.

Bara M, Guiet-Bara A (2001) Magnesium regulation of Ca^{2+} channels in smooth muscle and endothelial cells of human allantochorial placental vessels. *Magnes Res* 14:11-18.

Barbagallo M, Dominguez LJ (2007) Magnesium metabolism in type 2 diabetes mellitus, metabolic syndrome and insulin resistance. *Arch Biochem Biophys* 458:40-47.

Barnes PJ (1995) Beta-adrenergic receptors and their regulation. *Am J Respir Crit Care Med* 152:838-860.

Beavis AD, Powers M (2004) Temperature dependence of the mitochondrial inner membrane anion channel: the relationship between temperature and inhibition by magnesium. *J Biol Chem* 279:4045-4050.

Bednarczyk P, Dolowy K, Szewczyk A (2005) Matrix Mg^{2+} regulates mitochondrial ATP-dependent potassium channel from heart. *FEBS Lett* 579:1625-1630.

Belge H, Gailly P, Schwaller B, Loffing J, Debaix H, Riveira-Munoz E, Beauwens R, Devogelaer JP, Hoenderop JG, Bindels RJ, Devuyst O (2007) Renal expression of parvalbumin is critical for NaCl handling and response to diuretics. *Proc Natl Acad Sci USA* 104:14849-14854.

Bessac BF, Fleig A (2007) TRPM7 channel is sensitive to osmotic gradients in human kidney cells. *J Physiol* 582:1073-1086.

Bird SJ, Maguire ME (1978) The agonist-specific effect of magnesium ion on binding by β-adrenergic receptors of S49 lymphoma cells: Interactions of GTP and magnesium in magnesium in adenylate cyclase activation. *J Biol Chem* 253:8826-8834.

Bogucka K, Wojtczak L (1971) Intramitochondrial distribution of magnesium. *Biochem Biophys Res Commun* 44: 1330-1337.

Brauchi S, Krapivinsky G, Krapivinsky L, Clapham DE (2008) TRPM7 facilitates cholinergic vesicle fusion with the plasma membrane. *Proc Natl Acad Sci U S A* 105:8304-8308.

Brierley GP, Davis M, Jung DW (1987) Respiration-dependent uptake and extrusion of Mg^{2+} by isolated heart mitochondria. *Arch Biochem Biophys* 253: 322-332.

Brown EM, Gamba G, Riccardi D, Lombardi M, Butters R, Kifor O, Sun A, Hediger MA, Lytton J, Herbert SC (1993) Cloning and characterization of an extracellular Ca^{2+}-sensing from bovine parathyroid. *Nature* 366:575-580.

Brunet S, Scheuer T, Klevit R, Catterall WA (2006) Modulation of $Ca_v1.2$ channels by Mg^{2+} acting at an EF-hand motif in the COOh-terminal domain. *J Gen Physiol* 126:311-323.

Bui DM, Gregan J, Jarosch E, Ragnini A, Schweyen RJ (1999) The bacterial magnesium transporter CorA can functionally substitute for its putative homologue Mrs2p in the Yeast inner mitochondrial membrane. *J Biol Chem* 274:20438-20443.

Butler MG (1990) Prader-Willi syndrome: current understanding of cause and diagnosis. *Am J Med Genet* 35:319-332.

Cao G, Thébault S, van der Wijst J, van der Kemp A, Lasonder E, Bindels RJ, Hoenderop JG (2008) RACK1 inhibits TRPM6 activity via phosphorylation of the fused alpha-kinase domain. *Curr Biol* 18:168-176.

Cao G, van der Wijst J, van der Kemp A, van Zeeland F, Bindels RJ, Hoenderop JG (2009) Regulation of the epithelial Mg^{2+} channel TRPM6 by estrogen and the associated repressor protein of estrogen receptor activity (REA). *J Biol Chem* 284:14788-14795.

Cefaratti C, McKinnis A, Romani A (2004) Altered Mg^{2+} transport across liver plasma membrane from streptozotocin-treated rats. *Mol Cell Biochem* 262:145-154.

Cefaratti C, Romani A (2007) Functional characterization of two distinct Mg^{2+} extrusion mechanisms in cardiac sarcolemmal vesicles. *Mol Cell Biochem* 303:63-72.

Cefaratti C, Romani A (2011) Modulation of Na^{+}/Mg^{2+} exchanger stoichiometry ratio by Cl^{-} ions in basolateral rat liver plasma membrane vesicles. *Mol Cell Biochem* 351:133-142.

Cefaratti C, Romani A, Scarpa A (1998) Characterization of two Mg^{2+} transporters in sealed plasma membrane vesicles from rat liver. *Am J Physiol* 275:C995-C1008.

Cefaratti C, Romani A, Scarpa A (2000) Differential localization and operation of distinct Mg^{2+} transporters in Apical and Basolateral Sides of Rat Liver Plasma Membrane. *J Biol Chem* 275:3772-3780.

Cefaratti C, Ruse C (2007) Protein kinase A dependent phosphorylation activates Mg^{2+} efflux in the basolateral region of the liver. *Mol Cell Biochem* 297:209-214.

Chen H-S, Xie J, Zhang Z, Su L-T, Yue L, Runnels LW (2010) Blockade of TRPM7 channel activity and cell death by inhibitors of 5-lipoxygenase. *PLoS One* 5:e11161.

Chubanov V, Gudermann T, Schlingmann KP (2005) Essential role for TRPM6 in epithelial magnesium transport and body magnesium homeostasis. *Pflugers Arch* 451:228-234.

Chubanov V, Waldegger S, Mederos y Schnitzler M, Vitzthum H, Sassen MC, Seyberth HW, Konrad M , Gudermann T (2004) Disruption of TRPM6/TRPM7 complex formation by a mutation in the TRPM6 gene causes hypomagnesemia with secondary hypocalcemia. *Proc Natl Acad Sci U S A* 101:2894-2899.

Clark K, Langeslag M, van Leeuwen B, Ran L, Ryazanov AG, Figdor CG, Moolenaar WH, Jalink K, van Leeuwen FN (2006) TRPM7, a novel regulator of actomyosin contractility and cell adhesion. *EMBO J* 25:290-301.

Clark K, Middelbeek J, Lasonder E, Dulyaninova NG, Morrice NA, Ryazanov AG, Bresnick AR, Figdor CG, van Leeuwen FN (2008a) TRPM7 regulates myosin IIA filament stability and protein localization by heavy chain phosphorylation. *J Mol Biol* 378:790-803.

Clark K, Middelbeek J, Morrice NA, Figdor CG, Lasonder E, van Leeuwen FN (2008b) Massive autophosphorylation of the Ser/Thr-rich domain controls protein kinase activity of TRPM6 and TRPM7. *PLoS One* 3:e1876 (1-10).

Corkey BE, Duszynski J, Rich TL, Matchinsky B, Williamson JR (1986) Regulation of free and bound magnesium in rat hepatocytes and isolated mitochondria. *J Biol Chem* 261:2567-2574.

Covacci V, Bruzzese N, Sgambato A, Di Francesco A, Russo MA, Wolf FI, Cittadini A (1998) Magnesium restriction induces granulocytic differentiation and expression of p27Kip1 in human leukemic HL-60 cells. *J Cell Biochem* 70:313-322.

Csermely P, Fodor P, Somogyi J (1987) The tumor promoter tetradecanoylphorbol-13-acetate elicits the redistribution of heavy metal in subcellular fractions of rabbit thymocytes as measured by plasma emission spectroscopy. *Carcinogenesis* 8:1663-1666.

Cunningham D, Humblet Y, Siena S, Khayat D, Bleiberg H, Santoro A, Bets D, Mueser M, Harstrick A, Verslype C, Chau I, van Cutsem E (2004) Cetuximab monotherpay and cetuximab plus irinotecan in irinotecan-refractory metastatic colorectal cancer. *N Engl J Med* 351:337-345.

Dai L-J, Friedman PA, Quamme GA (1991) Cellular Mechanism of chlorothiazide and cellular potassium depletion on Mg^{2+} uptake in mouse distal convoluted tubule cells. *Kidney Inter* 51:1008-1017.

Dai L-J, Friedman PA, Quamme GA (1997) Phosphate depletion diminishes Mg^{2+} uptake in mouse distal convoluted tubule cells. *Kidney Inter* 51:1710-1718.

Dalal P, Romani A (2010) Adenosine triphosphate depletion by cyanide results in a Na^{+}-dependent Mg^{2+} extrusion from liver cells. *Metabolism* 59:1663-1671.

Di Francesco A, Desnoyer RW, Covacci V, Wolf FI, Romani A, Cittadini A, Bond M (1998) Changes in magnesium content and subcellular distribution during retinoic acid-induced differentiation of HL60 cells. *Arch Biochem Biophys* 360:149-157.

Di Polo R, Beauge' L (1988) An ATP-dependent Na^{+}/Mg^{2+} countertransport is the only mechanism for Mg^{2+} extrusion in squid axons. *Biochim Biophys Acta* 946:424-428.

Dimke H, van der Wjist J, Alexander TR, Mejier IM, Mulder GM, van Goor H, Tejpar S, Hoenderop JG, Bindels RJ (2010) Effects of the EGFR inhibitor erlotinib on magnesium handling. *J Am Soc Nephrol* 21:1309-1316.

Dipette DJ, Simpson K, Guntupalli J (1987) Systemic and regional hemodynamic effect of acute magnesium administration in the normotensive and hypertensive state. *Magnesium* 6:136-149.

Dolder M, Walzel B, Speer O, Schlattner U, Wallimann T (2003) Inhibition of the mitochondrial permeability transition by creatine kinase substrates. *J Biol Chem* 278:17760-17766.

Doleh L, Romani A (2007) Biphasic effect of extra-reticular Mg^{2+} on hepatic G6P transport and hydrolysis. *Arch Biochem Biophys* 467:283-290.

Dorovkov MV, Ryazanov AG (2004) Phosphorylation of annexin I by TRPM7 channel-kinase. *J Biol Chem* 279:50643-50646.

Ebel H, Gunther T (2003) Stimulation of Na^{+}/Mg^{2+} antiport in rat erythrocytes by intracellular Cl^{-}. *FEBS Lett* 543:103-107.

Ebel H, Hollstein M, Gunther T (2002) Role of the choline exchanger in Na^{+}-independent Mg^{2+} efflux from rat erythrocytes. *Biochim Biophys Acta* 1559:135-144.

Ebel H, Hollstein M, Günther T (2004) Differential effect of imipramine and related compounds on Mg^{2+} efflux from rat erythrocytes. *Biochim Biophys Acta* 1667:132-140.

Efrati E, Arsentiev-Rozenfeld J, Zelikovic I (2005) The human paracellin-1 gene (hPCLN-1): renal epithelial cell specific expression and regulation. *Am J Physiol* 288:F272-F283.

Elliot DA, Rizack MA (1974) Epinephrine and adrenocorticotrophic hormone-stimulated magnesium accumulation in adipocytes and their plasma membranes. *J Biol Chem* 249:3985-3990.

Erdos JJ, Maguire ME (1980) Independent desensitization of β-adrenergic receptor regulated magnesium transport and cyclic AMP accumulation. *Mol Pharmacol* 18:379-383.

Erdos JJ, Maguire ME (1983) Hormone-sensitive magnesium transport in murine S49 lymphoma cells: Characterization and specificity for magnesium. *J Physiol* 337:351-371.

Fagan TE, Cefaratti C, Romani A (2004) Streptozotocin-induced diabetes impairs Mg^{2+} homeostasis and uptake in rat liver cells. *Am J Physiol* 286:E184-E193.

Fagan TE, Romani A (2000) Activation of Na^{+}- and Ca^{2+}-dependent Mg^{2+} extrusion by a_1- and b_1-adrenergic agonists in rat liver cells. *Am J Physiol* 279:G943-G950.

Fagan TE, Romani A (2001) a_1-adrenoceptor-induced Mg^{2+} extrusion from rat hepatocytes occurs via Na^{+}-dependent transport mechanism. *Am J Physiol* 280:G1145-G1156.

Fatholahi M, Lanoue K, Romani A, Scarpa A (2000) Relationship between total and free cellular Mg^{2+} during metabolic stimulation of rat cardiac myocytes and perfused hearts. *Arch Biochem Biophys* 374:395-401.

Feray J-C, Garay R (1986) An Na^{+}-stimulated Mg^{2+} transport system in human red blood cells. *Biochim Biophys Acta* 856: 76-84.

Feray J-C, Garay R (1988) Demonstration of a Na^{+}:Mg^{2+} exchange in human red cells by its sensitivity to tricyclic antidepressant drugs. *Naunyn-Schmied Arch Pharmacol* 338:332-337.

Ferreira A, Rivera A, Romero JR (2004) Na^{+}/Mg^{2+} exchange is functionally coupled to the insulin receptor. *J Cell Physiol* 199:434-440.

Flatman PW (1984) Magnesium transport across cell membrane. *J Membr Biol* 80:1-14.

Flatman PW, Lew VL (1981) The magnesium dependence of sodium-pump-mediated sodium-potassium and sodium-sodium exchange in intact human red cells. *J Physiol* 315:421-446.

Flatman PW, Smith LM (1990) Magnesium transport in ferret red cells. *J Physiol* 431:11-25.

Garfinkel D, Garfinkel L (1988) Magnesium and regulation of carbohydrate metabolism at the molecular level. *Magnesium* 7:249-261.

Gasbarrini A, Borle AB, Farghali H, Bender C, Francavilla A, van Thiel D (1992) Effect of anoxia on intracellular ATP, Na^{+}_{i}, Ca^{2+}_{i}, Mg^{2+}_{i}, and cytotoxicity in rat hepatocytes. *J Biol Chem* 267:6654-6663.

Gaussin V, Gailly P, Gillis J-M, Hue L(1997) Fructose-induced increase in intracellular free Mg^{2+} ion concentration in rat hepatocytes: relation with the enzymes of glycogen metabolism. *Biochem J* 326:823-827.

Geigy Scientific Tables. (1984) Ed.: Lentner C., Ciba-Geigy, Basel, Switzerland.

Goytain A, Hines RM, El-Husseini A, Quamme GA (2007) NIPA1(SPG6), the basis for autosomal dominant form of hereditary spastic paraplegia, encodes a functional Mg^{2+} transporter. *J Biol Chem* 282:8060-8068.

Goytain A, Hines RM, Quamme GA (2008a) Functional characterization of NIPA2, a selective Mg^{2+} transporter. *Am J Physiol* 295:C944-C953.

Goytain A, Hines RM, Quamme GA (2008b) Huntingtin-interacting proteins, HIP14 and HIP14L, mediate dual functions, palmitoyl acyltransferase and Mg^{2+} transport. *J Biol Chem* 283:33365-33374.

Goytain A, Quamme GA (2005a) Identification and characterization of a novel mammalian Mg^{2+} transporter with channel-like properties. *BMC Genomics* 6:48.

Goytain A, Quamme GA (2005b) Functional characterization of human SLC41A1, a Mg^{2+} transporter with similarity to prokaryotic MgtE Mg^{2+} transporters. *Physiol Genomics* 21:337-342.

Goytain A, Quamme GA (2005c) Functional characterization of the human solute carrier, SLC41A2. *Biochem Biophys Res Commun* 330:701-705.

Goytain A, Quamme GA (2005d) Functional characterization of ACDP2 (ancient conserved domain protein), a divalent metal transporter. *Physiol Genomics* 22:382-389.

Goytain A, Quamme GA (2008) Identification and characterization of a novel family of membrane magnesium transporters, MMgT1 and MMgT2. *Am J Physiol* 294:C495-502.

Groenestege WM, Hoenderop JG, van den Heuvel L, Knoers N, Bindels RJ (2006) The epithelial Mg^{2+} channel transient receptor potential melastatin 6 is regulated by dietary Mg^{2+} content and estrogens. *J Am Soc Nephrol* 17:1035-1043.

Groenestege WM, Thébault S, van der Wijst J, van den Berg D, Janssen R, Tejpar S, van den Heuvel LP, van Cutsem E, Hoenderop JG, Knoers NV, Bindels RJ (2007) Impaired basolateral sorting of pro-EGF causes isolated recessive renal hypomagnesemia. *J Clin Invest* 117:2260-2267.

Grubbs RD, Collins SD, Maguire ME (1985) Differential compartmentation of magnesium and calcium in murine S49 lymphoma cells. *J Biol Chem* 259:12184-12192.

Grubbs RD, Maguire ME (1986) Regulation of magnesium but not calcium by phorbol esters. *J Biol Chem* 261:12550-12554.

Grubbs RD, Maguire ME (1987) Magnesium as a regulatory cation: Criteria and evaluation. *Magnesium* 6:113-127.

Grubbs RD, Wetherill CA, Kutschke K, Maguire ME (1984) Magnesium transport in murine S49 lymphoma cells: pharmacology and divalent cation selectivity. *Amer J Physiol* 248:C51-C57.

Guideri G (1992) Catecholamine modulation of Mg^{2+} plasma levels in the rat. *Arch Intern Pharmacodyn Therap* 14:122-125.

Gunther T (1986) Functional compartmentation of intracellular magnesium. *Magnesium* 5:53-59.

Günther T (1993) Mechanisms and regulation of Mg^{2+} efflux and Mg^{2+} influx. *Miner Electrolyte Metab* 19:259-265.

Gunther T (1996) Putative mechanism of Mg^{2+}/Mg^{2+} exchange and Na^{+}/Mg^{2+} antiport. *Magnes Bull* 18:2-6.

Günther T, Höllriegl V (1993) Na^{+}- and anion-dependent Mg^{2+} influx in isolated hepatocytes. *Biochim Biophys Acta* 1149:49-54.

Gunther T, Vormann J (1985) Mg^{2+} efflux is accomplished by an amiloride-sensitive Na^{+}/Mg^{2+} antiport. *Biochem Biophys Res Commun* 130:540-545.

Günther T, Vormann J (1990a) Induction of Mn^{2+}/H^{+} antiport in chicken erythrocytes by intracellular Mg^{2+} and Mn^{2+}. *FEBS Lett* 265:55-58.

Günther T, Vormann J (1990b) Na^{+}-dependent Mg^{2+} efflux from Mg^{2+}-loaded rat thymocytes and HL 60 cells. *Magnes Trace Elem* 9:279-282.

Gunther T, Vormann J (1992a) Activation of Na^{+}/Mg^{2+} antiport in thymocytes by cAMP. *FEBS Lett* 297:132-134.

Gunther T, Vormann J (1992b) Mechanism of beta-agonist-induced hypermagnesemia. *Magnes Bull* 14:122-125.

Günther T, Vormann J (1995) Reversibility of Na^{+}/Mg^{2+} antiport in rat erythrocytes. *Biochim Biophys Acta* 1234:105-110.

Gunther T, Vormann J, Forster R (1984) Regulation of intracellular magnesium by Mg^{2+} efflux. *Biochem Biophys Res Commun* 119:124-131.

Günther T, Vormann J, Höllriegl V (1990) Characterization of Na^{+}-dependent Mg^{2+} efflux from Mg^{2+}-loaded rat erythrocytes. *Biochim Biophys Acta* 1023:455-461.

Gunther T, Vormann J, Hollriegl V (1991) Noradrenaline-induced Na^{+}-dependent Mg^{2+} efflux from rat liver. *Magnes Bull* 13:122-124.

Günther T, Vormann J, McGuigan JA (1995) Buffering and activity coefficient of intracellular free magnesium concentration in human erythrocytes. *Biochem Mol Biol Int* 37:871-875.

Günzel D, Schlue WR (1996) Sodium-magnesium antiport in Retzius neurones of the leech *Hirudo medicinalis*. *J Physiol* 491:595-608.

Gusev K, Niggli E (2008) Modulation of the local SR Ca^{2+} release by intracellular Mg^{2+} in cardiac myocytes. *J Gen Physiol*. 132:721-730.

Gwanyanya A, Amuzescu B, Zakharov SI, Macianskiene R, Sipido KR, Bolotina VM, Vereecke J, Mubagwa K (2004) Magnesium-inhibited, TRPM6/7-like channel in cardiac myocytes: permeation of divalent cations and pH-mediated regulation. *J Physiol* 559:761-776.

Gwanyanya A, Sipido KR, Vereecke J, Mubagwa K (2006) ATP and PIP2 dependence of the magnesium-inhibited, TRPM7-like cation channel in cardiac myocytes. *Am J Physiol* 291:C627-C635.

Hansford RG (1994) Physiological role of mitochondrial Ca^{2+} transport. *J Bioenerg Biomembr* 26:495-508.

Harman AW, Nieminen AL, Lemasters JJ, Herman B (1990) Cytosolic free magnesium, ATP and blebbing during chemical hypoxia in cultured rat hepatocytes. *Biochem Biophys Res Commun* 170:477–483.

Henquin JC, Tamagawa T, Nenquin M, Cogneau M (1983) Glucose modulates Mg^{2+} fluxes in pancreatic islet cells. *Nature* 301:73-74.

Hofer AM, Machen TE (1993) Technique for in situ measurement of calcium in intracellular inositol 1,4,5-trisphosphate-sensitive stores using the fluorescent indicator mag-fura-2. *Proc Natl Acad Sci USA*. 90:2598-2602.

Hou J, Paul DL, Goodenough DA (2005). Paracellin-1 and the modulation of ion selectivity of tight junctions. *J Cell Sci* 118:5109-118.

Hou J, Renigunta A, Gomes AS, Hou M, Paul DL, Waldegger S, Goodenough DA (2009) Claudin-16 and claudin-19 interaction is required for their assembly into tight junctions and for renal reabsorption of magnesium. *Proc Natl Acad Sci U S A.* 106:15350-15355.

Howarth FC, Waring J, Hustler BI, Singh J (1994) Effects of extracellular magnesium and beta adrenergic stimulation on contractile force and magnesium mobilization in the isolated rat heart. *Magnes Res* 7:187-197.

Hwa J, Romani A, Marfella C, Scarpa A (1993) Mg^{2+} transport in erythrocytes: Regulation by intracellular pH or cAMP. *Biophys J* 63,A307.

Hwang DL, Yen CF, Nadler JL (1993) Insulin increases intracellular magnesium transport in human platelets. *J Clin Endocrinol Metab* 76:549-553.

Ikari A, Matsumoto S, Harada H, Takagi K, Hayashi H, Suzuki Y, Degawa M, Miwa M (2006) Phosphorylation of paracellin-1 at Ser217 by protein kinase A is essential for localization in tight junctions. *J Cell Sci* 119:1781-1789.

Ikari A, Okude C, Sawada H, Yamazaki Y, Sugatani J, Miwa M (2008) TRPM6 expression and cell proliferation are up-regulated by phosphorylation of Erk1/2 in renal epithelial cells. *Biochem Biophys Res Commun* 369:1129-1133.

Ikari A, Sanada A, Okude C, Sawada H, Yamazaki Y, Sugatani J, Miwa M (2010) Up-regulation of TRPM6 transcriptional activity by AP-1 in renal epithelial cells. *J Cell Physiol* 222:481-487.

Ishijima S, Tatibana M (1994) Rapid mobilization of intracellular Mg^{2+} by bombesin in Swiss 3T3 cells: Mobilization through external Ca^{2+}- and tyrosine kinase-dependent mechanism. *J Biochem* 115:730-737.

Jakob A, Becker J, Schottli G, Fritzsch G (1989) alpha$_1$-adrenergic stimulation causes Mg^{2+} release from perfused rat liver. *FEBS Lett* 246:127-130.

James MFM, Cork RC, Harlen GM, White JF (1988) Interaction of adrenaline and magnesium in the cardiovascular system of the baboon. *Magnesium* 7:37-43.

Jiang H, Tian SL, Zeng Y, Li LL, Shi J (2008) TrkA pathway(s) is involved in regulation of TRPM7 expression in hippocampal neurons subjected to ischemic-reperfusion and oxygen-glucose deprivation. *Brain Res Bull* 76:124-130.

Jiang J, Li M, Yue L (2005) Potentiation of TRPM7 inward current by protons. *J Gen Physiol* 126:137-150.

Jin J, Desai BN, Navarro B, Donovan A, Andrews NC, Clapham DE (2008) Deletion of Trpm7 disrupts embryonic development and thymopoiesis without altering Mg^{2+} homeostasis. *Science* 322:756-760.

Joborn H, Akerstrom G, Ljunghall S (1985) Effects of exogenous catecholamines and exercise on plasma magnesium concentrations. *Clin Endocrinol* 23:219-226.

Jung DW, Apel L, Brierley GP (1990) Matrix free Mg^{2+} changes with metabolic state in isolated heart mitochondria. *Biochemistry* 29:4121-4128.

Juttner R, Ebel H (1998) Characterization of Mg^{2+} transport in brush border membrane vesicles of rabbit ileum studied with mag-fura-2. *Biochim Biophys Acta* 1370:51-63.

Karoor V, Baltensperger K, Paul H, Czech MC, Malbon CC (1995) Phosphorylation of tyrosyl residues 350/354 of the beta-adrenergic receptor is obligatory for counterregulatory effects of insulin. *J Biol Chem* 270:25305-25308.

Kausalya PJ, Amasheh S, Gunzel D, Wurps H, Muller D, Fromm M, Hunziker W (2006) Disease-associated mutations affect intracellular traffic and paracellular Mg^{2+} transport function of Claudin-16. *J Clin Invest* 116:878-891.

Keenan D, Romani A, Scarpa A (1995) Differential regulation of circulating Mg^{2+} in the rat by b$_1$- and b$_2$-adrenergic receptor stimulation. *Circ Res* 77:973-983.

Keenan D, Romani A, Scarpa A (1996) Regulation of Mg^{2+} homeostasis by insulin in perfused rat livers and isolated hepatocytes. *FEBS Lett* 395:241-244.

Kehres DG, Lawyer CH, Maguire ME (1998) The CorA magnesium transporter gene family. *Microb Comp Genomics* 3:151-159.

Khan MA, Conigrave AD (2010) Mechanisms of multimodal sensing by extracellular Ca^{2+}-sensing receptors: a domain-based survey of requirements for binding and signalling. *Br J Pharmacol* 159:1039-1050

Kim SJ, Kang HS, Kang MS, Yu X, Park SY, Kim IS, Kim NS, Kim SZ, Kwak YG, Kim JS (2005) $alpha_1$-Agonists-induced Mg^{2+} efflux is related to MAP kinase activation in the heart, *Biochem Biophys Res Commun* 333:1132-1138.

Kolisek M, Launay P, Beck A, Sponder G, Serafini N, Brenkus M, Froschauer EM, Martens H, Fleig A, Schweigel M (2008) SLC41A1 is a novel mammalian Mg^{2+} carrier. *J Biol Chem* 283:16235-16247.

Kolisek M, Zsurka G, Samaj J, Weghuber J, Schweyen RJ, Schweigel M (2003) Mrs2p is an essential component of the major electrophoretic Mg^{2+} influx system in mitochondria. *EMBO J* 22:1235-1244.

Konno Y, Ohno S, Akita Y, Kawasaki H, Suzuki K (1989) Enzymatic properties of a novel phorbol ester receptor / protein kinase, nPKC. *J Biochem* 106:673–678.

Kubota T, Shindo Y, Tokuno K, Komatsu H, Ogawa H, Kudo S, Kitamura Y, Suzuki K, Oka K (2005) Mitochondria are intracellular magnesium stores: investigation by simultaneous fluorescent imaging in PC12 cells. *Biochim Biophys Acta* 1744:19-28.

Lal-Nag M, Morin PJ (2009) The claudins. *Genome Biol* 10(8):235.

Langeslag M, Clark K, Moolenaar WH, van Leeuwen FN, Jalink K (2007) Activation of TRPM7 channels by phospholipase C-coupled receptor agonists. *J Biol Chem* 282:232-239.

Laver DR, Honen BN (2008) Luminal Mg^{2+}, a key factor controlling RYR2-mediated Ca^{2+} release: cytoplasmic and luminal regulation modeled in a tetrameric channel. *J Gen Physiol* 132:429-446.

Li M, Du J, Jiang J, Ratzan W, Su LT, Runnels LW, Yue L (2007) Molecular determinants of Mg^{2+} and Ca^{2+} permeability and pH sensitivity in TRPM6 and TRPM7. *J Biol Chem* 282:25817-25830.

Li M, Jiang J, Yue L (2006) Functional characterization of homo- and heteromeric channel kinases TRPM6 and TRPM7. *J Gen Physiol* 127:525-537.

Li, S-H, Li, X-J (2004) Huntingtin–protein interactions and the pathogenesis of Huntington's disease. *Trends Genet* 20:146-152.

Ludi H, Schatzmann HJ (1987) Some properties of a system for sodium-dependent outward movement of magnesium from metabolizing human red blood cells. *J Physiol* 390:367-382.

Lüthi D, Günzel D, McGuigan JA (1999) Mg-ATP binding: its modification by spermine, the relevance to cytosolic Mg^{2+} buffering, changes in the intracellular ionized Mg2+ concentration and the estimation of Mg^{2+} by 31P-NMR. *Exp Physiol* 84:231-252.

Macianskiene R, Gwanyanya A, Vereecke J, Mubagwa K (2008) Inhibition of the magnesium-sensitive TRPM7-like channel in cardiac myocytes by nonhydrolysable GTP analogs: involvement of phosphoinositide metabolism. *Cell Physiol Biochem* 22:109-118.

Maguire ME (1984) Hormone-sensitive magnesium transport and magnesium regulation of adenylate cyclase. *Trends Pharmacol Sci* 5:73-77.

Maguire ME (1988) Magnesium and cell proliferation. *Ann NY Acad Sci* 551: 215-217.

Maguire ME, Erdos JJ (1978) Magnesium but not calcium accumulation is inhibited by β-adrenergic stimulation in S49 lymphoma cells. *J Biol Chem* 253:6633-6636.

Maguire ME, Erdos JJ (1980) Inhibition of magnesium uptake by β-adrenergic agonists and prostaglandin E_1 is not mediated by cyclic AMP. *J Biol Chem* 255:1030-1035.

Matsuda H (1991) Magnesium gating of the inwardly rectifying K^+ channel. *Annu Rev Physiol* 53:289-298.

Matsuura T, Kanayama Y, Inoue T, Takeda T, Morishima I (1993) cAMP-induced changes of intra-cellular Mg^{2+} levels in human erythrocytes. *Biochim Biophys Acta* 1220:31-36.

McCormack JG, Halestrap A, Denton RM (1990) Role of calcium ions in regulation of mammalian intramitochondrial metabolism. *Physiol Rev* 70:391-425.

Middelbeek J, Clark K, Venselaar HV, Huynen MA, van Leeuwen FN (2010) The alpha-kianse family: an exceptional branch on the protein kinase tree. *Cell Mol Life Sci* 67:875-890.

Molinoff PB (1984) Alpha- and beta-adrenergic receptor subtypes, properties, distribution and regulation. *Drugs* 28:1-14.

Moncrief MB, Maguire ME (1999) Magnesium transport in prokaryotes. *J Biol Inorg Chem* 4:523-527.

Mondon CE, Dolkas CB, Olefsky JM, Reaven GM (1974) Insulin sensitivity of isolated perfused rat liver. *Diabetes* 24: 225-229.

Monteilh-Zoller MK, Hermosura MC, Nadler MJ, Scharenberg AM, Penner R, Fleig A (2003) TRPM7 provides an ion channel mechanism for cellular entry of trace metal ions. *J Gen Physiol* 121:49-60.

Moore EW (1990) Biliary calcium and gallstone formation. *Hepatology* 12:206S-214S.

Moravec CS, Bond M (1991) Calcium is released from the junctional sarcoplasmic reticulum during cardiac muscle contraction. *Am J Physiol* 260:H989-H997.

Moravec CS, Bond M (1992) Effect of inotropic stimulation on mitochondrial calcium in cardiac muscle. *J Biol Chem* 267:5310-5316.

Mudge GH (1989) Agents affecting volume and composition of body fluids. In: *The Pharmacological Basis of Therapeutics* (Goodman Gilman A, Godman LS, Rall TW, Murad F, eds.) MacMillian, NY.

Muller D, Kausalya PJ, Claverie-Martin F, Meij IC, Eggert P, Garcia-Nieto V, Hunziker W (2003) A novel claudin 16 mutation associated with childhood hypercalciuria abolishes binding to ZO-1 and results in lysosomal mistargeting. *Am J Hum Genet* 73:1293-1301.

Nadler MJ, Hermosura MC, Inabe K, Perraud AL, Zhu Q, Stokes AJ, Kurosaki T, Kinet JP, Penner R, Scharenberg AM, Fleig A (2001) LTRPC7 is a Mg.ATP-regulated divalent cation channel required for cell viability. *Nature* 411:590-595.

Nemeth EF, Scarpa A (1987) Rapid mobilization of cellular Ca^{2+} in bovine parathyroid cells by external divalent cations. *J Biol Chem* 262:5188-5196.

Ogoma Y, Kobayashi H, Fujii T, Kondo Y, Hachimori A, Shimizu T, Hatano M (1992) Binding study of metal ions to S100 protein: ^{43}Ca, ^{25}Mg, ^{67}Zn and ^{39}K N.M.R.. *Int J Biol Macromol* 14:279-286.

Okahira M, Kubota M, Iguchi K, Usui S, Hirano K (2008) Regulation of aquaporin 3 expression by magnesium ion. *Eur J Pharmacol* 588:26-32.

Oki S, Ikura M, Zhang M (1997) Identification of Mg^{2+} binding sites and role of Mg^{2+} on target recognition by calmodulin. *Biochemistry* 36; 4309-4316.

Otto M, Heinrich R, Kuhn B, Jacobasch G (1974) A mathematical model for the influence of fructose 6-phosphate, ATP, potassium, ammonium and magnesium on the phosphofructo-kinase from rat erythrocytes. *Eur J Biochem* 49:169-178.

Panov A, Scarpa A (1996a) Independent modulation of the activity of alpha-ketoglutarate dehydrogenase complex by Ca^{2+} and Mg^{2+}. *Biochemistry* 35:427-432.

Panov A, Scarpa A (1996b) Mg^{2+} control of respiration in isolated rat liver mitochondria. *Biochemistry* 35:12849-12856.

Paravicini TM, Yogi A, Mazur A, Touyz RM (2009) Dysregulation of vascular TRPM7 and annexin-1 is associated with endothelial dysfunction in inherited hypomagnesemia. *Hypertension* 53:423-429.

Parente L, Solito E (2004) Annexin 1: more than an anti-phospholipase protein. *Inflamm Res* 53:125–132.

Piskacek M, Zotova L, Zsurka G, Schweyen RJ (2009) Conditional knockdown of hMRS2 results in loss of mitochondrial Mg^{2+} uptake and cell death. *J Cell Mol Med* 13:693-700.

Polimeni PI, Page E (1974) In: *Recent advances in study in cardiac cells and metabolism*. Ed.: Dhalle N S, vol IV, pp. 217-232, University Park Press, Baltimore.

Prakriya M, Lewis RS (2002) Separation and characterization of currents through store-operated CRAC channels and Mg^{2+}-inhibited cation (MIC) channels. *J Gen Physiol* 119:487-507.

Preston RR (1990) A magnesium current in *Paramecium*. *Science* 250:285-288.

Quamme GA (2010) Molecular identification of ancient and modern mammalian magnesium transporters. *Am J Physiol* 298:407-429.

Quamme GA, Dai L-S (1990) Presence of a novel influx pathway for Mg2+ in MDCK cells. *Am J Physiol* 259:C521-C525.

Quamme GA, Dirks JH (1980) Effect of intraluminal and contraluminal magnesium on magnesium and calcium transfer in the rat nephron. *Am J Physiol* 238:F187-F198.

Quamme GA, Rabkin SW (1990) Cytosolic free magnesium in cardiac myocytes: Identification of a Mg^{2+} influx pathway. *Biochem Biophys Res Commun* 167:1406-1412.

Quednau BD, Nicoll DA, Philipson KD (2004) The sodium/calcium exchanger family - SLC8. *Pflugers Arch* 447:543-548.

Raftos JE, Lew VL, Flatman PW (1999) Refinement and evaluation of a model of Mg^{2+} buffering in human red cells. *Eur J Biochem* 263:635-45.

Rainier S, Chai JH, Tokarz D, Nicholls RD, Fink JK (2003) NIPA1 gene mutations cause autosomal dominant hereditary spastic paraplegia (SPG6). *Am J Hum Gene*t 73:967-971.

Rasgado-Flores H, Gonzalez-Serratos H, DeSantiago J (1994) Extracellular Mg^{2+}-dependent Na^+, K^+, and Cl^- efflux in squid giant axons. *Am J Physiol* 266:C1112-C1117.

Rayssiguier Y (1977) Hypomagnesemia resulting from adrenaline infusion in ewes: its relation to lipolysis. *Horm Metab Res* 9:309-314.

Reed G, Cefaratti C, Berti-Mattera LN, Romani A (2008) Lack of insulin impairs Mg^{2+} homeostasis and transport in cardiac cells of streptozotocin-injected diabetic rats.*J Cell Biochem* 104:1034-1053.

Resnick LM (1993) Ionic basis of hypertension, insulin resistance, vascular disease, and related disorders. The mechanism of "syndrome X". *Am J Hypertens* 6:123S-134S.

Resnick LM, Altura BT, Gupta RK, Laragh JH, Alderman MH, Altura BM (1993) Intracellular and extracellular magnesium depletion in type 2 (non-insulin-dependent) diabetes mellitus. *Diabetologia* 36:767-770.

Rogers TA (1961) The exchange of radioactive magnesium in erythrocytes. *J Cell Comp Physiol* 57:119-121.

Rogers TA, Haven FL, Mahan PE (1960) Exchange of magnesium in the rat. *J Natl Cancer Inst* 25:887-888.

Romani A (2007) Regulation of magnesium homeostasis and transport in mammalian cells. *Arch Biochem Biophys* 458:90-102.

Romani A, Dowell E, Scarpa A (1991) Cyclic AMP-induced Mg^{2+} release from rat liver hepatocytes, permeabilized hepatocytes, and isolated mitochondria. *J Biol Chem* 266:24376-24384.

Romani A, Marfella C, Scarpa A (1992) Regulation of Mg^{2+} uptake in isolated rat myocytes and hepatocytes by protein kinase C. *FEBS Lett* 296:135-140.

Romani A, Marfella C, Scarpa A (1993a) Regulation of magnesium uptake and release in the heart and in isolated ventricular myocytes. *Circ Res* 72:1139-1148.

Romani A, Marfella C, Scarpa A (1993b) Hormonal stimulation of Mg^{2+} uptake in hepatocytes. Regulation by plasma membrane and intracellular organelles. *J Biol Chem* 268:15489-15495.

Romani A, Scarpa A (1990a) Hormonal control of Mg^{2+} in the heart. *Nature* 346:841-844.

Romani A, Scarpa A (1990b) Norepinephrine evokes a marked Mg^{2+} efflux from liver cells. *FEBS Lett* 269:37-40.

Romani A, Scarpa A (1992) Regulation of cell magnesium. *Arch Biochem Biophys* 298:1-12.

Romani A, Scarpa A (2000) Regulation of cellular magnesium. *Front Biosci* 5:D720-D734.

Romani AM, Maguire ME (2002) Hormonal regulation of Mg^{2+} transport and homeostasis in eukaryotic cells. *Biometals* 15:271-283.

Romani AM, Matthews VD, Scarpa A (2000) Parallel stimulation of glucose and Mg^{2+} accumulation by insulin in rat hearts and cardiac ventricular myocytes. *Circ Res* 86:326-333.

Rondón LJ, Groenestege WM, Rayssiguier Y, Mazur A (2008) Relationship between low magnesium status and TRPM6 expression in the kidney and large intestine. *Am J Physiol* 294:R2001-R2007.

Rubin H (2005) Central roles of Mg^{2+} and $MgATP^{2-}$ in the regulation of protein synthesis and cell proliferation: significance for neoplastic transformation. *Adv Cancer Res* 93:1-58.

Runnels LW, Yue L, Clapham DE (2001) TRP-PLIK, a bifunctional protein with kinase and ion channel activities, *Science* 291:1043-1047.

Runnels LW, Yue L , Clapham DE (2002) The TRPM7 channel is inactivated by PIP(2) hydrolysis. *Nat Cell Biol* 4:329-336.

Rutter GA, Osbaldeston NJ, McCormack JG, Denton RM (1990) Measurement of matrix free Mg^{2+} concentration in rat heart mitochondria by using entrapped fluorescent probes. *Biochem J* 271:627-634.

Ryazanov AG (2002) Elongation factor-2 kinase and its newly discovered relatives. *FEBS Lett* 514:26-29.

Ryazanova LV, Pavur KS, Petrov AN, Dorovkov MV, Ryazanov AG (2001) [Novel type of signaling molecules: protein kinases covalently linked to ion channels]. *Mol Biol* (Mosk) 35:321-332.

Sahni J, Nelson B, Scharenberg AM (2007) SLC41A2 encodes a plasma-membrane Mg^{2+} transporter. *Biochem* J 401:505-513.

Sahni J, Scharenberg AM (2008) TRPM7 ion channels are required for sustained phosphoinositide 3-kinase signaling in lymphocytes. *Cell Metab* 8:84-93.

Scarpa A, Brinley FJ (1981) In situ measurements of free cytosolic magnesium ions. *Fed Proc* 40:2646-252.

Schatzmann HJ (1993) Asymmetry of the magnesium sodium exchange across the human red cell membrane. *Biochim Biophys Acta* 1148:15-18.

Schlingmann KP, Weber S, Peters M, Niemann NL, Vitzthum H, Klingel K, Kratz M, Haddad E, Ristoff E, Dinour D, Syrrou M, Nielsen S, Sassen M, Waldegger S, Seyberth HW, Konrad M (2002) Hypomagnesemia with secondary hypocalcemia is caused by mutations in TRPM6, a new member of the TRPM gene family. *Nat Genet* 31:166–170.

Schmitz C, Deason F, Perraud A-L (2007) Molecular components of vertebrate Mg^{2+} homeostasis regulation. *Magnes Res* 20:6-18.

Schmitz C, Dorovkov MV, Zhao X, Davenport BJ, Ryazanov AG, Perraud A-L (2005) The channel kinases TRPM6 and TRPM7 are functionally nonredundant. *J Biol Chem* 280:37763-37771.

Schmitz C, Perraud AL, Johnson CO, Inabe K, Smith MK, Penner R, Kurosaki T, Fleig A, Scharenberg AM (2003) Regulation of vertebrate cellular Mg^{2+} homeostasis by TRPM7. *Cell* 114:191-200.

Schweigel M, Lang I, Martens H (1999) Mg^{2+} transport in sheep rumen epithelium: evidence for an electrodiffusive uptake mechanism. *Am J Physiol* 277:G976-G982.

Schweigel M, Martens H (2003) Anion-dependent Mg^{2+} influx and a role for a vacuolar H^+-ATPase in sheep rumianl epithelial cells. *Am J Physiol* 285:G45-G53.

Schweigel M, Vormann J, Martens H (2000) Mechanisms of Mg^{2+} transport in cultured ruminal epithelial cells. *Am J Physiol* 278:G400-G408.

Serrano J, Dashti SR, Perez-Reyes E, Jones SW (2000) Mg^{2+} block unmasks Ca^{2+}/Ba^{2+} selectivity of alpha1G T-type calcium channels. *Biophys J* 79:3052-3062.

Sgambato A, Wolf FI, Faraglia B, Cittadini A (1999) Magnesium depletion causes growth inhibition, reduced expression of cyclin D1, and increased expression of P27Kip1 in normal but not in transformed mammary epithelial cells. *J Cell Physiol* 180:245-254.

Shafik IM, Quamme GA (1989) Early adaptation of renal Mg^{2+} reabsorption in response to magnesium restriction. *Am J Phyiol* 257:F974-F977.

Shaul O, Hilgemann DW, de-Almeida-Engler J, Van Montagu M, Inz D, Galili G (1999) Cloning and characterization of a novel Mg^{2+}/H^+ exchanger, *EMBO J* 18:3973-3980.

Shi J, Krishnamoorthy G, Wang Y, Hu L, Chaturvedi N, Harilal D, Qin J, Cui J (2002) Mechanism of magnesium activation of calcium-activated potassium channels. *Nature* 418:876-880.

Shibatani T, David LL, McCormack AL, Frueh K, Skach WR (2005) Proteomic analysis of mammalian oligosaccharyltransferase reveals multiple subcomplexes that contain Sec61, TRAP, and two potential new subunits. *Biochemistry* 44:5982-5992.

Simon DB, Lu Y, Choate KA, Velazquez H, Al-Sabban E, Praga M, Casari G, Bettinelli A, Colussi G, Rodrigues-Soriano J, McCredie D, Milford D, Sanjad S, Lifton RP (1999) Paracellin-1, a renal tight junction protein required for paracellular Mg^{2+} resorption. *Science* 285:103-1106.

Smith RL, Thompson LJ, Maguire ME (1995) Cloning and characterization of MgtE, a putative new class of Mg^{2+} transporter from Bacillus firmus OF4. *J Bacteriol* 177:1233-1238.

Smoake JA, Moy G-MM, Fang B, Solomon SS (1995) Calmodulin-dependent cyclic AMP phospho-diesterase in liver plasma membranes: Stimulated by insulin. *Arch Biochem Biophys* 323:223-232.

Somlyo AV, McClellan G, Gonzalez-Serratos H, Somlyo AP (1985) Electron probe X-ray microanalysis of post-tetanic Ca^{2+} and Mg^{2+} movements across the sarcoplasmic reticulum *in situ*. *J Biol Chem* 260:6801-6807.

Stanbury JB (1948) The blocking action of magnesium on sympathetic ganglia. *J Pharmacol Exp Ther* 93:52-62.

Su L-T, Agapito M A, Li M, Simpson W, Huttenlocher A, Habas R, Yue L , Runnels LW (2006) Trpm7 regulates cell adhesion by controlling the calcium dependent protease calpain. *J Biol Chem* 281:11260-11270.

Suarez A, Pulido N, Casla A, Casanova B, Arrieta FJ, Rovira A (1995) Impaired tyrosine-kinase activity of muscle insulin receptors from hypomagnesaemic rats. *Diabetologia* 38:1262–1270.

Takezawa R, Schmitz C, Demeuse P, Scharenberg AM, Penner R, Fleig A (2004) Receptor-mediated regulation of the TRPM7 channel through its endogenous protein kinase domain. *Proc Natl Acad Sci USA* 101:6009-6014.

Tammaro P, Smith AL, Crowley BL, Smirnov SV (2005) Modulation of the voltage-dependent K^+ current by intracellular Mg^{2+} in rat aortic smooth muscle cells. *Cardiovasc Res* 65:387-396.

Tang EY, Parker PJ, Beattie J, Houslay MD (1993) Diabetes induces selective alterations in the expression of protein kinase C isoforms in hepatocytes. *FEBS Lett* 326:117–123.

Tashiro M, Konishi M (1997) Na^+ gradient-dependent Mg^{2+} transport in smooth muscle cells of guinea pig tenia cecum. *Biophys J* 73:3371-3384.

Tashiro M, Tursun P, Miyazaki T, Watanabe M, Konishi M (2002) Effects of membrane potential on Na^+-dependent Mg^{2+} extrusion from rat ventricular myocytes. *Jpn J Physiol* 52:541-551.

Taylor R., Agius L (1988) The biochemistry of diabetes. *Biochem J* 250:625-640.

Tessman PA, Romani A (1998) Acute effect of EtOH on Mg^{2+} homeostasis in liver cells: Evidence for the activation of an Na^+/Mg^{2+} exchanger. *Am J Physiol* 275:G1106-G1116.

Thebault S, Alexander RT, Tiel Groenestege WM, Hoenderop JG, Bindels RJ (2009) EGF increases TRPM6 activity and surface expression. *J Am Soc Nephrol* 20:78-85.

Thébault S, Cao G, Venselaar H, Xi Q, Bindels RJ, Hoenderop JG (2008) Role of the alpha-kinase domain in transient receptor potential melastatin 6 channel and regulation by intracellular ATP. *J Biol Chem* 283:19999-20007.

Torres LM, Cefaratti C, Perry B, Romani A (2006) Involvement of ERK1/2 and p38 in Mg^{2+} accumulation in liver cells. *Mol Cell Biochem* 288:191-199.

Torres LM, Konopnika B, Berti-Mattera LN, Liedtke C, Romani A (2010) Defective Translocation of PKCepsilon in EtOH-Induced Inhibition of Mg Accumulation in Rat Hepatocytes. *Alcohol Clin Exp Res* 34:1659-1669.

Torres LM, Youngner J, Romani A (2005) Role of glucose in modulating Mg^{2+} homeostasis in liver cells from starved rats. *Am J Physiol* 288:G195-G206.

Touyz RM, He Y, Montezano ACI, Yao G, Chubanov V, Gudermann T, Callera GE (2006) Differential regulation of transient receptor potential melastatin 6 and 7 cation channels by ANG II in vascular smooth muscle cells from spontaneously hypertensive rats. *Am J Physiol* 290:R73-R78.

Touyz RM, Schiffrin EL (1996) Angiotensin II and vasopressin modulate intracellular free magnesium in vascular smooth muscle cells through Na^+-dependent protein kinase C pathways. *J Biol Chem* 271:24353-24358.

Touyz RM, Yao G (2003) Modulation of vascular smooth muscle cell growth by magnesium-role of mitogen-activated protein kinases. *J Cell Physiol* 197:326-335.

Trache A, Trzeciakowski JP, Meininger GA (2010) Mg^{2+} modulates integrin-extracellular matrix interaction in vascular smooth muscle cells studied by atomic force microscopy. *J Mol Recognit* 23:316-321.

van der Wjist J, Hoenderop JG, Bindels RJ (2009) Epithelial Mg^{2+} channel TRPM6: insight into the molecular regulation. *Magnes Res* 22:127-132.

Voets T, Nilliues B, Hoefs S, van der Kemp AW, G Droogmans, Bindels RJ, Hoenderop JG (2004) TRPM6 forms the Mg^{2+} influx channel involved in intestinal and renal Mg^{2+} absorption. *J Biol Chem* 279:19-25.

Volpe P, Alderson-Lang BH, Nickols GA (1990) Regulation of inositol 1,4,5-trisphosphate-induced Ca^{2+} release. I. Effect of Mg^{2+}. *Am J Physiol* 258:C1077-C1085.

Volpe P, Vezú L (1993) Intracellular magnesium and inositol 1,4,5-trisphosphate receptor: molecular mechanisms of interaction, physiology and pharmacology. *Magnes Res* 6:267-274.

Vormann J, Gunther T (1987) Amiloride sensitive net Mg^{2+} efflux from isolated perfused rat hearts. *Magnesium* 6:220-224.

Vormann J, Magdorf K, Günther T, Wahn U (1994) Increased Na^+/Mg^{2+} antiport in erythrocytes of patients with cystic fibrosis. *Eur J Clin Chem Clin Biochem* 32:833-836.

Waas WF, Dalby KN (2003) Physiological concentrations of divalent magnesium ion activate the

Serine/Threonine specific protein kinase ERK2. *Biochemistry* 42:2960-2970.

Wabakken T, Rian E, Kveine M, Aasheim H-C (2003) The human solute carrier SLC41A1 belongs to a novel eukaryotic subfamily with homology to prokaryotic MgtE Mg^{2+} transporters. *Biochem Biophys Res Commun* 306:718-724.

Walder RY, Landau D, Meyer P, Shalev H, Tsolia M, Borochowitz Z, Boettger MB, Beck GE, Englehardt RK, Carmi R, Sheffield VC (2002) Mutation of TRPM6 causes familial hypomagnesemia with secondary hypocalcemia. *Nat Genet* 31:171-174.

Walder RY, Yang B, Stokes JB, Kirby PA, Cao X, Shi P, Searby CC, Husted RF, Sheffield VC (2009) Mice defective in Trpm6 show embryonic morality and neural tube defects, *Human Mol Gen* 18:4367-4375.

Wang CY, Davoodi-Semiromi A, Shi JD, Yang P, Huang YQ, Agundez JA, Moran JM, Ochoa B, Hawkins-Lee B, She JX (2003) High resolution mapping and mutation analyses of candidate genes in the urofacial syndrome (UPS) critical region. *Am J Med Genet A* 119:9-14.

Wang CY, Shi JD, Yang P, Kumar PG, Li QZ, Run QG, Su YC, Scott HS, Kao KJ, She JX (2003) Molecular cloning and characterization of a novel gene family of four ancient conserved domain proteins (ACDP). *Gene* 306:37-44.

Wang CY, Yang P, Chi JD, Purohit S, Guo D, An H, Gu JG, Ling J, Dong Z, She JX (2004) Molecular cloning and characterization of the mouse Acdp gene family. *BMC Genomics* 5:7.

Wang M, Berlin JR (2006) Channel phosphorylation and modulation of L-type Ca^{2+} currents by cytosolic Mg^{2+} concentration. *Am J Physiol* 291:C83-C92.

Wang S, George SE, Davis JP, Johnson JD (1998) Structural determinants of Ca^{2+} exchange and affinity in the C terminal of cardiac troponin C. *Biochemistry* 37:14539-14544.

Wei WL, Sun HS, Olah ME, Sun X, Czerwinska E, Czerwinski W, Mori Y, Orser BA, Xiong ZG, Jackson MF, Tymianski M, MacDonald JF (2007) TRPM7 channels in hippocampal neurons detect levels of extracellular divalent cations. *Proc Natl Acad Sci U SA* 104:16323-16328.

White RE, Hartzell HC (1988) Effects of intracellular free magnesium on calcium current in isolated cardiac myocytes. *Science* 239:778-780.

Wiesenberger G, Waldherr M, Schweyen RJ (1992) The nuclear gene MRS2 is essential for the excision of group II introns from yeast mitochondrial transcripts in vivo. *J Biol Chem* 267:6963-6969.

Wolf FI, Cittadini A (2003) Chemistry and biochemistry of magnesium. *Mol Aspects Med* 24:3-9.
Wolf FI, Cittadini AR, Maier JA (2009a) Magnesium and tumors: ally or foe? *Cancer Treat Rev* 35:378-382.

Wolf FI, Covacci V, Bruzzese N, Di Francesco A, Sachets A, Cord D, Cittadini A (1998) Differentiation of HL-60 promyelocytic leukemia cells is accompanied by a modification of magnesium homeostasis. *J Cell Biochem* 71:441-448.

Wolf FI, Di Francesco A, Cittadini A (1994) Characterization of magnesium efflux from Ehrlich ascites tumor cells. *Arch Biochem Biophys* 308:335-341.

Wolf FI, Di Francesco A, Covacci V, Cittadini A (1997) Regulation of magnesium efflux from rat spleen lymphocytes. *Arch Biochem Biophys* 344:397-403.

Wolf FI, Di Francesco A, Covacci V, Corda D, Cittadini A (1996) Regulation of intracellular magnesium in ascites cells: involvement of different regulatory pathways. *Arch Biochem Biophys* 331:194-200.

Wolf FI, Torsello A, Fasanella S Cittadini A (2003) Cell physiology of magnesium. *Mol Asp Med* 24:11-26.
Wolf FI, Trapani V, Simonacci M, Boninsegna A, Mazur A, Maier JA (2009b) Magnesium deficiency affects mammary epithelial cell proliferation: involvement of oxidative stress. *Nutr Cancer* 61:131-136.

Xu W, Willis JS (1994) Sodium transport through the amiloride-sensitive Na-Mg pathway of hamster red cells. *J Membr Biol* 141:277-287.

Yamaguchi S, Ishikawa T (2008) The electgrogenic Na^{+}-HCO_3^{-} cotransporter NBCe1-B is regulated by cellular Mg^{2+}. *Biochem Biophys Res Commun* 376:100-104.

YamaguchiH, Matsushita M, Nairn A, Kuriyan J (2001) Crystal structure of the atypical protein kinase domain of a TRP channel with phosphotransferase activity. *Mol Cell* 7:1047-1057.

Yanai A, Huang K, Kang R, Singaraja RR, Arstikaitis P, Gan L, Orban PC, Mullard A, Cowan CM, Raymond LA, Drisdel RC, Green WN, Ravikumar B, Rubinsztein DC, El-Husseini A, Hayden MR (2006) Palmitoylation of huntingtin by HIP14 is essential for its trafficking and function. *Nat. Neurosci* 9:824-831.

Yang Z, Wang J, Altura BT, Altura BM (2000) Extracellular magnesium deficiency induces contraction of arterial muscle: role of PI3-kinases and MAPK signaling pathways. *Pflugers Arch* 439:240-247.

Yang ZW, Wang J, Zheng T, Altura BT, Altura BM (2001) Ethanol-induced contractions in cerebral arteries: role of tyrosine and mitogen-activated protein kinases. *Stroke* 32:249-257.

Zhang GH, Melvin JE (1992) Secretagogue-induced mobilization of an intracellular Mg^{2+} pool in rat sublingual mucous acini. *J Biol Chem* 267:20721-20727.

Zhang GH, Melvin JE (1996) Na^{+}-dependent release of Mg^{2+} from an intracellular pool in rat sublingual mucous acini. *J Biol Chem 271*:29067-29072.

Zhang J, Wier G, Blaustein MP (2002) Mg^{2+} blocks myogenic tone but not K^{+}-induced constriction: Role for SOCs in small arteries. *Am J Physiol* 283:H2692-H2705.

Zhou H, Clapham DE (2009) Mammalian MagT1 and TUSC3 are required for cellular magnesium uptake and vertebrate embryonic development. *Proc Natl Acad Sci U S A* 106:15750-15755.

Zsurka G, Gregan J, Schweyen RJ (2001) The human mitochondrial Mrs2p protein functionally substitutes for its yeast homologue, a candidate magnesium transporter. *Genomics* 72:158-168.

Magnesium transport across the blood-brain barriers

Mounir N. Ghabriel ✉ *and Robert Vink*

Discipline of Anatomy and Pathology & Adelaide Centre for Neuroscience Research, School of Medical Sciences, The University of Adelaide, Adelaide, South Australia 5005, Australia.
✉ mounir.ghabriel@adelaide.edu.au

Abstract

The finding that magnesium levels are reduced in acute and chronic brain diseases has led to a recent surge in interest in the role of magnesium in the normal and injured nervous system, although the mechanisms of magnesium decline in pathological conditions and its availability in the neural tissue after administration are not fully understood. The brain has two main barrier systems: (1) the blood-brain barrier (BBB) formed by brain capillary endothelial cells which separate the blood from the extracellular fluid in the neuropil; and (2) the blood-CSF barrier (BCSFB) formed by choroidal epithelial cells which separate the blood from the CSF. Genetic studies in families with hereditary hypomagnesemia have identified mutations in two genes encoding claudin-16 (paracellin-1) and claudin-19, both localized at tight junctions between nephron epithelial cells and providing passive paracellular conductance for magnesium in the kidney. Endothelial cells of the BBB also express claudins, although whether members of the claudin family expressed at the BBB and BCSFB have similar conductance for magnesium akin to the role of claudin-16 and -19 in the nephron remains to be confirmed. Recently, the transient receptor potential melastatin (TRPM) members TRPM6 and TRPM7 have been identified as cation channels for magnesium transport. Although it is not known if choroidal epithelial cells express TRPM6 and TRPM7, these molecules are expressed by brain endothelial cells and may play a role in magnesium transport. While it is evident that magnesium enters the CNS through the BBB and is actively transported by choroidal epithelial cells into the CSF, the mechanisms of its entry into the brain will require further investigation.

Introduction

Magnesium is a critical cation and an essential nutrient for normal body functions; hence mechanisms exist in the body for its homeostasis through a highly integrated feedback system involving intestinal absorption, renal excretion, bone metabolism and the parathyroid gland (Dai *et al,* 2001). Magnesium is involved in a myriad of biochemical processes including acting as a cofactor in the activation of many intracellular enzymes (Aikawa, 1976; Ebel and Gunther, 1980; Gunther, 2008) and is important for protein synthesis (Terasaki and Rubin 1985) and cell membrane stabilization (Bara and Guiet-Bara 1984). Magnesium deficiency reduces protein synthesis, serum antibody activity and the immune response (McCoy and Kenney, 1975), and induces CNS epileptiform activity (Morris, 1992) and hypomagnesemic tetany (Fontenot *et al,* 1989). There is an inverse correlation between dietary magnesium and the level of C-reactive protein (a marker of inflammation) and the level of E-selectin (a marker of endothelial cell dysfunction) (Song *et al,* 2007). Recent technical developments have allowed better assessment of the levels of magnesium in the body, although the blood, which is used in routine testing, contains only 0.3% of the total body magnesium (Elin, 1987). Approximately one half of the magnesium contained in the body is stored in the bone, while the rest exists in the soft tissues, mainly in the intracellular compartment, with less that 1% being present in the extracellular compartment (Elin, 1988). Indeed, magnesium is the second most common cation in the intracellular compartment after potassium. More than one half of the plasma content of magnesium is bound to plasma proteins, and the remaining free ionized magnesium (Mg^{2+}), the metabolically active fraction, is held within a narrow range (0.53-0.67mM) in normal healthy controls (Altura and Altura, 1991). The recommended daily allowance ranges from 320 to

420mg/day for women and men, respectively (Bergman *et al,* 2009).

There has been a recent surge in interest in the dynamics and role of magnesium in the normal and injured brain due to accumulating evidence of a reduction in the level of total and free Mg^{2+} in the brain in acute and chronic neurological diseases (Vink *et al,* 1987; Vink *et al,* 2009). In intensive care patients with traumatic brain injury (TBI) reduction of serum ionized Mg^{2+} correlates with the severity of TBI as determined by the Glasgow Coma Scale Score (Kahraman *et al,* 2003). In experimental TBI in the rat there is a sustained decline in intracellular Mg^{2+}, detected by phosphorus magnetic resonance spectroscopy, that correlates with motor deficit (Cernak *et al,* 2004; Heath and Vink, 1996), while magnesium administration significantly improves motor outcome (Heath and Vink 1999; Turner *et al,* 2004). Magnesium administration reduces TBI-induced brain edema (Feldman *et al,* 1996) and restores blood-brain barrier (BBB) effectiveness to Evans blue tracer when compared to injured non-treated rats (Esen *et al,* 2003; Imer *et al,* 2009). Magnesium also reduces brain edema after cold-induced brain injury (Turkoglu *et al,* 2008). However, the mechanisms of magnesium decline in pathological conditions and its availability in the neural tissue after administration are still unclear (Vink *et al,* 2009).

Therapeutically, magnesium can be administered orally, intravenously or intramuscularly (Elin, 1988). It is most commonly used used as magnesium chloride, sulphate, gluconate, acetate (Fine *et al,* 1991) or lactate (Fine *et al,* 1991; Simoes Fernandes *et al,* 1985). Magnesium therapy has been utilized in numerous experimental and clinical settings including migraine (Peikert *et al,* 1996), asthma (Cheuk *et al,* 2005), depression (Eby and Eby, 2006), anxiety (Kara *et al,* 2002), diabetes (Resnick *et al,* 1993; Wester and Dyckner, 1987), hypertension (Wester and Dyckner, 1987), atrial fibrillation (Fanning *et al,* 1991), sleep disorders, insomnia and chronic fatigue (Takahashi *et al,* 1992), dementia (Glick, 1990), osteoporosis (Sojka and Weaver, 1995), fibromyalgia (Porter *et al,* 2010), pain (Soave *et al,* 2009), eclampsia (Euser and Cipolla, 2009), constipation (Guerrera *et al,* 2009), cerebral palsy (Rouse, 2009), lacunar stroke (Muir *et al,* 2004), TBI (McIntosh *et al,* 1988) and aneurysmal subarachnoid hemorrhage (van den Bergh, 2009; Yahia *et al,* 2005).

The current review will briefly outline the status of magnesium in the body, then will summarize current knowledge of its distribution in the CNS and discuss its transport across barrier membranes in the brain compared to its transport in other organs such as the kidney.

Magnesium absorption and excretion

Much of our knowledge about magnesium absorption and excretion was gained in the latter part of the twentieth century and particularly in the nineties. Studies of normal subjects showed that magnesium bioavailability from high magnesium containing food sources such as almonds is equal to that obtained from soluble magnesium acetate, but enteric coating of magnesium chloride impairs magnesium bioavailability (Fine *et al,* 1991). Magnesium absorption occurs mainly in the small intestine (Brannan *et al,* 1976; Graham *et al,* 1960; Schroeder *et al,* 1969). The kinetics and rate of magnesium absorption are not dependant on calcium intake (Brannan *et al,* 1976). Under basal conditions the small intestine absorbs 30–50% of the magnesium intake, although this percentage diminishes with senescence, chronic renal disease and increasing intake (Musso 2009). The fractional magnesium absorption appears to fall progressively so that absorption as a function of intake is curvilinear (Fine *et al,* 1991). The fecal magnesium appears to be primarily derived from material that is not absorbed by the body rather than magnesium secreted by the intestine (Aikawa, 1976). Approximately 80% of the absorbed magnesium passes in the glomerular filtrate (Dai *et al,* 2001; Quamme and de Rouffignac, 2000).

More that 95% of the magnesium filtered by the glomerulus is reclaimed mainly in the thick ascending loop of Henle (60-70%) and to a lesser extent (10-15%) in the proximal convoluted tubules (Brunette *et al,* 1974; Dai *et al,* 2001; Quamme 1997; Quamme and de Rouffignac, 2000). A further 10% of magnesium in the filtrate is claimed in the distal convoluted tubule (de Rouffignac and Quamme, 1994) and this segment contributes to magnesium conservation (Quamme 1997). Magnesium reabsorption within the thick ascending loop appears to be passive and occurs via the paracellular route (de Rouffignac and Quamme, 1994), being driven by the trans-epithelial voltage (Quamme, 1997; Quamme and de Rouffignac, 2000), where positive luminal charge favors movement of magnesium from the luminal to the abluminal side of nephron epithelium (Quamme, 1997). On the other hand magnesium transport in the distal convoluted tubule is active and transcellular (Quamme, 1 997). While the mechanisms of magnesium transport were unclear and speculative (Dai *et al,* 2001; Quamme and Dirks, 1980) more recent reports point to specific paracellular (Efrati *et al,* 2005; Simon *et al,* 1999) and transcellular (Hoenderop and Bindels, 2005) routes across barrier membranes.

Barriers between the blood and the CNS

Two main fluid compartments are associated with the brain, the extracellular fluid (ECF) that bathes neurons and glial cells, and the cerebrospinal fluid (CSF) located in the subarachnoid space and ventricles of the brain (Figure 1).

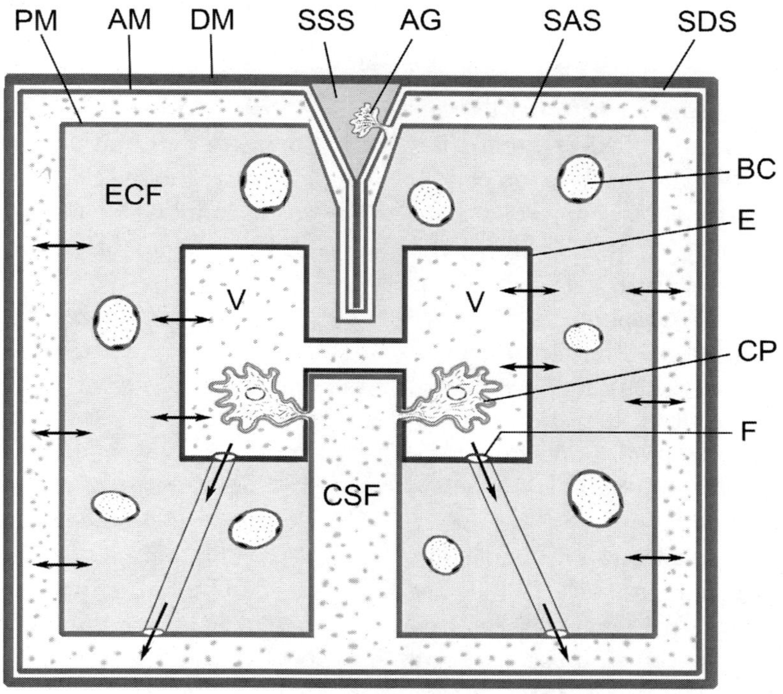

Figure 1. Diagram showing locations of the blood-brain barrier (BBB), the blood-CSF barrier (BCSFB) and the meninges. The cranial dura mater (DM) encloses all intracranial contents, and is formed of two fused layers that separate at certain places to enclose dural venous sinuses, such as the superior sagittal sinus (SSS). The subdural space (SDS) is a potential space as the dura and arachnoid mater (AM) are closely apposed. The arachnoid mater is impermeable to CSF contained in the subarachnoid space (SAS). The arachnoid mater forms the arachnoid granulations (AG) that pierce the dural wall of the superior sagittal sinus and drain the CSF into the venous blood. Brian capillaries (BC) are lined with endothelial cells joined by tight junctions and form the BBB, thus they control the composition of the extracellular fluid (ECF). Ventricles (V) of the brain contain CSF produced mainly by the choroidal epithelium, which covers the choroid plexuses (CP) and form the BCSFB. The ventricles are lined with ependymal cells (E), which are continuous with the choroidal epithelium at the neck of the choroid plexus. The core of the choroid plexus is formed of pia mater and contains fenestrated capillaries. CSF leaves the ventricular system via the three foramina of the fourth ventricle, represented here by two channels (F). The CSF and ECF of the brain equilibrate through the pia mater on the surface of the brain, and the ependyma lining the ventricles (double-headed arrows).

Exchange between the blood and these fluid compartments can potentially occur at four sites, which have barrier mechanisms: (1) brain capillary endothelial cells, which separate the ECF from the blood and form the BBB; (2) the choroidal epithelial cells at the ventricular surface of the choroid plexuses, which interface between the blood and the CSF and form the blood-CSF barrier (BCSFB); (3) the arachnoid mater, which surrounds the CSF contained within the subarachnoid space; (4) the circumventricular organs of the brain, which have fenestrated capillaries. The four sites form potential entry routes for water, molecules, electrolytes, toxins, pathogens and drugs (Segal, 2000).

The arachnoid mater and circumventricular organs

The arachnoid mater forms an external barrier, the morphological substrates of which are the flat tightly packed mesothelial cells (the arachnoid barrier cell layer) with their numerous tight junctions. They separate the CSF from the subdural space and the dura (Fig.1), which has fenestrated capillaries (Nabeshima *et al,* 1975; Vandenabeele *et al,* 1996). The arachnoid is avascular (Alcolado *et al,* 1988) and, relative to brain capillaries, has a much less surface area, thus its contribution to transport from the subdural space to the CSF and brain is negligible. Also the circumventricular organs of the brain, although they have fenestrated capillaries (McKinley *et al,* 2003; Sunn *et al,* 2003), they are provided with an internal mechanism that contributes to a barrier between these sites and the surrounding brain. They have rapid venous return systems, which compensates for the leaky capillaries, effectively preventing the spread of marker molecules to the surrounding brain tissue (Hashimoto, 1988; Segal, 2000). Therefore, the two main routes that are likely to have greater involvement in the regulation of the ECF and CSF environments are the BBB and BCSFB (Abbott *et al,* 2010).

The blood-brain barrier (BBB)

The concept of a BBB has been proposed over a century ago (Bradbury 1979) and is still being developed (Wolburg *et al,* 2009). The BBB is formed by endothelial cells of brain capillaries, the characteristics of which are influenced by the surrounding microenvironment, including astrocytes and pericytes (Wolburg *et al,* 2009). Apart from capillaries in the circumventricular organs which have fenestrated endothelial cells, those in the rest of the brain are lined with specialized endothelial cells which show few endocytotic vesicles, have no fenestrations and are rich in mitochondria (Brightman and Reese, 1969; Fenstermacher *et al,* 1988; Reese and Karnovsky, 1967; Rubin and Staddon, 1999; Sedlakova *et al,* 1999). Brain endothelial cells have high electrical resistance (Butt *et al,* 1990) and are joined by tight junctions (TJs) (Begley and Brightman, 2003; Rubin and Staddon, 1999). These TJs have long been recognized as the sites of exclusion of protein tracers as detected by electron microscopy (Brightman and Reese 1969; Reese and Karnovsky 1967; Sedlakova *et al,* 1999). Freeze-fracture electron microscopy revealed that these tight junctions have an elaborate and complex arrangement of network of interconnecting strands of intramembranous particles, that particularly cleave with the P-face leaving corresponding grooves on the E-face of replicas of the split membrane (Sedlakova *et al,* 1999).

The BBB therefore plays a pivotal role in the tight regulation and rigorous stabilization of the chemical composition of brain ECF against fluctuations in the plasma chemistry, thus promoting normal neuronal signaling. The privileged status of the brain being protected by the BBB has a downside, in restricting access by drugs and therapeutic agents into the brain when needed (Abbott and Romero, 1996). Although the barrier nature of the BBB has been emphasized, it is obviously a selective barrier, as it should allow passage of nutrients and electrolytes. Thus endothelial cells of brain vessels are endowed with a host of receptors, enzymes and carriers in a polarized distribution to promote selective transport (Abbott *et al,* 2010; Betz *et al,* 1980; Ohtsuki and Terasaki, 2007; Roberts *et al,* 2008). Brain endothelial cells express the glucose transporter Glut-1 protein (Dick *et al,* 1984; Harik *et al,* 1994; Ohtsuki and Terasaki, 2007; Pardridge *et al,* 1990; Pardridge, 1991), which is coupled to neuronal demand (Leybaert, 2005) and its expression increases in hypoxia (Harik *et al,* 1994). Rat brain endothelial cells express a barrier antigen (Sternberger and Sternberger, 1987), neutralization of which leads to reversible opening of the BBB to exogenous and endogenous proteins (Ghabriel *et al,* 2000; Ghabriel *et al,* 2004). Lipophilic molecules can penetrate endothelial cell membranes by diffusion, although some of these may be effluxed via ABC transporters, such as P-glycoprotein (Begley 2004; Miller, 2010; Shen and Zhang, 2010). Macromolecules may cross the BBB via receptor-mediated transcytosis (Descamps *et al,* 1996), or adsorptive-mediated transcytosis (Villegas and Broadwell, 1993; Zlokovic *et al,* 1990). Water-soluble nutrients and metabolites can to a limited degree pass passively across the BBB, but greater bulks of water, hydrophilic molecules and electrolytes have to be transported via carrier systems and channels (Zhang *et al,* 2002). Amino acids, nucleosides, small peptides, organic anions and organic cations are transported via solute carriers (Abbott *et al,* 2010; Koepsell *et al,* 2003; Ohtsuki and Terasaki, 2007).

Unlike in other organs, such as the intestinal wall where the extracellular space is large and is occupied by loose connective tissue, that of the brain is very narrow as neuronal and glial membranes are closely apposed leaving a gap of 20-50 nm (Vanharreveld *et al,* 1965) with a small volume of ECF. A small change in the ECF volume may lead to large alterations in electrolyte concentrations, deleteriously affecting neuronal excitability (Amiry-Moghaddam and Ottersen, 2003). Hence water transport across the BBB is intricately linked to ions transport. Brain perivascular astrocytic foot processes, sub-pial astrocytes and the ependyma, which lines the ventricles, express the water channels AQP-4 (Amiry-Moghaddam and Ottersen, 2003; Li *et al,* 2009; Nielsen *et al,* 1997). More recent studies demonstrated that brain endothelial cells also express AQP-4 at their luminal and abluminal membranes, albeit at a much lower density than in astrocytic foot processes (Amiry-Moghaddam and Ottersen, 2003; Kobayashi *et al,* 2001). The link between water movements and electrolyte concentrations is further strengthened by the co-expression of AQP4 and Kir-4.1 potassium channels, and the discovery that water movement is associated with potassium fluxes in the same direction (Amiry-Moghaddam and Ottersen, 2003; Niermann *et al,* 2001). The BBB is relatively permeable to water, allowing a slow bulk flow (Abbott, 2004) but less so to ions (Go, 1997). Electrolytes homeostasis in the ECF is actively maintained by the BBB, as evidenced by a high Na^+, K^+-ATPase activity in brain endothelial cells (Bauer *et al,* 1990; Go, 1997; Seda *et al,* 1984). Potassium concentration in the ECF is kept at a lower level than that of plasma (Hansen, 1985).

The blood-CSF barrier (BCSFB)

The brain has four choroid plexuses that project into the two lateral ventricles and the third and fourth ventricles. Each choroid plexus contains a core of loosely arranged stroma derived from the leptomeninges. Their ventricular surface is extremely fringed (Fig.1). The core of the plexus is richly supplied with capillaries, the endothelial cells of which have fenestrations and leaky tight junctions (Wolburg and Paulus, 2010). Large molecules such as peroxidase penetrate the choroid plexus capillaries and enter the interstitial space in the core of the plexus (Brightman, 1968). As the plexus invaginates the ventricle it acquires a covering of ependyma, the cell layer that forms the lining of the ventricle (Fig.1). This ependymal covering is known as the choroidal epithelium, which, although continuous with the rest of the ependyma at the neck of the choroid plexus, is structurally and functionally different, as it becomes modified and specialized to form the BCSFB (Brightman 1968; Redzic and Segal 2004; Tripathi 1973). The choroidal epithelium therefore separates the CSF from the milieu of the plexus core with its leaky capillaries. Choroidal epithelial cells are joined by tight junctions, which occlude the paracellular route (Wolburg and Lippoldt, 2002; Wolburg and Paulus, 2010). Choroidal epithelial cells actively produce the CSF and regulate its electrolyte, protein and water content (Bradbury *et al,* 1963). Choroidal epithelial cells express the water channels AQP-1 (Agre *et al,* 1993; Nielsen *et al,* 1993). In addition to their main function of CSF secretion choroidal epithelial cells transport some substances from the blood to the CSF, for example, nucleotides and ascorbic acid, and actively removes other substances from the CSF (Go, 1997).

There is no barrier between the brain and CSF located in the subarachnoid space, as the cells of the pia mater on the brain surface have gap junctions and no tight junctions (Alcolado *et al,* 1988). Peroxidase perfused into the subarachnoid space penetrates between pia mater cells, through the basement membrane of astrocytes at the brain surface and between astrocytes (outer glia limitans) to enter the neuropil

(Brightman and Reese, 1969). Also free exchange occurs between the CSF located in the ventricles and the brain ECF across the ependymal lining of the ventricles, as peroxidase injected into the ventricles enter the neuropil (Brightman and Reese, 1969), thus the CSF and the ECF of the brain equilibrate.

Magnesium transport across barrier membranes including the BBB and BCSFB

Magnesium transport in the kidney

The kidney is the main contributor to magnesium homeostasis, thus it is not surprising that research efforts to understand magnesium transport were focused on epithelial cells of the nephron. During the last decade greater understanding of the transport of magnesium across cell membranes was gained through genetic studies in families with hereditary abnormal magnesium balance, positional cloning and knockout mice investigations (Hoenderop and Bindels, 2005). Such studies led to the identification of genes encoding proteins involved in the transport of magnesium. One human gene, the *paracellin-1* (*PCLN-1)*, encodes the protein paracellin-1. *PCLN-1* mRNA was detected using RT-PCR in the thick ascending limb of Henle's loop and the distal convoluted tubule of the kidney in the rabbit (Simon *et al,* 1999) and rodents (Weber *et al,* 2001). The PCLN-1 protein was also detected using immunocytochemistry in the same segments in rabbit kidney using an antibody to PCLN-1 (Simon *et al,* 1999). Using confocal microscopy and double immuno-fluorescence for PCLN-1 and occuldin, a tight junction ubiquitous protein (Furuse *et al,* 1993), demonstrated colocalisation of the two proteins to intercellular tight junction at both segments of rabbit nephrons (Simon *et al,* 1999). The paracellin-1 protein is a member of the claudin family (claudin 16) (Simon *et al,* 1999). Families with mutation in *PCLN-1* gene show hypo-magnesemia and renal magnesium wasting (Simon *et al,* 1999). The paracellin-1 located in the tight junction between epithelial cells in the nephron acts as a passive channel for reabsorbing magnesium along the paracellular route being favored by the positive luminal charge. Because these families also show hypercalciurea and urinary calculi, it was suggested that PCLN-1 is also a conductance for calcium (Simon *et al,* 1999). Such discovery modified the previously prevalent view that tight junctions exist to prevent passage of molecules and are static; rather, they do provide selective barriers. Further studies on human recessive renal magnesium loss mapped a second locus on chromosome 1p34.2 and have identified mutations in *CLDN19*, which encodes the TJ protein claudin-19 expressed in the nephron tubules (Konrad *et al,* 2006).

Recently plasma membrane cation channels that belong to the transient receptor potential (TRP) superfamily have been described and were classified into 7 subfamilies. The closely related subfamilies TRPC, TRPV, TRPM, TRPN and TRPA are classified as group 1, while group 2 includes TRPML and TRPP (Montell 2005). The TRPM subfamily includes 8 members, of which TRPM6 and TRMP7 have been recognized as highly permeable Mg^{2+} transporters into cells, and have been particularly studied in epithelial cells of the nephron (Aikawa 1976; Dai *et al,* 2001). In familial autosomal-recessive hypomagnesemia with sec-ondary hypocalcemia, affected infants suffer from seizures and tetany due to abnormal handling of Mg^{2+} in intestinal absorption and renal reabsorption. Genetic analysis pointed to a gene, *TRPM6*, which was mutated in these patients (Schlingmann *et al,* 2002; Walder *et al,* 2002). Using immunocytochemistry, it was shown that TRPM6 protein is localized to the apical membrane of renal distal convoluted tubules epithelium, the site of active reclaiming of magnesium, and also at the brush border of apical membranes of intestinal epithelium, the main site of magnesium absorption (Voets *et al,* 2004). Patch-clamp analysis and measurement of intracellular magnesium indicated that TRPM6 forms all or at least part of the magnesium channel in absorbing epithelia (Voets *et al,* 2004). It has been suggested that mammary epithelial cells in culture, with high and low magnesium content, adapt to low magnesium availability by upregulating magnesium influx via TRPM6, and to high magnesium availability by increasing magnesium efflux primarily via Na^{+}/Mg^{2+} exchange (Wolf *et al,* 2010). The TRPM7 also has a central role in Mg^{2+} homeostasis, because TRPM7-deficient cells become Mg^{2+} deficient, and cannot survive (Schmitz *et al,* 2003).

Magnesium transport across the BBB

Magnesium entry into the brain correlates with maturation of the BBB. In fetal sheep and the guinea pig, there is a drop in the concentration of Mg^{2+} in the cerebral hemispheres, which corresponds approximately to the minimum in potassium content and the maximum in chloride and sodium contents (Bradbury *et al,* 1972). During rat postnatal development, brain content of magnesium shows regional variations. At day 5, magnesium is most marked in the pons and medulla and least marked in the cerebral cortex. Magnesium levels in all regions decline after day 5, in parallel with the decrease in water content and the increase in tissue weight, suggesting that the maturation of the BBB plays an important role in brain magnesium homeostasis (Chan *et al,* 1992).

Magnesium is able to cross the BBB (Sacco *et al,* 2007), and it is transported via the barrier with a net flux from the blood into the parenchyma. Active magnesium transport from blood to the extracellular fluid of the brain is evidenced by its higher concentration in the cortical extracellular fluid than its concentration in the plasma-dialysate or cisternal CSF (Bito, 1969). Magnesium administration attenuates cell death due to cytoskeletal alteration (Saatman *et al,* 2001) and reduces apoptosis and the expression of p53 following TBI (Lee *et al,* 2004). Thus its administration rectifies the decline in intracellular Mg^{2+} levels and cellular functions (Saatman *et al,* 2001). In experimental closed head trauma, treatment with magnesium restores the polarity of astrocytes, in terms of aquaporin-4 distribution, to a preinjury state (Ghabriel *et al,* 2006). A similar protective effect for magnesium was demonstrated in induced hypoglycemia (Kaya *et al,* 2001). This indicates replenishing of magnesium in the extracellular space of the brain. However, the question remains, how does magnesium cross endothelial cells of the BBB? Is magnesium transport across the BBB similar to its transport across nephron epithelial cells? If so, does Mg^{2+} cross the BBB via a paracellular route or a transcellular route or both?

Concerning the paracellular route, the proposed role for PCLN-1 (claudin-16) in the nephron (Simon *et al,* 1999), acting as a conductance for Mg^{2+}, and its exclusive location in the kidney (Efrati *et al,* 2005; Weber *et al,* 2001), raise the possibility that other members of the claudin family may play a similar role for paracellular conductance across other barrier membranes. Members of the claudin family are involved in the formation of TJ strands in various tissues (Morita *et al,* 1999). There is tissue-specific expression of claudin members in tight junctions, with a specific colocalisation of occludin with some but not all claudins (Peppi and Ghabriel, 2004). Magnesium is important for cell membrane stabilization. In the CNS, the myelin sheath is an elaboration of the cell membrane of oligodendrocytes, which express claudin-11. In claudin-11-deficient mice, the TJs are absent in the myelin sheath of oligodendrocytes and mice show demyelination (Gow *et al,* 1999). This indicates that claudin-11 is an important component in the stability and formation of the myelin tight junctions. Also endothelial cells of brain microvessels express several claudins, including claudin-1, -3, -5 and -12 (Coisne *et al,* 2005; Liebner *et al,* 2000; Matter and Balda, 2003; Morita *et al,* 1999; Tsukita and Furuse, 1999; Wolburg *et al,* 2003). Breakdown of the BBB in experimental autoimmune encephalomyelitis in the mouse and the leaky vessels in human glioblastoma multiforme are accompanied by selective loss of claudin-3 in BBB TJs (Wolburg *et al,* 2003). Although direct link between Mg^{2+} permeability and claudins has not been established in the CNS similar to the link between claudin-16 and epithelial cells of the nephron, it is tempting to speculate that, in addition to their supporting role in the morphology the BBB TJs, claudins in TJs of brain endothelial cells may contribute to Mg^{2+} conductance at the BBB. It is also speculated here that claudin-11 in the CNS myelin, in addition to its morphological supporting role, may act as a conductance for Mg^{2+} across the consecutive myelin lamellae, providing a faster access route from the ECF to the periaxonal space.

Concerning the transport of Mg^{2+} across the BBB via a transcellular route, it may also be prudent to compare the BBB to other barrier membranes. As stated above, TRPM6 transporter protein has been localized to the apical membrane of renal distal convoluted tubules epithelium, the site of active reclaiming of magnesium (Voets *et al,* 2004), and TRPM7 in the kidney also has a central role in Mg^{2+} homeostasis (Schmitz *et al,* 2003). In mouse brain, using quantitative RT-PCR, TRPM3 and TRPM7 mRNA were detected at high levels, and 19 other isoforms were also present (Brown *et al,* 2008; Kunert-Keil *et al,* 2006). Also in human brain TRPM1, 2, 3, 6 and 7 have been detected using RT-PCR (Fonfria *et al,* 2006). Evidence of TRPM presence in brain endothelial cells was obtained from endothelial cell cultures. Immortalized mouse brain microvessel endothelial cells, freshly isolated cerebral microvessels and primary cultured rat brain endothelial cells express multiple TRPC and TRPV isoforms, and also TRPM2, M3, M4, and M7 mRNA (Brown *et al,* 2008). We would like to suggest therefore that the TRPM6 and TRPM7, the gatekeepers of magnesium (Schlingmann *et al,* 2007), are likely to play a main role in brain endothelial cell transport of magnesium via the transcellular route. Western blotting and immunofluorescence assays for TRPM6 and TRPM7 similar to those performed for TRPV4 in mouse cerebral microvascular endothelial cells (Ma *et al,* 2008) would support this suggestion. Also direct evidence may be obtained from measuring intracellular magnesium in endothelial cell culture similar to previous reports on mammary epithelial cells in culture (Voets *et al,* 2004)

Magnesium transport across the blood-CSF barrier

What has become apparent from experimental research and human studies is that magnesium concentration in the CSF is actively maintained above that of the plasma, and changes in CSF magnesium lag behind changes in its concentration in the plasma and are less pronounced (Bradbury and Sarna, 1977; Morris, 1992). Thus electrolyte composition in the CSF of adult mammals is different from that of plasma and is more stable, suggesting the existence of mechanisms for electrolyte homeostasis in the CSF, necessary for normal brain function (Bradbury *et al,* 1972; Somjen, 2002). The mechanisms determining the concentrations of ions in CSF appear to develop at different and largely independent rates (Bradbury *et al,* 1972). In the dog (Oppelt *et al,* 1963) and human (Nischwitz *et al,* 2008) the concentration of magnesium is higher in the CSF compared to plasma. Also in fetal sheep and guinea pigs magnesium concentration in the CSF is slightly higher than that of plasma (Amtorp and Sorensen, 1974; Bradbury *et al,* 1972). An investigation of the permeability of the human BCSFB to magnesium carried out in 29 individuals, using paired serum and CSF samples, showed a mean CSF/serum ratio of 1.3 (Nischwitz *et al,* 2008). This study also compared magnesium to other metals, and suggested that low molecular weight species such as magnesium and calcium cross the BCSFB through less specific ion channels compared to high molecular weight metals such as iron, copper and zinc, which can pass the barrier only via well controlled receptor mediated pathways (Nischwitz *et al,* 2008)

The choroidal epithelium plays an active role in maintaining the level of magnesium in the CSF by sensing changes in the CSF and altering the rate of active magnesium secretion (Oppelt *et al,* 1963; Reed and Yen 1978). Physiological studies of isolated choroid plexus of sheep (Allsop 1986) and cat (Reed and Yen 1978) showed that the choroid plexus is able to transfer magnesium against a concentration gradient. An in vivo study demonstrated a directional flow of magnesium into the CNS (Allsop and Pauli, 1985). In normal cows the magnesium concentration in the ventricular CSF was found to be higher than its concentration in the lumbar CSF (Allsop and Pauli, 1985). Under hypomagnesemic conditions, magnesium concentration in the ventricle decreased more rapidly than that of the lumbar CSF, while intravenous infusion of magnesium led to increased magnesium in the ventricular CSF before changes in the lumbar CSF (Allsop and Pauli, 1985). This study indicates that the access of magnesium from the blood to the brain is mainly via the choroid plexus to CSF, which equilibrates with the CNS parenchyma. Transport of magnesium in the choroid plexus is influenced by other selective electrolytes. For example, high levels of potassium in the perfusate of the choroid plexus leads to a reduction in the transfer rate of magnesium, but higher levels of calcium does not have a similar effect on the transfer of magnesium (Allsop, 1986).

A recent clinical trial on the protective role of magnesium in traumatic brain injury (Temkin *et al,* 2007) failed to replicate the improved outcome detected in experimental studies on rodents (Temkin *et al,* 2007; Vink and Cernak, 2000). In this clinical trial, plasma magnesium was maintained at higher levels compared to the placebo group and normal plasma level, to counteract the reported decline in Mg^{2+} in TBI patients (Kahraman *et al,* 2003). Since under normal conditions choroidal epithelial cells actively transport magnesium into the CSF, it is likely that such activity was disrupted in TBI cases in humans leading and failure of magnesium entry to the CNS. It is relevant here to state that in the rat, TBI induces severe morphological changes in choroidal epithelial cells detected by scanning and transmission electron microscopy that were still evident 4 weeks after trauma (Ghabriel *et al,* 2010).

Although one cannot dismiss the possibility that new channels may be involved in the transport of magnesium at the choroid plexus, it is natural to look at other systems for similar magnesium transport mechanisms. As stated above the strongest evidence for magnesium transport was obtained from genetic studies in familial hypomagnesemia, positional cloning and knockout mice investigations (Konrad *et al,* 2006; Schlingmann *et al,* 2005; Schlingmann *et al,* 2007; Simon *et al,* 1999; Walder *et al,* 2002) which identified TRPM6 and TRPM7 as candidates for transcellular transport, and Claudin16 (Efrati *et al,* 2005; Simon *et al,* 1999) for paracellular transport in the kidney. Recently TRPM7 has also been identified in smooth muscle cells in the vasculature (Callera *et al,* 2009). Although TRPM6 and TRPM7 were detected in the brain using RT-PCR it is not clear if these channels are expressed in choroidal epithelial cells. The role of claudin-16 and claudin-19 in magnesium reabsorption from the kidney filtrate has been discussed in previous sections, and the role of claudins as selective conductance to ions through tight junction has been stated. The choroidal epithelial cells show selective expression of claudin-1, -2 and -5 at and near to their tight junctions. Also the endothelial cells within the choroid plexus show stronger expression of claudin-5 than claudin-1 and -2 (Lippoldt *et al,* 2000). However, claudin-16 and claudin-19 have not been reported in the choroid plexus. Whether other claudin members may contribute to magnesium conductance in the choroid plexus is speculative. Thus it appears that the channels for magnesium transport in the choroid plexus remain to be clarified.

Acknowledgement
Supported, in part, by funding from the Neurosurgical Research Foundation (Australia).

References

Abbott NJ, Romero IA (1996) Transporting therapeutics across the blood-brain barrier. *Mol Med Today* 2:106-13.

Abbott NJ (2004) Evidence for bulk flow of brain interstitial fluid: significance for physiology and pathology. *Neurochem Int* 45:545-52.

Abbott NJ, Patabendige AA, Dolman DE, Yusof SR, Begley DJ (2010) Structure and function of the blood-brain barrier. *Neurobiol Dis* 37:13-25.

Agre P, Preston GM, Smith BL, Jung JS, Raina S, Moon C, Guggino WB, Nielsen S (1993) Aquaporin CHIP: the archetypal molecular water channel. *Am J Physiol* 265:F463-76.

Aikawa (1976) Biochemistry and physiology of magnesium. In: *Trace elements in human health* (D PASaO, ed). New York: Academic Press, 47-78.

Alcolado R, Weller RO, Parrish EP, Garrod D (1988) The cranial arachnoid and pia mater in man: anatomical and ultrastructural observations. *Neuropathol Appl Neurobiol* 14:1-17.

Allsop TF, Pauli JV (1985) Magnesium concentrations in the ventricular and lumbar cerebrospinal fluid of hypomagnesaemic cows. *Res Vet Sci* 38:61-4.

Allsop TF (1986) Transfer of magnesium across the perfused choroid plexus of sheep. *Aust J Biol Sci* 39:161-9.

Altura BT, Altura BM (1991) Measurement of ionized magnesium in whole blood, plasma and serum with a new ion-selective electrode in healthy and diseased human subjects. *Magnes Trace Elem* 10:90-8.

Amiry-Moghaddam M, Ottersen OP (2003) The molecular basis of water transport in the brain. *Nat Rev Neurosci* 4:991-1001.

Amtorp O, Sorensen SC (1974) The ontogenetic development of concentration differences for protein and ions between plasma and cerebrospinal fluid in rabbits and rats. *J Physiol* 243:387-400.

Bara M, Guiet-Bara A (1984) Potassium, magnesium and membranes. Review of present status and new findings. *Magnesium* 3:215-25.

Bauer HC, Tontsch U, Amberger A, Bauer H (1990) Gamma-glutamyl-transpeptidase (GGTP) and NA+K(+)-ATPase activities in different subpopulations of cloned cerebral endothelial cells: responses to glial stimulation. *Biochem Biophys Res Commun* 168:358-63.

Begley DJ, Brightman MW (2003) Structural and functional aspects of the blood-brain barrier. *Prog Drug Res* 61:39-78.

Begley DJ (2004) ABC transporters and the blood-brain barrier. *Curr Pharm Des* 10:1295-312.

Bergman C, Gray-Scott D, Chen JJ, Meacham S (2009) What is next for the Dietary Reference Intakes for bone metabolism related nutrients beyond calcium: phosphorus, magnesium, vitamin D, and fluoride? *Crit Rev Food Sci Nutr* 49:136-44.

Betz AL, Firth JA, Goldstein GW (1980) Polarity of the blood-brain barrier: distribution of enzymes between the luminal and antiluminal membranes of brain capillary endothelial cells. *Brain Res* 192:17-28

Bito LZ (1969) Blood-Brain Barrier: Evidence for Active Cation Transport between Blood and the Extraceliular Fluid of Brain. *Science* 165:81-3.

Bradbury MW, Stubbs J, Hughes IE, Parker P (1963) The Distribution of Potassium, Sodium, Chloride and Urea between Lumbar Cerebrospinal Fluid and Blood Serum in Human Subjects. *Clin Sci* 25:97-105.

Bradbury MW, Crowder J, Desai S, Reynolds JM, Reynolds M, Saunders NR (1972) Electrolytes and water in the brain and cerebrospinal fluid of the foetal sheep and guinea-pig. *J Physiol* 227:591-610.

Bradbury MW, Sarna GS (1977) Homeostasis of the ionic composition of the cerebrospinal fluid. *Exp Eye Res* 25 Suppl:249-57.

Bradbury MWB (1979). *The concept of a blood-brain barrier*. Wiley: Chichester; New York.

Brannan PG, Vergne-Marini P, Pak CY, Hull AR, Fordtran JS (1976) Magnesium absorption in the human small intestine. Results in normal subjects, patients with chronic renal disease, and patients with absorptive hypercalciuria. *J Clin Invest* 57:1412-8

Brightman MW (1968) The intracerebral movement of proteins injected into blood and cerebrospinal fluid of mice. *Prog Brain Res* 29:19-40

Brightman MW, Reese TS (1969) Junctions between intimately apposed cell membranes in the vertebrate brain. *J Cell Biol* 40:648-77.

Brown RC, Wu L, Hicks K, O'Neil R G (2008) Regulation of blood-brain barrier permeability by transient receptor potential type C and type v calcium-permeable channels. *Microcirculation* 15:359-71.

Brunette MG, Vigneault N, Carriere S (1974) Micropuncture study of magnesium transport along the nephron in the young rat. *Am J Physiol* 227:891-6.

Butt AM, Jones HC, Abbott NJ (1990) Electrical resistance across the blood-brain barrier in anaesthetized rats: a developmental study. *J Physiol* 429:47-62.

Callera GE, He Y, Yogi A, Montezano AC, Paravicini T, Yao G, Touyz RM (2009) Regulation of the novel Mg2+ transporter transient receptor potential melastatin 7 (TRPM7) cation channel by bradykinin in vascular smooth muscle cells. *J Hypertens* 27:155-66.

Cernak I, Vink R, Zapple DN, Cruz MI, Ahmed F, Chang T, Fricke ST, Faden AI (2004) The pathobiology of moderate diffuse traumatic brain injury as identified using a new experimental model of injury in rats. *Neurobiol Dis* 17:29-43.

Chan AW, Minski MJ, Lim L, Lai JC (1992) Changes in brain regional manganese and magnesium levels during postnatal development: modulations by chronic manganese administration. *Metab Brain Dis* 7:21-33.

Cheuk DK, Chau TC, Lee SL (2005) A meta-analysis on intravenous magnesium sulphate for treating acute asthma. *Arch Dis Child* 90:74-7.

Coisne C, Dehouck L, Faveeuw C, Delplace Y, Miller F, Landry C, Morissette C, Fenart L, Cecchelli R, Tremblay P, Dehouck B (2005) Mouse syngenic in vitro blood-brain barrier model: a new tool to examine inflammatory events in cerebral endothelium. *Lab Invest* 85:734-46.

Dai LJ, Ritchie G, Kerstan D, Kang HS, Cole DE, Quamme GA (2001) Magnesium transport in the renal distal convoluted tubule. *Physiol Rev* 81:51-84.

de Rouffignac C, Quamme G (1994) Renal magnesium handling and its hormonal control. *Physiol Rev* 74:305-22.

Descamps L, Dehouck MP, Torpier G, Cecchelli R (1996) Receptor-mediated transcytosis of transferrin through blood-brain barrier endothelial cells. *Am J Physiol* 270:H1149-58.

Dick AP, Harik SI, Klip A, Walker DM (1984) Identification and characterization of the glucose transporter of the blood-brain barrier by cytochalasin B binding and immunological reactivity. *Proc Natl Acad Sci U S A* 81:7233-7.

Ebel H, Gunther T (1980) Magnesium metabolism: a review. *J Clin Chem Clin Biochem* 18:257-70.

Eby GA, Eby KL (2006) Rapid recovery from major depression using magnesium treatment. *Med Hypotheses* 67:362-70.

Efrati E, Arsentiev-Rozenfeld J, Zelikovic I (2005) The human paracellin-1 gene (hPCLN-1): renal epithelial cell-specific expression and regulation. *Am J Physiol Renal Physiol* 288:F272-83.

Elin RJ (1987) Assessment of magnesium status. *Clin Chem* 33:1965-70.

Elin RJ (1988) Magnesium metabolism in health and disease. *Dis Mon* 34:161-218.

Esen F, Erdem T, Aktan D, Kalayci R, Cakar N, Kaya M, Telci L (2003) Effects of magnesium administration on brain edema and blood-brain barrier breakdown after experimental traumatic brain injury in rats. *J Neurosurg Anesthesiol* 15:119-25.

Euser AG, Cipolla MJ (2009) Magnesium sulfate for the treatment of eclampsia: a brief review. *Stroke* 40:1169-75.

Fanning WJ, Thomas CS, Jr., Roach A, Tomichek R, Alford WC, Stoney WS, Jr. (1991) Prophylaxis of atrial fibrillation with magnesium sulfate after coronary artery bypass grafting. *Ann Thorac Surg* 52:529-33.

Feldman Z, Gurevitch B, Artru AA, Oppenheim A, Shohami E, Reichenthal E, Shapira Y (1996) Effect of magnesium given 1 hour after head trauma on brain edema and neurological outcome. *J Neurosurg* 85:131-7.

Fenstermacher J, Gross P, Sposito N, Acuff V, Pettersen S, Gruber K (1988) Structural and functional variations in capillary systems within the brain. *Ann N Y Acad Sci* 529:21-30.

Fine KD, Santa Ana CA, Porter JL, Fordtran JS (1991) Intestinal absorption of magnesium from food and supplements. *J Clin Invest* 88:396-402.

Fonfria E, Murdock PR, Cusdin FS, Benham CD, Kelsell RE, McNulty S (2006) Tissue distribution profiles of the human TRPM cation channel family. *J Recept Signal Transduct Res* 26:159-78.

Fontenot JP, Allen VG, Bunce GE, Goff JP (1989) Factors influencing magnesium absorption and metabolism in ruminants. *J Anim Sci* 67:3445-55.

Furuse M, Hirase T, Itoh M, Nagafuchi A, Yonemura S, Tsukita S (1993) Occludin: a novel integral membrane protein localizing at tight junctions. *J Cell Biol* 123:1777-88.

Ghabriel MN, Zhu C, Hermanis G, Allt G (2000) Immunological targeting of the endothelial barrier antigen (EBA) in vivo leads to opening of the blood-brain barrier. *Brain Res* 878:127-35.

Ghabriel MN, Lu JJ, Tadros R, Hermanis G (2004) A narrow time-window for access to the brain by exogenous protein after immunological targeting of a blood-brain barrier antigen. *J Comp Pathol* 131:52-60.

Ghabriel MN, Thomas A, Vink R (2006) Magnesium restores altered aquaporin-4 immunoreactivity following traumatic brain injury to a pre-injury state. *Acta Neurochir Suppl* 96:402-6.

Ghabriel MN, Zdziarski IM, Leigh C, Vink R (2010) Changes in the blood-CSF barrier in experimental traumatic brain injury. *Acta Neurochir Suppl* 106:239-45.

Glick JL (1990) Dementias: the role of magnesium deficiency and an hypothesis concerning the pathogenesis of Alzheimer's disease. *Med Hypotheses* 31:211-25.

Go KG (1997) The normal and pathological physiology of brain water. *Adv Tech Stand Neurosurg* 23:47-142.

Gow A, Southwood CM, Li JS, Pariali M, Riordan GP, Brodie SE, Danias J, Bronstein JM, Kachar B, Lazzarini RA (1999) CNS myelin and sertoli cell tight junction strands are absent in Osp/claudin-11 null mice. *Cell* 99:649-59.

Graham LA, Caesar JJ, Burgen AS (1960) Gastrointestinal absorption and excretion of Mg 28 in man. *Metabolism* 9:646-59.

Guerrera MP, Volpe SL, Mao JJ (2009) Therapeutic uses of magnesium. *Am Fam Physician* 80:157-62.

Gunther T (2008) Comment on the number of Mg2+ -activated enzymes. *Magnes Res* 21:185-7.

Hansen AJ (1985) Effect of anoxia on ion distribution in the brain. *Physiol Rev* 65:101-48.

Harik SI, Behmand RA, LaManna JC (1994) Hypoxia increases glucose transport at blood-brain barrier in rats. *J Appl Physiol* 77:896-901.

Hashimoto PH (1988) Tracer in cisternal cerebrospinal fluid is soon detected in choroid plexus capillaries. *Brain Res* 440:149-52.

Heath DL, Vink R (1996) Traumatic brain axonal injury produces sustained decline in intracellular free magnesium concentration. *Brain Res* 738:150-3.

Heath DL, Vink R (1999) Improved motor outcome in response to magnesium therapy received up to 24 hours after traumatic diffuse axonal brain injury in rats. *J Neurosurg* 90:504-9.

Hoenderop JG, Bindels RJ (2005) Epithelial Ca2+ and Mg2+ channels in health and disease. *J Am Soc Nephrol* 16:15-26.

Imer M, Omay B, Uzunkol A, Erdem T, Sabanci PA, Karasu A, Albayrak SB, Sencer A, Hepgul K, Kaya M (2009) Effect of magnesium, MK-801 and combination of magnesium and MK-801 on blood-brain barrier permeability and brain edema after experimental traumatic diffuse brain injury. *Neurol Res* 31:977-81.

Kahraman S, Ozgurtas T, Kayali H, Atabey C, Kutluay T, Timurkaynak E (2003) Monitoring of serum ionized magnesium in neurosurgical intensive care unit: preliminary results. *Clin Chim Acta* 334:211-5.

Kara H, Sahin N, Ulusan V, Aydogdu T (2002) Magnesium infusion reduces perioperative pain. *Eur J Anaesthesiol* 19:52-6.

Kaya M, Kucuk M, Kalayci RB, Cimen V, Gurses C, Elmas I, Arican N (2001) Magnesium sulfate attenuates increased blood-brain barrier permeability during insulin-induced hypoglycemia in rats. *Can J Physiol Pharmacol* 79:793-8.

Kobayashi H, Minami S, Itoh S, Shiraishi S, Yokoo H, Yanagita T, Uezono Y, Mohri M, Wada A (2001) Aquaporin subtypes in rat cerebral microvessels. *Neurosci Lett* 297:163-6.

Koepsell H, Schmitt BM, Gorboulev V (2003) Organic cation transporters. *Rev Physiol Biochem Pharmacol* 150:36-90.

Konrad M, Schaller A, Seelow D, Pandey AV, Waldegger S, Lesslauer A, Vitzthum H, Suzuki Y, Luk JM, Becker C, Schlingmann KP, Schmid M, Rodriguez-Soriano J, Ariceta G, Cano F, Enriquez R, Juppner H, Bakkaloglu SA, Hediger MA, Gallati S, Neuhauss SC, Nurnberg P, Weber S (2006) Mutations in the tight-junction gene claudin 19 (CLDN19) are associated with renal magnesium wasting, renal failure, and severe ocular involvement. *Am J Hum Genet* 79:949-57.

Kunert-Keil C, Bisping F, Kruger J, Brinkmeier H (2006) Tissue-specific expression of TRP channel genes in the mouse and its variation in three different mouse strains. *BMC Genomics* 7:159.

Lee JS, Han YM, Yoo DS, Choi SJ, Choi BH, Kim JH, Kim YH, Huh PW, Ko YJ, Rha HK, Cho KS, Kim DS (2004) A molecular basis for the efficacy of magnesium treatment following traumatic brain injury in rats. *J Neurotrauma* 21:549-61.

Leybaert L (2005) Neurobarrier coupling in the brain: a partner of neurovascular and neurometabolic coupling? *J Cereb Blood Flow Metab* 25:2-16.

Li X, Kong H, Wu W, Xiao M, Sun X, Hu G (2009) Aquaporin-4 maintains ependymal integrity in adult mice. *Neuroscience* 162:67-77.

Liebner S, Kniesel U, Kalbacher H, Wolburg H (2000) Correlation of tight junction morphology with the expression of tight junction proteins in blood-brain barrier endothelial cells. *Eur J Cell Biol* 79:707-17.

Lippoldt A, Liebner S, Andbjer B, Kalbacher H, Wolburg H, Haller H, Fuxe K (2000) Organization of choroid plexus epithelial and endothelial cell tight junctions and regulation of claudin-1, -2 and -5 expression by protein kinase C. *Neuroreport* 11:1427-31.

Ma YY, Huo HR, Li CH, Zhao BS, Li LF, Sui F, Guo SY, Jiang TL (2008) Effects of cinnamaldehyde on PGE2 release and TRPV4 expression in mouse cerebral microvascular endothelial cells induced by interleukin-1beta. *Biol Pharm Bull* 31:426-30.

Matter K, Balda MS (2003) Holey barrier: claudins and the regulation of brain endothelial permeability. *J Cell Biol* 161:459-60.

McCoy JH, Kenney MA (1975) Depressed immune response in the magnesium-deficient rat. *J Nutr* 105:791-7.

McIntosh TK, Faden AI, Yamakami I, Vink R (1988) Magnesium deficiency exacerbates and pretreatment improves outcome following traumatic brain injury in rats: 31P magnetic resonance spectroscopy and behavioral studies. *J Neurotrauma* 5:17-31.

McKinley MJ, McAllen RM, Davern P, Giles ME, Penschow J, Sunn N, Uschakov A, Oldfield BJ (2003) The sensory circumventricular organs of the mammalian brain. *Adv Anat Embryol Cell Biol* 172:III-XII, 1-122.

Miller DS (2010) Regulation of P-glycoprotein and other ABC drug transporters at the blood-brain barrier. *Trends Pharmacol Sci* 31:246-54.

Montell C (2005) The TRP superfamily of cation channels. *Sci STKE* 2005:re3.

Morita K, Furuse M, Fujimoto K, Tsukita S (1999) Claudin multigene family encoding four-transmembrane domain protein components of tight junction strands. *Proc Natl Acad Sci U S A* 96:511-6.

Morris ME (1992) Brain and CSF magnesium concentrations during magnesium deficit in animals and humans: neurological symptoms. *Magnes Res* 5:303-13.

Muir KW, Lees KR, Ford I, Davis S (2004) Magnesium for acute stroke (Intravenous Magnesium Efficacy in Stroke trial): randomised controlled trial. *Lancet* 363:439-45.

Musso CG (2009) Magnesium metabolism in health and disease. *Int Urol Nephrol* 41:357-62.

Nabeshima S, Reese TS, Landis DM, Brightman MW (1975) Junctions in the meninges and marginal glia. *J Comp Neurol* 164:127-69.

Nielsen S, Smith BL, Christensen EI, Agre P (1993) Distribution of the aquaporin CHIP in secretory and resorptive epithelia and capillary endothelia. *Proc Natl Acad Sci U S A* 90:7275-9.

Nielsen S, Nagelhus EA, Amiry-Moghaddam M, Bourque C, Agre P, Ottersen OP (1997) Specialized membrane domains for water transport in glial cells: high-resolution immunogold cytochemistry of aquaporin-4 in rat brain. *J Neurosci* 17:171-80.

Niermann H, Amiry-Moghaddam M, Holthoff K, Witte OW, Ottersen OP (2001) A novel role of vasopressin in the brain: modulation of activity-dependent water flux in the neocortex. *J Neurosci* 21:3045-51.

Nischwitz V, Berthele A, Michalke B (2008) Speciation analysis of selected metals and determination of their total contents in paired serum and cerebrospinal fluid samples: An approach to investigate the permeability of the human blood-cerebrospinal fluid-barrier. *Anal Chim Acta* 627:258-69.

Ohtsuki S, Terasaki T (2007) Contribution of carrier-mediated transport systems to the blood-brain barrier as a supporting and protecting interface for the brain; importance for CNS drug discovery and development. *Pharm Res* 24:1745-58.

Oppelt WW, MacIntyre I, Rall DP (1963) Magnesium exchange between blood and cerebrospinal fluid. *Am J Physiol* 205:959-62.

Pardridge WM, Boado RJ, Farrell CR (1990) Brain-type glucose transporter (GLUT-1) is selectively localized to the blood-brain barrier. Studies with quantitative western blotting and in situ hybridization. *J Biol Chem* 265:18035-40.

Pardridge WM (1991) Advances in cell biology of blood-brain barrier transport. *Semin Cell Biol* 2:419-26.

Peikert A, Wilimzig C, Kohne-Volland R (1996) Prophylaxis of migraine with oral magnesium: results from a prospective, multi-center, placebo-controlled and double-blind randomized study. *Cephalalgia* 16:257-63.

Peppi M, Ghabriel MN (2004) Tissue-specific expression of the tight junction proteins claudins and occludin in the rat salivary glands. *J Anat* 205:257-66.

Porter NS, Jason LA, Boulton A, Bothne N, Coleman B (2010) Alternative medical interventions used in the treatment and management of myalgic encephalomyelitis/chronic fatigue syndrome and fibromyalgia. *J Altern Complement Med* 16:235-49.

Quamme GA, Dirks JH (1980) Magnesium transport in the nephron. *Am J Physiol* 239:F393-401.

Quamme GA (1997) Renal magnesium handling: new insights in understanding old problems. *Kidney Int* 52:1180-95.

Quamme GA, de Rouffignac C (2000) Epithelial magnesium transport and regulation by the kidney. *Front Biosci* 5:D694-711.

Redzic ZB, Segal MB (2004) The structure of the choroid plexus and the physiology of the choroid plexus epithelium. *Adv Drug Deliv Rev* 56:1695-716.

Reed DJ, Yen MH (1978) The role of the cat choroid plexus in regulating cerebrospinal fluid magnesium. *J Physiol* 281:477-85.

Reese TS, Karnovsky MJ (1967) Fine structural localization of a blood-brain barrier to exogenous peroxidase. *J Cell Biol* 34:207-17.

Resnick LM, Altura BT, Gupta RK, Laragh JH, Alderman MH, Altura BM (1993) Intracellular and extracellular magnesium depletion in type 2 (non-insulin-dependent) diabetes mellitus. *Diabetologia* 36:767-70.

Roberts LM, Black DS, Raman C, Woodford K, Zhou M, Haggerty JE, Yan AT, Cwirla SE, Grindstaff KK (2008) Subcellular localization of transporters along the rat blood-brain barrier and blood-cerebral-spinal fluid barrier by in vivo biotinylation. *Neuroscience* 155:423-38.

Rouse DJ (2009) Magnesium sulfate for the prevention of cerebral palsy. *Am J Obstet Gynecol* 200:610-2.

Rubin LL, Staddon JM (1999) The cell biology of the blood-brain barrier. *Annu Rev Neurosci* 22:11-28.

Saatman KE, Bareyre FM, Grady MS, McIntosh TK (2001) Acute cytoskeletal alterations and cell death induced by experimental brain injury are attenuated by magnesium treatment and exacerbated by magnesium deficiency. *J Neuropathol Exp Neurol* 60:183-94.

Sacco RL, Chong JY, Prabhakaran S, Elkind MS (2007) Experimental treatments for acute ischaemic stroke. *Lancet* 369:331-41.

Schlingmann KP, Weber S, Peters M, Niemann Nejsum L, Vitzthum H, Klingel K, Kratz M, Haddad E, Ristoff E, Dinour D, Syrrou M, Nielsen S, Sassen M, Waldegger S, Seyberth HW, Konrad M (2002) Hypomagnesemia with secondary hypocalcemia is caused by mutations in TRPM6, a new member of the TRPM gene family. *Nat Genet* 31:166-70.

Schlingmann KP, Sassen MC, Weber S, Pechmann U, Kusch K, Pelken L, Lotan D, Syrrou M, Prebble JJ, Cole DE, Metzger DL, Rahman S, Tajima T, Shu SG, Waldegger S, Seyberth HW, Konrad M (2005) Novel TRPM6 mutations in 21 families with primary hypomagnesemia and secondary hypocalcemia. *J Am Soc Nephrol* 16:3061-9.

Schlingmann KP, Waldegger S, Konrad M, Chubanov V, Gudermann T (2007) TRPM6 and TRPM7--Gatekeepers of human magnesium metabolism. *Biochim Biophys Acta* 1772:813-21.

Schmitz C, Perraud AL, Johnson CO, Inabe K, Smith MK, Penner R, Kurosaki T, Fleig A, Scharenberg AM (2003) Regulation of vertebrate cellular Mg2+ homeostasis by TRPM7. *Cell* 114:191-200.

Schroeder HA, Nason AP, Tipton IH (1969) Essential metals in man. Magnesium. *J Chronic Dis* 21:815-41.

Seda HW, Hughes RD, Gove CD, Williams R (1984) Inhibition of rat brain Na+,K+-ATPase activity by serum from patients with fulminant hepatic failure. *Hepatology* 4:74-9.

Sedlakova R, Shivers RR, Del Maestro RF (1999) Ultrastructure of the blood-brain barrier in the rabbit. *J Submicrosc Cytol Pathol* 31:149-61.

Segal MB (2000) The choroid plexuses and the barriers between the blood and the cerebrospinal fluid. *Cell Mol Neurobiol* 20:183-96.

Shen S, Zhang W (2010) ABC transporters and drug efflux at the blood-brain barrier. *Rev Neurosci* 21:29-53.

Simoes Fernandes J, Pereira T, Carvalho J, Franca A, Andrade R, Nogueira Pereira J, Rodrigues JC, Laires MJ, Halpern MJ (1985) Therapeutic effect of a magnesium salt in patients suffering from mitral valvular prolapse and latent tetany. *Magnesium* 4:283-90.

Simon DB, Lu Y, Choate KA, Velazquez H, Al-Sabban E, Praga M, Casari G, Bettinelli A, Colussi G, Rodriguez-Soriano J, McCredie D, Milford D, Sanjad S, Lifton RP (1999) Paracellin-1, a renal tight junction protein required for paracellular Mg2+ resorption. *Science* 285:103-6.

Soave PM, Conti G, Costa R, Arcangeli A (2009) Magnesium and anaesthesia. *Curr Drug Targets* 10:734-43.

Sojka JE, Weaver CM (1995) Magnesium supplementation and osteoporosis. *Nutr Rev* 53:71-4.

Somjen GG (2002) Ion regulation in the brain: implications for pathophysiology. *Neuroscientist* 8:254-67.

Song Y, Li TY, van Dam RM, Manson JE, Hu FB (2007) Magnesium intake and plasma concentrations of markers of systemic inflammation and endothelial dysfunction in women. *Am J Clin Nutr* 85:1068-74.

Sternberger NH, Sternberger LA (1987) Blood-brain barrier protein recognized by monoclonal antibody. *Proc Natl Acad Sci U S A* 84:8169-73.

Sunn N, McKinley MJ, Oldfield BJ (2003) Circulating angiotensin II activates neurones in circumventricular organs of the lamina terminalis that project to the bed nucleus of the stria terminalis. *J Neuroendocrinol* 15:725-31.

Takahashi H, Imai K, Katanuma A, Sugaya T, Hisano K, Motoya S, Aoki S, Sugiyama T, Yachi A (1992) [A case of chronic fatigue syndrome who showed a beneficial effect by intravenous administration of magnesium sulphate]. *Arerugi* 41:1605-10.

Temkin NR, Anderson GD, Winn HR, Ellenbogen RG, Britz GW, Schuster J, Lucas T, Newell DW, Mansfield PN, Machamer JE, Barber J, Dikmen SS (2007) Magnesium sulfate for neuroprotection after traumatic brain injury: a randomised controlled trial. *Lancet Neurol* 6:29-38.

Terasaki M, Rubin H (1985) Evidence that intracellular magnesium is present in cells at a regulatory concentration for protein synthesis. *Proc Natl Acad Sci U S A* 82:7324-6.

Tripathi RC (1973) Ultrastructure of the arachnoid mater in relation to outflow of cerebrospinal fluid. A new concept. *Lancet* 2:8-11.

Tsukita S, Furuse M (1999) Occludin and claudins in tight-junction strands: leading or supporting players? *Trends Cell Biol* 9:268-73.

Turkoglu OF, Eroglu H, Okutan O, Tun MK, Bodur E, Sargon MF, Oner L, Beskonakli E (2008) A comparative study of treatment for brain edema: magnesium sulphate versus dexamethasone sodium phosphate. *J Clin Neurosci* 15:60-5.

Turner RJ, Dasilva KW, O'Connor C, van den Heuvel C, Vink R (2004) Magnesium gluconate offers no more protection than magnesium sulphate following diffuse traumatic brain injury in rats. *J Am Coll Nutr* 23:541S-4S.

van den Bergh WM (2009) Magnesium in subarachnoid haemorrhage: proven beneficial? *Magnes Res* 22:121-6.

Vandenabeele F, Creemers J, Lambrichts I (1996) Ultrastructure of the human spinal arachnoid mater and dura mater. *J Anat* 189 (Pt 2):417-30.

Vanharreveld A, Crowell J, Malhotra SK (1965) A Study of Extracellular Space in Central Nervous Tissue by Freeze-Substitution. *J Cell Biol* 25:117-37.

Villegas JC, Broadwell RD (1993) Transcytosis of protein through the mammalian cerebral epithelium and endothelium. II. Adsorptive transcytosis of WGA-HRP and the blood-brain and brain-blood barriers. *J Neurocytol* 22:67-80.

Vink R, McIntosh TK, Demediuk P, Faden AI (1987) Decrease in total and free magnesium concentration following traumatic brain injury in rats. *Biochem Biophys Res Commun* 149:594-9.

Vink R, Cernak I (2000) Regulation of intracellular free magnesium in central nervous system injury. *Front Biosci* 5:D656-65.

Vink R, Cook NL, van den Heuvel C (2009) Magnesium in acute and chronic brain injury: an update. *Magnes Res* 22:158S-62S.

Voets T, Nilius B, Hoefs S, van der Kemp AW, Droogmans G, Bindels RJ, Hoenderop JG (2004) TRPM6 forms the Mg2+ influx channel involved in intestinal and renal Mg2+ absorption. *J Biol Chem* 279:19-25.

Walder RY, Landau D, Meyer P, Shalev H, Tsolia M, Borochowitz Z, Boettger MB, Beck GE, Englehardt RK, Carmi R, Sheffield VC (2002) Mutation of TRPM6 causes familial hypomagnesemia with secondary hypocalcemia. *Nat Genet* 31:171-4.

Weber S, Schlingmann KP, Peters M, Nejsum LN, Nielsen S, Engel H, Grzeschik KH, Seyberth HW, Grone HJ, Nusing R, Konrad M (2001) Primary gene structure and expression studies of rodent paracellin-1. *J Am Soc Nephrol* 12:2664-72.

Wester PO, Dyckner T (1987) Magnesium and hypertension. *J Am Coll Nutr* 6:321-8.

Wolburg H, Lippoldt A (2002) Tight junctions of the blood-brain barrier: development, composition and regulation. *Vascul Pharmacol* 38:323-37.

Wolburg H, Wolburg-Buchholz K, Kraus J, Rascher-Eggstein G, Liebner S, Hamm S, Duffner F, Grote EH, Risau W, Engelhardt B (2003) Localization of claudin-3 in tight junctions of the blood-brain barrier is selectively lost during experimental autoimmune encephalomyelitis and human glioblastoma multiforme. *Acta Neuropathol* 105:586-92.

Wolburg H, Noell S, Wolburg-Buchholz K, Mack A, Fallier-Becker P (2009) Agrin, aquaporin-4, and astrocyte polarity as an important feature of the blood-brain barrier. *Neuroscientist* 15:180-93.

Wolburg H, Paulus W (2010) Choroid plexus: biology and pathology. *Acta Neuropathol* 119:75-88.

Wolf FI, Trapani V, Simonacci M, Mastrototaro L, Cittadini A, Schweigel M (2010) Modulation of TRPM6 and Na(+)/Mg(2+) exchange in mammary epithelial cells in response to variations of magnesium availability. *J Cell Physiol* 222:374-81.

Yahia AM, Kirmani JF, Qureshi AI, Guterman LR, Hopkins LN (2005) The safety and feasibility of continuous intravenous magnesium sulfate for prevention of cerebral vasospasm in aneurysmal subarachnoid hemorrhage. *Neurocrit Care* 3:16-23.

Zhang EY, Knipp GT, Ekins S, Swaan PW (2002) Structural biology and function of solute transporters: implications for identifying and designing substrates. *Drug Metab Rev* 34:709-50.

Zlokovic BV, Skundric DS, Segal MB, Lipovac MN, Mackic JB, Davson H (1990) A saturable mechanism for transport of immunoglobulin G across the blood-brain barrier of the guinea pig. *Exp Neurol* 107:263-70.

Intracellular free Mg^{2+} and $MgATP^{2-}$ in coordinate control of protein synthesis and cell proliferation

Harry Rubin✉

Department of Molecular and Cell Biology, Life Sciences Addition, University of California, Berkeley, CA 94720-3200, USA.
✉ hrubin@berkeley.edu

Abstract

Specific and non-specific mitogens stimulate the proliferation of cultured fibroblasts. They also stimulate other responses that are part of a coordinate response, some members of which are essential for proliferation and others that are not. The synthesis of protein is an early response to mitogens and its continuation through the G1 period drives the accumulation of protein which is required for the initiation of DNA synthesis hours later. The parabola-like curve for dependence of protein synthesis on intracellular Mg^{2+} concentration is similar to that of cell-free ribosome preparations, and is later reflected in the initiation of DNA synthesis. Hence, DNA synthesis is dependent on the rate of protein synthesis which is regulated by the concentration of intracellular Mg^{2+}. Presumably free Mg^{2+} is an indicator of the fraction of ATP^{4-} that is complexed with Mg^{2+} as $MgATP^{2-}$, which is the immediate regulatory form. Uridine uptake is determined by its phosphorylation which is also dependent on intracellular Mg^{2+} in the coordinate response, but unlike protein synthesis, neither influences DNA synthesis nor exhibits downturn at a high Mg^{2+} concentration. Intracellular free Mg^{2+} determines the onset of protein synthesis in activated frog oocytes and its rate in lymphocytes. Mg^{2+} regulation of protein synthesis is effected through the PI 3-K pathway at mTOR phosphorylation of two translation-regulating proteins. Regulation of proliferation by Mg^{2+} is lost in transformed cells. Mg^{2+} and $MgATP^{2-}$ apparently play a central role in the regulation of metabolism in a wide variety of cells and developmental stages across the animal kingdom.

Introduction

The study of the regulation of cell proliferation was greatly facilitated in the 1960s and 1970s by the development of monolayer cell culture. This permitted direct microscopic examination of cell populations including cellular morphology and behavior. Techniques were also developed for suspending and accurately counting the cells. It was also possible to vary the cell population size, change the constituents of the medium, and uniformly label the cells with radioactive chemicals to study their metabolism. Some general features of cell growth stimulation have to be considered before delving into the possible mechanism(s) of its control. Most of the experiments to be described here were conducted in cell culture with fibroblasts obtained directly from chicken embryos, or with established lines of mouse fibroblasts. In most cases they were allowed to grow into confluent sheets to establish contact inhibition with low levels of DNA synthesis that represented the small proportion of cells in the S-period, and no net proliferation. Fresh medium containing serum or other growth stimulants was added and measurements of various cellular parameters were made at intervals thereafter.

After application of a stimulus to a growth-inhibited culture, increase in DNA synthesis, representing the increased proportion of cells in the S-period, does not begin for 4 hours in *ex vivo* chicken embryo cells (Rubin and Steiner, 1975) or 10 hours in an established line of mouse cells (Rubin *et al,* 1978). This indicates that multiple metabolic processes are required to produce that response. These include increases in the rates of uptake of glucose analogs, and uridine prior to its incorporation into RNA (Rubin, 1975b). Although neither of these responses is required for the increased DNA synthesis, they are clearly part of a coordinate response of the cells to the growth stimulants, and have to be taken into account in understanding the intracellular mechanism of growth regulation. Most significant, there is also a fractional increase in the rate of protein synthesis that must be maintained throughout the period preceding DNA synthesis, and is essential for its initiation (Rubin, 2005). Small decreases of protein synthesis in cells treated with a specific inhibitor of protein synthesis result in large decreases in the fraction of cells that later initiate DNA synthesis (Brooks, 1977; and Figure 1).

Another aspect of growth stimulation concerns treatments other than serum growth factors that produce the same constellation of responses. Certain hormones such as insulin produce the coordinate response in some cell types, indicating that a specific interaction between proteins and their receptors at the cell surface can initiate the coordinate response. However, the same effects are produced by removing a strip of cells from a confluent monolayer, which allows migration and multiplication of the cells at the margin. This indicates that the coordinate response is not limited to specific receptors. A similar conclusion is suggested by the finding that subtoxic concentrations of heavy metals including zinc, cadmium, and mercury initiate the coordinate response in chick embryo fibroblasts (Rubin, 1975b). Lead stimulated DNA synthesis in some experiments, and in other experiments did not (Sanui and Rubin, 1984). Those cultures in which DNA was not stimulated showed no increase in cellular Mg^{2+}, whereas those that were significantly stimulated exhibited a 10 - 13% increase in intracellular Mg^{2+}. Stimulation of DNA synthesis by lead coincided with the formation of lead precipitate in the medium.

A striking finding made with a permanent line of cells originating from mouse embryo fibroblasts was that increasing concentrations of inorganic pyrophosphate initiated the coordinate response at precisely the concentration (about 0.2 mM in standard medium) at which it first formed a flocculent precipitate with calcium (Rubin and Sanui, 1977). The stimulation required contact of the precipitate with the cell surface as shown by the failure of stimulation when the culture dish was inverted so that the precipitate did not contact the cells (Bowen-Pope and Rubin, 1983). The stimulation was terminated when the pH of the medium was slightly lowered and the precipitate dissolved, showing that the effect required the precipitate and was exerted at the surface of the cell.

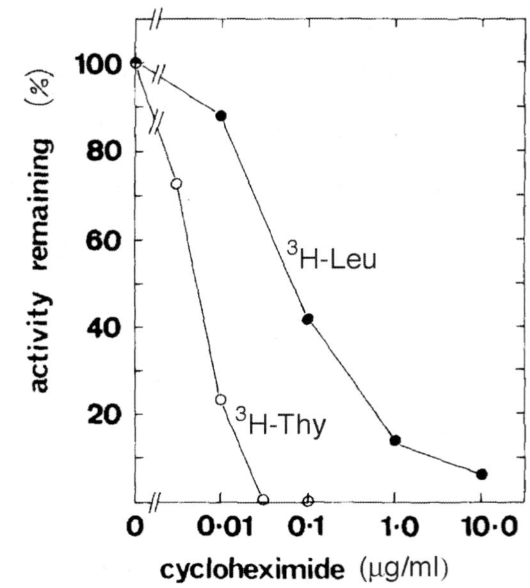

Figure 1. Inhibition of protein synthesis by cycloheximide and its effect on the initiation of DNA synthesis in mouse 3T3 cells. Quiescent cells were stimulated with serum in the presence of the indicated concentrations of cycloheximide. Cultures were pulse-labeled for protein synthesis with ^{3}H-leucine at 2 hours (●) and continuously labeled with ^{3}H-thymidine for 24 hours (O). Ordinate: radioactivity incorporated as percentage of control (no cycloheximide) (Brooks, 1977).

In the absence of pyrophosphate, supranormal concentrations of either Ca^{2+} or orthophosphate caused graded increases in DNA synthesis (Rubin and Sanui, 1977). The effect of supranormal Ca^{2+} depended on orthophosphate and *vice versa*. The stimulation was associated with increasing turbidity of the medium, consistent with the involvement of a precipitate interacting with the cell membrane. Several other non-physiological, non-specific treatments could initiate the coordinate response, although most of them could not maintain multiple rounds of cell multiplication. One exception was the wound-healing experiment, which allowed continued cell multiplication until the cleared strip was completely covered with cells. The sum total of these experiments indicates that perturbation of the cell membrane, which could be brought about by specific or non-specific means, is involved in growth stimulation, and raises the question of what intracellular response(s) or second messenger(s) mediate the diverse reactions of the coordinate response.

Variations of intracellular K^+, Na^+ or Ca^+ failed to reproduce the coordinate response in a balanced manner (Moscatelli *et al,* 1979) nor did changes in the pH of the medium (Rubin, 2005). Intracellular Mg^{2+} was considered a logical candidate as a second messenger for regulating the coordinate response to membrane perturbation because it is required for every phosphoryl transfer in the cell. Drastic reduction in Mg^{2+} concentration in the medium reduced the number of cells in the S-period of the cell cycle, but the effect was erratic (Rubin, 1975a). Phosphorylated compounds that bind Mg^{2+} were more reproducible, especially inorganic pyrophosphate in concentrations that exceeded the concentration of Mg^{2+} in the medium. Unlike the very low concentrations of pyrophosphate that stimulated mouse fibroblasts via a precipitate with Ca^{2+} (Bowen-Pope and Rubin, 1983), the inhibition of fibroblast growth was most efficient in low concentrations of Ca^{2+} in which there was no precipitate. Mg^{2+} deprivation, further lowered by its binding with pyrophosphate, suppressed all elements of the coordinate response in a balanced manner (Rubin, 1975a).

Changes in total and free Mg^{2+} after stimulation of cells with mitogens

The major cellular cations were measured in confluent chick embryo fibroblasts 16 hours after a fresh change of medium with insulin substituting for serum (Sanui and Rubin, 1978). There was more than a 16-fold increase in the overall rate of DNA synthesis in the optimal concentration of insulin, with a 22% increase in total Mg^{2+} of the cells as measured by atomic absorption spectrophotometry. There was no change in total cell Ca^{2+}, negligible change in Na^+ and a 14% increase in K^+, an element that plays an adjunct role to Mg^{2+} in the synthesis of protein in cell-free systems (Schreier and Staehelin, 1973). In an experiment with a contact –inhibited and serum-limited line of mouse fibroblasts, the addition of fresh medium containing serum induced a 15-fold increase of DNA synthesis at 17 hours, associated with a 15% increase in total Mg^{2+} (Sanui and Rubin, 1982). There was only a marginal increase in K^+, and decreases in Na^+ and Ca^{2+}. These results were consistent with a central role for Mg^{2+} in supporting cell proliferation.

It seemed likely to us that intracellular free Mg^{2+} combined with ATP^{4-} is its regulatory form, possibly made available by cation exchange with intracellular K^+ that releases bound Mg^{2+} from the inner surface of the cell membrane (Rubin, 1976; Sanui and Rubin, 1978). The free Mg^{2+} would combine with ATP^{4-} to form $MgATP^{2-}$,which would stimulate phosphoryl transfer reactions throughout the cell, and reduce the inhibitory $KATP^{3-}$ form. However, we did not have an efficient means at the time of measuring free Mg^{2+} in the cell. The development of a Mg^{2+}-sensitive fluorescent dye, mag-fura-2, made it possible to quantify intracellular free Mg^{2+} (Murphy *et al,* 1989; Raju *et al,* 1989). It was used to monitor free Mg^{2+} in a quiescent, confluent line of mouse fibroblasts stimulated by insulin or by insulin combined with epidermal growth factor (Ishijima *et al,* 1991). The combination of the two growth factors led to a significant increase of intracellular free Mg^{2+} from a basal level of 0.22 mM to 0.29 mM at 30 minutes, and to 0.35 mM at 60 minutes. After 60 minutes the free Mg^{2+} levels seemed to decline, but the measurements were no longer reliable because of leakage of the dye. Epidermal growth factor produced a 50-fold increase in DNA synthesis when added to a serum-starved line of differentiated myocytes (Grubbs, 1991). Free Mg^{2+} increased after a 5-minute lag period, rising gradually from an initial 0.32 mM to as high as 1.4 mM at 20 minutes, and then leveled off. There was no change in the cellular pH or free Ca^{2+} during the 20-minute period. The dose-response to epidermal growth factor was the same for free Mg^{2+} and the synthesis of DNA, strengthening the case for the dependence of the proliferative response on the rise of free Mg^{2+}.

Correlations between cellular Mg^{2+}, protein synthesis and the onset of DNA synthesis

A series of experiments was carried out in which external Mg^{2+} was varied over a wide range (1-48 mM) in a medium containing only 0.02 Ca^{2+} (Rubin *et al* 1979). The low Ca^{2+} concentration increased the permeability of the cells for entry of Mg^{2+}. Intracellular Mg^{2+} content and the rate of protein synthesis were measured at 3 and 17 hours and the rate of DNA synthesis at 17 hours.

The results showed that the intracellular Mg^{2+} concentration increased as the external Mg^{2+} concentration was increased, but the rate of protein synthesis at 3 hours peaked at 20 mM external Mg^{2+} concentration, and declined with higher (30 – 48 mM) Mg^{2+} concentrations (Figure 2A, B). The rate of DNA synthesis at 17 hours peaked at the same Mg^{2+} concentration as protein synthesis at 3 hours (Figure 2A), consistent with the dependence of the onset of the S-period on the rate of protein synthesis during the preceding G1-period.

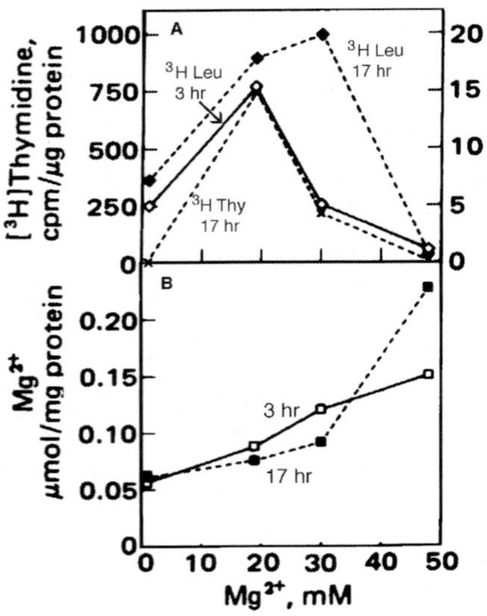

Figure 2. Effects of extracellular Mg^{2+} on intracellular Mg^{2+} and on protein and DNA synthesis. Quiescent mouse 3T3 cells were stimulated with 10% dialyzed serum in Ca^{2+}-deprived medium with varying concentrations of Mg^{2+}. At 3 hours some of the cultures were A) labeled with ^{3}H-leucine; and at 17 hours with ^{3}H-leucine or ^{3}H-thymidine; B) processed for measurement of intracellular Mg^{2+} at 3 and 17 hours (Rubin *et al,* 1979).

Protein synthesis at 17 hours showed a stimulation at 30 mM external Mg^{2+} which had first inhibited protein synthesis at 3 hours, and consequently reduced DNA synthesis at 17 hours (Figure 2A). The increased protein synthesis at 17 hours was associated with a decrease of cellular Mg^{2+} from its inhibitory level at 3 hours to a physiological stimulatory level at 17 hours (Figure 2A, B), indicating the cells were able to reduce Mg^{2+} content to functional levels. If the external Mg^{2+} levels were carried to even higher external levels (48 mM), the cellular Mg^{2+} rose to very high levels at 17 hours and both protein and DNA synthesis remained close to zero, indicating toxic damage of the cells. The overall results provided strong evidence of Mg^{2+} as an indirect regulator of the onset of DNA synthesis through its direct effect on the rate of preceding protein synthesis. It should be recalled however that the free Mg^{2+} level is an indicator of the fraction of ATP^{4-} that is complexed to Mg^{2+} as $MgATP^{2-}$ which is the true regulator (Rubin, 2005).

Figure 3 plots the rate of protein synthesis at 3 hours against the intracellular concentration of Mg^{2+}, showing the sharp increase in protein synthesis with small increases of intracellular Mg^{2+} in the physiological range (0.05 – 0.08 µmole/mg protein). At high concentrations of Mg^{2+}, protein synthesis is reduced both in cultured cells and in cell free systems (Schreier and Staehelin, 1973; and Figure 4). The same concentration dependence is exhibited by DNA synthesis in cells at 17 hours (Rubin *et al,* 1978, and Figure 5), which is consistent with the dependence of DNA synthesis on prior protein synthesis. The increase of protein synthesis with ascending Mg^{2+} at physiological intracellular levels has to be maintained through the G-1 period in order to get the full response of DNA

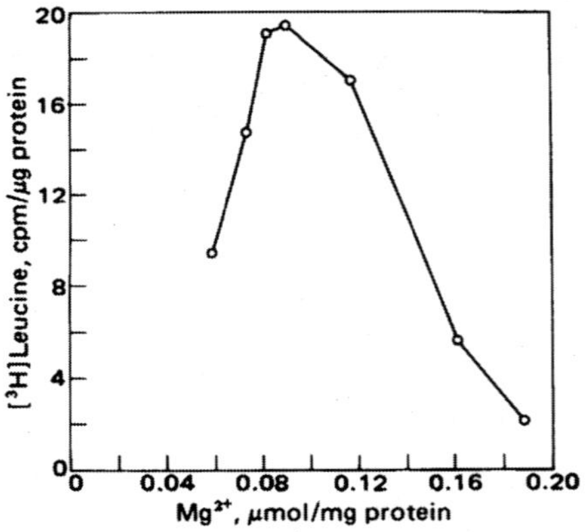

Figure 3. Relationship between intracellular Mg^{2+} and protein synthesis. Quiescent mouse 3T3 cultures were stimulated with 10% dialyzed serum in Ca^{2+}-deprived medium and varying concentrations of Mg^{2+}. At 3 hours some of the cultures were labeled with ^{3}H-leucine, or processed for measurement of intracellular Mg^{2+} (Rubin *et al,* 1979).

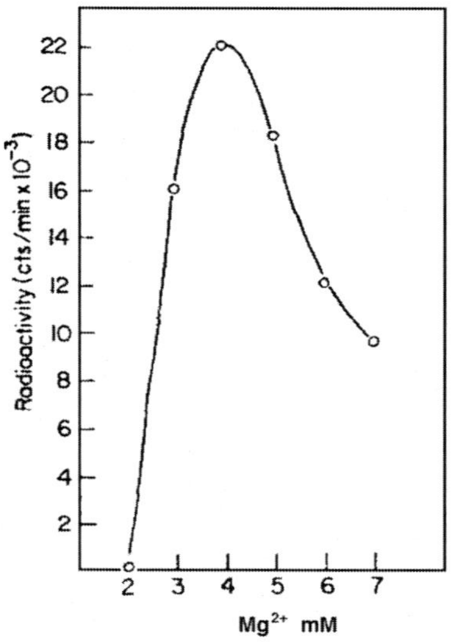

Figure 4. Mg^{2+}dependency of globin synthesis by mouse liver polysomes in a cell-free system, with labeling by ^{14}C-leucine. After correction for chelation of Mg^{2+} by ATP and GTP, the effective Mg^{2+} concentration is 1.4 mM lower than that indicated (Schreier and Staehelin, 1973). The correction does not take into account that 32% of cytosolic Mg^{2+} is bound to low affinity, non-diffusible sites (Corkey *et al,* 1986). Note the steep increase in globin synthesis with Mg^{2+} at lower levels, closer to an estimated intracellular free Mg^{2+}, if account is taken of all the low affinity binding sites.

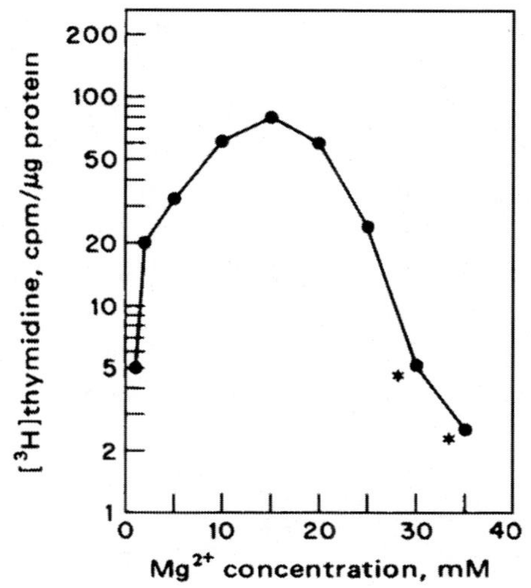

Figure 5. DNA synthesis as a function of extra-cellular Mg^{2+}. Quiescent mouse 3T3 cells were stimulated with 10% dialyzed serum in Ca^{2+}-deprived medium with varying concentrations of Mg^{2+}. At 17 hours the cultures were labeled with ^{3}H-thymidine. The asterisks associated with the two highest concentrations of Mg^{2+} in the medium and greatly reduced incorporation in DNA indicate many foci of degenerated cells (Rubin *et al,* 1978).

synthesis. The high concentration of total Mg^{2+} in cells, and the low affinity of Mg^{2+} binding sites, results in rather large changes of free Mg^{2+} with small variations in total cell Mg^{2+}. This makes Mg^{2+} an unlikely short-term regulatory molecule like Ca^{2+}, but long term change in total Mg^{2+}, as exhibited in mitogen stimulation, may have profound effects on metabolic regulation given the sensitivity of free Mg^{2+} to alterations in total Mg^{2+} (Corkey *et al,* 1986).

Response of protein synthesis in frog oocytes to injection of Mg^{2+} resembles that of stimulation by gonadotropin

Frog oocytes are large enough (850-950 micrometers in diameter) to allow microinjection of materials, and to measure cations and protein synthesis in single cells (Horowitz and Lau, 1988). When stimulated by gonadotropin these quiescent cells begin to synthesize protein that drives their growth and maturation into eggs. Exposing oocytes in saline to gonadotropin that acts via cell surface receptors increases cytoplasmic K^+ activity and protein synthesis for at least 10 days (Lau *et al,* 1988). These effects are mimicked by microinjection of K^+ into oocytes immersed in paraffin oil to prevent contributions from external sources. The results suggested that K^+ activity is critical to activate and perpetuate protein synthesis.

Further analysis of the results showed that there was a greater effect of K^+ on translation in the oocytes than expected from its effect on cell-free translation (Horowitz and Tluczek, 1989). Also, injection of Na^+ into the oocytes stimulated protein synthesis to the same extent as K^+, despite the fact that Na^+ has no effect on cell-free translation systems. These results indicated that Na^+ and K^+ compete with each other for binding to high affinity anions such as phosphate groups on membranes. Ca^{2+} was ruled out as the displaced cation, but Mg^{2+} stimulated protein synthesis at much lower and narrower concentrations than did K^+. It was concluded that Mg^{2+}, presumably as $MgATP^{2-}$, is the effector directly controlling translation rates in oocytes. There was also evidence that stimulation of the oocytes by gonadotropin, which was necessarily done in saline medium containing Mg^{2+}, added extracellular Mg^{2+} to that contributed by intracellular cation exchange (Horowitz and Tluczek, 1989).

Role of Mg^{2+} in regulating uridine uptake

The uptake rate of uridine into the acid soluble fraction of the cytoplasm increases several fold within a few minutes after stimulating cells with serum (Bowen-Pope and Rubin, 1977), and is sensitive to the concentration of Mg^{2+} in the medium (Rubin, 1976). External uridine is not required for growth of the cells, and its increased uptake does not require protein synthesis (Bowen-Pope and Rubin, 1977). The regulation of uridine uptake by Mg^{2+} occurs at its phosphorylation, which is the same step at which serum modulates uridine uptake (Vidair and Rubin, 1981).

Phosphorylation of uridine is catalyzed by uridine kinase, which responds to Mg^{2+} in cell-free systems in a manner similar to that exhibited by uridine uptake in living cells. Unlike protein synthesis, uridine uptake is not inhibited by high concentrations of Mg^{2+} in the cells, which is consistent with its simpler dependence on initial phosphorylation *vs* the many steps at which net protein synthesis may be affected by Mg^{2+} (Bowen-Pope *et al,* 1979). Thymidine uptake does not respond to mitogenic stimulation, nor does it require Mg^{2+} at the concentrations required by uridine (Vidair and Rubin, 1981). This is presumably because the Km of uridine kinase for Mg^{2+} is higher than that of thymidine kinase and within the normal range of intracellular Mg^{2+} variation (Vidair and Rubin, 2005). The divalent cation ionophore A23187 facilitates the manipulation of intracellular Mg^{2+} concentration without increasing the generalized permeability of the cell. In high concentrations of extracellular Mg^{2+}, the ionophore-treated cells take up uridine in the absence of protein growth factors at the same high rate as in their presence. The results support the thesis that increased uridine uptake in cells treated with growth factors is determined by a membrane-activated increase in intracellular free Mg^{2+}.

Molecular studies of Mg^{2+} regulation in lymphocytes

TRPM7 is a membrane protein with intrinsic ion channel and protein kinase domains (Schmitz *et al,* 2003). An established line of chicken lymphocytes deficient in TRPM7 entered a quiescent phase when cultured in standard concentrations (0.4 mM) of Mg^{2+} similar to that of lymphocytes in the organism. Raising the Mg^{2+} concentration in the medium to 15 mM resulted in an increase in both the viability and proliferation of the cells, implying increased protein accumulation accompanying progress through the cell cycle. This activation indicated that TRPM7 has an essential role in regulating physiological concentrations of Mg^{2+} by an uptake pathway with functional coupling between its channel and kinase domains. TRPM7 channels are required for PI 3-K function as a central regulator of growth in lymphocytes (Sahni and Scharenberg, 2008), as had been hypothesized from studies of Mg^{2+} regulation in fibroblasts (Rubin, 2005). The PI 3-K pathway leads through a protein kinase cascade to mTOR kinase which is a central regulator of protein synthesis (Schmelzle and Hall, 2000). mTOR accomplishes this role by phosphorylating serines and threonines on two proteins which drive further steps that initiate translation (Terada *et al,* 1994; Sahni and Scharenberg, 2008). The mTOR phosphorylations have a high Km for $MgATP^{2-}$, which is in the physiological range of free Mg^{2+}. Total Mg^{2+} in the TRPM7-deficient lymphocytes in standard medium underwent a significant decrease, but no change in free Mg^{2+} was detected, which contrasts with the increase in free Mg^{2+} in mitogen-stimulated fibroblasts (Ishijima *et al,* 1991) and in myocytes (Grubbs, 1991).

A number of the known properties of quiescent, *ex-vivo* lymphocytes were also measured in the TRPM7-deficient lymphocytes in standard medium containing 0.4 mM Mg^{2+} (Sahni *et al,* 2010). The DNA content and size of the two cell sources were similar, and suggested that TRPM7 and Mg^{2+} are involved in the activation of normal quiescent lymphocytes. The TRPM7-deficient lymphocytes increased in size and entered rapid proliferation when the concentration of Mg^{2+} in the medium was increased. The key cell regulator *p27* was elevated in both normal, quiescent lymphocytes and in TRPM7-deficient cells in standard medium. A reduction in RNA, store-operated Ca^{2+} entry and altered energy metabolism was found in the quiescent TRPM7-deficient cells and in normal quiescent lymphocytes. The addition of excess Mg^{2+} to the deficient cells altered all these processes in a characteristic manner of activation of normal lymphocytes, just as it activated the coordinate response of fibroblasts in Ca^{2+}-deficient medium (Rubin *et al,* 1979). The implication of these and foregoing results is that cytosolic free Mg^{2+} and $MgATP^{2-}$ play a central role in the regulation of all cell types and stages of development across the animal kingdom.

Loss of Mg^{2+} regulation in neoplastically transformed cells

Neoplastically transformed cells have the capacity to proliferate in lower concentrations of serum and to higher saturation densities than non-transformed cells (Rubin, 1981). Cell transformation causes a selective loss of the regulatory role of Mg^{2+} in cellular multiplication (McKeehan and Ham, 1978). Deprivation of Mg^{2+} caused transformed cells to flatten and to assume a regularly patterned, non-overlapping relationship to one another (Rubin *et al,* 1981). After 3 days of Mg^{2+} deprivation, the rate of DNA synthesis became highly dependent on both serum concentration and population density, thus resembling the growth behavior of non-transformed cells. The capacity of the normalized transformed cells to produce colonies in agar in normal Mg^{2+} is greatly reduced after 7 days of Mg^{2+} deprivation in monolayer culture (Rubin and Chu, 1982).

The Ca^{2+} content of transformed cells is only one-third that of non-transformed cells, but it increases to that of the non-transformed cells in Mg^{2+}-deprived medium (Rubin *et al,* 1981). The normalization of these parameters in Mg^{2+}-deprived transformed cells is reversed a few days after their subculture in Mg^{2+}-adequate medium. The results support the suggestion that a defect in Mg^{2+} regulation of the multiplication of transformed cells is a basic feature of neoplastic transformation (McKeehan and Ham, 1978) which could be exerted at the level of protein synthesis (Rubin, 2005; Sahni and Scharenberg, 2008). Nothing has been established about the cause of the postulated loss of Mg^{2+} control in transformed cells but one possibility has to do with their actively moving surface membranes (Abercrombie and Ambrose, 1958), which could result in lowering of the binding of Mg^{2+} to anionic groups on their internal surface, and its release into the cytosol (Rubin, 2005). This, of course, would shift the question to what causes the excessive membrane activity, which gets into the somatic cell genetics of neoplastic transformation, and is beyond the scope of this article.

Conclusions

There were several lines of thought that led to the suspicion that Mg^{2+} plays a central role in regulation of growth and replication. Among them were the observations that a variety of unrelated and non-specific substances could initiate at least one round of DNA synthesis and cell replication (Rubin, 1975b; Rubin and Sanui, 1977). Another was that a number of reactions were activated by mitogenic substances that were essential for cell replication and others that were not, but all responded directly to the mitogens hours before the synthesis of DNA was initiated (Bowen-Pope and Rubin, 1977). These early responses were considered part of a coordinate response and drove a search for a second messenger that could regulate all members of that response. That search was pursued by depriving confluent, contact-inhibited cultures of each extracellular candidate in turn, and determining the capacity of its removal to inhibit both the early responses and later increases in DNA synthesis of freshly stimulated cultures (Rubin, 1976; Rubin *et al,* 1979). The most significant early response of the cells for controlling later DNA synthesis was the synthesis of proteins, and the only measured cation that correlated quantitatively with both reactions was total intracellular Mg^{2+} concentration produced by variation in extracellular Mg^{2+}. In order to reliably produce a change of intracellular Mg^{2+} over a wide range, it was necessary to drastically lower the concentration of Ca^{2+} in the medium while varying the extracellular concentration of Mg^{2+}. The deprivation of Ca^{2+} increased the permeability of the cells for Mg^{2+} as well as for other small molecules. It was concluded that the concentration of free Mg^{2+} in the cells determined the level of the coordinate response, and most significantly of protein synthesis.

This conclusion was in part based on small increases in total Mg^{2+} assuming that there were accompanying increases in free Mg^{2+}. Supporting evidence for this conclusion was provided by experiments in *Xenopus* oocytes which allowed direct injection and measurement of free Mg^{2+} (Horowitz and Tluczek, 1989). However, there was a failure to demonstrate an increase in free Mg^{2+} by indicator measurements in activated lymphocytes (Rink *et al,* 1982), despite the reported increase in total Mg^{2+} (Sahni *et al,* 2010). It should be noted that although Mg^{2+} is a co-factor in all phosphoryl transfers in cells, the actual regulatory substrate is $MgATP^{2-}$ in which the Mg^{2+} is chelated by ATP^{4-}, and therefore would not be registered by indicators of free Mg^{2+}.

The PI 3-K pathway is essential for the regulation of protein synthesis (Richardson *et al,* 2004). It leads through a protein kinase cascade to mTOR kinase, which is considered a central regulator of protein synthesis (Schmelzle and Hall, 2000). mTOR accomplishes this role by phosphorylating serines and threonines on two protein substrates which regulate the initiation of translation, mainly of ribosomal proteins and elongation factors (Terada *et al,* 1994). The mTOR phosphorylations have a high Km for $MgATP^{2-}$ (Dennis *et al,* 2001; Jaeschke *et al,* 2004). It may be significant for the coordination of protein synthesis with energy production that the kinases of carbohydrate metabolism which phosphorylate low molecular substrates have a Km for $MgATP^{2-}$ similar to that of mTOR (Edelman *et al,* 1987; Garner and Rosett, 1973). Hence $MgATP^{2-}$ may have as important a role in regulating energy production as it does in regulating protein and DNA synthesis.

One aspect of Mg^{2+} regulation that needs more investigation is the putative role of the loss of its function in cell transformation (McKeehan and Ham, 1978; Rubin *et al,* 1981). A major target for mTOR phosphorylation is the eukaryotic initiation factor 4E (eIF4E). Enhanced phosphorylation of eIF4E up-regulates several proteins implicated in tumorigenesis (Furic *et al,* 2010). Since mTOR is itself regulated by $MgATP^{2-}$ (Rubin, 2005; Sahni and Scharenberg, 2008), the loss of regulation by Mg^{2+} in tumorigenesis, if confirmed, should lead to increased activity of eIF4E and could account for its frequent involvement in human cancer (Hay, 2010). Hence, the measurement of free Mg^{2+} in neoplastic transformation would be a logical next step.

Acknowledgements

I am grateful to Dorothy M. Rubin for editing the manuscript. The meticulous preparation of material and measurements of cations by the late Dr. Hisashi Sanui in cells and media by atomic absorption spectrophotometry lent great accuracy and reliability to the results. The work of graduate students Dan Bowen-Pope, Dave Moscatelli, Mark Terasaki and Charlie Vidair contributed much in their day to an under-standing of the role of Mg^{2+} in the coordinate response of cells to mitogenic stimuli.

References

Abercrombie M, Ambrose EJ (1958) Interference microscope studies of cell contacts in tissue culture. *Exp Cell Res* 15:332-45.

Bowen-Pope DF, Rubin H (1977) Magnesium and calcium effects on uptake of hexoses and uridine by chick embryo fibroblasts. *Proc Natl Acad Sci USA* 74:1585-9.

Bowen-Pope DF, Vidair C, Sanui H, Rubin H (1979) Separate roles for calcium and magnesium in their synergistic effect on uridine uptake by cultured cells. *Proc Natl Acad Sci USA* 76:1308-12.

Bowen-Pope DF, Rubin H (1983) Growth stimulatory precipitates of Ca^{2+} and pyrophosphate. *J Cell Physiol* 117:51-61.

Brooks RF (1977) Continuous protein synthesis is required to maintain the probability of entry into S phase. *Cell* 12:311-7.

Corkey BE, Duszynski J, Rich TL, Matschinsky B, Williamson JR (1986) Regulation of free and bound magnesium in rat hepatocytes and isolated mitochondria. *J Biol Chem* 261:2567-74.

Dennis PB, Jaeschke A, Saitoh M, Fowler B, Kozma SC, Thomas G (2001) Mammalian TOR: a homeostatic ATP sensor. *Science* 294:1102-5.

Edelman AM, Blumenthal DK, Krebs EG (1987) Protein serine/threonine kinases. *Ann Rev Biochem* 56:567-93.

Furic L, Rong L, Larsson O, Koumakpayi IH, Yoshida K, Brueschke A, Petroulakis E, Bobichaud N, Pollak M, Gaboury LA, Pandolfi PP, Saad F, Sonenberg N (2010) eIF4E phosphorylation promotes tumorigenesis and is associated with prostate cancer progression. *Proc Natl Acad Sci USA* 107:14134-9.

Garner P, Rosett T (1973) The influence of Mg^{2+}/adenine nucleotide ratios and absolute concentration of Mg^{2+}/adenine nucleotide on the observed velocity of some kinase reactions. *FEBS Lett* 34:243-6.

Grubbs RD (1991) Effect of epidermal growth factor on Mg^{2+} homeostasis in BC3H-1 myocytes. *Am J Physiol* 260:C1158-C64.

Hay N (2010) Mnk earmarks eIF4E for cancer therapy. *Proc Natl Acad Sci USA* 107:13975-6.

Horowitz SB, Lau Y-T (1988) A function that relates protein synthetic rates to potassium activity *in vivo*. *J Cellular Physiol* 135:425-34.

Horowitz SB, Tluczek LJM (1989) Gonadotropin stimulates oocyte translation by increasing magnesium activity through intracellular potassium-magnesium exchange. *Proc Natl Acad Sci USA* 86:9652-6.

Ishijima S, Sonoda T, Tatibana M (1991) Mitogen-induced early increase in cytosolic free Mg^{2+} concentration in single Swiss 3T3 fibroblasts. *Am J Physiol* 261:C1074-C80.

Jaeschke A, Dennis PB, Thomas G (2004) mTOR: a mediator of intracellular homeostasis. In: *TOR, Target of Rapamycin* (Thomas G, Sabatini DM, Hall MN, eds), Vol. 279, Berlin: Springer Verlag, 283-98.

Lau Y-T, Yassin RR, Horowitz SB (1988) Potassium salt microinjection into *Xenopus* oocytes mimics gonadotropin treatment. *Science* 240:1231-323.

McKeehan W, Ham RG (1978) Calcium and magnesium ions and the regulation of multiplication in normal and transformed cells. *Nature* 275:756-8.

Moscatelli D, Sanui H, Rubin H (1979) Effects of depletion of K^{+}, Na^{+}, or Ca^{2+}, on DNA synthesis and cell cation content in chick embryo fibroblasts. *J Cell Physiol* 101:117-28.

Murphy E, Freudenrich CC, Levy LA, London RE (1989) Monitoring cytosolic free magnesium in cultured chicken heart cells by use of the fluorescent indicator Furaptra. *Proc Natl Acad Sci USA* 86:2981-4.

Raju B, Murphy E, Levy LA, Hall RD, London RE (1989) A fluorescent indicator for measuring cytosolic free magnesium. *Am J Physiol* 256:C540-C8.

Richardson CJ, Schalm SS, Blenis J (2004) PI3-kinase and TOR: PIKTORing cell growth. *Seminars in Dev Biol* 15:147-59.

Rink TJ, Tsien RY, Pozzan T (1982) Cytoplasmic pH and free Mg^{2+} in lymphocytes. *J Cell Biol* 95:189-96.

Rubin H (1975a) Central role for magnesium in coordinate control of metabolism and growth in animal cells. *Proc Natl Acad Sci USA* 72:3551-5.

Rubin H (1975b) Nonspecific nature of the stimulus to DNA synthesis in cultures of chick embryo cell. *Proc Natl Acad Sci USA* 72:1676-80.

Rubin H, Steiner R (1975) Reversible alteration in the mitotic cycle of chick embryo cells in various states of growth regulation. *J Cell Physiol* 85:261-70.

Rubin H (1976) Magnesium deprivation reproduces the coordinate effects of serum removal or cortisol addition on transport and metabolism in chick embryo fibroblasts. *J Cell Physiol* 89:613-26.

Rubin H, Sanui H (1977) Complexes of inorganic pyrophosphate, orthophosphate and calcium as stimulants of 3T3 cells multiplication. *Proc Natl Acad Sci USA* 74:5025-30.

Rubin H, Terasaki M, Sanui H (1978) Magnesium reverses inhibitory effects of calcium deprivation on coordinate response of 3T3 cells to serum. *Proc Natl Acad Sci USA* 75:4379-83.

Rubin H, Terasaki M, Sanui H (1979) Major intracellular cations and growth control: Correspondence among magnesium content, protein synthesis, and the onset of DNA synthesis in Balb/c 3T3 cells. *Proc Natl Acad Sci USA* 76:3917-21.

Rubin H (1981) Growth regulation, reverse transformation, and adaptability of 3T3 cells in decreased Mg^{2+} concentration. *Proc Natl Acad Sci USA* 78:328-32.

Rubin H, Vidair C, Sanui H (1981) Restoration of normal appearance, growth behavior and calcium content to transformed 3T3 cells by magnesium deprivation. *Proc Natl Acad Sci USA* 78:2350-4.

Rubin H, Chu B (1982) Self-normalization of highly transformed 3T3 cells through maximized contact interaction. *Proc Natl Acad Sci USA* 79:1903-7.

Rubin H (2005) Central roles of Mg^{2+} and of $MgATP^{2-}$ in the regulation of protein synthesis and cell proliferation: significance for neoplastic transformation. *Adv Cancer Res* 93:1-58.

Sahni J, Scharenberg AM (2008) TRPM7 ion channels are required for sustained phosphoinositide 3-kinase signaling in lymphocytes. *Cell Metabolism* 8:84-93.

Sahni J, Tamura R, Sweet I, Scharenberg AM (2010) TRPM7 regulates quiescent/proliferative metabolic transitions in lymphocytes. *Cell Cycle* 9:3565-74.

Sanui H, Rubin H (1978) Membrane bound and cellular cationic changes associated with insulin stimulation of cultured cells. *J Cell Physiol* 96:265-78.

Sanui H, Rubin H (1982) Changes of intracellular and externally bound cations accompanying serum stimulation of mouse Balb/c3T3 cells. *Exp Cell Res* 139:15-25.

Sanui H, Rubin H (1984) Ionic changes associated with lead stimulation of DNA synthesis in Balb/c3T3 cells. *Biological Trace Element Research* 6:289-307.

Schmelzle T, Hall MN (2000) TOR, a central controller of cell growth. *Cell* 103:253-62.

Schmitz C, Perraud A-L, Johnson CO, Inabe K, Smith MK, Penner R, Kurosaki T, Fleig A, Scharenberg A (2003) Regulation of vertebrate cellular Mg^{2+} homeostasis by TRPM7. *Cell* 114:191-200.

Schreier MH, Staehelin T (1973) Initiation of mammalian protein synthesis: the importance of ribosome and initiation factor quality for the efficiency of *in vitro* systems. *J Mol Biol* 73:329-49.

Terada N, Patel HR, Takase K, Kohno K, Nairns AC (1994) Rapamycin selectively inhibits translation of mRNAs encoding elongation factors and ribosomal proteins. *Proc Natl Acad Sci USA* 91:11477-81.

Vidair C, Rubin H (1981) Evaluation of Mg^{2+} as an intracellular regulator of uridine uptake. *J Cell Physiol* 108:317-25.

Vidair C, Rubin H (2005) Mg^{2+} as activator of uridine phosphorylation and other cellular responses to growth factors. *Proc Natl Acad Sci USA* 102:662-6.

Magnesium and the Yin-Yang interplay in apoptosis

Valentina Trapani, Lucia Mastrototaro and Federica I. Wolf ✉

Istituto di Patologia Generale e Centro di Ricerche Oncologiche Giovanni XXIII, Università Cattolica del Sacro Cuore, Rome, Italy.
✉ fwolf@rm.unicatt.it

Abstract

Apoptosis is a distinctive feature in the physiology of the developing brain, but also a key event in pathological conditions of the adult brain. The basic mechanisms executing cell death by apoptosis are conserved among different tissues and in different conditions, while the initiating event(s) may be more specific. Magnesium appears to be an important player in the process, though it might exert opposite actions depending on extra/intracellular availability. Extracellular magnesium deficiency induces apoptosis, mainly through increased oxidative stress, while intracellular magnesium mobilization from intracellular stores and consequent increase of cytosolic free magnesium seem to act in the effector phase. The molecular mechanism and the physio-pathological meaning of these findings await further characterization. The issue is even more complex in the context of the brain, where many concurring factors may determine a pro- or anti-apoptotic environment. A deeper understanding of the yin-yang role of magnesium in apoptosis may cast light on the basic processes that regulate cell fate, and consequently may open up novel opportunities for a successful therapeutic intervention for all the pathological conditions where excessive and undue apoptosis takes place.

Cell death by apoptosis

Multicellular organisms maintain their homeostasis thanks to a tightly regulated mode of cell death. Programmed cell death, or apoptosis, is an internally controlled suicide program consisting in a stereotyped sequence of biochemical and morphological changes that allow the cell to die without adversely affecting its neighbors, *i.e.* without causing inflammation. As such, apoptosis is distinct from necrosis, the traumatic form of cell death whereby massive disruption of the surrounding tissue takes place. A cell may be doomed to die either by apoptosis or necrosis depending on the intensity and duration of the stimulus, the rapidity of the death process, and the extent of ATP depletion suffered by the cell.

Apoptosis occurs in numerous physiological, adaptive and pathological events: 1) during development; 2) as a homeostatic mechanism to maintain cell populations in proliferating tissues; 3) as a defense mechanism such as in immune reactions; 4) following cell injury from various agents; and 5) in aging. There is general agreement that this form of cell death is an energy-dependent cascade of molecular events leading to cell shrinkage with maintenance of organelle integrity; long recognized features of apoptosis are protein cleavage and cross-linking, chromatin condensation, DNA fragmentation and, ultimately, phagocytic recognition and engulfment of the dying cell. The process of apoptosis is triggered by a diverse range of cell signals, which may originate either extracellularly (*i.e.* death receptor ligation with their cognate ligands, extrinsic pathway) or intracellularly (*e.g.* DNA damage or organelle dysfunction, intrinsic pathway).

The apoptotic cascade consists of three parts: first, cells process the receptor-mediated death signal (initiation phase, somewhat more cell-specific), then get ready to implement apoptosis (effector phase, more conserved among different tissues) and finally commit suicide (degradation phase). During the initiation phase, the receptor-mediated death signal activates an intracellular cascade of events including: *i)* activation of initiator caspases (caspase-8, for example), that can act early in the cell death process before, or independently of, mitochondrial changes; *ii)* increase in levels of oxyradicals and Ca^{2+}; *iii)* transcription and translocation of pro-apoptotic Bcl-2 family members (Bax and Bad) to the mitochondrial membrane. The execution phase involves: *i)* increased mitochondrial Ca^{2+} and oxyradical levels; *ii)* opening of permeability transition pores (PTP) in the mitochondrial membrane; *iii)* release of cytochrome *c* and many other apoptosis-inducing factors from the mitochondrial matrix into the cytosol; *iv)* formation of a molecular complex (the apoptosome) between cytochrome *c* and apoptotic protease-activating factor 1 (Apaf-1), that recruits and activates pro-caspase-9. Activated caspase-9, in turn, activates caspase-3, which begins the degradation phase: proteins are cleaved by various caspases and packed by transglutaminases, while nucleic acids are cleaved by activated Ca^{2+}/Mg^{2+} endonucleases, which results in the formation of apoptotic bodies and subsequent phagocytosis by elicited macrophages or neighboring cells. It is interesting to underline the role of mitochondria in triggering apoptosis. Whether or not a direct injury jeopardizing the efficiency of these energy producing organelles occurs, mitochondria play a pivotal role in the cell death decision, as apoptotic factors are released by active mechanisms which can be unrelated to mitochondrial damage (Tait and Green, 2010).

Role of Magnesium in Apoptosis

In the attempt to review the role of magnesium in apoptosis, one should first of all keep in mind that the effects of extracellular magnesium availability may differ from those due to intracellular magnesium fluxes or mobilization. In fact, decreased extracellular magnesium availability does not necessarily reflect an intracellular depletion, as demonstrated by the fact that *in vivo* serum magnesium levels are not a reliable marker of pathological hypomagnesemia. Sensitivity to extracellular magnesium availability is highly tissue-specific, and can be translated in molecular terms by considering the expression and activity of magnesium-specific cation channels, such as the transient receptor potential melastatin (TRPM) -6 and -7 channels, which, by modulating transmembrane cation fluxes, regulate the intracellular ion concentration (Schlingmann *et al*, 2007). Furthermore, intracellular magnesium is tightly buffered to meet specific metabolic requirements. As discussed elsewhere in this book, large changes in total cell magnesium occur with little or no change in cytosolic free magnesium, suggesting that the changes in total magnesium are due to changes in bound or sequestered magnesium (Murphy, 2000). ATP is the most important intracellular magnesium buffer. Following massive ATP hydrolysis intracellular free magnesium transiently increases and is subsequently released into the extracellular environment. As a consequence, in a dying cell an increase in ionized magnesium occurs. Therefore, caution should be used also when investigating the role of intracellular magnesium as a player in the apoptotic program, in order to discriminate coincidental from causative events.

In conclusion, whether considering extracellular magnesium availability or intracellular magnesium concentration, the story is more complicated than it appears at first glance. We will attempt to discuss the issue by reviewing the latest available data in view of the complex cellular physiology of magnesium.

Extracellular magnesium and apoptosis

Several important aspects of magnesium biochemistry and physiology point to a possible role for this cation in the apoptotic process. As discussed in other chapters of this book, magnesium is a key modulator of cell proliferation and metabolism and, most importantly, magnesium availability appears to affect the occurrence of oxidative stress. Many studies are available in the literature on the subject, but the most convincing ones investigate the effects of hypomagnesemia *in vivo*. In these circumstances, however, other factors, including inflammation, cytokine production and activation of phagocyte oxidative burst, concur to what is referred to as the pro-oxidant effect of hypomagnesemia (Mazur *et al*, 2007). Induction of apoptosis mediated by oxidative stress following magnesium deprivation has been documented in several tissues. Accelerated thymus involution, a classical example of apoptosis, was found in magnesium-deficient rats (Malpuech-Brugère *et al*, 1999). Dietary magnesium deficiency also induced apoptosis in cardiovascular tissues (Altura *et al*, 2009; Tejero-Taldo *et al*, 2007) and in the liver (Martin *et al*, 2003; Martin *et al*, 2008). In addition to the induction of reactive oxygen species, low magnesium availability could in principle trigger apoptosis by affecting DNA structure. This occurs not only by promoting oxidative DNA damage, but also by impairing DNA repair mechanisms, since magnesium is required for several crucial DNA repair enzyme activities, *e.g.* endonucleases, ligases, topoisomerases (Hartwig, 2001).

Intracellular magnesium and apoptosis

As to intracellular events, several *in vitro* studies have suggested a promoting role for magnesium in apoptosis. An early increase in intracellular magnesium seems to follow both extrinsic and intrinsic induction of apoptosis (Patel *et al*, 1994; Chien *et al*, 1999; Zhang *et al*, 2005). The most straightforward explanation is that the increase in intracellular magnesium concentration is necessary for stimulating the activity of Ca^{2+}/ Mg^{2+}dependent endonucleases, which perform the apoptotic event *par excellence*, *i.e.* nucleosomal DNA fragmentation. Interestingly, however, the source of intracellular magnesium was hypothesized to be in the mitochondria (Chien *et al*, 1999), which is particularly appealing, as it is well established that mitochondria play a central role in the onset of the apoptotic program. Other lines of evidence point to the same direction. While the opening of the permeability transition pores appears to be dispensable for the release of cytochrome c, this is not the case for the presence of magnesium, which instead seems an absolute requirement (Eskes *et al*, 1998; Kim *et al*, 2000). Another study (Salvi *et al*, 2004) indicated that an apoptotic compound, gliotoxin, can specifically activate a magnesium efflux system from mitochondria in conditions of preserved mitochondrial integrity (*i.e.* high membrane potential, no swelling and retention of other ions). Most importantly, it has been shown that mitochondria act in fact as magnesium stores, and Mg^{2+} release can occur following Ca^{2+} release and prior to ATP hydrolysis (Kubota *et al*, 2005). It is noteworthy that the same Authors have recently demonstrated that glutamate administration to rat hippocampal neurons triggers the same pathway, whereby Ca^{2+} accumulation in the mitochondria is required for Mg^{2+} release from the organelles (Shindo *et al*, 2010). The presence of a specific mitochondrial channel for magnesium, Mrs2, (Kolisek *et al*, 2003) corroborates these findings; as the activity of Mrs2 is dependent from membrane potential, it can be speculated that stored magnesium might be released through the channel upon depolarization. Intriguingly, in a recent paper Mrs2 expression has been associated with resistance to drug-induced apoptosis in cancer cells (Chen *et al*, 2009): by upregulating magnesium uptake into mitochondria, Mrs2 might counteract the increase in cytosolic magnesium that seems to be necessary for the execution of the apoptotic program *via* the mitochondrial pathway (Wolf and Trapani, 2009). In conclusion, the latest findings seem to concur to suggest a finer involvement of magnesium in the apoptotic cascade: not just a biochemical factor, but rather a crucial control element in life *vs.* death decisions (see Table I for a summary). At present, these are only attractive speculations; most importantly, it has to be clarified whether the increase in intracellular magnesium occurring following an apoptotic stimulus is just a coincidental event (for example, due to mitochondrial depolarization) or rather a causative determinant in the downstream signaling cascade.

Table1: Magnesium and apoptosis

EXTRACELLULAR	INTRACELLULAR
DECREASED MAGNESIUM Impaired trophic signaling factor Increased oxidative stress Increased DNA damage Decreased DNA repair 🡻 **EXTRINSIC AND INTRINSIC PATHWAY**	**INCREASED MAGNESIUM** Mitochondrial damage Mitochondrial dysfunction Ca^{2+} signals Excitotoxicity 🡻 **INTRINSIC PATHWAY**

Neuronal Apoptosis

In contrast to the rapid turnover of cells in proliferative/renewing tissues, neurons commonly survive for the entire lifetime of the organism — this enduring nature of neurons is necessary for maintaining the function of those cells within neuronal circuits. However, during development of the central and peripheral nervous systems, many neurons undergo apoptosis during a time window that coincides with the process of synaptogenesis (Oppenheim, 1991). Initial overproduction of neurons, followed by death of some, is probably an adaptive process that provides enough neurons to form nerve cell circuits that are precisely matched to their functional specifications. However, the persistence of neurons throughout life to preserve brain function implies that a consider-able evolutionary pressure was placed on the development of mechanisms that guarded against neuronal death and/or promoted neuronal survival and plasticity.

Trophic factors

Like all cells, neuronal survival requires trophic support. Viktor Hamburger and Rita Levi-Montalcini described in a seminal paper that the survival of developing neurons is directly related to the availability of their innervating targets (Hamburger and Levi-Montalcini, 1949). This laid the foundation for the neurotrophin hypothesis, which proposed that immature neurons compete for target-derived trophic factors that are in limited supply. Neurotrophins, which include nerve growth factor (NGF), brain-derived neurotrophic factor (BDNF), and neurotrophins 3 and 4/5 (Lewin and Barde, 1996), generally activate and ligate the Trk receptors (TrkA, TrkB and TrkC), which are cell-surface receptors with intrinsic tyrosine kinase activity. They can autophosphorylate; for instance, after the binding of NGF to TrkA, the receptor phosphorylates several tyrosine residues within its own cytoplasmic tail. These phosphotyrosines in turn serve as docking sites for other molecules such as phospholipase Cg, phosphoinositide 3-kinase (PI(3)K) and adaptor proteins such as Shc, and these signal transduction molecules coordinate neuronal survival through the Akt and MAP kinase signaling pathways (Hennigan *et al*, 2007). Several neurotrophic factors and cytokines use a survival pathway involving the transcription factor NF-κB (Mattson and Camandola, 2000). The neurotrophin hypothesis predicts correctly that neuronal survival requires a positive survival signal; it did not, however, provide a concrete hypothesis as to how neurons die in the absence of trophic support; it was assumed that neurons die simply of passive starvation. In 1988, using cultured sympathetic neurons as a model system, Johnson and colleagues showed that inhibition of RNA and protein synthesis blocked sympathetic neuronal cell death induced by nerve growth factor (NGF) deprivation (Martin *et al*, 1988), providing the first tangible evidence that neurons might actually actively instigate their own demise.

Glutamate receptors

Lack of neurotrophic support is undeniably the best-studied signal which may trigger apoptosis during development of the nervous system. However, most neurons in the mammalian central nervous system possess receptors for another trigger of apoptosis, glutamate.

Glutamate is a major excitatory neurotransmitter with a crucial role in neural development, synaptic plasticity, and learning and memory under physiological conditions (Riedel *et al*, 2003). Glutamate receptors are classified into several classes. In this context, we will go into some detail only for N-methyl-D-aspartate (NMDA) receptors. NMDA receptors are tetra-heteromeric ligand-gated ion channels that open upon the binding of glutamate. Magnesium binds the channel pore in a voltage-dependent manner; thus, at normal physiological resting membrane potential, the NMDA receptor is blocked by Mg^{2+}. Synaptic release of glutamate causes Na^{+} influx through α-amino-3-hydroxy-5-methyl-4-isoxazole-propionate (AMPA) receptors in the postsynaptic cell, resulting in partial membrane depolarization sufficient to lift the Mg^{2+} block and activate the channel. The activated NMDA receptor is permeable to Na^{+} but, crucially, also to Ca^{2+}. This Ca^{2+} influx mediates most of the physiological effects of NMDA receptor activity, leading to postsynaptic depolarization and action potential in the postsynaptic neuron.

Physiological levels of synaptic NMDA receptor activity are essential for neuronal survival (Hetman and Kharebava, 2006). However, regulation of glutamatergic neurotransmission is critical, as improper management of glutamate levels and glutamate receptor activity may impair not only its signaling properties, but can lead to cell death. The concept of excitotoxicity was first proposed by John Olney in 1969 as a toxic effect of excessive or prolonged activation of receptors by excitatory amino acids (Olney, 1969). Although the molecular pathways involved in excitotoxicity are still not fully understood at the present, there is a wealth of evidence suggesting that over-stimulation of glutamate receptors produces multiple adverse effects including impairment of intracellular calcium homeostasis, dysfunction of mitochondria and endoplasmic reticulum, increase in nitric oxide (NO) production and free radicals, persistent activation of proteases and kinases, increases in expression of pro-death transcription factors and immediate early genes (IEGs), ultimately leading to apoptosis (Wang and Qin, 2010). Excitotoxicity might mediate neuronal damage in various neurological disorders including ischemia and traumatic brain injury (Arundine and Tymianski, 2004) and neurodegenerative diseases (Lipton and Rosenberg, 1994; Rego and Oliveira, 2003); it has also been implicated in neonatal brain injury (Johnston, 2005). NMDA receptors are important mediators of glutamate-induced excitotoxicity, as calcium entering through over-activated NMDA receptors results in more cell death as opposed to calcium entering through non-NMDA glutamate receptors or voltage-gated calcium channels (Cristofanilli and Akopian, 2006), which maybe due in part to their high permeability to Ca^{2+} and incomplete desensitization.

Thus, responses to NMDA receptor activity follow a classical hormetic dose-response curve: both too much and too little can be harmful (Hardingham, 2009).

Pathological stimuli

Another trigger of neuronal death is increased oxidative stress, whereby free radicals (such as the superoxide anion radical and the hydroxyl radical) damage cellular lipids, proteins and nucleic acids by disrupting chemical bonds in those molecules. Metabolic stress, in which levels of glucose, oxygen and other molecules required for ATP (energy) production are decreased, and environmental toxins may also initiate neuronal apoptosis (Mattson, 2000). These stimuli are mostly involved in aging and pathological conditions, such as acute or chronic neuro-degenerative diseases. The classical and most studied pathway of oxidation-induced apoptosis consists in cell-damage triggered phosphorylation of p53 and transcription of pro-apoptotic factors like Bid or Bad leading to mitochondrial-dependent activation of caspase 9.

The genetic and environmental factors that trigger neuronal apoptosis may be different in various physiological and pathological settings and can vary from those active in other tissues, but most of the subsequent biochemical events that execute the cell death process are highly conserved and shared with all other cell types. Thus, the key components of the apoptosis program in neurons, like that of other cell types, are Apaf-1 and proteins in the Bcl-2 and caspase families. Nevertheless, different types of neurons, and neurons at different developmental stages, express different combinations of Bcl-2 and caspase family members, which is one way of providing the specificity of regulation (Yuan and Yankner, 2000).

Tissue specific factors

An alternative way to control cell death or survival is through the expression of tissue-specific proteins that affect signal transduction reactions and may be either pro-apoptotic or pro-survival.

The prostate apoptosis response-4 (Par-4) protein was identified as being upregulated in prostate tumor cells undergoing apoptosis, but is now known to be essential in developmental and pathological neuronal death (Guo *et al*, 1998). Levels of Par-4 increase rapidly in response to various apoptotic stimuli through enhanced translation of Par-4 messenger RNA. Par-4 acts at an early stage of the apoptotic cascade prior to caspase activation and mitochondrial dys-function, by a mechanism that may involve inhibition of the antiapoptotic transcription factor NF-kβ and suppression of Bcl-2 expression and/or function (Mattson *et al*, 1999).

Rai is an Shc-related adaptor protein whose expression is exclusively restricted to the nervous system. It exerts a prosurvival function in neuronal cells by activating the PI3K/Akt signaling pathway (Pelicci *et al*, 2002).

A neuron-specific splice variant of the variable subunit Bβ was characterized, which is induced upon neuronal differentiation, targets protein phosphatase 2A to mitochondria and accelerates neuronal cell apoptosis after survival factor deprivation (Dagda *et al*, 2003).

Lately, a brain-specific isoform of mitochondrial apoptosis-inducing factor, AIF2, has been isolated (Hangen *et al*, 2010). AIF2 dimerizes with AIF1 and has a stronger membrane anchorage; therefore it is conceivable the neuron-specific AIF2 may have been 'designed' to be retained in mitochondria and to minimize its potential neurotoxic activity.

In conclusion, although mature neurons are among the most long-lived cell types in mammals, immature neurons die in large numbers and the regulation of apoptosis has a major role in sculpting the developing brain. Furthermore, not only is apoptosis important in regulating neuronal development, but it might also be a cardinal feature in the adult brain in several pathological conditions that will be detailed in the section on neurodegenerative diseases.

Role of Magnesium in Neuronal Apoptosis

Deciphering the role of magnesium in the apoptotic process is further complicated in the nervous system, as the blood brain barrier may restrain serum magnesium availability within the CNS. Indeed, this has been advocated as the cause for the failure of clinical trials assessing magnesium therapy in acute and chronic brain injury (Vink *et al*, 2009).

A significant part of the literature on the effects of magnesium on apoptosis in the brain is related to perinatal brain, as magnesium is often used as a treatment for pre-eclampsia/eclampsia and preterm labor. The basis for its use as a tocolytic is due to its observed effects in reducing myometrial contractility through extra- and intracellular mechanisms of action (Fomin *et al*, 2006). However, the use of magnesium sulphate as a drug in obstetrical medicine for both mother and fetus is highly controversial. A recent meta-analysis of all trials has recommended the use of magnesium for neuroprotection in the preterm fetus, as it resulted both safe and effective (Doyle *et al*, 2009). Nevertheless, some caution is mandatory, as several reports point to detrimental effects of magnesium for the fetal brain, depending on the dose (Mittendorf *et al*, 2006; Dribben *et al*, 2009), on the period of neurodevelopment when the exposure occurred (Dribben *et al*, 2009) or on the level of stress experienced (Krueger *et al*, 2001). In addition, some papers report a pro-apoptotic action of magnesium in placental tissues (Black *et al*, 2001; Gude *et al*, 2000). The major hurdle to establishing protective or deleterious effects of tocolytic magnesium to the developing brain is that magnesium's effects on preterm infant's brains, and the mechanisms of those effects, are not understood.

As discussed earlier, neuronal apoptosis can be triggered by three main mechanisms: 1) lack of growth factors; 2) overstimulation of glutamate receptors; and 3) oxidative stress. Magnesium could play a (different) role in each of these signaling pathways.

First, most growth factors work through receptor tyrosine kinases (RTKs) which require two magnesium ions for maximal activity. Kinases downstream of these RTKs, such as PI -kinase and the anti-apoptotic kinase Akt require magnesium both for their activation and activity. Therefore extracellular magnesium could modulate the effect of growth factors on CNS cells, or activate their second messenger systems directly, ultimately affecting viability, proliferation, and apoptosis in these cells.

Secondly, under conditions of normal membrane polarization magnesium is known to block the NMDA glutamate receptor and prevent ion flow through the channel. Therefore, in principle, magnesium should protect against excitotoxicity-induced apoptosis. Nevertheless, as already discussed, normal physiological patterns of NMDA receptor activity promote neuroprotection against both apoptotic and excitotoxic insults; *vice versa*, NMDA receptor blockade can promote neuronal death outright or render neurons vulnerable to secondary trauma (Hardingham, 2009). Indeed, most NMDA antagonists have miserably failed as neuroprotective agents in clinical trials, in large part because of intolerable side effects (Lipton, 2006). Moreover, it has been shown that various drugs that inhibit neuronal activity, including NMDA antagonists, trigger widespread apoptotic neurodegeneration in the developing brain and cause long-term neurobehavioral deficits; in the infant rodent brain, peak sensitivity to this effect is in the P3 to P7 period (Ikonomidou *et al*, 1999). Thus, although other mechanisms may play a role, it seems likely that the neuroapoptogenic action demonstrated for magnesium in some studies could be mediated by its action at NMDA receptors.

Third, as mentioned earlier on, magnesium deprivation may induce or exacerbate oxidative stress, another trigger of neuronal death, especially in pathological conditions; on this regard magnesium supplementation might well have a neuroprotective action.

Apoptosis in neurodegenerative diseases

As already mentioned, neuronal death by apoptosis is a distinctive physiological feature of the developing brain; once synaptogenesis is over, the remaining neurons will usually survive throughout life to preserve brain function. Unfortunately, however, many people experience excessive death of specific neuronal sub-populations as a result of chronic diseases including Alzheimer's disease, Parkinson's disease, Huntington's disease and amyotrophic lateral sclerosis. Neuronal death may also occur as a consequence of acute conditions, such as stroke or traumatic brain and spinal cord injury. For each of these disorders, apoptosis has been implicated as the main form of cell death, though it is very difficult to demonstrate it for both technical and ethical reasons. Much of the evidence supporting an apoptotic mode of neuronal death comes from studies of animal and cell-culture models of neurodegenerative disorders (Mattson, 2000).

Physiological apoptosis in the developing brain and pathological apoptosis in the adult brain share similar molecular mechanisms in the effector phase, but may differ in the initiation. Whereas trophic factor withdrawal has a prominent role in apoptosis during development, toxic insults resulting from biochemical or genetic accidents seem to be the triggering event in neurodegenerative disorders. An emerging theme is the toxicity of abnormal protein structures or aggregates (Yuan and Yankner, 2000). Indeed, a defining feature of Alzheimer's disease is accumulation of amyloid plaques formed by aggregates of amyloid-β peptide (Aβ), Parkinson's disease is characterized by the appearance of α-synuclein oligomers, Huntington's disease is caused by expansions of a trinucleotide (CAG) sequence in the huntingtin gene producing a protein containing increased polyglutamine repeats, and the neuropathological signature of amyotrophic lateral sclerosis (ALS) is the presence of ubiquitinated inclusions immuno-reactive for the proteins TDP-43 and/or FUS/TLS in the cytoplasm of motor neurons. Moreover, mutations in specific genes may predispose to neuronal degeneration, *e.g.* presenilin in Alzheimer's disease, parkin in Parkinson's disease, huntingtin in Huntington's disease, and Cu/Zn-superoxide dismutase (SOD) in ALS (please refer to the dedicated chapters in this book for further details).

The identification of specific genetic and environmental factors responsible for chronic neurodegenerative disorders has bolstered evidence for a shared pathway of neuronal apoptosis involving oxidative stress, perturbed calcium homeostasis and mitochondrial dysfunction ultimately converging on caspase activation (Zündorf and Reiser, 2010; Gibson *et al*, 2010).

In Alzheimer's disease, toxic forms of Aβ may induce Ca^{2+} influx into neurons by formation of an oligomeric pore in the plasma membrane, thereby rendering neurons vulnerable to excitotoxicity and apoptosis (Supnet and Bezprozvanny, 2010). Aβ also generates hydrogen peroxide and hydroxyl radicals, producing membrane lipid peroxidation and consequently membrane depolarization and excitotoxicity through NMDA receptor channels and voltage-gated Ca^{2+} channels (Sultana and Butterfield, 2010; Butterfield *et al*, 2010). In addition, Aβ accumulates in mitochondria, impairs the activity of complexes III and IV of the respiratory chain, causes elevated cytoplasmic Ca^{2+} levels and oxidative stress, and reduces ATP synthesis, further increasing Ca^{2+} overload and oxidative stress (Moreira *et al*, 2010).

Mitochondrial dysfunction is a defect occurring early in the pathogenesis of both sporadic and familial Parkinson's disease. Mitochondrial association of α-synuclein in cells was linked to impairment of respiratory complex I activity, oxidative modification of mitochondrial proteins, and increased levels of Ca^{2+} and nitric oxide (Navarro and Boveris, 2009).

Mitochondrial Ca^{2+} overload is also a decisive commitment step for Huntington's disease. Mutant huntingtin facilitates opening of the PTP and directly impairs the mitochondrial function. Furthermore, huntingtin forms a ternary complex with other proteins, which causes Ca^{2+} release from the ER and renders neurons more sensitive to Ca^{2+}-mediated cellular dysfunction (Damiano *et al*, 2010).

The mutations in SOD responsible for ALS do not decrease antioxidant activity of the enzyme, but result in the gain of an adverse pro-apoptotic activity that may involve increased peroxidase activity. Through interactions with hydrogen peroxide or superoxide anion, the mutant enzyme may induce oxidative damage to membranes and disturbances in mitochondrial function that make neurons vulnerable to excitotoxic apoptosis (Vucic and Kiernan, 2009). Also stroke and trauma, and the consequent brain ischemia, initiate biochemical and molecular events involving many of the same neurodegenerative cascades that occur in the chronic neurodegenerative diseases described above, namely excitotoxicity, calcium overload and oxidative stress (Arundine and Tymianski, 2004).

In conclusion, despite the concurrence of diverse genetic and environmental factors for acute and chronic neurodegenerative disorders, such conditions possess a common denominator as to the ultimate mechanisms executing neuronal death, which are identical to those involved in normal brain development and all converge to mitochondrial dysfunction. On one hand, these findings testify the evolutionary importance of conserving fundamental processes; on the other hand, they call for further research to understand the basic mechanisms and the key regulators of neuronal fate, as novel opportunities for targeted therapeutic intervention may arise.

Role of magnesium in neurodegenerative diseases

As detailed above, there is increasing evidence that neuronal death by apoptosis is associated with both acute and chronic neurodegenerative disorders. Interestingly, brain free magnesium levels have been shown to decline in a number of such pathologies (Vink *et al*, 2009). As a consequence, a considerable research effort has been directed toward establishing the mechanisms of such decline and the potential for magnesium administration as a neuroprotective agent.

Brain magnesium decline is a ubiquitous feature of traumatic brain injury and is associated with the development of motor and cognitive deficits. Experimentally, parenteral administration of magnesium up to 12 h post trauma restores brain magnesium homeostasis and profoundly improves both motor and cognitive outcome. Although the mechanism of action is unclear, magnesium has been shown to attenuate a variety of secondary injury factors, including brain edema, cerebral vasospasms, glutamate excitotoxicity, calcium-mediated events, lipid peroxidation, mitochondrial permeability transition, and apoptosis. Disappointingly, magnesium therapy has failed in clinical trials. Increase in brain free magnesium concentration seems to be essential to confer neuroprotection, and intravenous magnesium administration only marginally increases CSF magnesium concentration, which suggests that the integrity of the blood-brain barrier and the regulation of magnesium in the cerebrospinal fluid are largely maintained following acute brain injury and limit magnesium bioavailability in the brain (Vink and Nimmo, 2009).

Magnesium therapy has also been described in the clinical stroke literature, with similar negative results, though magnesium was shown to be beneficial in a subgroup of patients with noncortical, or lacunar strokes (Ginsberg, 2008). Magnesium may protect via multiple mechanisms, including NMDA receptor blockade, inhibition of excitatory neurotransmitter release, blockade of calcium channels, as well as vascular smooth muscle relaxation, and may be more bioavailable, as it is well known that the blood brain barrier around infarcted tissue is highly permeable, thus potentially facilitating local magnesium entry to the injured tissues.

Intriguingly, the cation channel TRPM7, which is crucial for Mg^{2+} homeostasis and cell survival (Schmitz *et al*, 2003), seems to be a critical mediator of anoxic cell death. It appears that TRPM7 gating lies downstream of NMDA receptor-mediated NO free-radical production. In this paradigm, excitotoxicity is likely the initiating signal in a cell death cascade that involves nNOS activation with subsequent peroxynitrite production, which in turn activates TRPM7 channels. Calcium influx through TRPM7 then creates a positive feedback loop of ROS production, which eventually kills the cell (Aarts and Tymianski, 2005). TRPM7 suppression made neurons resistant to ischemic death after brain ischemia and preserved neuronal morphology and function; also, it prevented ischemia-induced deficits in long-term potentiation and preserved performance in memory tasks (Sun *et al*, 2009). The role of the magnesium-specific channel TRPM6 in these processes is currently unclear, but, given its localization in the brain, its permeability to Mg^{2+} and its functional interaction with TRPM7, it may be involved in neuronal death as well (Cook *et al*, 2009). At present, the role of TRPM6/7 channels in magnesium transport seems less important than their facilitation of other cation fluxes, but it cannot be ruled out, especially considering the known involvement of magnesium in excitotoxicity and oxidative stress, as discussed earlier.

With respect to chronic brain degeneration, the first connection between magnesium and three apparently dissimilar neurodegenerative disorders (ALS, Parkinson's and Alzheimer's diseases) came from the observation that those conditions occurred at extraordinarily high rates in geographically separate foci among three genetically different, homogenous Western Pacific populations (Durlach *et al*, 1997). Intensive research conducted over the years led to the identification of two candidate environmental factors: *i*) severely low levels of Ca^{2+} and Mg^{2+} in the soil and drinking water coupled with abnormal mineral metabolism; and *ii*) the putative neurotoxin b-methylamino-L-alanine (L-BMAA), derived from the cycad plant, a traditional food source in Guam. Experimental findings supported this hypothesis: animals fed diets that mimic the mineral composition in the disease foci environment showed signs of neuronal damage; of the various combinations of Ca^{2+} and Mg^{2+} contents tested, exposure to low Mg^{2+} (one-fifth of the normal level), was more deleterious, causing significant loss of dopaminergic neurons in the substantia nigra (Oyanagi *et al*, 2006). Furthermore, motor neurons are selectively more vulnerable to L-BMAA toxicity, and these toxic effects are mediated through $[Ca^{2+}]_i$ rises via Ca-A/K channels and other pathways, and subsequent reactive oxygen species generation (Rao *et al*, 2006).

In the hyperendemic foci in the Western Pacific, the unique mineral composition of the environment creates a condition of increased oxidative stress because low Mg^{2+} levels cause lipid peroxidation while transition metals act as redox catalysts causing increased ROS production. Therefore, the genes whose function is most likely to be affected are ion channels expressed in the CNS and modulated by oxidative stress. TRPM7 and TRPM2 fulfill these conditions; their functional properties are interconnected with calcium and magnesium homeostasis, oxidative stress, mitochondrial dysfunction, and immune mechanisms, all principal suspects in neurodegeneration (Hermosura and Garruto, 2007). Indeed, variants of both genes have been found in Guamanian neurodegenerative disorders and may contribute to their pathogenesis (Hermosura *et al*, 2008; Hermosura *et al*, 2005).

Despite the evidence implicating magnesium in the etiology of neurodegenerative diseases, the therapeutic effects of magnesium supplementation are not well documented. Magnesium administration proved beneficial in an *in vitro* model of Parkinson's disease, where in particular magnesium concentration seems critical in the onset of the disease (Hashimoto *et al*, 2008), but there is still much to be done to fully appreciate the therapeutic potential of magnesium.

Conclusion

An extensive and up-to-date review of the literature shows that drawing a clear-cut conclusion on the role of magnesium in neuroapoptosis is not an easy task. Magnesium may play pleiotropic roles in different stages of

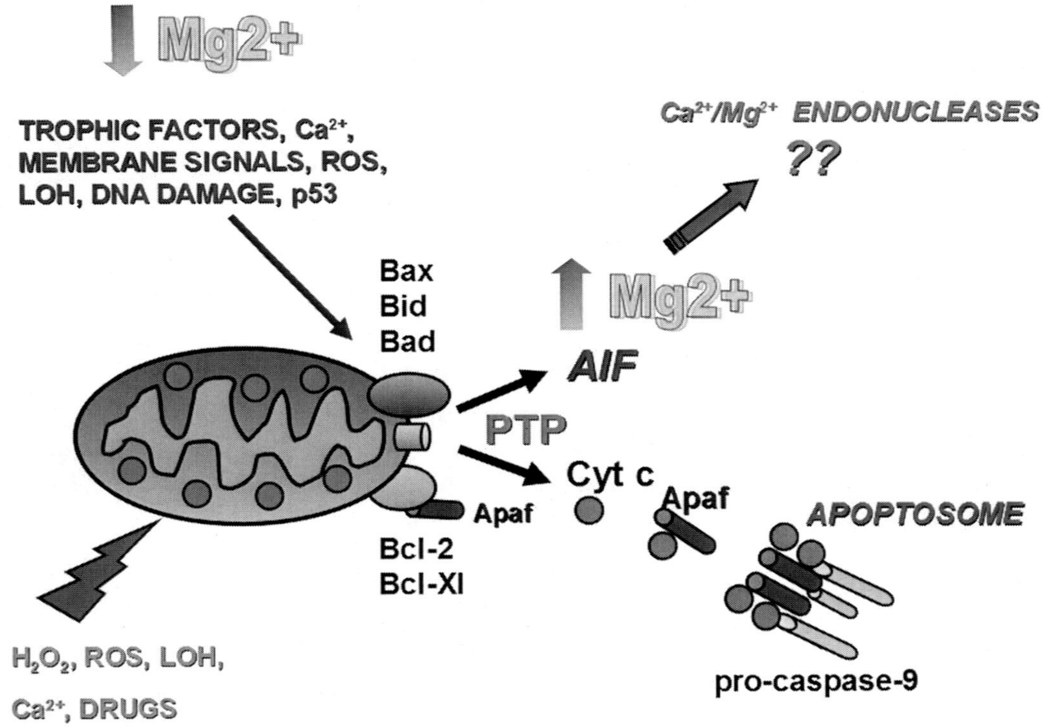

Figure 1. Potential points of interaction between magnesium and apoptotic factors.

the apoptotic process, that range from modulating growth factor- and Ca^{2+}-dependent signal transduction to affecting oxidative stress-related reactions. From this point of view, increased extracellular magnesium availability should in principle be considered anti-apoptogenic. On the other hand, an increase in cytosolic free magnesium, which seems to be released from mitochondrial stores, appears to accompany the intrinsic apoptotic process. The pathophysiological meaning of this occurrence in the context of apoptosis induction/execution awaits to be defined (see Figure 1 for a summary).

On a more physiological ground, in the brain magnesium availability should be considered within a more complex and interconnected picture, where other conditions, such as developmental stage, inflammation, acute or chronic injuries, blood brain barrier integrity, *etc.* may concur in determining a pro or anti-apoptotic environment.

We believe that further investigation into the role of magnesium in the molecular mechanisms of apoptosis is warranted for a deeper understanding of the basic processes that regulate cell fate, and ultimately for a successful therapeutic intervention when these processes go awry.

Acknowledgments
Supported by the Italian Ministry of Education, University and Research PRIN 2007ZT39FN and Linea D1 2004-2009.

References

Aarts MM, and Tymianski M (2005) TRPM7 and ischemic CNS injury. *Neuroscientist* 11:116-123.

Altura BM, Shah NC, Jiang XC, Li Z, Perez-Albela JL, Sica AC, Altura BT (2009) Short-term magnesium deficiency results in decreased levels of serum sphingomyelin, lipid peroxidation, and apoptosis in cardiovascular tissues. *Am J Physiol Heart Circ Physiol* 297:H86-92.

Arundine M, Tymianski M (2004) Molecular mechanisms of glutamate-dependent neurodegeneration in ischemia and traumatic brain injury. *Cell Mol Life Sci* 61:657-68.

Black S, Yu H, Lee J, Sachchithananthan M, Medcalf RL (2001) Physiologic concentrations of magnesium and placental apoptosis: prevention by antioxidants. *Obstet Gynecol* 98:319-24.

Butterfield DA, Bader Lange ML, Sultana R (2010) Involvements of the lipid peroxidation product, HNE, in the pathogenesis and progression of Alzheimer's disease. Biochim Biophys Acta 1801(8):924-9.

Chen Y, Wei X, Yan P, Han Y, Sun S, Wu K, Fan D (2009) Human mitochondrial Mrs2 protein promotes multidrug resistance in gastric cancer cells by regulating p27, cyclin D1 expression and cytochrome C release. *Cancer Biol Ther* 8:607-14.

Chien MM, Zahradka KE, Newell MK, Freed JH (1999) Fas-induced B cell apoptosis requires an increase in free cytosolic magnesium as an early event. *J Biol Chem* 274:7059-66.

Cook NL, van den Heuvel C, Vink R (2009) Are the transient receptor potential melastatin (TRPM) channels important in magnesium homeostasis following traumatic brain injury? *Magnes Res* 22:225-234.

Cristofanilli M, Akopian A (2006) Calcium channel and glutamate receptor activities regulate actin organization in salamander retinal neurons. *J Physiol* 575:543–554

Dagda RK, Zaucha JA, Wadzinski BE, Strack S (2003) A developmentally regulated, neuron-specific splice variant of the variable subunit Bbeta targets protein phosphatase 2A to mitochondria and modulates apoptosis. *J Biol Chem* 278:24976-85.

Damiano M, Galvan L, Déglon N, Brouillet E (2010) Mitochondria in Huntington's disease. *Biochim Biophys Acta* 1802:52-61.

Deshmukh M, Johnson EM (1997) Programmed cell death in neurons: focus on the pathway of nerve growth factor deprivation-induced death of sympathetic neurons. *Mol Pharmacol* 51:897-906.

Doyle LW, Crowther CA, Middleton P, Marret S, Rouse D (2009) Magnesium sulphate for women at risk of preterm birth for neuroprotection of the fetus. *Cochrane Database Syst Rev* (1):CD004661.

Durlach J, Bac P, Durlach V, Durlach A, Bara M, Guiet-Bara A (1997) Are age-related neurodegenerative diseases linked with various types of magnesium depletion? *Magnes Res* 10:339-53.

Eskes R, Antonsson B, Osen-Sand A, Montessuit S, Richter C, Sadoul R, Mazzei G, Nichols A, Martinou JC (1998) Bax-induced cytochrome C release from mitochondria is independent of the permeability transition pore but highly dependent on Mg^{2+} ions. *J Cell Biol* 143:217-24.

Fomin VP, Gibbs SG, Vanam R, Morimiya A, Hurd WW (2006) Effect of magnesium sulfate on contractile force and intracellular calcium concentration in pregnant human myometrium. *Am J Obstet Gynecol* 194:1384–1390.

Gibson GE, Starkov A, Blass JP, Ratan RR, Beal MF (2010) Cause and consequence: mitochondrial dysfunction initiates and propagates neuronal dysfunction, neuronal death and behavioral abnormalities in age-associated neurodegenerative diseases. *Biochim Biophys Acta* 1802:122-34.

Ginsberg MD (2008) Neuroprotection for ischemic stroke: past, present and future. *Neuropharmacology* 55:363-89.

Gude NM, Stevenson JL, Moses EK, King RG (2000) Magnesium regulates hypoxia-stimulated apoptosis in the human placenta. *Clin Sci (Lond)* 98:375-80.

Guo Q, Fu W, Xie J, Luo H, Sells SF, Geddes JW, Bondada V, Rangnekar VM, Mattson MP (1998) Par-4 is a mediator of neuronal degeneration associated with the pathogenesis of Alzheimer disease. *Nature Med* 4:957–962.

Hamburger V, Levi-Montalcini R (1949) Proliferation, differentiation and degeneration in the spinal ganglia of the chick embryo under normal and experimental conditions. *J Exp Zool* 111:457–502.

Hangen E, De Zio D, Bordi M, Zhu C, Dessen P, Caffin F, Lachkar S, Perfettini JL, Lazar V, Benard J, Fimia GM,

Piacentini M, Harper F, Pierron G, Vicencio JM, Bénit P, de Andrade A, Höglinger G, Culmsee C, Rustin P, Blomgren K, Cecconi F, Kroemer G, Modjtahedi N (2010) A brain-specific isoform of mitochondrial apoptosis-inducing factor: AIF2. *Cell Death Differ* 17:1155-66.

Hardingham GE (2009) Coupling of the NMDA receptor to neuroprotective and neurodestructive events. *Biochem Soc Trans* 37(Pt 6):1147-60.

Hartwig A (2001) Role of magnesium in genomic stability. *Mutat Res* 475:113-21.

Hashimoto T, Nishi K, Nagasao J, Tsuji S, Oyanagi K (2008) Magnesium exerts both preventive and ameliorating effects in an in vitro rat Parkinson disease model involving 1-methyl-4-phenylpyridinium (MPP+) toxicity in dopaminergic neurons. *Brain Res* 1197:143-51.

Hennigan A, O'Callaghan RM, Kelly AM (2007) Neurotrophins and their receptors: roles in plasticity, neurodegeneration and neuroprotection. *Biochem Soc Trans* 35(Pt 2):424-7.

Hermosura MC, Cui AM, Go RC, Davenport B, Shetler CM, Heizer JW, Schmitz C, Mocz G, Garruto RM, Perraud AL (2008) Altered functional properties of a TRPM2 variant in Guamanian ALS and PD. *Proc Natl Acad Sci USA* 105:18029-34.

Hermosura MC, Garruto RM (2007) TRPM7 and TRPM2-Candidate susceptibility genes for Western Pacific ALS and PD? *Biochim Biophys Acta* 1772:822-35.

Hermosura MC, Nayakanti H, Dorovkov MV, Calderon FR, Ryazanov AG, Haymer DS, Garruto RM (2005) A TRPM7 variant shows altered sensitivity to magnesium that may contribute to the pathogenesis of two Guamanian neurodegenerative disorders. *Proc Natl Acad Sci USA* 102:11510-5

Hetman M, Kharebava G (2006) Survival signaling pathways activated by NMDA receptors. *Curr Top Med Chem* 6:787-99.

Ikonomidou C, Bosch F, Miksa M, Bittigau P, Vockler J, Dikranian K, Tenkova TI, Stefovska V, Turski L, Olney JW (1999) Blockade of NMDA receptors and apoptotic neurodegeneration in the developing brain. *Science* 283:70–74.

Johnston MV (2005) Excitotoxicity in perinatal brain injury. *Brain Pathol* 15:234-40.

Kim TH, Zhao Y, Barber MJ, Kuharsky DK, Yin XM (2000) Bid-induced cytochrome c release is mediated by a pathway independent of mitochondrial permeability transition pore and Bax. *J Biol Chem* 275:39474-81.

Kolisek M, Zsurka G, Samaj J, Weghuber J, Schweyen RJ, Schweigel M (2003) Mrs2p is an essential component of the major electrophoretic Mg^{2+} influx system in mitochondria. *EMBO J* 22:1235-44.

Krueger RC Jr, Santore MT, Dawson G, Schwartz NB (2001) Increased extracellular magnesium modulates proliferation in fetal neural cells in culture. *Brain Res Dev Brain Res* 127:99-109.

Kubota T, Shindo Y, Tokuno K, Komatsu H, Ogawa H, Kudo S, Kitamura Y, Suzuki K, Oka K (2005) Mitochondria are intracellular magnesium stores: investigation by simultaneous fluorescent imagings in PC12 cells. *Biochim Biophys Acta* 1744:19-28.

Lewin GR, Barde YA (1996) Physiology of the neurotrophins. *Annu Rev Neurosci* 19:289–317.

Lipton SA (2006) Paradigm shift in neuroprotection by NMDA receptor blockade: memantine and beyond. *Nat Rev Drug Discov* 5:160-70.

Lipton SA, Rosenberg PA (1994) Excitatory amino acids as a final common pathway for neurologic disorders. *N Engl J Med* 330:613-22.

Malpuech-Brugère C, Nowacki W, Gueux E, Kuryszko J, Rock E, Rayssiguier Y, Mazur A (1999) Accelerated thymus involution in magnesium-deficient rats is related to enhanced apoptosis and sensitivity to oxidative stress. *Br J Nutr* 81:405-11.

Martin DP, Schmidt RE, Di Stefano PS, Lowry OH, Carter JG, Johnson EM Jr (1988) Inhibitors of protein synthesis and RNA synthesis prevent neuronal death caused by nerve growth factor deprivation. *J Cell Biol* 106:829–844.

Martin H, Richert L, Berthelot A (2003) Magnesium deficiency induces apoptosis in primary cultures of rat hepatocytes. *J Nutr* 133:2505-11.

Martin H, Uring-Lambert B, Adrian M, Lahlou A, Bonet A, Demougeot C, Devaux S, Laurant P, Richert L, Berthelot A (2008) Effects of long-term dietary intake of magnesium on oxidative stress, apoptosis and ageing in rat liver. *Magnes Res* 21:124-30.

Mattson MP (2000) Apoptosis in neurodegenerative disorders. *Nat Rev Cell Mol Biol* 1:120-9.

Mattson MP, Camandola S (2000) NF-κB in neurodegenerative disorders. *J Clin Invest* 61:134–139.

Mattson MP, Duan W, Chan SL, Camandola S (1999) Par-4: an emerging pivotal player in neuronal apoptosis and neurodegenerative disorders. *J Mol Neurosci* 13:17-30.

Mazur A, Maier JA, Rock E, Gueux E, Nowacki W, Rayssiguier Y (2007) Magnesium and the inflammatory response: potential physiopathological implications. *Arch Biochem Biophys* 458:48-56.

Mittendorf R, Dammann O, Lee KS (2006) Brain lesions in newborns exposed to high-dose magnesium sulfate during preterm labor. *J Perinatol* 26:57-63.

Moreira PI, Carvalho C, Zhu X, Smith MA, Perry G (2010) Mitochondrial dysfunction is a trigger of Alzheimer's disease pathophysiology. *Biochim Biophys Acta* 1802:2-10.

Murphy E (2000) Mysteries of magnesium homeostasis. *Circ Res* 86:245-8.

Navarro A, Boveris A (2009) Brain mitochondrial dysfunction and oxidative damage in Parkinson's disease. *J Bioenerg Biomembr* 41:517-21.

Olney JW (1969) Brain lesions, obesity, and other disturbances in mice treated with monosodium glutamate. *Science* 164:719–721.

Oppenheim RW (1991) Cell death during development of the nervous system. *Annu Rev Neurosci* 14:453–501.

Oyanagi K, Kawakami E, Kikuchi-Horie K, Ohara K, Ogata K, Takahama S, Wada M, Kihira T, Yasui M (2006) Magnesium deficiency over generations in rats with special references to the pathogenesis of the Parkinsonism-dementia complex and amyotrophic lateral sclerosis of Guam. *Neuropathology* 26:115–28.

Patel T, Bronk SF, Gores GJ (1994) Increases of intracellular magnesium promote glycodeoxycholate-induced apoptosis in rat hepatocytes. *J Clin Invest* 94:2183-92.

Pelicci G, Troglio F, Bodini A, Melillo RM, Pettirossi V, Coda L, De Giuseppe A, Santoro M, Pelicci PG (2002) The neuron-specific Rai (ShcC) adaptor protein inhibits apoptosis by coupling Ret to the phosphatidylinositol 3-kinase/Akt signaling pathway. *Mol Cell Biol* 22:7351-63.

Rao SD, Banack SA, Cox PA, Weiss JH (2006) BMAA selectively injures motor neurons via AMPA/kainate receptor activation. *Exp Neurol* 201:244–52.

Rego AC, Oliveira CR (2003) Mitochondrial dysfunction and reactive oxygen species in excitotoxicity and apoptosis: implications for the pathogenesis of neurodegenerative diseases. *Neurochem Res* 28:1563–1574.

Riedel G, Platt B, Micheau J (2003) Glutamate receptor function in learning and memory. *Behav Brain Res* 140:1-47.

Salvi M, Bozac A, Toninello A (2004) Gliotoxin induces Mg^{2+} efflux from intact brain mitochondria. *Neurochem Int* 45:759-64.

Schlingmann KP, Waldegger S, Konrad M, Chubanov V, Gudermann T (2007) TRPM6 and TRPM7--Gatekeepers of human magnesium metabolism. *Biochim Biophys Acta* 1772:813-21.

Schmitz C, Perraud AL, Johnson CO, Inabe K, Smith MK, Penner R, Kurosaki T, Fleig A, Scharenberg AM (2003) Regulation of vertebrate cellular Mg^{2+} homeostasis by TRPM7. *Cell* 114:191-200.

Shindo Y, Fujimoto A, Hotta K, Suzuki K, Oka K (2010) Glutamate-induced calcium increase mediates magnesium release from mitochondria in rat hippocampal neurons. *J Neurosci Res* 88:3125-32.

Sultana R, Butterfield DA (2010) Role of oxidative stress in the progression of Alzheimer's disease. J *Alzheimers Dis* 19:341-53.

Sun HS, Jackson MF, Martin LJ, Jansen K, Teves L, Cui H, Kiyonaka S, Mori Y, Jones M, Forder JP, Golde TE, Orser BA, Macdonald JF, Tymianski M (2009) Suppression of hippocampal TRPM7 protein prevents delayed neuronal death in brain ischemia. *Nat Neurosci* 12:1300-7.

Supnet C, Bezprozvanny I (2010) The dysregulation of intracellular calcium in Alzheimer disease. *Cell Calcium* 47:183-9.

Tait SW, Green DR (2010) Mitochondria and cell death: outer membrane permeabilization and beyond. *Nat Rev Mol Cell Biol* 11:621-32.

Tejero-Taldo MI, Chmielinska JJ, Weglicki WB (2007) Chronic dietary Mg^{2+} deficiency induces cardiac apoptosis in the rat heart. *Magnes Res* 20:208-12.

Vink R, Cook NL, van den Heuvel C (2009) Magnesium in acute and chronic brain injury: an update. *Magnes Res* 22:158S-162S.

Vink R, Nimmo AJ (2009) Multifunctional drugs for head injury. *Neurotherapeutics* 6:28-42.
Vucic S, Kiernan MC (2009) Pathophysiology of neurodegeneration in familial amyotrophic lateral sclerosis. *Curr Mol Med* 9:255-72.

Wang Y, Qin ZH (2010) Molecular and cellular mechanisms of excitotoxic neuronal death. *Apoptosis* 15:1382-402.

Wolf FI, Trapani V (2009) Multidrug resistance phenotypes and MRS2 mitochondrial magnesium channel: two players from one stemness? *Cancer Biol* Ther 8:615-7.

Yuan J, Yankner BA (2000) Apoptosis in the nervous system. *Nature* 407:802-9.

Zhang XY, Bai DC, Wu YJ, Li WG, Liu NF (2005) Proanthocyanidin from grape seeds enhances anti-tumor effect of doxorubicin both in vitro and in vivo. *Pharmazie* 60:533-8.

Zhang XY, Li WG, Wu YJ, Bai DC, Liu NF (2005) Proanthocyanidin from grape seeds enhances doxorubicin-induced antitumor effect and reverses drug resistance in doxorubicin-resistant K562/DOX cells. *Can J Physiol Pharmacol* 83:309-18.

Zündorf G, Reiser G (2010) Calcium dysregulation and homeostasis of neural calcium in the molecular mechanisms of neurodegenerative diseases provide multiple targets for neuroprotection. *Antioxid Redox Signa* 14:1275-88.

Brain free magnesium homeostasis as a target for reducing cognitive aging

Jean-Marie Billard ✉

Université Paris Descartes, Faculté de Médecine René Descartes, Centre de Psychiatrie et Neurosciences, UMR 894, Paris, France.
✉ jean-marie.billard@inserm.fr

Abstract

In the general deterioration of physiological functions that takes place in aging, the prevalence of cognitive impairments, and particularly of those related to learning and memory, makes these deficits a major concern of public health. Although the exact nature of cellular and molecular substrates underlying learning and memory still remains an open issue for the neurobiologist, the current hypothesis views it is determined by the capacity of brain neuronal networks to express short- and long-term changes in synaptic strength. Accordingly, the capacity of functional plasticity is impaired in the brain of aged memory-deficient animals. Short-term changes in synaptic transmission closely depend on transmitter release and neuronal excitability while long-term modifications are mainly related to the activation of the N-methyl-D-aspartate receptor (NMDA-R), a subtype of glutamate receptors. Because transmitter release, neuronal excitability and NMDA-R activation are modulated by magnesium (Mg^{2+}), a change in brain Mg^{2+} homeostasis could affect synaptic strength and plasticity in neuronal networks and consequently could alter memory capacities. In addition, alteration of brain Mg^{2+} levels could be regarded as a possible mechanism contributing to cognitive aging. According to these postulates, long-term increase in Mg^{2+} levels facilitates the conversion of synapses to a plastic state while learning and memory capacities are enhanced in adult animals fed with a diet enriched in Mg^{2+}-L-threonate, a treatment that significantly elevates brain Mg^{2+} levels. Because Mg^{2+}-L-threonate also improves learning and memory in aged animals, the regulation of brain Mg^{2+} homeostasis may therefore be regarded as a relevant target for the development of new pharmacological strategies aimed at minimizing cognitive aging.

Introduction

Alterations in brain anatomy and physiology are frequent features that gradually take place in the course of aging, to finally impair cognitive functions, such as learning and memory. In the last decades, extensive behavioral experiments performed in animal models of aging confirm that the efficient learning and memory in young individuals is slowed down with age, while forgetfulness is accelerated (Barnes and McNaughton, 1985; Gallagher and Rapp, 1997; Lanahan *et al,* 1997; Norris and Foster, 1999; Ward *et al,* 1999), and like in humans, deficits concern several forms of memory, including spatial, associative and long-term memory (Clayton *et al,* 2002; Gruart *et al,* 2008; Houston *et al,* 1999; Rosenzweig and Barnes, 2003; Sykova *et al,* 2002; Winocur and Moscovitch, 1990; Zornetzer *et al,* 1982). Neuronal or synaptic loss is unlikely to significantly account for the senescent-associated cognitive deficits (Eriksen *et al,* 2009; Geinisman *et al,,* 2004; Luebke *et al,,*; Morrison and Hof 2007; Rapp and Gallagher 1996) and a wealth of data now rather indicate that changes in functional properties within neuronal networks are mainly concerned (Billard 2006; Burke and Barnes, 2006; Craik and Bialystok, 2006; Disterhoft *et al,,* 1994; Driscoll *et al,* 2003; Erickson and Barnes, 2003; Foster 2007; Grady and Craik, 2000; Hsu *et al,* 2002; Kelly *et al,* 2006; Lister and Barnes, 2009; Magnusson, 1998; Mora *et al,* 2007; Sykova *et al,* 1998; Toescu and Verkhratsky, 2004). In particular, studies of long-lasting modifications of glutamatergic neurotransmission, such as long-term potentiation (LTP) and long-term depression (LTD) of synaptic strength, now considered as functional substrates of memory encoding (Bear and Malenka, 1994; Bliss 1990; Collingridge and Bliss, 1995; Eichenbaum, 1996; Izquierdo, 1991; Kim and Linden, 2007; Lisman and McIntyre,

2001; Martin *et al,* 2000; Teyler and DiScenna, 1987), show substantial changes with age (Barnes, 2003; Billard, 2006; Burke and Barnes, 2006; Foster, 2006; Norris *et al,* 1996). Among the different mechanisms that may account for these age-associated impairment of synaptic plasticity (Foster 2007; Rosenzweig and Barnes 2003), the activation of the N-methyl-D-aspartate subtype of glutamate receptors (NMDA-R) has received particular attention. Indeed, these receptors are pivotal for the regulation of synaptic strength, by means of their high permeability to calcium (Ca^{2+}), which triggers the activation of specific intracellular protein kinases and phosphatases (Wang *et al,* 1997). Although it is obvious that NMDA-R activation is impaired in aging (Barnes *et al,* 1997; Junjaud *et al,* 2006; Potier *et al,* 2000), all of the underlying mechanisms have yet to be definitely characterized and it remains to be determined to what extent they are involved in age-related deficits in synaptic plasticity and of memory capacities.

Among the different mechanisms possibly involved in cognitive aging is a change in ion homeostasis (Roberts 1999) since transmitter release, cellular excitability and expression of synaptic plasticity closely depend on ion flux across neuronal membranes. Although Ca^{2+} regulation has initially gathered the largest interest in aging studies (Thibault *et al,* 2007; Toescu *et al,* 2004; Verkhratsky and Toescu, 1998), the role of magnesium (Mg^{2+}), which is found in a relative large concentration in the central nervous system (CNS) (Chutkow, 1974; Poenaru *et al,* 1997), is now much more considered. Indeed, aging is a risk factor for Mg^{2+} deficit (Wakimoto and Block, 2001) [for a review see (Durlach *et al,* 1998) and brain Mg^{2+} levels are significantly reduced in age-associated neurodegenerative diseases (Andrasi *et al,* 2000; Andrasi *et al,* 2005; Basun *et al,* 1991). On the other hand, the well-known regulation of NMDA-R activation by Mg^{2+} (Mayer and Westbrook, 1987; Nowak *et al,* 1984) and the fact that altered Mg^{2+} levels impair memory functions (Bardgett *et al,* 2005; Bardgett *et al,* 2007; Landfield and Morgan, 1984), strongly suggest that a change in Mg^{2+} homeostasis could contribute to the physiopathology of cognitive aging.

After reviewing the different roles of Mg^{2+} in the regulation of synaptic mechanisms at glutamatergic synapses, the present report will consider whether Mg^{2+} could be involved in deficits of these mechanisms that occur in the aging brain, and finally recent data will be presented suggesting Mg^{2+} as a relevant dietary component that could help in reducing age-associated memory impairments.

The impact of brain Mg^{2+} levels on synaptic mechanisms contributing to cognitive functions

Although Mg^{2+} is the second most abundant intracellular mineral after potassium and is present at large amount in the cerebrospinal fluid of both rodents (0.8 mM; (Chutkow, 1974) and humans (1.0 to 1.2 mM; (Basun *et al,* 1991; Kapaki *et al,* 1989), its role on neural activity and synaptic plasticity has been much less considered compared to other divalent cations such as calcium (Ca^{2+}). This is rather surprising regarding that Mg^{2+} is a cofactor for more than 300 enzymes and also tightly interacts with phospholipids and nucleic acids (Hofmann *et al,* 2000; Wolf and Cittadini, 2003), suggesting that the mineral should be able to modulate brain activity on a broad scale. Initially, the role of Mg^{2+} has mainly been evaluated *in vitro* by lowering extracellular levels ($[Mg^{2+}]_e$), a procedure that increases spontaneous firing rate of neurons through membrane depolarization (Furukawa *et al,* 2009; Stone *et al,* 1992). This decrease in $[Mg^{2+}]_e$ can lead to paroxysmal events in slice preparations from both animals and humans, which resemble abnormal activities occurring during sustained seizures *in vivo* (Armand *et al,* 1998; Jones and Heinemann, 1988; Stanton *et al,* 1987). Using high performance liquid chromatography, quantification of basal efflux of amino acids indicates that only levels of glutamate, the neurotransmitter involved in most of excitatory synapses in the CNS, are significantly enhanced in low $[Mg^{2+}]_e$ medium (Furukawa *et al,* 2009; Smith *et al,* 1989). These data point out a first contribution of Mg^{2+} regarding the activity of excitatory synapses in the brain, that is the regulation of the probability of transmitter release (Figure 1, left), as initially characterized at neuromuscular junctions (Kelly and Robbins, 1983; Kuno and Takahashi, 1986). But several lines of evidence show that beside this ubiquitous control on the probability of glutamate release at presynaptic terminals, $Mg^{2+}$is also able to influence

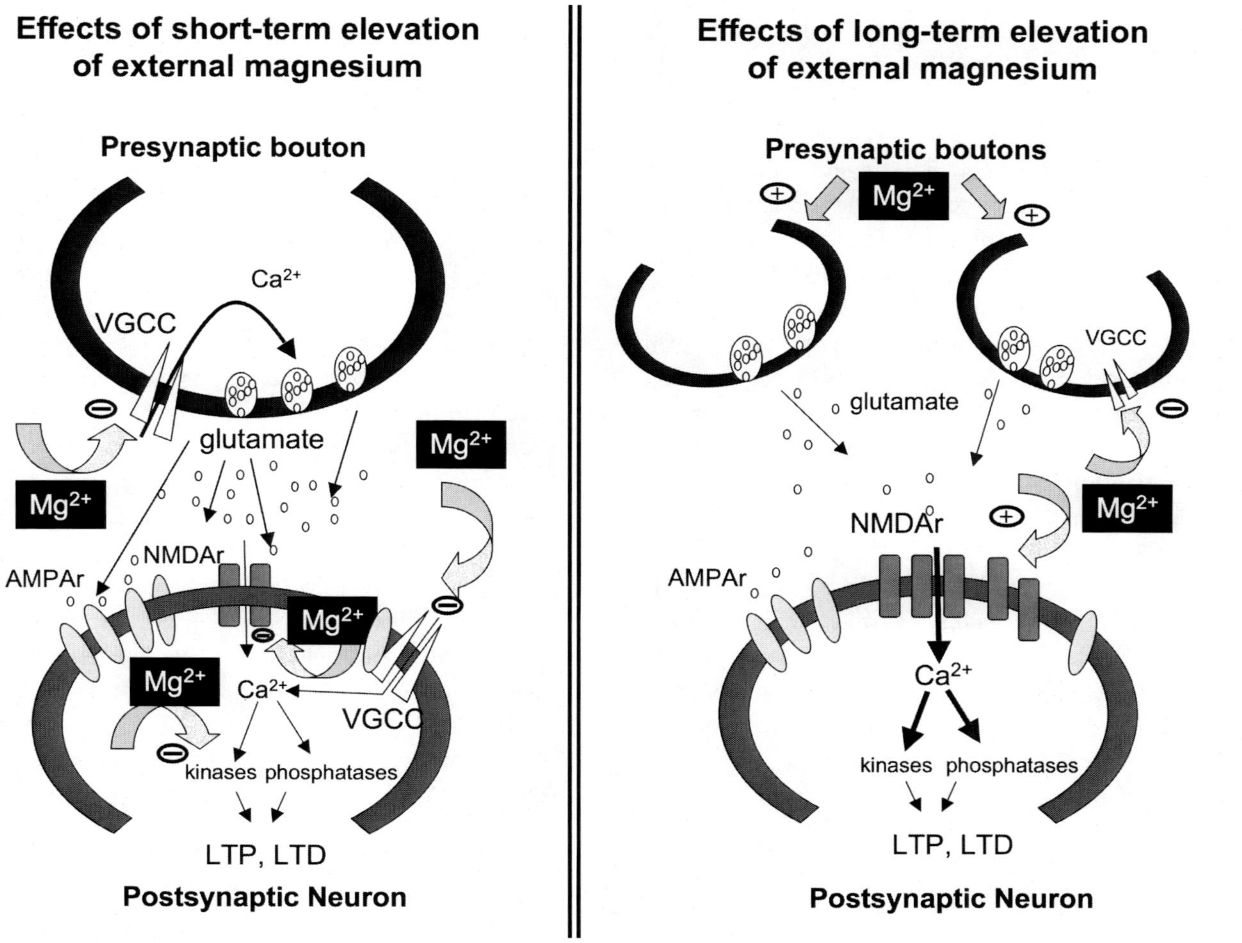

Figure 1. Schematic representation of the positive and negative effects of short-term (left) and long-term (right) elevation of brain Mg^2 levels on neurotransmission and synaptic plasticity at an excitatory glutamatergic synapse. AMPAr: α-amino-3-hydroxy-5-methyl-4-isoxazolepropionic acid receptor; NMDAr: N-methyl-D-aspartate receptor, VGCC: voltage-gated calcium channels.

synaptic activity by acting at postsynaptic level (Figure 1, left). For instance, frequency potentiation (FP), which represents an increase in synaptic strength rapidly developing during repetitive activation of glutamatergic afferent fibers (Anderson and Lomo, 1966; Andreasen and Lambert, 1998), is greater after elevating $[Mg^{2+}]_e$ (Landfield and Morgan, 1984). This is mainly due to the ability of Mg^{2+} to reduce the calcium-dependent post-burst afterhyper-polarization (AHP) of membrane potential, which is normally induced in depolarized neurons to limit excessive firing (Hotson and Prince, 1980; Lorenzon and Foehring, 1992; Madison and Nicoll, 1984). AHPs are reversibly reduced by the acquisition of learning-dependent behavioral tasks such as trace eyeblink conditioning or spatial water maze (Moyer *et al*, 2000; Thompson *et al,* 1996). Thus, by controlling the initial postsynaptic depolarization through the regulation of AHP amplitude and duration, Mg^{2+} is able to modulate synaptic strength and to alter cognitive abilities (Disterhoft and Oh, 2006).

Although there is no doubt that Mg^{2+} may be considered as firmly involved in the regulation of synaptic activity through the pre- and post-synaptic mechanisms described above, an additional and essential role for the mineral has emerged at the end of the eighties from electrophysiological studies demonstrating that Mg^{2+} inhibits currents through channels associated with the N-methyl-D-aspartate subtype of glutamate receptors (NMDA-R) by directly blocking the ion pore (Bekkers and Stevens, 1993; Jahr and Stevens, 1990; Mayer and Westbrook, 1987; Nowak *et al,* 1984). A transient rise in $[Mg^{2+}]_e$ within physiological range, i.e. from 0.8 to 1.2

mM, rapidly reduces the current amplitude mediated by NMDA-R by more than 60% in cultured neurons clamped at potentials below -50 mV while further increase in $[Mg^{2+}]_e$ is significantly less effective (Slutsky *et al,* 2004). Importantly, this depression effect does not occur at depolarized potentials, revealing a voltage dependency for the block of NMDA-R by Mg^{2+}, which underlies the pivotal role of NMDA-R in the induction of synaptic plasticity such as long-term potentiation (LTP) and long-term depression (LTD). Indeed, following high-frequency activation of presynaptic terminals, the glutamate-induced depolarization of membrane potential releases NMDA-R from Mg^{2+} block allowing Ca^{2+} to enter the cells (Figure 1, left). As a consequence, activation of specific kinases or phosphatases is triggered thus modifying synaptic strength (Wang *et al,* 1997). Several lines of evidence show effects of transient changes in Mg^{2+} levels on the induction of synaptic plasticity. For instance, a rapid rise in $[Mg^{2+}]_e$ selectively antagonizes LTP by reducing the depolarization-induced Ca^{2+} influx (Dunwiddie and Lynch, 1979; Malenka *et al,* 1992; Malenka and Nicoll, 1993). Interestedly, LTP is also suppressed in slices bathed with a Mg^{2+}-free medium (Frankiewicz and Parsons, 1999; Jouvenceau *et al,* 2002), a loss that is independent of NMDA-R activation but rather due to changes in signaling cascades in post-synaptic neurons that remain to be characterized (Hsu *et al,* 2000). At intracellular level, Mg^{2+} also regulates the activity of Ca^{2+}-dependent protein kinases governing NMDA-dependent LTP. For instance, it controls the subcellular localization of protein kinase C (PKC), which closely determines the function of the enzyme (Tanimura *et al,* 2002) and stimulates the dephosphorylation and deactivation of Calmodulin Kinase II (CaMKII) (Easom *et al,* 1998).

Despite much of data underline that a transient increase in Mg^{2+} levels unables synapses to remain highly plastic, an unexpected opposite result has been reported *in vitro* after studying the effects of long-term elevation of the mineral (Figure 1, right). Indeed, when $[Mg^{2+}]_e$ is increased within physiological range in neuronal cultures for more than several hours, NMDA-R-mediated currents are enhanced and the expression of LTP significantly facilitated (Slutsky *et al,* 2004). In the same conditions, synaptic strength is not modified following a single action potential but increased after a burst of inputs. These long-term facilitation effects of Mg^{2+} on neurotransmission and synaptic plasticity also occur *in vivo* since they are found in young rats fed with a diet enriched in Mg^{2+}-L-threonate (Mg^{2+}-T), a new highly bioavailable compound that enhances loading of Mg^{2+} into the brain (Slutsky *et al,* 2010). The increase in the density of functional presynaptic boutons (Slutsky *et al,* 2010) coupled with the weaker glutamate release at synapses found after chronic Mg^{2+} elevation (Slutsky *et al,* 2004) indicate that long lasting changes in Mg^{2+} homeostasis are able to modify the pattern of synaptic assemblies within neuronal networks, from a limited number of synapses with high probability of release to a larger density with low probability of release (Figure 1, right). In addition, both the increase in $[Mg^{2+}]_e$ *in vitro* and the elevation of brain Mg^{2+} *in vivo* up-regulate the expression of NR2B-containing NMDA-R (Slutsky *et al,* 2004; Slutsky *et al,* 2010). This increase, proposed to counterbalance the higher blockade of NMDA-R opening associated with chronic elevation of $[Mg^{2+}]_e$, contributes to the greater capacity of synapses to be highly plastic.

Because the pattern and strength of synaptic transmission are widely believed to code memory traces (Bear and Malenka, 1994; Bliss, 1990; Collingridge and Bliss, 1995; Eichenbaum, 1996; Izquierdo, 1991; Kim and Linden, 2007; Lisman and McIntyre, 2001; Martin *et al,* 2000; Neves *et al,* 2008; Teyler and DiScenna, 1987), their susceptibility to short- and long-term changes in Mg^{2+} homeostasis described above predict that cognitive abilities would also be modulated by altering Mg^{2+} levels. Accordingly, Mg^{2+} deficiency impairs fear-conditioning (Bardgett *et al,* 2005; Bardgett *et al,* 2007) while chronically elevating plasma Mg^{2+} over several days improves reversal learning in the hippocampus-dependent T-maze task (Landfield and Morgan, 1984). However, whether brain Mg^{2+} levels are really altered in these studies has been questioned considering that Mg^{2+} loading into the brain is tightly regulated by active transport processes that maintain a concentration gradient between the cerebrospinal fluid (CSF) and the plasma. In fact, Mg^{2+} levels are poorly affected in the brain after long lasting increase in plasma Mg^{2+} induced by intravenous injection of $MgSO_4$ both in animals and humans (Kim *et al,* 1996; McKee *et al,* 2005). Nevertheless, this rigorous control of brain Mg^{2+}

levels has recently been overcome using the highly bioavailable compound Mg^{2+}-T which increases Mg^{2+} concentrations in CSF by at least 15% (Slutsky *et al,* 2010). Behavioral characterization of the Mg^{2+}-T-treated rats indicates significant improvements of learning abilities, working memory as well as short- and long-term memory compared to control animals (Slutsky *et al,* 2010), confirming that even moderate, changes in brain Mg^{2+} homeostasis are capable to alter cognitive performances.

The impact of brain Mg^{2+} levels on impaired synaptic mechanisms underlying cognitive aging

Although a link between Mg^{2+}deficiency and cellular senescence has been proposed for the age-related deterioration of a large range of physiological functions (Killilea and Maier, 2008), a causal effect on deficits of cognitive functions is still questioned, even aging is thought as a general risk factor for Mg^{2+} deficit (Durlach *et al,* 1993; Wakimoto and Block, 2001). In fact, Mg^{2+}concentrations determined in various brain structures only slightly decrease in healthy aging (Morita *et al,* 2001; Takahashi *et al,* 2001). However, since even a very small disturbance of $[Mg^{2+}]_e$ is able to substantially modify synaptic assemblies supporting cognitive performances as reported above, it may be postulated that age-related changes in Mg^{2+} levels, even of very weak amplitude, could contribute to the physiopathology of cognitive aging.

Regarding the regulation of transmitter release at presynaptic terminals, the increase in basal release of glutamate determined in the brain of aged rats and monkeys *in vivo* (Massieu and Tapia, 1997; Quintero *et al,* 2007) suggests a possible role for Mg^{2+}. According to this postulate, spontaneous miniature end-plate potentials increase in amplitude at neuromuscular junctions in aging, that has been shown to reflect an impaired regulation of transmission release by Mg^{2+} (Kelly and Robbins, 1983). Nevertheless, whether a similar effect of Mg^{2+} also occurs at central synapses still remains to be demonstrated.

Age-related decrease in neuronal excitability is well documented, indicating that the amplitude and duration of AHPs are enhanced with age (Disterhoft and Oh, 2006; Disterhoft and Oh, 2007; Power *et al,* 2002; Thibault *et al,* 2007). AHP amplitude inversely correlates with both acquisition and probe performance in learning behaviors among aged animals (Tombaugh *et al,* 2005) and pharmacological treatments that rescue the age-related alteration of AHPs, also minimize memory deficits (Oh *et al,* 1999; Weiss *et al,* 2000). These data strongly suggest that a decrease in neuronal excitability is a potent mechanism contributing to the physiopathology of cognitive aging (Disterhoft and Oh, 2006). Although the fact that Mg^{2+} is involved in this functional deficit has not yet been formally demonstrated, some indirect experimental data suggest that this may be probably the case. Frequency potentiation, which is negatively correlated to AHP magnitude (Thibault *et al,* 2001), is reduced by age (Diana *et al,* 1994; Landfield and Lynch, 1977; Landfield *et al,* 1986; Thibault *et al,* 2001) and this alteration is prevented by elevating $[Mg^{2+}]_e$ (Landfield and Morgan, 1984; Landfield *et al,* 1986). From these results, it may be hypothesized that the age-related facilitation of Ca^{2+} conductances supporting the increase in AHPs is not only due to a greater density of Ca^{2+} channels on neuronal membranes (Campbell *et al,* 1996; Thibault and Landfield, 1996; Thibault *et al,* 2001; Veng *et al,* 2003) but also for some extent, to a weaker competition between cations following Mg^{2+} depletion.

Regarding the expression of long-lasting synaptic plasticity, extensive electrophysiological studies report age-related deficits of both LTP and LTD in aged memory-impaired animals, that reflects a shift in Ca^{2+} sources with a weaker role for NMDA-R and an increased contribution of voltage-gated Ca^{2+} channels and intracellular stores with different kinetic properties (Foster and Kumar, 2002; Gant *et al,* 2006; Junjaud *et al,* 2006; Kumar and Foster, 2005; Shankar *et al,* 1998; Thibault *et al,* 2007). NMDA-R activation is impaired in aged animals (Barnes *et al,* 1997; Burke and Barnes, 2010; Clayton *et al,* 2002; Eckles-Smith *et al,* 2000; Fontan-Lozano *et al,* 2007; Kollen *et al,* 2010; Magnusson, 1998; Ontl *et al,* 2004; Potier *et al,* 2000), that is not due to a reduced receptor density but rather to changes in pharmacological properties of the glutamatergic receptor (Billard and Rouaud, 2007; Junjaud *et al,* 2006; Kollen *et al,* 2010; Kuehl-Kovarik *et al,* 2003; Mothet *et al,* 2006; Turpin *et al,* 2009). Among the possible mechanisms affecting

NMDA-R activation in aging, a role for Mg^{2+} has been evaluated. No significant alteration of NMDA-R susceptibility to Mg^{2+} block occurs during aging since the percent decrease in NMDA-R-mediated synaptic potentials is comparable in young and aged animals after transient $[Mg^{2+}]_e$ elevation (Barnes *et al*, 1997; Potier *et al*, 2000). Also altering $[Mg^{2+}]_e$ affects NMDA-R-dependent LTP as well as short-term potentiation (STP) in a similar way in the two groups of animals indicating that a change in Mg^{2+} block of NMDA-R is unlikely to contribute to the age-related impairment of synaptic plasticity (Potier *et al*, 2000). However, a role for Mg^{2+} in LTP deficits occurring in aged animals does not definitively be discarded. For instance, a weaker activation of NMDA-R by its co-agonist D-serine has been shown to underlie LTP impairment in aged rodents, that is due to a weaker production of the amino acid by its synthesizing enzyme serine racemase (SR) (Junjaud *et al*, 2006; Mothet *et al*, 2006; Potier *et al*, 2010; Turpin *et al*, 2009). Because SR activity is potently stimulated by Mg^{2+}, which increases 5- to 10-fold the rate of racemization of L- to D-serine, an impaired activation of SR by Mg^{2+} may therefore be possibly regarded as a potent mechanism linking lower brain Mg^{2+} levels to deficits of NMDA-R activation and related synaptic plasticity in aging.

Regarding the effects of long-lasting elevation of $[Mg^{2+}]_e$, functional improvements also occur at synapses of the aging brain (Slutsky *et al*, 2010). The density of synaptophysin- and synaptobrevin-immunostained puncta is decreased in the hippocampal dentate gyrus of aged animals whereas synaptic loss in the *stratum radiatum* of CA1 subfield is less pronounced and even remains controversial (Burke and Barnes, 2006; Geinisman *et al*, 2004; Smith *et al*, 2000). However, in aged Mg^{2+}-T treated rats, the number of functional synaptic connections is significantly increased in both hippocampal areas compared to aged controls (Slutsky *et al*, 2010). As in young animals, a treatment with Mg^{2+}-T also up-regulatesNR2B-containing NMDA-R, thus improving LTP expression in slices from aged animals (Slutsky *et al*, 2010). Interestingly, both the increase in functional synaptic connections and the facilitated induction of synaptic plasticity (Figure 2A) (see (Slutsky *et al*, 2010)). In addition, it is worth noting in these aged treated animals that the density of synaptophysin- puncta returns to

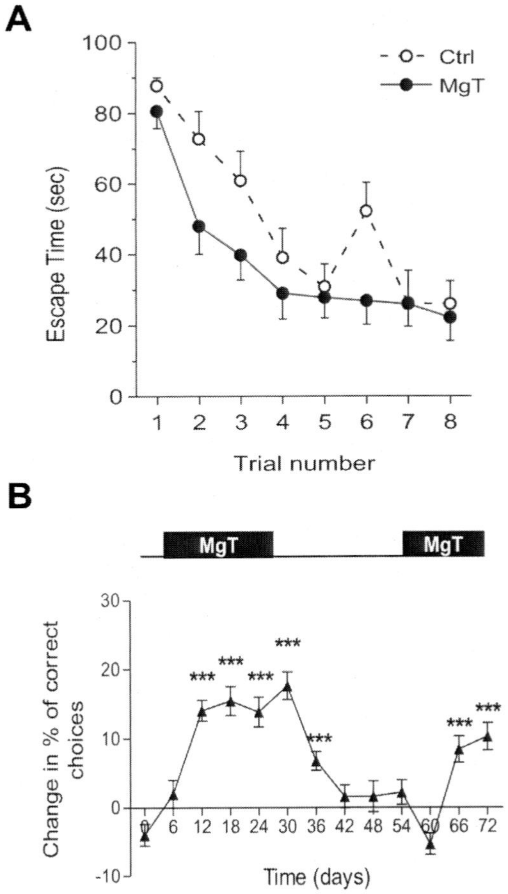

Figure 2. Elevation of brain Mg^{2} levels by Mg^{2+}-T improves memory in aged rats. (A). Mg^{2+}-T aged treated rats show shorter escape time in the water maze task indicating faster learning. (B). Time course of the reversible benefit effect of Mg^{2+}-T treatment on spatial working memory in aged rats. Modified from (Slutsky *et al*, 2010).

the control level after the end of Mg^{2+}-T supplementation and the time course of this decrease matches that of the reinstallation of impairment in memory scores (Figure 2B).

Other possible routes involving brain Mg^{2+} in cognitive aging

The basal forebrain cholinergic complex including the medial septum/diagonal band, the substantia innominata, and the nucleus basalis of Meynert of Broca, represents a second major excitatory pathway of the CNS (Dutar *et al*, 1995; McKinney *et al*, 1983; Mesulam *et al*, 1983; Mesulam *et al*, 1984; Woolf *et al*, 1984). During the past fifty years, many experiments were directed at testing whether this cholinergic pathway is involved in aspects of cognition and a significant role in learning and memory has been firmly debated (see (McKinney and Jacksonville, 2005) for a review). Electrically-induced release of acetylcholine generates slow and long-lasting excitatory postsynaptic potentials involving the activation of muscarinic receptors (Dutar and Nicoll, 1988; Misgeld *et al,* 1989; Muller and Misgeld, 1986). These responses are impaired in aging (Lippa *et al,* 1985; Potier *et al,* 1993; Segal 1982; Shen and Barnes 1996; Taylor and Griffith, 1993), that reflects a decreased transmitter release from cholinergic terminals (Aubert *et al,* 1995; Birthelmer *et al,* 2003; Scali *et al,* 1994; Takei *et al,* 1989; Vannucchi *et al,* 1997) but also a weaker activation of postsynaptic receptors (Calhoun *et al,* 2004; Lippa *et al,* 1985; Potier *et al,* 1992; Potier *et al,* 1993; Segal 1982; Vannucchi *et al,* 1997). However, it is worth noting that the degree of memory deficit does not appear to closely correlate with changes in cholinergic synaptic activity (Calhoun *et al,* 2004; Potier *et al,* 1993; Shen and Barnes, 1996), suggesting that acetylcholine should not play a critical role in cognitive aging as initially proposed (Bartus *et al,* 1982; Bartus *et al,* 1985; Pepeu, 1988).

In addition to reduce acetylcholine release (Jope, 1981; Vickroy and Schneider, 1991), Mg^{2+} also acts on postsynaptic muscarinic receptors through several distinct mechanisms. First, Mg^{2+} is able to bind to the allosteric region of the M2 subtype of receptors, decreasing the inhibitory effects of some modulators on the dissociation of orthosteric ligands (Burgmer *et al,* 1998). Second, Mg^{2+} reduces a non-selective cationic conductance activated by muscarinic agonists (Guerineau *et al,* 1995), and finally the cation is necessary for activating G-proteins coupled to muscarinic receptors (Cladman and Chidiac, 2002; Shiozaki and Haga, 1992; Zhang *et al,* 2004). Regarding these multiple interactions, it is obvious that changes in Mg^{2+} levels are likely to contribute to the alteration of cholinergic neurotransmission that occurs in aging. Although direct evidence is still lacking, several data of the literature argue for the possibility that changes in brain Mg^{2+} may contribute to the age-associated impairment of acetylcholine-dependent synaptic activity. For instance, hypomagnesia significantly weakens responses of cortical neurons to iontophoretically applied acetylcholine (El-Beheiry and Puil, 1990) while the high-affinity binding at the muscarinic receptor in Alzheimer's disease is closely regulated by Mg^{2+} (Ladner and Lee, 1999).

Conclusion

Although it is obvious that additional studies are necessary to unravel the mechanisms connecting brain Mg^{2+} homeostasis and cognitive aging, experimental data progressively accumulate showing that even moderate changes in the concentration of the mineral are able to significantly affect the assembly and functionality of neuronal networks involved in cognition. Recently, the World Health Organization reaches consensus that in a majority of the world's population, the dietary Mg^{2+} intake is lower than recommended, especially in the aging population (see also (Ford and Mokdad, 2003; Galan, 1997). Based on the results summarized in the present review, there is no doubt that elevating Mg^{2+} levels in the brain of the elderly could represent a promising strategy to minimize or even prevent cognitive deficits that take place with age.

References

Anderson P, Lomo T (1966) Mode of activation of hippocampal pyramidal cells by excitatory synapses on dendrites. *Exp Brain Res* 2:247-60.

Andrasi E, Igaz S, Molnar Z, Mako S (2000) Disturbances of magnesium concentrations in various brain areas in Alzheimer's disease. *Magnes Res* 13:189-96.

Andrasi E, Pali N, Molnar Z, Kosel S (2005) Brain aluminum, magnesium and phosphorus contents of control and Alzheimer-diseased patients. *J Alzheimers Dis* 7:273-84.

Andreasen M, Lambert JD (1998) Factors determining the efficacy of distal excitatory synapses in rat hippocampal CA1 pyramidal neurones. *J Physiol* 507 (Pt 2):441-62.

Armand V, Louvel J, Pumain R, Heinemann U (1998) Effects of new valproate derivatives on epileptiform discharges induced by pentylenetetrazole or low Mg2+ in rat entorhinal cortex-hippocampus slices. *Epilepsy Res* 32:345-55.

Aubert I, Rowe W, Meaney MJ, Gauthier S, Quirion R (1995) Cholinergic markers in aged cognitively impaired Long-Evans rats. *Neuroscience* 67:277-92.

Bardgett ME, Schultheis PJ, McGill DL, Richmond RE, Wagge JR (2005) Magnesium deficiency impairs fear conditioning in mice. *Brain Res* 1038:100-6.

Bardgett ME, Schultheis PJ, Muzny A, Riddle MD, Wagge JR (2007) Magnesium deficiency reduces fear-induced conditional lick suppression in mice. *Magnes Res* 20:58-65.

Barnes CA, McNaughton BL (1985) An age comparison of the rates of acquisition and forgetting of spatial information in relation to long-term enhancement of hippocampal synapses. *Behav Neurosci* 99:1040-8.

Barnes CA, Rao G, Shen J (1997) Age-related decrease in the N-methyl-D-aspartateR-mediated excitatory postsynaptic potential in hippocampal region CA1. *Neurobiol Aging* 18:445-52.

Barnes CA (2003) Long-term potentiation and the ageing brain. *Philos Trans R Soc Lond B Biol Sci* 358:765-72.

Bartus RT, Dean RL, 3rd, Beer B, Lippa AS (1982) The cholinergic hypothesis of geriatric memory dysfunction. *Science* 217:408-14.

Bartus RT, Dean RL, Pontecorvo MJ, Flicker C (1985) The cholinergic hypothesis: a historical overview, current perspective, and future directions. *Ann N Y Acad Sci* 444:332-58.

Basun H, Forssell LG, Wetterberg L, Winblad B (1991) Metals and trace elements in plasma and cerebrospinal fluid in normal aging and Alzheimer's disease. *J Neural Transm Park Dis Dement Sect* 3:231-58.

Bear MF, Malenka RC (1994) Synaptic plasticity: LTP and LTD. *Curr Opin Neurobiol* 4:389-99.

Bekkers JM, Stevens CF (1993) NMDA receptors at excitatory synapses in the hippocampus: test of a theory of magnesium block. *Neurosci Lett* 156:73-7.

Billard JM (2006) Ageing, hippocampal synaptic activity and magnesium. *Magnes Res* 19:199-215.

Billard JM, Rouaud E (2007) Deficit of NMDA receptor activation in CA1 hippocampal area of aged rats is rescued by D-cycloserine. *Eur J Neurosci* 25:2260-8.

Birthelmer A, Stemmelin J, Jackisch R, Cassel JC (2003) Presynaptic modulation of acetylcholine, noradrenaline, and serotonin release in the hippocampus of aged rats with various levels of memory impairments. *Brain Res Bull* 60:283-96.

Bliss TV (1990) Long-term potentiation. *Science* 249:973.

Burgmer U, Schulz U, Trankle C, Mohr K (1998) Interaction of Mg2+ with the allosteric site of muscarinic M2 receptors. *Naunyn Schmiedebergs Arch Pharmacol* 357:363-70.

Burke SN, Barnes CA (2006) Neural plasticity in the ageing brain. *Nat Rev Neurosci* 7:30-40.

Burke SN, Barnes CA (2010) Senescent synapses and hippocampal circuit dynamics. *Trends Neurosci* 33:153-61.

Calhoun ME, Mao Y, Roberts JA, Rapp PR (2004) Reduction in hippocampal cholinergic innervation is unrelated to recognition memory impairment in aged rhesus monkeys. *J Comp Neurol* 475:238-46.

Campbell LW, Hao SY, Thibault O, Blalock EM, Landfield PW (1996) Aging changes in voltage-gated calcium currents in hippocampal CA1 neurons. *J Neurosci* 16:6286-95.

Chutkow JG (1974) Metabolism of magnesium in central nervous system. Relationship between concentrations of magnesium in cerebrospinal fluid and brain in magnesium deficiency. *Neurology* 24:780-7.

Cladman W, Chidiac P (2002) Characterization and comparison of RGS2 and RGS4 as GTPase-activating proteins for m2 muscarinic receptor-stimulated G(i). *Mol Pharmacol* 62:654-9.

Clayton DA, Mesches MH, Alvarez E, Bickford PC, Browning MD (2002) A hippocampal NR2B deficit can mimic age-related changes in long-term potentiation and spatial learning in the Fischer 344 rat. *J Neurosci* 22:3628-37.

Collingridge GL, Bliss TV (1995) Memories of NMDA receptors and LTP. *Trends Neurosci* 18:54-6.

Craik FI, Bialystok E (2006) Cognition through the lifespan: mechanisms of change. *Trends Cogn Sci* 10:131-8.

Diana G, Scotti de Carolis A, Frank C, Domenici MR, Sagratella S (1994) Selective reduction of hippocampal dentate frequency potentiation in aged rats with impaired place learning. *Brain Res Bull* 35:107-11.

Disterhoft JF, Moyer JR, Jr., Thompson LT (1994) The calcium rationale in aging and Alzheimer's disease. Evidence from an animal model of normal aging. *Ann N Y Acad Sci* 747:382-406.

Disterhoft JF, Oh MM (2006) Learning, aging and intrinsic neuronal plasticity. *Trends Neurosci* 29:587-99.

Disterhoft JF, Oh MM (2007) Alterations in intrinsic neuronal excitability during normal aging. *Aging Cell* 6:327-36.

Driscoll I, Hamilton DA, Petropoulos H, Yeo RA, Brooks WM, Baumgartner RN, Sutherland RJ (2003) The aging hippocampus: cognitive, biochemical and structural findings. *Cereb Cortex* 13:1344-51.

Dunwiddie TV, Lynch G (1979) The relationship between extracellular calcium concentrations and the induction of hippocampal long-term potentiation. *Brain Res* 169:103-10.

Durlach J, Durlach V, Bac P, Rayssiguier Y, Bara M, Guiet-Bara A (1993) Magnesium and ageing. II. Clinical data: aetiological mechanisms and pathophysiological consequences of magnesium deficit in the elderly. *Magnes Res* 6:379-94.

Durlach J, Bac P, Durlach V, Rayssiguier Y, Bara M, Guiet-Bara A (1998) Magnesium status and ageing: an update. *Magnes Res* 11:25-42.

Dutar P, Nicoll RA (1988) Classification of muscarinic responses in hippocampus in terms of receptor subtypes and second-messenger systems: electro-physiological studies in vitro. *J Neurosci* 8:4214-24.

Dutar P, Bassant MH, Senut MC, Lamour Y (1995) The septohippocampal pathway: structure and function of a central cholinergic system. *Physiol Rev* 75:393-427.

Easom RA, Tarpley JL, Filler NR, Bhatt H (1998) Dephosphorylation and deactivation of Ca2+/ calmodulin-dependent protein kinase II in betaTC3-cells is mediated by Mg2+- and okadaic-acid-sensitive protein phosphatases. *Biochem J* 329 (Pt 2):283-8.

Eckles-Smith K, Clayton D, Bickford P, Browning MD (2000) Caloric restriction prevents age-related deficits in LTP and in NMDA receptor expression. *Brain Res Mol Brain Res* 78:154-62.

Eichenbaum H (1996) Learning from LTP: a comment on recent attempts to identify cellular and molecular mechanisms of memory. *Learn Mem* 3:61-73.

el-Beheiry H, Puil E (1990) Effects of hypomagnesia on transmitter actions in neocortical slices. *Br J Pharmacol* 101:1006-10.

Erickson CA, Barnes CA (2003) The neurobiology of memory changes in normal aging. *Exp Gerontol* 38:61-9.

Eriksen N, Stark AK, Pakkenberg B (2009) Age and Parkinson's disease-related neuronal death in the substantia nigra pars compacta. *J Neural Transm Suppl*:203-13.

Fontan-Lozano A, Saez-Cassanelli JL, Inda MC, de los Santos-Arteaga M, Sierra-Dominguez SA, Lopez-Lluch G, Delgado-Garcia JM, Carrion AM (2007) Caloric restriction increases learning consolidation and facilitates synaptic plasticity through mechanisms dependent on NR2B subunits of the NMDA receptor. *J Neurosci* 27:10185-95.

Ford ES, Mokdad AH (2003) Dietary magnesium intake in a national sample of US adults. *J Nutr* 133:2879-82.

Foster TC, Kumar A (2002) Calcium dysregulation in the aging brain. *Neuroscientist* 8:297-301.

Foster TC (2006) Biological markers of age-related memory deficits: treatment of senescent physiology. *CNS Drugs* 20:153-66.

Foster TC (2007) Calcium homeostasis and modulation of synaptic plasticity in the aged brain. *Aging Cell* 6:319-25.

Frankiewicz T, Parsons CG (1999) Memantine restores long term potentiation impaired by tonic N-methyl-D-aspartate (NMDA) receptor activation following reduction of Mg2+ in hippocampal slices. *Neuropharmacology* 38:1253-9.

Furukawa Y, Kasai N, Torimitsu K (2009) Effect of Mg2+ on neural activity of rat cortical and hippocampal neurons in vitro. *Magnes Res* 22:174S-81S.

Galan p, Preziosi P, Durlach V, Valeix P, Ribas L, Bouzid D, Favier A, Hercberg S (1997) Dietary magnesium intake in a French adult population. *Magnes Res* 10:321-28.

Gallagher M, Rapp PR (1997) The use of animal models to study the effects of aging on cognition. *Annu Rev Psychol* 48:339-70.

Gant JC, Sama MM, Landfield PW, Thibault O (2006) Early and simultaneous emergence of multiple hippocampal biomarkers of aging is mediated by Ca2+-induced Ca2+ release. *J Neurosci* 26:3482-90.

Geinisman Y, Ganeshina O, Yoshida R, Berry RW, Disterhoft JF, Gallagher M (2004) Aging, spatial learning, and total synapse number in the rat CA1 stratum radiatum. *Neurobiol Aging* 25:407-16.

Grady CL, Craik FI (2000) Changes in memory processing with age. *Curr Opin Neurobiol* 10:224-31.

Gruart A, Lopez-Ramos JC, Munoz MD, Delgado-Garcia JM (2008) Aged wild-type and APP, PS1, and APP + PS1 mice present similar deficits in associative learning and synaptic plasticity independent of amyloid load. *Neurobiol Dis* 30:439-50.

Guerineau NC, Bossu JL, Gahwiler BH, Gerber U (1995) Activation of a nonselective cationic conductance by metabotropic glutamatergic and muscarinic agonists in CA3 pyramidal neurons of the rat hippocampus. *J Neurosci* 15:4395-407.

Hofmann K, Tomiuk S, Wolff G, Stoffel W (2000) Cloning and characterization of the mammalian brain-specific, Mg2+-dependent neutral sphingomyelinase. *Proc Natl Acad Sci U S A* 97:5895-900.

Hotson JR, Prince DA (1980) A calcium-activated hyperpolarization follows repetitive firing in hippocampal neurons. *J Neurophysiol* 43:409-19.

Houston FP, Stevenson GD, McNaughton BL, Barnes CA (1999) Effects of age on the generalization and incubation of memory in the F344 rat. *Learn Mem* 6:111-9.

Hsu KS, Ho WC, Huang CC, Tsai JJ (2000) Transient removal of extracellular Mg(2+) elicits persistent suppression of LTP at hippocampal CA1 synapses via PKC activation. *J Neurophysiol* 84:1279-88.

Hsu KS, Huang CC, Liang YC, Wu HM, Chen YL, Lo SW, Ho WC (2002) Alterations in the balance of protein kinase and phosphatase activities and age-related impairments of synaptic transmission and long-term potentiation. *Hippocampus* 12:787-802.

Izquierdo I (1991) Role of NMDA receptors in memory. *Trends Pharmacol Sci* 12:128-9.

Jahr CE, Stevens CF (1990) Voltage dependence of NMDA-activated macroscopic conductances predicted by single-channel kinetics. *J Neurosci* 10:3178-82.

Jones RS, Heinemann U (1988) Synaptic and intrinsic responses of medical entorhinal cortical cells in normal and magnesium-free medium in vitro. *J Neurophysiol* 59:1476-96.

Jope RS (1981) Acetylcholine turnover and compartmentation in rat brain synaptosomes. *J Neurochem* 36:1712-21.

Jouvenceau A, Potier B, Poindessous-Jazat F, Dutar P, Slama A, Epelbaum J, Billard JM (2002) Decrease in calbindin content significantly alters LTP but not NMDA receptor and calcium channel properties. *Neuropharmacology* 42:444-58.

Junjaud G, Rouaud E, Turpin F, Mothet JP, Billard JM (2006) Age-related effects of the neuromodulator D-serine on neurotransmission and synaptic potentiation in the CA1 hippocampal area of the rat. *J Neurochem* 98:1159-66.

Kapaki E, Segditsa J, Papageorgiou C (1989) Zinc, copper and magnesium concentration in serum and CSF of patients with neurological disorders. *Acta Neurol Scand* 79:373-8.

Kelly KM, Nadon NL, Morrison JH, Thibault O, Barnes CA, Blalock EM (2006) The neurobiology of aging. *Epilepsy Res* 68 Suppl 1:S5-20.

Kelly SS, Robbins N (1983) Progression of age changes in synaptic transmission at mouse neuromuscular junctions. *J Physiol* 343:375-83.

Killilea DW, Maier JA (2008) A connection between magnesium deficiency and aging: new insights from cellular studies. *Magnes Res* 21:77-82.

Kim SJ, Linden DJ (2007) Ubiquitous plasticity and memory storage. *Neuron* 56:582-92.

Kim YJ, McFarlane C, Warner DS, Baker MT, Choi WW, Dexter F (1996) The effects of plasma and brain magnesium concentrations on lidocaine-induced seizures in the rat. *Anesth Analg* 83:1223-8.

Kollen M, Stephan A, Faivre-Bauman A, Loudes C, Sinet PM, Alliot J, Billard JM, Epelbaum J, Dutar P, Jouvenceau A (2010) Preserved memory capacities in aged Lou/C/Jall rats. *Neurobiol Aging* 31:129-42.

Kuehl-Kovarik MC, Partin KM, Magnusson KR (2003) Acute dissociation for analyses of NMDA receptor function in cortical neurons during aging. *J Neurosci Methods* 129:11-7.

Kumar A, Foster TC (2005) Intracellular calcium stores contribute to increased susceptibility to LTD induction during aging. *Brain Res* 1031:125-8.

Kuno M, Takahashi T (1986) Effects of calcium and magnesium on transmitter release at Ia synapses of rat spinal motoneurones in vitro. *J Physiol* 376:543-53.

Ladner CJ, Lee JM (1999) Reduced high-affinity agonist binding at the M(1) muscarinic receptor in Alzheimer's disease brain: differential sensitivity to agonists and divalent cations. *Exp Neurol* 158:451-8.

Lanahan A, Lyford G, Stevenson GS, Worley PF, Barnes CA (1997) Selective alteration of long-term potentiation-induced transcriptional response in hippocampus of aged, memory-impaired rats. *J Neurosci* 17:2876-85.

Landfield PW, Lynch G (1977) Impaired monosynaptic potentiation in in vitro hippocampal slices from aged, memory-deficient rats. *J Gerontol* 32:523-33.

Landfield PW, Morgan GA (1984) Chronically elevating plasma Mg2+ improves hippocampal frequency potentiation and reversal learning in aged and young rats. *Brain Res* 322:167-71.

Landfield PW, Pitler TA, Applegate MD (1986) The effects of high Mg2+-to-Ca2+ ratios on frequency potentiation in hippocampal slices of young and aged rats. *J Neurophysiol* 56:797-811.

Lippa AS, Loullis CC, Rotrosen J, Cordasco DM, Critchett DJ, Joseph JA (1985) Conformational changes in muscarinic receptors may produce diminished cholinergic neurotransmission and memory deficits in aged rats. *Neurobiol Aging* 6:317-23.

Lisman JE, McIntyre CC (2001) Synaptic plasticity: a molecular memory switch. *Curr Biol* 11:R788-91.

Lister JP, Barnes CA (2009) Neurobiological changes in the hippocampus during normative aging. *Arch Neurol* 66:829-33.

Lorenzon NM, Foehring RC (1992) Relationship between repetitive firing and afterhyperpolarizations in human neocortical neurons. *J Neurophysiol* 67:350-63.

Luebke J, Barbas H, Peters A Effects of normal aging on prefrontal area 46 in the rhesus monkey. *Brain Res Rev* 62:212-32.

Madison DV, Nicoll RA (1984) Control of the repetitive discharge of rat CA 1 pyramidal neurones in vitro. *J Physiol* 354:319-31.

Magnusson KR (1998) The aging of the NMDA receptor complex. *Front Biosci* 3:e70-80.

Malenka RC, Lancaster B, Zucker RS (1992) Temporal limits on the rise in postsynaptic calcium required for the induction of long-term potentiation. *Neuron* 9:121-8.

Malenka RC, Nicoll RA (1993) NMDA-receptor-dependent synaptic plasticity: multiple forms and mechanisms. *Trends Neurosci* 16:521-7.

Martin SJ, Grimwood PD, Morris RG (2000) Synaptic plasticity and memory: an evaluation of the hypothesis. *Annu Rev Neurosci* 23:649-711.

Massieu L, Tapia R (1997) Glutamate uptake impairment and neuronal damage in young and aged rats in vivo. *J Neurochem* 69:1151-60.

Mayer ML, Westbrook GL (1987) Permeation and block of N-methyl-D-aspartic acid receptor channels by divalent cations in mouse cultured central neurones. *J Physiol* 394:501-27.

McKee JA, Brewer RP, Macy GE, Borel CO, Reynolds JD, Warner DS (2005) Magnesium neuroprotection is limited in humans with acute brain injury. *Neurocrit Care* 2:342-51.

McKinney M, Coyle JT, Hedreen JC (1983) Topographic analysis of the innervation of the rat neocortex and hippocampus by the basal forebrain cholinergic system. *J Comp Neurol* 217:103-21.

McKinney M, Jacksonville MC (2005) Brain cholinergic vulnerability: relevance to behavior and disease. *Biochem Pharmacol* 70:1115-24.

Mesulam MM, Mufson EJ, Wainer BH, Levey AI (1983) Central cholinergic pathways in the rat: an overview based on an alternative nomenclature (Ch1-Ch6). *Neuroscience* 10:1185-201.

Mesulam MM, Mufson EJ, Levey AI, Wainer BH (1984) Atlas of cholinergic neurons in the forebrain and upper brainstem of the macaque based on monoclonal choline acetyltransferase immunohistochemistry and acetylcholinesterase histochemistry. *Neuroscience* 12:669-86.

Misgeld U, Muller W, Polder HR (1989) Potentiation and suppression by eserine of muscarinic synaptic transmission in the guinea-pig hippocampal slice. *J Physiol* 409:191-206.

Mora F, Segovia G, del Arco A (2007) Aging, plasticity and environmental enrichment: structural changes and neurotransmitter dynamics in several areas of the brain. *Brain Res Rev* 55:78-88.

Morita A, Abdireyim D, Kimura M, Itokawa Y (2001) The effect of aging on the mineral status of female SAMP1 and SAMR1. *Biol Trace Elem Res* 80:53-65.

Morrison JH, Hof PR (2007) Life and death of neurons in the aging cerebral cortex. *Int Rev Neurobiol* 81:41-57.

Mothet JP, Rouaud E, Sinet PM, Potier B, Jouvenceau A, Dutar P, Videau C, Epelbaum J, Billard JM (2006) A critical role for the glial-derived neuromodulator D-serine in the age-related deficits of cellular mechanisms of learning and memory. *Aging Cell* 5:267-74.

Moyer JR, Jr., Power JM, Thompson LT, Disterhoft JF (2000) Increased excitability of aged rabbit CA1 neurons after trace eyeblink conditioning. *J Neurosci* 20:5476-82.

Muller W, Misgeld U (1986) Slow cholinergic excitation of guinea pig hippocampal neurons is mediated by two muscarinic receptor subtypes. *Neurosci Lett* 67:107-12.

Neves G, Cooke SF, Bliss TV (2008) Synaptic plasticity, memory and the hippocampus: a neural network approach to causality. *Nat Rev Neurosci* 9:65-75.

Norris CM, Korol DL, Foster TC (1996) Increased susceptibility to induction of long-term depression and long-term potentiation reversal during aging. *J Neurosci* 16:5382-92.

Norris CM, Foster TC (1999) MK-801 improves retention in aged rats: implications for altered neural plasticity in age-related memory deficits. *Neurobiol Learn Mem* 71:194-206.

Nowak L, Bregestovski P, Ascher P, Herbet A, Prochiantz A (1984) Magnesium gates glutamate-activated channels in mouse central neurones. *Nature* 307:462-5.

Oh MM, Power JM, Thompson LT, Moriearty PL, Disterhoft JF (1999) Metrifonate increases neuronal excitability in CA1 pyramidal neurons from both young and aging rabbit hippocampus. *J Neurosci* 19:1814-23.

Ontl T, Xing Y, Bai L, Kennedy E, Nelson S, Wakeman M, Magnusson K (2004) Development and aging of N-methyl-D-aspartate receptor expression in the prefrontal/frontal cortex of mice. *Neuroscience* 123:467-79.

Pepeu G (1988) Acetylcholine and brain aging. *Pharmacol Res Commun* 20:91-7.

Poenaru S, Manicom R, Rouhani S, Aymard P, Bajenaru O, Rayssiguier Y, Emmanouillidis E, Gueux E, Nkanga N, Durlach J, Dall'ava J (1997) Stability of brain content of magnesium in experimental hypomagnesemia. *Brain Res* 769:329-32.

Potier B, Rascol O, Jazat F, Lamour Y, Dutar P (1992) Alterations in the properties of hippocampal pyramidal neurons in the aged rat. *Neuroscience* 48:793-806.

Potier B, Lamour Y, Dutar P (1993) Age-related alterations in the properties of hippocampal pyramidal neurons among rat strains. *Neurobiol Aging* 14:17-25.

Potier B, Poindessous-Jazat F, Dutar P, Billard JM (2000) NMDA receptor activation in the aged rat hippocampus. *Exp Gerontol* 35:1185-99.

Potier B, Turpin FR, Sinet PM, Rouaud E, Mothet JP, Videau C, Epelbaum J, Dutar P, Billard JM (2010) Contribution of the d-Serine-Dependent Pathway to the Cellular Mechanisms Underlying Cognitive Aging. *Front Aging Neurosci* 2:1.

Power JM, Wu WW, Sametsky E, Oh MM, Disterhoft JF (2002) Age-related enhancement of the slow outward calcium-activated potassium current in hippocampal CA1 pyramidal neurons in vitro. *J Neurosci* 22:7234-43.

Quintero JE, Day BK, Zhang Z, Grondin R, Stephens ML, Huettl P, Pomerleau F, Gash DM, Gerhardt GA (2007) Amperometric measures of age-related changes in glutamate regulation in the cortex of rhesus monkeys. *Exp Neurol* 208:238-46.

Rapp PR, Gallagher M (1996) Preserved neuron number in the hippocampus of aged rats with spatial learning deficits. *Proc Natl Acad Sci U S A* 93:9926-30.

Roberts EL, Jr. (1999) Using hippocampal slices to study how aging alters ion regulation in brain tissue. *Methods* 18:150-9.

Rosenzweig ES, Barnes CA (2003) Impact of aging on hippocampal function: plasticity, network dynamics, and cognition. *Prog Neurobiol* 69:143-79.

Scali C, Casamenti F, Pazzagli M, Bartolini L, Pepeu G (1994) Nerve growth factor increases extracellular acetylcholine levels in the parietal cortex and hippocampus of aged rats and restores object recognition. *Neurosci Lett* 170:117-20.

Segal M (1982) Changes in neurotransmitter actions in the aged rat hippocampus. *Neurobiol Aging* 3:121-4.

Shankar S, Teyler TJ, Robbins N (1998) Aging differentially alters forms of long-term potentiation in rat hippocampal area CA1. *J Neurophysiol* 79:334-41.

Shen J, Barnes CA (1996) Age-related decrease in cholinergic synaptic transmission in three hippocampal subfields. *Neurobiol Aging* 17:439-51.

Shiozaki K, Haga T (1992) Effects of magnesium ion on the interaction of atrial muscarinic acetylcholine receptors and GTP-binding regulatory proteins. *Biochemistry* 31:10634-42.

Slutsky I, Sadeghpour S, Li B, Liu G (2004) Enhancement of synaptic plasticity through chronically reduced Ca2+ flux during uncorrelated activity. *Neuron* 44:835-49.

Slutsky I, Abumaria N, Wu LJ, Huang C, Zhang L, Li B, Zhao X, Govindarajan A, Zhao MG, Zhuo M, Tonegawa S, Liu G (2010) Enhancement of learning and memory by elevating brain magnesium. *Neuron* 65:165-77.

Smith DA, Connick JH, Stone TW (1989) Effect of changing extracellular levels of magnesium on spontaneous activity and glutamate release in the mouse neocortical slice. *Br J Pharmacol* 97:475-82.

Smith TD, Adams MM, Gallagher M, Morrison JH, Rapp PR (2000) Circuit-specific alterations in hippocampal synaptophysin immunoreactivity predict spatial learning impairment in aged rats. *J Neurosci* 20:6587-93.

Stanton PK, Jones RS, Mody I, Heinemann U (1987) Epileptiform activity induced by lowering extracellular [Mg2+] in combined hippocampal-entorhinal cortex slices: modulation by receptors for norepinephrine and N-methyl-D-aspartate. *Epilepsy Res* 1:53-62.

Stone TW, Bartrup JT, Brooks PA, Connick JH, Smith DA (1992) Interactions of adenosine and magnesium on neuronal excitability and transmitter sensitivity in the hippocampal slice. *Epilepsy Res Suppl* 8:237-42.

Sykova E, Mazel T, Simonova Z (1998) Diffusion constraints and neuron-glia interaction during aging. *Exp Gerontol* 33:837-51.

Sykova E, Mazel T, Hasenohrl RU, Harvey AR, Simonova Z, Mulders WH, Huston JP (2002) Learning deficits in aged rats related to decrease in extracellular volume and loss of diffusion anisotropy in hippocampus. *Hippocampus* 12:269-79.

Takahashi S, Takahashi I, Sato H, Kubota Y, Yoshida S, Muramatsu Y (2001) Age-related changes in the concentrations of major and trace elements in the brain of rats and mice. *Biol Trace Elem Res* 80:145-58.

Takei N, Nihonmatsu I, Kawamura H (1989) Age-related decline of acetylcholine release evoked by depolarizing stimulation. *Neurosci Lett* 101:182-6.

Tanimura A, Nezu A, Morita T, Hashimoto N, Tojyo Y (2002) Interplay between calcium, diacylglycerol, and phosphorylation in the spatial and temporal regulation of PKCalpha-GFP. *J Biol Chem* 277:29054-62.

Taylor L, Griffith WH (1993) Age-related decline in cholinergic synaptic transmission in hippocampus. *Neurobiol Aging* 14:509-15.

Teyler TJ, DiScenna P (1987) Long-term potentiation. *Annu Rev Neurosci* 10:131-61.

Thibault O, Landfield PW (1996) Increase in single L-type calcium channels in hippocampal neurons during aging. *Science* 272:1017-20.

Thibault O, Hadley R, Landfield PW (2001) Elevated postsynaptic [Ca2+]i and L-type calcium channel activity in aged hippocampal neurons: relationship to impaired synaptic plasticity. *J Neurosci* 21:9744-56.

Thibault O, Gant JC, Landfield PW (2007) Expansion of the calcium hypothesis of brain aging and Alzheimer's disease: minding the store. *Aging Cell* 6:307-17.

Thompson LT, Moyer JR, Jr., Disterhoft JF (1996) Trace eyeblink conditioning in rabbits demonstrates heterogeneity of learning ability both between and within age groups. *Neurobiol Aging* 17:619-29.

Toescu EC, Verkhratsky A (2004) Ca2+ and mitochondria as substrates for deficits in synaptic plasticity in normal brain ageing. *J Cell Mol Med* 8:181-90.

Toescu EC, Verkhratsky A, Landfield PW (2004) Ca2+ regulation and gene expression in normal brain aging. *Trends Neurosci* 27:614-20.

Tombaugh GC, Rowe WB, Rose GM (2005) The slow afterhyperpolarization in hippocampal CA1 neurons covaries with spatial learning ability in aged Fisher 344 rats. *J Neurosci* 25:2609-16.

Turpin FR, Potier B, Dulong JR, Sinet PM, Alliot J, Oliet SH, Dutar P, Epelbaum J, Mothet JP, Billard JM (2009) Reduced serine racemase expression contributes to age-related deficits in hippocampal cognitive function. *Neurobiol Aging* [Epub ahead of print].

Vannucchi MG, Scali C, Kopf SR, Pepeu G, Casamenti F (1997) Selective muscarinic antagonists differentially affect in vivo acetylcholine release and memory performances of young and aged rats. *Neuroscience* 79:837-46.

Veng LM, Mesches MH, Browning MD (2003) Age-related working memory impairment is correlated with increases in the L-type calcium channel protein alpha1D (Cav1.3) in area CA1 of the hippocampus and both are ameliorated by chronic nimodipine treatment. *Brain Res Mol Brain Res* 110:193-202.

Verkhratsky A, Toescu EC (1998) Calcium and neuronal ageing. *Trends Neurosci* 21:2-7.

Vickroy TW, Schneider CJ (1991) Characterization of divalent cation-induced [3H]acetylcholine release from EGTA-treated rat hippocampal synaptosomes. *Neurochem Res* 16:1175-85.

Wakimoto P, Block G (2001) Dietary intake, dietary patterns, and changes with age: an epidemiological perspective. *J Gerontol A Biol Sci Med Sci* 56 Spec No 2:65-80.

Wang JH, Ko GY, Kelly PT (1997) Cellular and molecular bases of memory: synaptic and neuronal plasticity. *J Clin Neurophysiol* 14:264-93.

Ward MT, Stoelzel CR, Markus EJ (1999) Hippocampal dysfunction during aging II: deficits on the radial-arm maze. *Neurobiol Aging* 20:373-80.

Weiss C, Preston AR, Oh MM, Schwarz RD, Welty D, Disterhoft JF (2000) The M1 muscarinic agonist CI-1017 facilitates trace eyeblink conditioning in aging rabbits and increases the excitability of CA1 pyramidal neurons. *J Neurosci* 20:783-90.

Winocur G, Moscovitch M (1990) Hippocampal and prefrontal cortex contributions to learning and memory: analysis of lesion and aging effects on maze learning in rats. *Behav Neurosci* 104:544-51.

Wolf FI, Cittadini A (2003) Chemistry and biochemistry of magnesium. *Mol Aspects Med* 24:3-9.

Woolf NJ, Eckenstein F, Butcher LL (1984) Cholinergic systems in the rat brain: I. projections to the limbic telencephalon. *Brain Res Bull* 13:751-84.

Zhang Q, Okamura M, Guo ZD, Niwa S, Haga T (2004) Effects of partial agonists and Mg2+ ions on the interaction of M2 muscarinic acetylcholine receptor and G protein Galpha i1 subunit in the M2-Galpha i1 fusion protein. *J Biochem* 135:589-96.

Zornetzer SF, Thompson R, Rogers J (1982) Rapid forgetting in aged rats. *Behav Neural Biol* 36:49-60.

Section 2

Magnesium in Neurological Diseases

The role of magnesium therapy in learning and memory

Michael R. Hoane ✉

Restorative Neuroscience Laboratory, Brain and Cognitive Science Program, Department of Psychology, Southern Illinois University, Carbondale, IL, USA.
✉ mhoane@siu.edu

Abstract

The old saying "you are what you eat" is becoming increasingly important in the field of neuroscience these days. There is mounting evidence that nutritional factors are beginning to play a major role in cognitive status, or cognitive wellbeing. One of these emerging factors is magnesium (Mg^{2+}). Although the physiological investigation of Mg^{2+} has a long history, its role in cognitive function is just starting to emerge. The focus of this chapter is to review the available literature on the effects of Mg^{2+} on cognitive function in the healthy and diseased/injured brain. In addition, data from our laboratory will be presented that has investigated the effects of Mg^{2+} manipulation on learning and memory tasks in rodents, as well as the ability of Mg^{2+} therapy to improve cognitive performance in the damaged brain.

Introduction

The purpose of this chapter is to provide a review of the literature on the role of Mg^{2+} in cognitive function. Although the research on this topic is generally sparse, there is an accumulating body of evidence suggesting that Mg^{2+} is vitally important. The role that micronutrients play in maintaining and promoting cognitive ability and neural plasticity has started to receive a good deal of attention. A recent paper has provided an excellent review on how various nutrients promote cognitive performance and neural plasticity (Gómez-Pinilla, 2008). Although this review does not specifically discuss the role of Mg^{2+}, it is clear that this is a rapidly evolving area of research. Another review does address the role of Mg^{2+} and its relationship with other micronutrients on cognitive function and performance; it especially highlights the important role that Mg^{2+} has in interacting with other micronutrients (Huskisson *et al*, 2007). Recent evidence also suggests the Mg^{2+} plays an important role in age-related deficits in neurotransmitter release, neuronal excitability and synaptic plasticity related to cognition (Billard, 2006), and these topics will be reviewed in Chapter 6.

Additionally, there is ample evidence that Mg^{2+} plays an important role in the pathophysiological processes following traumatic brain injury (TBI) and that Mg^{2+} therapy is effective in promoting functional recovery in a variety of animal models (Hoane and Barth, 2001; Hoane, 2004; Sen and Gulati, 2010; van den Heuvel and Vink, 2004; Vink *et al*, 2009). Specifically, this chapter will focus on reviewing the literature on Mg^{2+} and cognitive function and review a series of studies conducted in our laboratory that have investigated the ability of Mg^{2+} therapy to alter cognitive function and to improve cognitive recovery following focal and traumatic brain injuries in the rat.

Introduction to rodent cognitive assessment

The Morris water maze (MWM) is a standard task for measuring cognitive/spatial performance in rodents. This task uses a water-filled tank with a submerged escape platform and many different aspects of memory can be assessed (Hoane *et al*, 2003; Hoane, 2005; Hoane *et al*, 2009; Kaufman *et al*, 2010; Lindner, 1997; Lindner *et al*, 1998; Quigley *et al*, 2009). Briefly, a reference memory trial consists of placing the rat into the water at one of 4 randomly chosen start locations. A computer-assisted video tracking system is used to measure the swim latency and distance to the submerged escape platform. On trials designed to measure working memory the escape platform is relocated to a new position in the tank every day. The first trial (in the new location) is considered an information trial and the subsequent 3 trials are test trials and are averaged to form the dependent variable. Additional paradigms can be used that incorporate various mazes or dividers that are placed into the tank that can test other aspects of learning and memory in the rodent.

Additionally, the Barnes spatial maze, a dry version of the MWM, can also be used to assess cognitive/spatial performance (Vink *et al*, 2003). Rats are placed on an elevated 1.2 m circular table top with 19 holes cut around the periphery. The rat learns the location of the hole that leads to an escape tunnel. The latency to find the correct hole is then analyzed. Operant chambers (Skinner boxes) can be used to assess appetitive conditioning of learning ratios under various conditions. In general, rats are shaped to bar-press for a reinforcer and then are shifted to more complicated reward paradigms. Thus, there are many ways in which rodent cognitive assessments can be made and many of these have been utilized to examine the role of Mg^{2+} in cognition.

Role of Mg^{2+} in health and cognition

The importance of Mg^{2+} in normal cellular functioning has been well documented, as has its importance in the pathophysiology following injury. Previously, several reviews have been written that address these issues (Hoane and Barth, 2001; Hoane, 2004; van den Heuvel and Vink, 2004) so only a brief synopsis will be provided in this paper. Mg^{2+} is involved in many critical cellular processes including cellular respiration, protein synthesis, membrane stability and regulation of vascular tone. A more detailed discussion on the physiology of Mg^{2+} is presented in several chapters within Section 1 of this book.

Although the main focus of this chapter is on animal models, there are some interesting human studies that have examined the role of Mg^{2+} in cognitive ability. A recent study examined the correlation between levels of several trace minerals (iron, Mg^{2+}, potassium and zinc) in the hair of adolescent girls and their academic record. Care must be taken with the interpretation of correlational studies of this nature, there was evidence that some trace minerals correlated more highly with increased academic performance. Specifically, it was found that Mg^{2+} and zinc demonstrated a strong positive correlation with academic performance (Wang *et al*, 2008). Furthermore, a recent case report of a patient presenting with anorexia nervosa and Wernicke-Korsakoff syndrome was found to have a low serum Mg^{2+} level (Saad *et al*, 2010). Although the main cause of this condition was thiamine deficiency, a major adjunct factor was believed to be Mg^{2+} deficiency. The results from this case study are supported by a review article on micronutrients and cognitive performance that details the inter-relationships between Mg^{2+} and other micronutrients such as the B-group vitamins and how deficiencies in these nutrients interact to produce cognitive deficits (Huskisson *et al*, 2007). Thus, there is an expanding literature that suggests that Mg^{2+} status plays an important role in cognitive performance.

A unique condition in which Mg^{2+} has been implicated in is TBI. McIntosh and colleagues have shown that Mg^{2+} homeostasis is disrupted following CNS injury (McIntosh *et al*, 1988; Vink *et al*, 1988). Fluid percussion injury (FPI) produced a rapid and severe decline in intra- and extracellular Mg^{2+} levels, which correlated significantly with the severity of the behavioral deficits observed following injury (McIntosh *et al*, 1988; Vink *et al*, 1988). Additional research on the role of Mg^{2+} and neurological diseases will be presented in Section 2 of the book; as well as, the role of Mg^{2+} in cognitive function following TBI later in this chapter. These findings suggest that Mg^{2+} plays an important role in normal physiology and in the pathophysiological events that occur following injury to the nervous system.

Recent laboratory data

Mg^{2+} therapy and learning

From a purely pharmacological standpoint, administration of Mg^{2+} immediately prior to the acquisition of a learning task should have a detrimental effect on that task given the non-competitive antagonistic properties of Mg^{2+} at the NMDA receptor. It has been shown that administration of other NMDA antagonists such as MK-801 and PCP have been shown to disrupt spatial learning in rodents (Kesner *et al*, 1993; McLamb *et al*, 1990; Murray and Ridley, 1997); however, in some cases a facilitative effect can be shown (Pussinen and Sirvio, 1999). In order to examine the biological activity of Mg^{2+} administration on the acquisition of learning, a $MgCl_2$ solution was administered (1 mmol/kg or 2 mmol/kg, *i.p.*) prior to the acquisition of learning a reference memory task in the MWM (Hoane, 2007). Intact rats received daily injections of $MgCl_2$, 30 min prior to the start of their MWM session and were tested for 5 consecutive days for 4 trials per day with an intertrial interval (ITI) of 15 min. The reference memory acquisition paradigm was used in the MWM. In this paradigm, the submerged escape platform stayed in the same location for every trial and the animals were released from 1 of 4 different starting points in the maze. As can be seen in Figure 1, the vehicle-treated (0.9% saline, *i.p.*) group showed steady acquisition of the task. In comparison, the $MgCl_2$-treated animals showed a more varied response. The initial acquisition of the 2 mmol group was slightly lengthened on day 1 compared to the other groups. On day 4, both groups of $MgCl_2$-treated animals started to show a lengthening of their escape latencies compared to vehicle-treated animals. On the last 2 test days the comparison of swim latencies between the 2 mmol and saline group was significantly different ($p < 0.01$) indicating a possible learning impairment on the task.

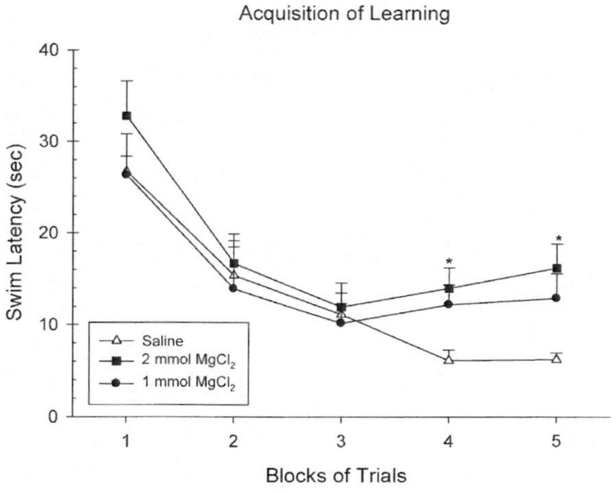

Figure 1. The effects of repeated pre-testing administration of $MgCl_2$ (1 or 2 mmol/kg) on the acquisition of a reference memory task in the MWM. Plotted are the mean (+SEM) swim latencies to find the submerged escape platform. The 2 mmol dose of $MgCl_2$ significantly impaired swim latencies starting on the 4th day of testing (* = $p < 0.05$).

Thus, it appears that daily dosing with the higher dose of $MgCl_2$ produced a significant degree of amnesia after 3 days. Unfortunately, testing was terminated after 5 days so it is unknown if this effect would have persisted or worsened with additional testing. It should be noted that, in general, the NMDA antagonists that work at the PCP site on the NMDA receptor (i.e., MK-801 and PCP) seem to have a greater amnesic effect than $MgCl_2$. This may raise some concerns for continued dosing regimens of Mg^{2+} therapy lasting more than a couple days. However, a longer window of time between administrations and testing may reveal different findings, because this effect is perceived to be state dependent. Thus, given these behavioral results it is clear that systemic injections of $MgCl_2$ did indeed exert behavioral effects in uninjured animals with an intact blood-brain barrier (BBB), and therefore give support to the ability of $MgCl_2$ to cross the BBB. This finding supports earlier research to this fact (Hallack *et al*, 1992).

We have also recently investigated the effect of dietary Mg^{2+} deficiency on learning acquisition in the MWM. Rats were placed on either a standard laboratory diet or a commercially available Mg^{2+} deficient diet for 14 days. Peripheral blood collections were performed for determination of serum Mg^{2+} levels and all animals were placed back on to the standard diet. The serum analysis indicated a significant loss in serum Mg^{2+} in the deficiency group ($p < 0.05$). One week later, animals were tested for the acquisition of a reference memory task over 4 days (4 trials per day, 15 min ITI). As can be seen in Figure 2A, the 14 days of Mg^{2+} deficiency significantly impaired the initial acquisition of the task on the first day ($p<0.05$). The animals were then switched to a more challenging working memory assessment in the MWM. As can be seen in Figure 2B, the animals that experienced Mg^{2+}-deficiency showed impaired learning on the task ($p<0.05$). Additionally, animals were trained to acquire a fixed ration (FR-10) schedule of reinforcement in an operant chamber. The total number of bar presses is shown in Figure 2C, the higher number of responses results in a greater number of reinforcers being delivered and can be equated to the learning of the reinforcement schedule. Animals on the Mg^{2+}-deficient diet responded at a significantly lower level ($p<0.05$) than those animals on the Mg^{2+}-normal diet, suggesting a learning impairment. A somewhat similar finding has been shown in mice exposed to a Mg^{2+} deficient diet (Bardgett *et al*, 2005; Bardgett *et al*, 2007).

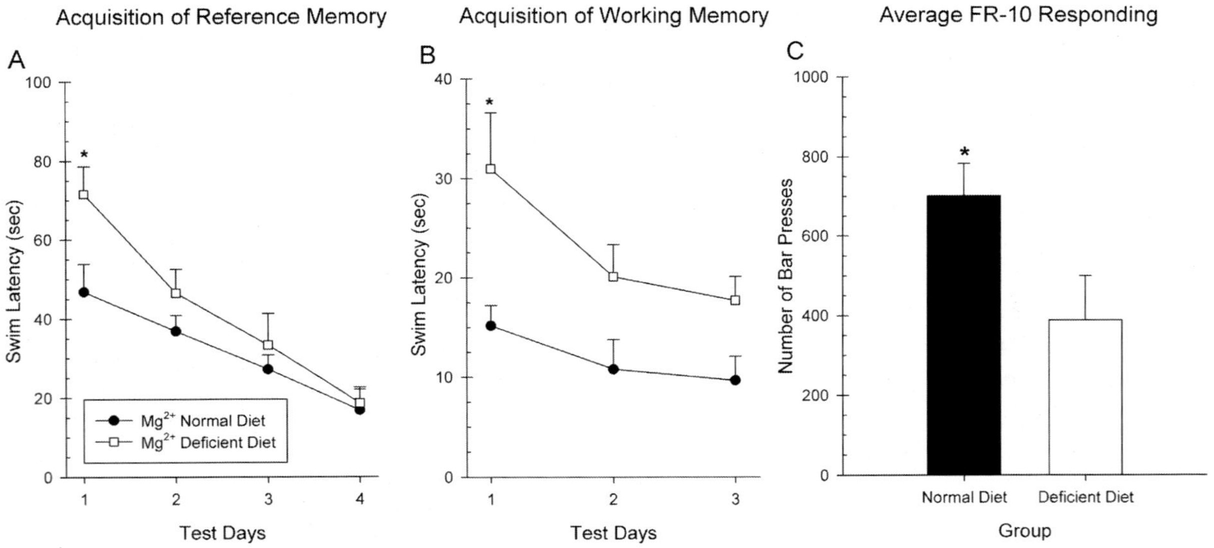

Figure 2. The effects of dietary restriction of Mg^{2+} on cognitive performance in the MWM. Plotted are the mean swim latencies (+SEM) on the acquisition of reference memory task (A), working memory (B) and the acquisition of a FR-10 reinforcement schedule in an operant chamber (C). A two week period of dietary Mg^{2+} deficiency, followed by reinstatement back to a Mg^{2+} normal diet resulted in significant impairments in cognitive performance on all measures (* = $p < 0.05$).

In this study, 10 days of Mg^{2+} deficiency resulted in impaired learning of a conditioned fear task; however, maze performance in the MWM was not impaired. Thus, these data suggest that even temporary Mg^{2+} deficiency may interfere with learning.

A newly formulated form of Mg^{2+}, magnesium-L-threonate (MgT) has been shown to increase cerebrospinal fluid levels of Mg^{2+} to a much greater degree than other Mg^{2+} preparations (e.g., $MgCl_2$) (Slutsky *et al*, 2010). Administration of MgT has also been shown to result in an enhancement of various forms of cognitive/ learning ability in rodents, including working memory. This effect was also evident in aged rats following which cognitive abilities were generally reduced. The beneficial behavioral effects were thought to be caused by beneficial changes in synaptic plasticity within the hippocampus (Slutsky *et al*, 2010).

Effects of Mg^{2+} therapy on cognitive function following brain injury

Several studies have investigated the ability of Mg^{2+} to improve acute cognitive function in animal models of TBI. It has been shown that administration of $MgCl_2$ following FPI improved cognitive outcome by reducing memory loss following injury (Smith *et al*, 1993). However, administration of $MgCl_2$ failed to improve the acquisition of a reference memory task in the MWM following injury (Bareyre *et al*, 1999). It has also been recently shown that administration of $MgSO_4$ (250 µmol/kg, *i.v.*), 30 min following diffuse axonal injury improved recovery of a spatial memory task on the Barnes maze (Vink *et al*, 2003). In addition, administration of an intravenous solution of $MgCl_2$ (150 µmol) prior to FPI prevented the occurrence of injury-induced impairments on working and reference memory tasks in a radial maze (Enomoto *et al*, 2005).

There have been very few attempts to examine the ability of Mg^{2+} therapy to resolve long-term cognitive dysfunction. A recent study has shown severe cognitive deficits in the acquisition of a reference memory task in the MWM when tested 8 months post-FPI (Browne *et al*, 2004). The administration of $MgSO_4$ (125 µmol, *i.v.*) or NPS 1506 (an NMDA antagonist) failed to improve the acquisition of the reference memory task compared to vehicle controls. However, it was found that $MgSO_4$ did reduce the amount of ipsilateral hippocampal cell loss; thus, preservation of the hippocampus failed to result in significant cognitive improvement (Browne *et al*, 2004). Given the limited number of studies and their mixed results, it is important to further investigate the effect of Mg^{2+} therapy on the recovery of cognitive function following injury.

Examination of Mg^{2+} therapy following focal injury

In our laboratory we have examined recovery of cognitive function in a bilateral focal cortical ablation model. Rats were given small (4 mm^2) electrolytic lesions aimed at the bilateral anterior medial cortex (bAMC) of the frontal lobe (Hoane *et al*, 2003). Administration of Mg^{2+} therapy occurred 15 min following injury with rats receiving either injections of $MgCl_2$ (1 or 2 mmol/kg, *i.p.*) or saline (1 ml/kg). This regimen was repeated again 24 and 72 hrs later, so that each rat received 3 injections within the first 72 hrs following injury. Behavioral testing began 5 days after injury and included the assessment of cognitive function. The MWM was used to investigate the acquisition of reference and working memory. In addition, the MWM tank was also used to examine spatial ability using a delayed matching-to-sample (DMTS) task, a very sensitive measure of spatial working memory.

As can be seen in Figure 3A&B, the results of the behavioral testing indicated that bAMC lesions produced severe deficits in cognitive function on both the reference and working memory tasks in the MWM. Mg^{2+} therapy with either the 1 or 2 mmol dose did not significantly facilitate the acquisition of reference memory in the MWM; however, the mean swim latencies for both $MgCl_2$ groups were greatly improved compared to saline in the last 2 blocks of trials. Although Mg^{2+} therapy did not demonstrate a statistically significant improvement on reference memory performance in the present study, it did improve working memory performance in the MWM. Administration of the 2 mmol dose of $MgCl_2$ significantly reduced the working memory deficit compared to saline treatment on the first 2 days of testing. The 1 mmol dose of $MgCl_2$ also reduced the working memory impairments on the first day of testing and significantly improved working memory performance on day 2 of testing. Severe cognitive impairments were also seen on the DMTS spatial memory test following injury. The 2 mmol dose of $MgCl_2$ significantly reduced the number of trials needed to reach the criterion of 80% correct choices compared to saline-treated rats, while the 1 mmol dose of $MgCl_2$ did not, although the number of trials was greatly reduced. Thus, Mg^{2+} therapy was effective in a task and dose-dependent manner in this study.

Mg^{2+} therapy in the traumatically injured brain

To examine the ability of Mg^{2+} therapy following TBI, groups of rats were prepared with a cortical contusion injury (CCI) or sham procedure and then assigned to either $MgCl_2$ (1.0 mmol/kg, i.p.) or saline treatment conditions (Hoane, 2005). Mg^{2+} therapy was administered 15 min and 24 hr following injury. Rats were then examined for cognitive/spatial performance in the MWM, investigating the acquisition of reference and working memory. Administration of $MgCl_2$ following CCI significantly reduced some of the behavioral impairments observed following injury (see Figure 3C&D). The acquisition of reference memory in the MWM was significantly improved compared to saline-treated rats. In contrast, $MgCl_2$ did not improve working memory performance.

In a second study, the ability of Mg^{2+} therapy to improve cognitive/spatial performance following unilateral CCI was examined. Groups of rats were given unilateral CCIs or sham surgeries of the left sensorimotor motor/frontal cortex. One hr following injury, rats were administered 1 mmol /kg $MgCl_2$ or saline. They were then tested for their ability to acquire a reference memory task in the MWM on 4 consecutive days (4 trials/day) starting 11 days after CCI. Their working memory performance was measured on days 16 and 17. It was found that the single 1 mmol/kg dose of $MgCl_2$ effectively facilitated the acquisition of the reference memory task compared to treatment with saline (see Figure 4). In a similar manner, the working memory performance was greatly enhanced following CCI in the Mg^{2+}-treated rats compared to the saline-treated rats. In fact, the working memory performance of the Mg^{2+}-treated rats could not be distinguished from the sham controls on either day of working memory testing (see working memory graph in Fig 4). Mg^{2+} treatment appeared to have prevented the occurrence of the working memory deficit following unilateral frontal injury.

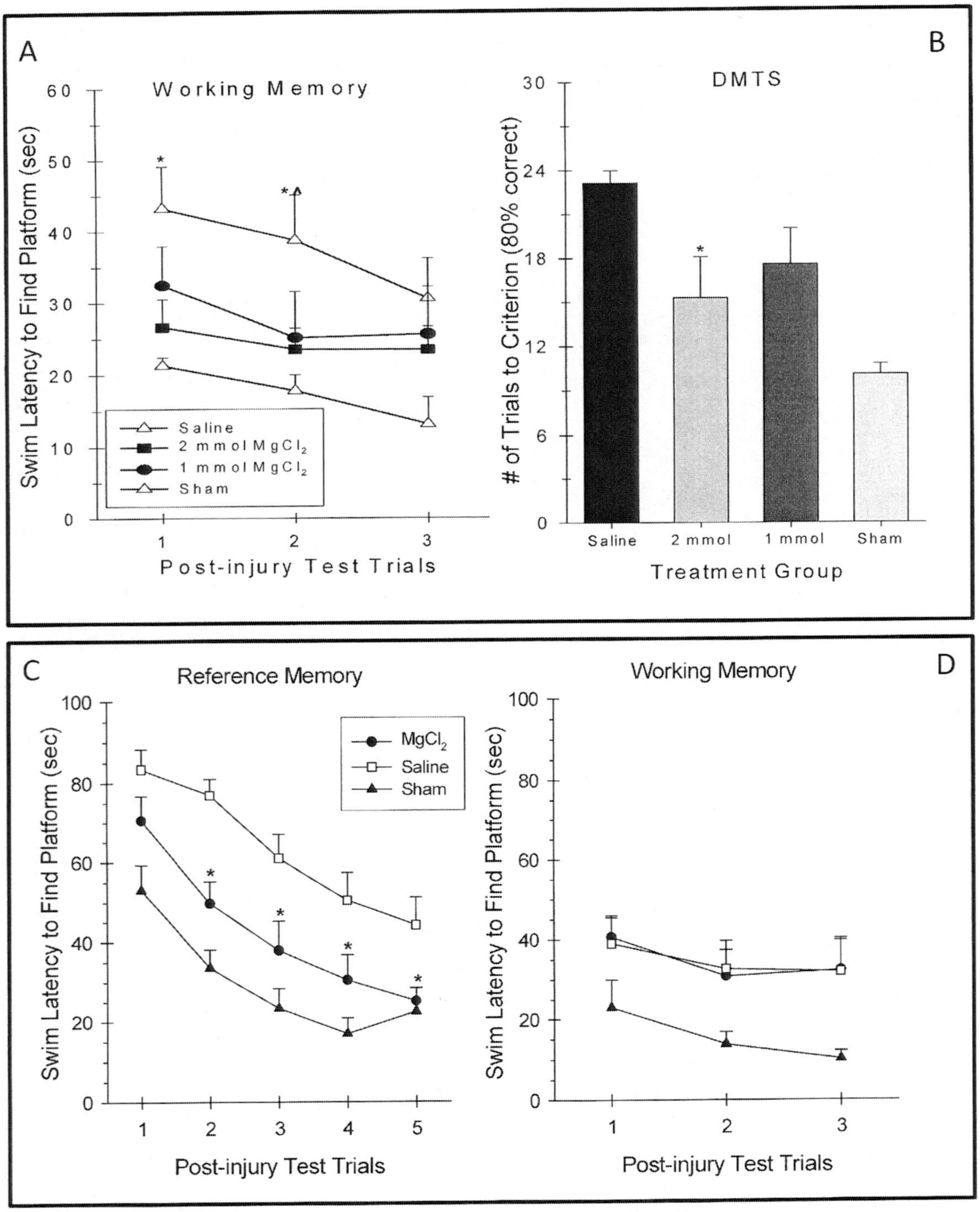

Figure 3. The effects of a regimen of $MgCl_2$ (1 or 2 mmol/kg) administered following bAMC focal lesions on cognitive performance in the MWM. Plotted are the mean swim latencies (+SEM) during the acquisition phase of a working memory task (A) and the mean number of trials to criterion in the DMTS test (B) is presented. There was a dose and task-dependent effect on recovery. The 2 mmol dose provided the greatest improvement on both measures of working memory (* = $p < 0.05$ comparing 2 mmol $MgCl_2$ to saline; ^ = $p < 0.05$ comparing 1 mmol $MgCl_2$ to saline). Adapted from (Hoane *et al*, 2003). The effects of a regimen of $MgCl_2$ (1 mmol/kg) administered 15 min following bilateral CCI of the frontal cortex. Plotted are the mean swim latencies (+SEM) on the acquisition of reference memory (C) and working memory (D) tasks in the MWM. Administration of $MgCl_2$ significantly improved the acquisition of a reference memory task, but not working memory following CCI (* = $p < 0.05$). Adapted from (Hoane *et al*, 2005).

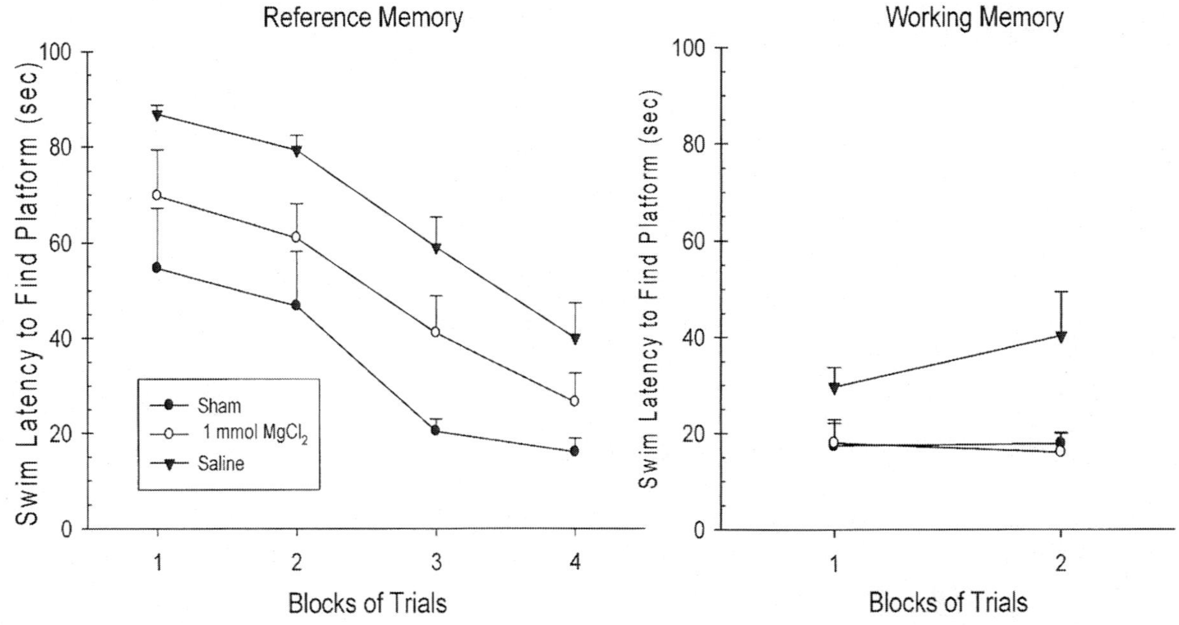

Figure 4. The effects of $MgCl_2$ (1 mmol/kg) administration 1 hr following unilateral CCI of the sensorimotor/frontal cortex. Plotted are the mean swim latencies (+SEM) on the acquisition of reference memory and working memory tasks in the MWM. Administration of $MgCl_2$ significantly improved the acquisition of a reference memory task and working memory following CCI. Adapted from (Hoane, 2007).

Discussion

The results of these studies have demonstrated a wide range of conditions in which Mg^{2+} therapy regulates cognitive function. It was first shown that daily injections of $MgCl_2$ administered 30 mins prior to training on the task worsened acquisition of the reference memory task. It was also demonstrated that a two-week regimen of dietary Mg^{2+} deficiency impaired learning on 3 different cognitive tasks. This finding is especially interesting because the animals had been placed back onto a normal laboratory diet prior to the assessment phase of the study.

Mg^{2+} therapy in several models of cortical ablation and TBI have demonstrated positive effects on cognitive recovery. However, these effects occurred in a task and dose-dependent manner. Following focal ablation of the bAMC, $MgCl_2$ improved working memory performance on several measures and slightly improved reference memory performance. The CCI studies performed in our laboratory have shown that $MgCl_2$ administration following injury improved cognitive performance in a task-dependent manner. Previous studies that have examined the ability of Mg^{2+} therapy to improve cognitive performance following injury have shown mixed results. For example, administration of $MgCl_2$ following FPI has been shown to improve cognitive outcome by reducing memory loss in the MWM (Smith *et al*, 1993), but administration of $MgCl_2$ failed to improve the acquisition of a reference memory task in the MWM following injury (Bareyre *et al*, 1999). Thus, in a similar manner the current series of studies has shown similar mixed results. That is, significant effects were seen in some cases and non-significant effects were seen in others. However, in general we saw significant improvements in cognitive function by $MgCl_2$ in each of our studies. The discrepant results mainly varied based on dose and task-dependent properties of the studies.

From a mechanistic standpoint, Mg^{2+} therapy has multiple routes by which it can disrupt the pathophysiological processes that occur following injury and enhance cognitive recovery. In addition to offsetting injury-induced Mg^{2+}

depletion (McIntosh *et al*, 1988; Vink *et al*, 1988) and preventing excitotoxic neuronal death (Nowak *et al*, 1984) mediated by the NMDA receptor, Mg^{2+} has been shown to have several other effects. For instance, administration of $MgSO_4$ has been shown to limit the generation of injury-induced edema following closed-head injury (Feldman *et al*, 1996) and it has been more recently shown that $MgSO_4$ (30 mg/kg) reduced aquaporin-4 immunoreactivity, thus contributing to edema reduction following injury (Ghabriel *et al*, 2006). Administration of $MgCl_2$ has also been shown to reduce the expression of p53 mRNA, a gene associated with the induction of cell death, following lateral FPI (Muir *et al*, 1999). In this study it was found that 750 µmol/kg of $MgCl_2$ reduced the expression of p53 mRNA in the injured cortex compared to saline-treated controls (Muir *et al*, 1999). High concentrations of Mg^{2+} (3 mM) have been shown to inhibit lipid peroxidation (Regan *et al*, 1998). Regardless of the mechanisms of action, the data presented in this review has shown that $MgCl_2$ has strong biological activity, appears to cross the BBB, and can improve cognitive performance following cortical ablation or TBI.

Conclusion

The studies presented in this book chapter have demonstrated a wide range of activities for Mg^{2+} therapy in relationship to cognitive function in the rodent. Daily injections of $MgCl_2$ prior to the acquisition of a learning task blocked the acquisition of a reference memory task and dietary deficiency of Mg^{2+} impaired learning on a number of different tasks. Using the damaged brain as a model to examine the ability of Mg^{2+} therapy to improve cognitive performance also demonstrated significant advantages with the therapy. Thus, it does appear that Mg^{2+} status and therapy have significant effects on cognitive performance in the brain and that further research is warranted. In addition, an accumulating body of research suggests that Mg^{2+} also plays an important role in human cognitive performance. Given the reported rates of magnesium deficiency in humans it is likely that this could impair cognitive performance (Barbagallo and Dominguez, 2010; Elin, 2010). In addition, the most intriguing factor related to Mg^{2+} therapy for cognitive wellbeing may reside in the use of Mg^{2+} as a co-therapy with other vital nutrients, which may produce the strongest effects.

Acknowledgements

A special thanks is given to Alicia Swan for critical reading of an earlier draft of this chapter. Partial support provided by ARRA funds from NINDS grant NS045647-04

References

Barbagallo M, Dominguez LJ (2010) Magnesium and aging. *Curr Pharm Des* 16:832-9.

Bardgett ME, Schultheis PJ, McGill DL, Richmond RE, Wagge JR (2005) Magnesium deficiency impairs fear conditioning in mice. *Brain Res* 1038:100-6.

Bardgett ME, Schultheis PJ, Muzny A, Riddle MD, Wagge JR (2007) Magnesium deficiency reduces fear-induced conditional lick suppression in mice. *Magnes Res* 20:58-65.

Bareyre FM, Saatman KE, Helfaer MA, Sinson GP, Weisser JD, Brown AL, McIntosh TK (1999) Alterations in ionized and total blood magnesium after experimental traumatic brain injury: Relationship to neurobehavioral outcome and neuroprotective efficacy of magnesium chloride. *J Neurochem* 73:271-80.

Billard JM (2006) Ageing, hippocampal synaptic activity and magnesium. *Magnes Res* 19:199-215.

Browne KD, Leoni MJ, Iwata A, Chen XH, Smith DH (2004) Acute treatment with MgSO4 attenuates long-term hippocampal tissue loss after brain trauma in the rat. *J Neurosci Res* 77:878-83.

Elin RJ (2010) Assessment of magnesium status for diagnosis and therapy. *Magnes Res*. 23:194-8.

Enomoto T, Osugi T, Satoh H, McIntosh TK, Nabeshima T (2005) Pre-Injury magnesium treatment prevents traumatic brain injury-induced hippocampal ERK activation, neuronal loss, and cognitive dysfunction in the radial-arm maze test. *J Neurotrauma* 22:783-92.

Feldman Z, Gurevitch B, Artru AA, Oppenheim A, Shohami E, Reichenthal E, Shapira Y (1996) Effect of magnesium given 1 hour after head trauma on brain edema and neurological outcome. *J Neurosurg* 85:131-7.

Ghabriel MN, Thomas A, Vink R (2006) Magnesium restores altered aquaporin-4 immunoreactivity following traumatic brain injury to a pre-injury state. *Acta Neurochir Suppl* 96:402-6.

Gómez-Pinilla F (2008) Brain foods: The effects of nutrients on brain function. *Nat Rev Neurosci* 9:568-78.

Hallack M, Berman RF, Ortemkauf SM, Evans MI, Cotton DB (1992) Peripheral magnesium sulfate enters the brain and increases the threshold for hippocampal seizures in rats. *Am J Obstet Gynecol* 167.

Hoane MR, Barth TM (2001) The behavioral and anatomical effects of $MgCl_2$ therapy in an electrolytic lesion model of cortical injury in the rat. *Magnes Res* 14:51-63.

Hoane MR, Knotts AA, Akstulewicz SL, Aquilano M, Means LW (2003) The behavioral effects of magnesium therapy on recovery of function following bilateral anterior medial cortex lesions in the rat. *Brain Res Bull* 60:105-14.

Hoane MR (2004) Magnesium therapy and recovery of function in experimental models of brain injury and neurodegenerative disease. *Clin Calcium* 14:65-70.

Hoane MR (2005) Treatment with magnesium improves reference memory but not working memory while reducing GFAP expression following traumatic brain injury. *Restor Neurol Neurosci* 23:67-77.

Hoane MR, Wolyniak J, Akstulewicz SL (2005) Administration of riboflavin improves behavioral outcome and reduces edema formation and GFAP expression following traumatic brain injury. *J Neurotrauma* 22:1112-22.

Hoane MR (2007) Assessment of cognitive function following magnesium therapy in the traumatically injured brain. *Magnes Res* 20:229-36.

Hoane MR, Kaufman NA, Vitek MP, McKenna SE (2009) COG1410 improves cognitive performance and reduces cortical neuronal loss in the traumatically injured brain. *J Neurotrauma* 26:1-10.

Huskisson E, Maggini S, Ruf M (2007) The influence of micronutrients on cognitive function and performance. *J Int Med Res* 35:1-19.

Kaufman NA, Beare JE, Tan AA, Vitek MP, McKenna SE, Hoane MR (2010) COG1410, an apolipoprotein E-based peptide, improves cognitive performance and reduces cortical loss following moderate fluid percussion injury in the rat. *Behav Brain Res* 214:395-401.

Kesner RP, Dakis M, Bolland BL (1993) Phencyclidine disrupts long- but not short-term memory within a spatial learning task. *Psychopharmacology* 111:85-90.

Lindner MD (1997) Reliability, distribution, and validity of age-related cognitive deficits in the Morris water maze. *Neurobiol Learn Mem* 68:203-20.

Lindner MD, Plone MA, Cain CK, Frydel BR, Francis JM, Emerich DF, Sutton RL (1998) Dissociable long-term cognitive deficits after frontal versus sensorimotor cortical contusions. *J Neurotrauma* 15:199-216.

McIntosh TK, Faden AI, Yamakami I, Vink R (1988) Magnesium deficiency exacerbates and pretreatment improves outcome following traumatic brain injury in rats: ^{31}P magnetic resonance spectroscopy and behavioral studies. *J Neurotrauma* 5:17-31.

McLamb RL, Williams LR, Nanry KP, Wilson WA, Tilson HA (1990) MK-801 impedes the acquisition of a spatial memory task in rats. *Pharmacol Biochem Behav* 37:41-5.

Muir JK, Raghupathi R, Emery DL, Bareyre FM, McIntosh TK (1999) Postinjury magnesium treatment attenuates traumatic brain injury-induced cortical induction of p53 mRNA in rats. *Exp Neurol* 159:584-93.

Murray TK, Ridley RM (1997) The effect of dizocilpine (MK-801) on conditional discrimination learning in the rat. *Behav Pharmacol* 8:383-8.

Nowak L, Bregestovski P, Ascher P, Herbert A, Prochiantz A (1984) Magnesium gates glutamate activated channels in mouse central neurones. *Nature* 307:462-5.

Pussinen R, Sirvio J (1999) Effects of D-cycloserine, a positive modulator of N-methyl-D-aspartate receptors, and ST 587, a putative alpha-1 adrenergic agonist, individually and in combination, on the non-delayed and delayed foraging behaviour of rats assessed in the radial arm maze. *J Psychopharmacol* 13:171-9.

Quigley A, Tan AA, Hoane MR (2009) The effects of hypertonic saline and nicotinamide on sensorimotor and cognitive function following cortical contusion injury in the rat. *Brain Res* 1304:138-48.

Regan RF, Jasper E, Guo Y, Panter SS (1998) The effect of magnesium on oxidative neuronal injury in vitro. *J Neurochem* 70:77-85.

Saad L, Silva L, Banzato C, Dantas C, Garcia C (2010) Anorexia nervosa and Wernicke-Korsakoff syndrome: a case report. *J Med Case Reports* 4:1-5.

Sen AP, Gulati A (2010) Use of magnesium in traumatic brain injury. *Neurotherapeutics* 7:91-9.

Slutsky I, Abumaria N, Wu LJ, Huang C, Zhang L, Li B, Zhao X, Govindarajan A, Zhao MG, Zhuo M, Tonegawa S, Liu G (2010) Enhancement of learning and memory by elevating brain magnesium. *Neuron* 65:165-77.

Smith DH, Okiyama K, Gennarelli TA, McIntosh TK (1993) Magnesium and ketamine attenuate cognitive dysfunction following experimental brain injury. *Neurosci Lett* 157:211-4.

Van Den Heuvel C, Vink R (2004) The role of magnesium in traumatic brain injury. *Clin Calcium* 14:9-14.

Vink R, McIntosh TK, Demediuk P, Weiner MW, Faden AI (1988) Decline in intracellular free Mg^{2+} is associated with irreversible tissue injury after brain trauma. *J Biol Chem* 263:757-61.

Vink R, O'Connor CA, Nimmo AJ, Heath DL (2003) Magnesium attenuates persistent functional deficits following diffuse traumatic brain injury in rats. *Neurosci Lett* 336:41-4.

Vink R, Cook NL, van de Heuvel C (2009) Magnesium in acute and chronic brain injury: an update. *Magnes Res* 22:158S-62S.

Wang C-T, Li Y, Wang F-J, Shi Y-M, Lee B-T (2008) Correlation between iron, magnesium, potassium and zinc content in adolescent girl's hair and their academic records. *Chang Gung Med J* 31:358-62.

Magnesium in headache

Lisa A. Yablon✉ *and Alexander Mauskop*

The New York Headache Center, 30 East 76th Street, New York, NY 10021, USA.
✉ drmauskop@nyheadache.com

Abstract

Magnesium's role in migraine pathogenesis is well-described, with deficiencies known to promote cortical spreading depression, alter nociceptive processing, and neurotransmitter release and encourage the hyperaggregation of platelets, all major elements of migraine development. Research on magnesium has found it to be a potentially well-tolerated, safe and inexpensive option for migraine prevention, while it may also be effective as an acute treatment option for headaches including migraines, tension-type headaches and cluster headaches, particularly in certain patient subsets. This chapter will review the various aspects of migraine in which magnesium plays a part, as well as numerous studies on the use of magnesium in both headache prophylaxis and in the acute treatment of headaches, offering recommendations in its use in clinical practice.

Magnesium in the Body

Magnesium (Mg), the second most abundant intracellular divalent cation, is a cofactor of many enzymes and is involved in a plethora of cellular functions. It plays a central role in both glucose metabolism and in ATP function. Over 300 enzymes require the presence of magnesium ions for their catalytic action, including all enzymes utilizing or synthesizing ATP, or those that use other nucleotides to synthesize DNA and RNA. ATP exists in cells as a chelate of ATP and a magnesium ion. Because of the important interaction between phosphate and magnesium ions, magnesium ions are essential to the basic nucleic acid chemistry of life, and thus are essential to all cells of all known living organisms.

Magnesium is involved in the formation of phospholipids and the insertion of proteins into the phospholipid membrane, and is therefore critical to membrane stabilization (Durlach *et al*, 1987). It also contributes to contraction of the cytoskeleton at the myoneural junction, playing a vital role in the function of both skeletal, cardiac and other smooth muscles.

Magnesium is absorbed in the gastrointestinal tract, via intestinal epithelial channels in the ileum as well as by the renal system's thick ascending limb, distal tubule, and loop of Henle of the nephron (Wagner, 2007). It facilitates calcium absorption via the thick ascending limb, and the absorption of both ions is regulated by the parathyroid hormone (PTH) secreting cells of the parathyroid gland (Bapty *et al*, 1998). The calcium/magnesium sensing receptor within the parathyroid gland regulates absorption of both ions by detecting their levels in ionized form, and then controlling PTH secretion, thereby maintaining calcium homeostasis (Brown *et al*, 1993). Dietarily, absorption is affected by protein intake as well as phosphate, phytate and fat. Absorbed dietary magnesium is largely excreted through the urine, although most iatrogenically administered oral magnesium is excreted through the feces.

Adult human bodies contain approximately 24 grams of magnesium, with 67% located in the skeleton, 31% intracellularly (20% in skeletal muscle), and only 1-2% extracellularly. Of this amount, one half is ionized, and 25-30% is protein bound. As a result, levels found on routine serum testing, which only reflects that magnesium found in the extracellular space, is not representative of true total body magnesium stores (Moe, 2008).

Serum levels are typically 0.7–1.0 mmol/L or 1.8–2.4 mEq/L. Serum magnesium levels may appear normal even in cases of underlying intracellular deficiency, and true hypomagnesemia is common, possibly due to decreased intake or absorption, increased loss via the urine or diarrhea, or genetic factors (Henrotte, 1982).

Primary and Secondary Hypomagnesemia

Familial hypomagnesemia with secondary hypocalcemia has been studied in various kindreds, and heredity has been found to be X linked in some families, and autosomal recessive in others (Walder *et al*, 1997). There are currently more than 30 known mutations in the TRPM6 gene that are associated with familial hypomagnesemia and hypocalcemia. Another hereditary form of hypomagnesemia, tubular hypomagnesemia/hypokalemia with hypocalciuria (Gitelman's syndrome), is hypothesized to be due to two different types of genetic transmission, one autosomal recessive and one autosomal dominant with high phenotype variability (Bettinelli *et al*, 1995).

A population study in Germany found the prevalence of serum hypomagnesemia to be 14.5%, with even higher frequencies in females (Schimatschek and Rempis, 2001). Additionally, chronic disease is associated with hypomagnesemia, including diabetes, asthma, cardiovascular disease, sickle cell anemia, preeclampsia and eclampsia (Laites *et al*, 2004). 10-20% of hospitalized patients are deficient in magnesium, and up to 65% of patients in intensive care units are hypomagnesemic. Alcoholism is also associated with inadequate magnesium levels, in part due to poor nutrition (Bohmer and Mathiesen, 1982). It has also been implicated in patients with end-stage renal disease suffering from hemodialysis headache (Goksel *et al*, 2006), and is often seen in conjunction with electrolyte abnormalities including hypokalemia, hyponatremia, hypocalcemia and hypophosphatemia (Whang *et al*, 1985). A number of medications such as diuretics, aminoglycosides and digoxin are associated with hypomagnesemia, and patients with refractory hypocalcemia and hypokalemia should be evaluated for hypomagnesemia (Innerarity, 2000).

Magnesium Imbalances

Clinical symptoms of hypomagnesemia include hallucinations, depression, delirium, lethargy, weakness, paresthesias, tremors, premenstrual syndrome, cold extremities, leg or foot cramps, seizures, ventricular arrhythmias and congestive heart failure (Douban *et al*, 1996). However, since total body stores are not accurately represented by serum levels, routine blood testing and even erythrocyte Mg concentrations, may reveal normal levels, particularly in patients with low free (ionized) magnesium levels. Urinary fractional excretion or the oral magnesium load test can estimate the total body magnesium status. Intravenous magnesium loading tests are likely the most accurate and practical assess-ment, whereby total excretion of urinary magnesium is calculated over a 24 hour period, following administration of a loading dose; a retention of 20% or more indicates deficiency (Arnaud, 2008).

Hypermagnesemia, on the other hand, is a rare condition due to the nephron's rapid response to increased levels. It usually develops only in people with kidney failure who are given magnesium salts or who take drugs that contain magnesium such as laxatives or antacids. Clinical symptoms include nausea, muscle weakness, lethargy, confusion, hypotension and arrhythmias. In mild cases, withdrawing magnesium supplementation is often sufficient. In more severe cases, intravenous calcium gluconate and diuretics or dialysis may be required.

Magnesium Levels in Migraineurs

For many decades, it was postulated that magnesium deficiency played a role in migraine pathogenesis. However the lack of simple and reliable measures of magnesium levels prevented further research to prove this theory. While low serum, cerebrospinal fluid and cerebral tissue levels of magnesium have been found to be low in patients with migraine (Jain *et al*, 1985; Ramadan *et al*, 1989; Schoenen *et al*, 1991), these results have been inconsistent, with both normal and low levels detected in the same tissues of some patients. The variability of results may be due to the need to measure ionized magnesium as a true reflection of magnesium metabolism, and the development of an ion selective electrode for ionized magnesium in whole blood, serum, plasma and aqueous samples has made an accurate and rapid measurement of ionized magnesium levels possible (Altura *et al*, 1992).

A study measuring ionized magnesium levels in 40 patients during an acute migraine attack found that 50% had levels below 0.54 mmol/l (normal adult range 0.54-0.65 mmol/l) (Mauskop *et al*, 1995), with all subjects having total serum magnesium levels within normal limits. Intravenous administration of 1g of magnesium sulfate was most effective in those with low ionized magnesium, with 86% of patients reporting sustained pain relief over 24 hours in those found to have low serum ionized magnesium, while this was the case in only 16% of patients with normal levels. This finding was extended to patients with various headache types including migraine without aura, cluster headache, chronic migraine and chronic tension type headache (Mauskop *et al*, 1996), with most patients demonstrating low ionized magnesium levels. In addition, high serum ionized calcium to magnesium ratios were found in all headache types except for in those patients with chronic tension type headaches. Based on these findings, it has been suggested that tension type headache may possibly be discriminated from chronic migraine based on serum ionized magnesium levels (Mauskop *et al*, 1994).

Migraine Pathogenesis

Migraine is the most common form of disabling primary headache that afflicts patients, affecting approximately 12% of Western populations (Lipton *et al*, 2007). It is clear that there is genetic transmission of the disorder, although specific genes for most forms of migraine have not yet been identified. Additionally, although the exact etiology remains to be defined, current theories center on hyperexcitability of the cortex and trigeminovascular complex. In migraineurs, headache triggers stimulate the release of neuropeptides from the trigeminovascular neurons, including calcitonin gene-related peptide and substance P. Additionally, stimulation of the trigeminal ganglion increases cerebral blood flow due to the release of vasoactive intestinal peptide by the facial nerve (Goadsby and Macdonald, 1985). The vasodilation is accompanied by mast cell degranulation, blood vessel edema and increased vascular permeability, resulting in meningeal neurogenic inflammation.

The trigeminal nerve transmits this information to the brainstem trigeminal nucleus caudalis, and then on to the thalamic nuclei and the cortex, where the pain is ultimately perceived (Moskowitz, 1984). Other structures, including the periaqueductal gray matter and the locus coeruleus and the dorsal raphe nuclei, modulate pain transmission and therefore its perception (Martin and Behbehani, 2001).

Recent research has elucidated the aura phase of migraine, which affects up to 5% of the adult population (Agostini and Aliprandi, 2006). Migraine aura is the presentation of characteristic neurological symptoms usually developing prior to the onset of the painful phase of a migraine headache, believed to be due to a phenomenon known as cortical spreading depression (CSD). CSD was originally described by Leao (Leao, 1944) and is an intense depolarization of neuronal and glial membranes, with alterations in membrane resistance and ion flow. There is subsequent massive release of glutamate and potassium as well as an increase in intracellular sodium and calcium. This results in a strong wave of depolarization that spreads across contiguous neuronal tissue. It can be triggered by depolarization of a small region of brain tissue or by direct application of excitatory amino acids, and activation of the N-methyl-D aspartate (NMDA) receptor can evoke CSD (Gorji *et al*, 2001). There are characteristic alterations in cerebral blood flow, with an initial brief oligemia followed by a profound hyperemia, and a mild, long-lasting oligemia (Otori *et al*, 2003). Precisely how the aura phase of a migraine evolves into the painful phase remains unknown, and it has been theorized that it is due to the action of a number of inflammatory proteins including calcitonin gene-related peptide (CGRP), nitric oxide and vasoactive peptide (Goadsby, 1990) which feed into the trigeminal nerve and generate pial artery dilation and CSD, and, ultimately, headache.

Using phosphorus nuclear magnetic resonance spectroscopy (MRS), low levels of magnesium have been found in the cerebral tissue of some migraineurs both during attacks and interictally (Ramadan *et al*, 1989). Another study utilized the same technology to assess the brain cytosolic free magnesium concentration and free energy released by the hydrolysis of adenosine triphosphate, an index of cellular bioenergetics in both migraineurs and patients with cluster headaches (Lodi *et al*, 2001). Cytosolic free magnesium and the free energy released by the reaction of ATP hydrolysis were significantly reduced in the occipital lobes of patients with all types of migraine as well as in cluster headache patients. The authors of this study took these results to lend support to their hypothesis that the reduction of free magnesium in tissue with mitochondrial dysfunction is due to a bioenergetics deficit, as magnesium is essential for mitochondrial membrane stability and the coupling of oxidative phosphorylation. Phosphorus nuclear MRS demonstrated reduced magnesium in the occipital cortices of patients with hemiplegic migraine, with decreases correlating with the severity of neurological complaints (Boska *et al*, 2003). Interestingly, this study also found increased magnesium in the brains of patients with migraine without aura, which the authors attributed to a possible decrease in intracellular potassium, which may occur in neuronal tissue prone to hyper-excitability.

Various hypotheses abound as to the reason behind the hypomagnesemia observed in migraineurs. Some suggest that during a migraine headache, excessive amounts of magnesium are excreted due to stress. Others propose that stress triggers excretion of magnesium, with secondary hypomagnesemia causing a migraine (Durlach, 1976). During attacks as well as interictally, magnesium levels in both serum and saliva are decreased (Gallai *et al*, 1992), perhaps an indicator of low cerebral magnesium levels and therefore a decreased threshold for migraine development (Ramadan *et al*, 1989). Interictal studies on intracellular and serum levels in patients with migraines and tension-type headaches have shown inconsistent results. However a study of migraineurs utilizing the magnesium load test found that after loading with magnesium lactate, there was retention of the magnesium, suggesting a systemic deficiency. Further, interictal levels of erythrocyte magnesium are lower in both adult (Schoenen *et al*, 1991) and juvenile migraineurs with and without aura (Soriani *et al*, 1995). In support of these studies, one in which migraineurs with low erythrocyte magnesium levels as well as decreased ionized lymphoycyte magnesium levels were given mineral water containing magnesium over a two week period. Both erythrocyte and lymphocyte magnesium levels rose (Thomas *et al*, 2000). These suggest that assays of erythrocyte magnesium may be a useful and easily available tool to assess magnesium deficiency in migraineurs.

Magnesium in Migraine Pathogenesis

Magnesium is believed to be involved in a number of the aspects of migraine pathophysiology, and deficiency has been linked to cortical spreading depression (Mody *et al*, 1987), platelet aggregation (Baudouin-Legros *et al*, 1986), release of substance P (Weglicki and Phillips, 1992), neurotransmitter release (Coan and Collingridge, 1985) and vasoconstriction (Altura and Altura, 1982).

NMDA receptors are associated with nociception and the resulting neuroplastic changes in the trigeminal nociceptive neurons, as well as with regulation of cerebral blood flow (Foster and Fagg, 1987). Magnesium ions may block the NMDA receptor, thereby preventing calcium ions from moving intracellularly, and stopping the calcium's effects on neurons and cerebral vasculature (Coan and Collingridge, 1985). Decreased magnesium levels therefore facilitate the NMDA receptor, increasing it's effects on CSD, as well as the effect of glutamate on the NMDA receptor. The NMDA receptor has been shown to have a part in both the initiation and spread of cortical depression (Ferrari, 1992). Magnesium has been shown to block CSD induced by glutamate, and CSD is more easily initiated with decreased magnesium levels (Mody *et al*, 1987).

Nitric oxide (NO) plays a role as a synaptic modulator, affecting nociceptive processing (Meller and Gebhart, 1993) in addition to its involvement in the regulation of blood flow both intracranially and extracranially. It augments the NMDA receptor-evoked currents, thereby facilitating glutaminergic transmission (Choi and Lipton, 2000), which, as previously discussed, can be inhibited by magnesium. Production of NO can be inhibited by decreased magnesium levels.

CGRP, a neuropeptide, is released from activated trigeminal sensory nerves, is involved in the dilation of intracranial blood vessels and may also increase nociceptive transmission in the brainstem and spinal cord. It is therefore believed to play a central part in the development of migraines. A positive correlation has been demonstrated between migraines and serum CGRP levels, and after the pain of a migraine subsides, levels are observed to return to normal (Coderre *et al*, 1993). It has hence been hypothesized that inhibition of the release of CGRP either centrally or from the trigeminal nerve, may inhibit intracranial vasodilation thereby aborting migraine attacks. CGRP antagonists lack vasoconstrictive properties and have an advantage over current acute migraine treatment, triptans, which are contraindicated in patients with cardiovascular risk factors due to their vasoconstrictive effects.

Circulating CGRP levels have been shown to be decreased by the administration of magnesium in patients with primary Raynaud's phenomenon (PRP). A study followed CGRP levels in 12 women with PRP and 12 controls before and after the administration of intravenous magnesium sulfate. While there was no significant difference between baseline circulating CGRP in the two groups, following the infusion of magnesium sulfate there was a significant reduction in CGRP levels in the women with PRP only as well as a significant increase in RBC magnesium levels in the women with PRP but not in the control subjects (Myrdal *et al*, 1994).

Serotonin, released from platelets during migraines, promotes cerebral vasoconstriction as well as triggering nausea and vomiting. Cerebral vascular muscle serotonin receptors may develop increased affinity if serum ionized magnesium falls and the ratio of serum ionized calcium to magnesium increases. This may lead to further cerebral vasoconstriction and facilitates the release of serotonin from neuronal storage sites (Altura and Turlapaty, 1982). Pretreatment with magnesium has been shown to reduce serotonin-induced vasoconstriction (Goldstein and Zsoter, 1978).

Oral Magnesium Supplementation

A double-blind placebo-controlled study was performed in which 24 women with menstrually-related migraine were given supplementation with 360 mg of magnesium pyrrolidone carboxylic acid, divided into 3 divided daily doses taken from ovulation to the first day of menstrual flow (Facchinetti *et al*, 1991). The treatment was well-tolerated, with only one patient dropping out of the study due to side effects (magnesium-induced diarrhea), and significant reductions were observed in number of days of headache, total pain index and in Menstrual Distress Questionnaire score.

A larger double-blind, placebo-controlled, randomized study on 81 migraineurs receiving 600 mg of trimagnesium dicitrate taken once daily, showed attack frequency reduction of 41.6% in the magnesium group and 15.8% in controls. Three patients dropped out of the study due to side effects, 18.6% of patients complained of diarrhea and 4.7% of gastric irritation (Peikert *et al*, 1996).

A third placebo-controlled double-blind trial showed no effect of magnesium on migraine (Pfaffenrath *et al*, 1996), possibly attributable to the use of poorly-absorbed magnesium salt, as almost half of the treatment group complained of diarrhea.

A recent double-blind placebo-controlled, randomized study investigated the effects of 600 mg of magnesium citrate supplementation per day in patients with migraine without aura. A combination of clinical assessments, visual-evoked potentials (VEPs) and brain single-photon emission computerized tomography (SPECT) were performed to assess neurogenic and vascular mechanisms of action (Koseoglu *et al*, 2008). Supplementation was associated with significant decrease in migraine attack frequency and severity, as well as decreased P1 amplitude on VEPs, and increased cortical blood flow to the inferolateral temporal, inferofrontal and insular regions seen on SPECT. The authors suggested that magnesium may interfere with both neurogenic and vascular mechanisms of migraine and may hence be an effective prophylactic treatment. Other studies using SPECT have shown conflicting results (Ramadan *et al*, 1991; Ferrari *et al*, 1995; Olesen *et al*, 1982).

Women with menstrually-related migraine (MRM) may be particularly prone to developing magnesium deficiency. A prospective study involving 270 women, 61 of whom had MRM, showed that 45% had ionized magnesium deficiency during MRM attacks, 15% during non-menstrual attacks, 14% during menstruation without migraine and 15% between menstruation without migraine (Mauskop *et al*, 2002). Serum ionized calcium/magnesium levels were elevated in MRM, with normal ionized calcium levels.

Magnesium deficiency has also been found in pediatric migraine, with decreased levels of serum, RBC and mononuclear blood cell magnesium found in pediatric migraineurs with or without aura compared with patients with tension type headache and controls (Soriani *et al*, 1995; Mazzotta *et al*, 1999). Magnesium supplementation may be a safe and well-tolerated option for migraine prophylaxis in the prevention of pediatric migraine. However, while a double-blind placebo-controlled, randomized trial of patients aged 3 to 17 years found a statistically significant downward trend in headache frequency in those treated with magnesium oxide, the difference in the slopes of the two lines were not statistically significant (Wang *et al*, 2003). It could therefore not be determined if oral magnesium was superior to placebo in preventing frequent migraines in children and adolescents.

While oral magnesium is generally well-tolerated, the most prominent side-effect is diarrhea. Magnesium toxicity leads to loss of deep tendon reflexes as well as generalized muscle weakness. Severe toxicity can manifest as cardiac muscle weakness, respiratory paralysis and death, and patients with renal disease are at greater risk for developing toxicity. Although the diarrhea itself may prevent the development of toxicity, patients should be cautioned regarding excessive intake.

Intravenous Magnesium

Studies examining the use of intravenous magnesium in the treatment of acute migraine have been conflicting. A study on 40 patients with acute migraine attacks showed an 85% correlation between levels of serum ionized magnesium (measured during an attack) and clinical response to 1g of intravenous magnesium sulfate (Mauskop *et al*, 1995). Although the study was neither double-blinded nor placebo-controlled, both researchers and subjects were blinded to ionized magnesium levels. A further study on various headache types found 1g of magnesium sulfate to provide rapid relief in patients with low serum ionized magnesium levels (Mauskop *et al*, 1996).

A single-blind placebo-controlled, randomized trial involved 30 patients with migraines who were randomized to receive either magnesium sulfate 1g or placebo (Demirkaya *et al*, 2001). After 30 minutes, patients in the placebo group who had ongoing pain, nausea or vomiting were given magnesium sulfate 1g. Treatment was superior to placebo in terms of both response rate (100% for magnesium sulfate vs 7% for placebo) and pain-free rate (87% for magnesium sulfate vs 0% for placebo) and those treated did not experience headache recurrence within 24 hours. 87% complained of flushing or a burning sensation in the face and neck.

A double-blind placebo-controlled, randomized study evaluated the efficacy of magnesium sulfate 1g on the pain and associated symptoms of migraine with and without aura (Bigal *et al*, 2002). In subjects with migraine without aura, although there was a significant decrease in the intensity of photophobia and phonophobia, no significant differences were observed in pain relief or nausea. However subjects with migraine with aura had significant improvement in pain and all associated symptoms.

An emergency room based double-blind placebo-controlled, randomized study of 44 subjects with acute migraines tested a combination of magnesium sulfate 2g and metoclopramide 20mg versus metoclopramide 20mg alone at 15 minute intervals for up to 3 doses, or until pain relief occurred (Corbo *et al*, 2001). Pain intensity was recorded using a standard visual analog scale (VAS). Although both groups experienced more than 50mm improvement in the VAS score, improvement was smaller in the magnesium group, both comparing VAS score improvements and evaluating normal functional status. The authors suggested that magnesium may diminish the efficacy of metoclopramide in decreasing migraine pain.

A study involving 22 patients with cluster headaches who were treated with magnesium sulfate 1g found that 41% of patients reported 'meaningful relief' (defined as complete cessation of attacks or relief for more than 3 days) after treament (Mauskop *et al*, 1995).

Conclusion

Magnesium is central to numerous physiological functions, and the role it plays in the various aspects of migraine pathogenesis is well described. Although some studies have shown an association between migraines and magnesium deficiency, it is difficult to assess this with routine blood testing and serum magnesium levels are a poor reflection of body stores of the cation. Therefore, treatment should be based on clinical suspicion, with both oral and intravenous magnesium available as simple, safe, inexpensive and well-tolerated options for the management of migraines. In patients with symptoms suggestive of hypomagnesemia such as pre-menstrual syndrome, cold extremities and foot or leg cramps, we suggest daily magnesium supplementation with 400mg of chelated magnesium, magnesium oxide or slow-release magnesium. While some patients may require doses of up to 1000mg, diarrhea and abdominal pain may be limiting factors. Intravenous magnesium may be used in patients who are unable to tolerate or absorb oral magnesium or who are non-compliant with daily dosing. It may also be used for the treatment of acute migraines, or as a monthly prophylactic infusion, often administered premenstrually.

References

Agostini E, Aliprandi A (2006) The complications of migraine with aura. *Neurol Sci* 27(Suppl. 2): S91-S95.

Altura BM, Turlapaty PDMV (1982) Withdrawal of magnesium enhances coronary atrerial spasm produced by vasoactive agents. *Br J Pharmacol* 77:649-659.

Altura BT, Altura BM (1982) The role of magnesium in etiology of strokes and cerebral vasospasm. *Magnesium* 1:277-291.

Altura BT, Shirley TL, Young CC, Dell'Ofrano K, Hiti J, Welsh R, Yeh Q, Barbour RL, Altura BM (1994) Characterization of a new ion selective electrode for ionized magnesium in whole blood, plasma, serum and aqueous samples. *Scan J Clin Lab Invest* 54 (Suppl. 217): 21-36.

Altura BT, Shirley T, Young CC, Dell-Ofrano K, Handwerker SM, Altura BM (1992) A new method for the rapid determination of ionized Mg^{2+} in whole blood, serum and plasma. *Meth Find Exp Clin Pharmacol* 14(4),297-304.

Arnaud MJ (2008) Update on the assessment of magnesium status. *Br J Nutr* 99 Suppl 3: S24–36.

Bigal ME, Bordini CA, Tepper SJ, Speciali JG (2002) Intravenous magnesium sulphate in the acute treatment of migraine without aura and migraine with aura. A randomized, double-blind, placebo-controlled study. *Cephalalgia* 22:345-353.

Bapty BW, Dai LJ, Ritchie G, Jirik F, Canaff L, Hendy GN, Quamme GA (1998) Activation of Mg^{2+} Ca^{2+} sensing inhibits hormone-stimulated Mg^{2+} uptake in mouse distal convoluted tubule cells. *Am J Physiol* 275: F353-F360.

Baudoiun-Legros N, Dard B, Guichency P (1986) Hyperactivity of platelets from spontaneously hypertensive rats. Role of external magnesium. *Hypertension* 8:694-699.

Bettinelli A, Bianchetti MG, Borella P, Volpini E, Metta MG, Basilico E, Selicorni A, Bargellini A, Grassi MR (1995) Genetic heterogeneity in tubular hypomagnesemia-hypokalemia with hypocalciuria (Gitelman's syndrome). *Kidney Int* Feb;47(2):547-51.

Bohmer T, Mathiesen B (1982) Magnesium deficiency in chronic alcoholic patients uncovered by an intravenous loading test. *Scand J Clin Lab Invest* 42(8):633-6.

Boska MD, Welch KMA, Barker PB, Nelson JA, Schultz L (2002) Contrasts in cortical magnesium, phospholipid and energy metabolism between migraine syndromes. *Neurology* 58:1227-1233.

Brown EM, Gamba G, Riccardi D *et al* (1993) Cloning and characterization of an extracellular Ca^{2+}-sensing receptor from bovine parathyroid. *Nature* 366: 575-580.

Choi YB, Lipton SA (2000) Redox modulation of the NMDA receptor. *Sal Mol Life Sci* 57:1535-1541.

Coan EJ, Collingridge GL (1985) Magnesium ions block an N-methyl-D-aspartate-mediated component of synaptic transmission in rat hippocampus. *Neurosci Lett* 53:21-26.

Coderre TI, Katz J, Faccerino AL, Melzack R (1993) Contribution of central neuroplasticity to pathological pain: review of clinical and experimental evidence. *Pain* 52,259-285.

Corbo J, Esses D, Bijur PE, Iannaccone R, Gallagher EJ (2001) Randomized clinical trial of intraveous magnesium sulfate as an adjunctive medication for emergency department treatment of migraine headache. *Ann Emerg Med* 38:621-627.

Demirkaya S, Vural O, Dora B, Topcuoglu MA. Efficacy of intravenous magnesium sulfate in the treatment of acute migraine attacks. *Headache* 41,171-177.

Douban S, Brodsky MA, Whang DD, Whang R (1996) Significance of magnesium in congestive heart failure. *Am Heart J* Sep;132(3):664-71.

Durlach J (1976) Neurological manifestations of magnesium imbalance. In: *Handbook of Clinical Neurology* (Vinken PJ, Bruyn GW, eds), Amsterdam, Holland 28, 454-579.

Durlach J, Poenaru S Rouhani S, Bara, M, Guiet-Bara, A (1987) The control of central neuronal hyperexcitability in magnesium deficiency. In: *Nutrients and Brain Function* (Essman WB, ed) Karger, Basel, Switzerland, 48-71.

Fachianetti F, Sances G, Borella P, Genazzeni AR, Nappi G (1991) Magnesium prophylaxis of menstrual migraine: effects on intracellular magnesium. *Headache* 31:298-301.

Ferrari MD, Haan J, Blokland JA, Arndt JW, Minnee P, Zwinderman AH, Pauwels EK, Saxena PR (1995) Cerebral blood flow during migraine attacks without aura and effect of sumatriptan. *Arch Neurol* 52:135-139.
Foster AC, Fagg GE (1987) Neurobiology. Taking apart NMDA receptors. *Nature* 329:395-396.

Gallai V, Sarchielli P, Coata G, Firenze C, Morucci P, Abbritti G (1992) Serum and salivary magnesium levels in migraine: Results in a group of juvenile patients. *Headache* 32:132-153.

Goadsby PJ, Edvinsson L, Elkman R (1990) Vasoactive peptide release in the extracerebral circulation of humans during migraine headache. *Ann Neurol* 28:183-187.

Goadsby PJ, Macdonald GJ (1985) Extracranial vasodilatation mediated by VIP (Vasoactive Polypeptide*). Brain Res* 329:285-288.

Goksel BK, Torun D, Karaca S, Karatas M, Tan M, Sezgin N, Benli S, Sezer S, Ozdemir, N (2006) Is low blood magnesium level associated with hemodialysis headache? *Headache* 46,40-45.

Goldstein S, Zsoter TT (1978) The effect of magnesium on the response of smooth muscle to 5-hydroxytryptamine. *Br J Pharmacol* 62:507-514.

Gorji A, Scheller D, Straub H, Tegtmeier F, Kohling R, Hohling JM, Tuxhorn I, Ebner A, Wolf P, Werner Panneck H, Oppel F, Speckmann EJ (2001) Spreading depression in human neocortical slices. *Brain Res* 906,74-83.

Henrotte JG (1982) Genetic regulation of red blood cell magnesium content and major histocompatibility complex. *Magnesium* 1:69-80.

Innerarity S (2000) Hypomagnesemia in acute and chronic illness. *Crit Care Nurs* Q23:1-19.

Jain AC, Sethi NC, Balbar PK (1985) A clinical electroencephalographic and trace element study with special reference to zinc, copper and magnesium in serum and cerebrospinal fluid (CSF) in cases of migraine. *J Neurol Suppl* 232,161.

Koseoglu E, Talashoglu A, Gonul AS, Kula M (2008) The effects of magnesium prophylaxis in migraine without aura. *Mag Res* 21:101-108.

Laires MJ, Monteiro CP, Bicho M (2004) Role of cellular magnesium in health and human disease. *Front Biosci* 1,262-276.

Lipton RB, Bigal ME, Diamon M. AMPP Advisory Group (2007) Migraine prevalence, disease burden, and the need for preventative therapy. *Neurology* 68 (5):343-349.
Lodi R, Iotti S, Cortelli P, Pierangeli G, Cevoli S, Clementi V,. Soriani S, Montagna P, Barbiroli B (2001) Deficient energy metabolism is associated with low free magnesium in the brains of patients with migraine and cluster headache. *Brain Res Bull* 54:437-441.

Mauskop A, Altura BT, Altura BM (2002) Serum ionized magnesium levels and serum ionized calcium/ionized magnesium ratios in women with menstrual migraine. *Headache* 42:242-248.

Mauskop A, Altura BT, Cracco RQ, Altura BM (1994) Chronic daily headache - one disease or two?

Diagnostic role of serum ionized magnesium. *Cephalalgia* 14:24-28.

Mauskop A, Altura BT, Cracco RQ, Altura BM (1996) Intravenous magnesium sulfate rapidly alleviates headahes of various types. *Headache* 36:156-160.

Mauskop A, Altura BT, Cracco RQ, Altura BM (1995) Intravenous magnesium sulphate relieves cluster headaches in patients with low serum ionized magnesium levels. *Headache* 35:597-600.

Mauskop A, Altura BT, Cracco RQ, Altura BM (1995) Intravenous magnesium sulphate relieves migraine attacks in patients with low serum ionized magnesium levels: a pilot study. *Clin Sci* 89:633-636.

Mazotta G, Strachielli P, ALberti A, Gallai V (1999) Intracellular Mg^{2+} concentration and electromyographical ischemic test in juvenile headache. *Cephalalgia* 19:802-809.

Meller ST, Gebhart GF (1993) Nitric oxide (NO) and nociceptive processing in the spinal cord. *Pain* 52:127-136.

Modi I, Lambert JD, Heinemann U (1987) Low extracellular magnesium induces epileptiform activity and spreading depression in rat hippocampal slices. *J Neurophysiol* 57,869-888.

Moe SM (2008) Disorders involving calcium, phosphorous and magnesium. *Prim Care* 35(2): 215-237, v-vi.

Moskowitz MA (1984) The neurobiology of vascular head pain. *Ann Neurol* 16:157-168.

Myrdal U, Leppert J, Edvinsson L, Ekman R, Hedner T, Nilsson H, Ringqvist I (1994), Magnesium sulphate infusion decreases circulating calcitonin gene-related peptide (CGRP) in women with primary Raynaud's phenomenon. *Clin Physiol* 14:539-546.

Olesen J, Laurtizen M, Tfelt-Hansen P, Herriksen L, Larsen B (1982) Spreading cerebral oligemia in classical and normal cerebral blood flow in common migraine. *Headache* 22:242-248.

Otori T, Greenberg JH and Welsh FA (2003) Cortical spreading depression causes a long-lasting decrease in cerebral blood flow and induces tolerance to permanent focal ischemia in the rat brain. *J Cereb Blood Flow Metab*, 23:43-50.

Peikert A, Wilmingzig C, Kohne-Volland R. Prophylaxis of migraine with oral magnesium: results from a prospective, multi-center, placebo-controlled and double-blind randomized study. *Cephalalgia* 16:257-263.

Pfaffenrath V, Wessley P, Meyer C, Isler HR, Evers S, Grotemeyer KH, Tanieri Z, Soyka D, Gobel H, Fisher M (1996) Magnesium in the prophylaxis of migraine: a double-bind, placebo-controlled study. *Cephalalgia* 16:436-440.

Ramadan NM, Halvorsan H, Vande-Linde A, Levine SR, Helpern JA, Welch KMA (1989) Low brain magnesium in migraine. *Headache* 29:590-593.

Ramadan NM, Levine SR, Welch KMA (1991) Interictal cerebral blood flow asymmetries in migraine with aura. *Cephalalgia* 11(Suppl):42-43.

Schimatschek HF, Rempis R (2001) Prevalence of hypomagnesemia in an unselected German population of 16,000 individuals. *Magnes Res* 14:283-290.

Schoenen J, Sianard-Gainko J, Lenaerts M (1991) Blood magnesium levels in migraine. *Cephalalgia* 11,97-99.

Soriani S, Arnaldi C, De Carlo L, Arcudi D, Mazzotta D, Battistella P, Sartori S Abbasciano V (1995), Serum and red blod cell magnesium levels in juvenile maigraine patients. *Headache* 35:14-16.

Thomas J, Millot JM, Sebille S, Delabroise AM, Thomas E, Manfait M, Arnaud MJ (2000) Free and total magnesium in lymphocytes of migraine patients - effects of magnesium-rich mineral water intake. *Clin Chim Ecta* 295:64-75.

Wagner CA (2007) Disorders of renal magnesium handling explain renal magnesium transport. *J Nephrol* 20: 507-510.

Walder RY, Shalev H, Brennan TMH, Carmi R, Elbeduor K, Scott DA, Hanauer A, Mark AL, Patil S, Stone EM and Sheffield VC (1997). Familial Hypomagnesemia Maps to Chromosome 9q, not to the X Chromosome: Genetic Linkage Mapping and Analysis of a Balanced Translocation Breakpoint. *Hum Mol Genet* 6 (9): 1491-1497.

Wang F, Van Den Eeden SK, Ackerson LM, Salk SE, Reince RH, Elin RJ (2003). Oral magnesium oxide prophylaxis of frequent migrainous headache in children: a randomized, double-blind, placebo-controlled trial. *Headache* 43: 601-610.

Weglicki WB, Phillips TM (1992) Pathobiology of magnesium deficiency: a cytokine/neurogenic inflammation hypothesis. *Am J Physiol* 263 (Pt 2): R734-R737.

Whang R, Oei TO, Watanabe A (1985) Frequency of hypomagnesemia in hospitalized patients receiving digitalis. *Arch Intern Med* 145: 655-656.

The role of magnesium in edema and blood brain barrier disruption

Mehmet Kaya ✉ *and Bulent Ahishali*

Departments of Physiology and of Histology and Embryology, Istanbul Faculty of Medicine, Istanbul University, Capa 34093 Istanbul, Turkey.
✉ mehkaya@istanbul.edu.tr

Abstract

The blood-brain barrier (BBB) is constituted primarily of brain capillary endothelial cells and is a pre-requisite for the maintenance of brain homeostasis that is essential for optimal brain function. However, a variety of pathological conditions, such as sepsis, multiple sclerosis and epilepsia disrupt the BBB integrity and lead to the development of brain edema. Ionized magnesium (Mg^{2+}) is a crucial cofactor that plays an essential role within the cell and regulates a variety of biochemical reactions. Changes in intra- and extracellular Mg^{2+} concentrations influence the functions of cells and tissues. A growing body of evidence suggests that Mg^{2+} plays a pivotal role in ameliorating BBB disruption via a number of mechanisms during certain neurological diseases. Systemic delivery of Mg^{2+} may constitute an alternative approach in the future, both to improve BBB integrity and to decrease brain edema in the course of a variety of diseases involving brain tissue.

Introduction

Blood-Brain Barrier

The blood-brain barrier (BBB) is composed mainly of brain capillary endothelial cells and represents a dynamic structure that regulates the trafficking of molecules between blood and brain tissue. The passage of many circulating substances from the capillary bed into the brain parenchyma is tightly controlled by physical and enzymatic barriers provided by the endothelial cells of capillaries in the brain parenchyma (Abbott *et al*, 2010; Cardoso *et al*, 2010). In this way, the BBB is equipped with regulating means that enable the maintenance of neuronal homeostasis. In addition, the BBB harbors transport mechanisms that provide bidirectional control of exchange of nutrients, electrolytes and neurotoxins, and thus establishes an optimum milieu that is strictly essential in neuronal survival. Although the BBB appears to possess a static structure, it has the ability to adapt readily to sudden changes.

About 95% of the microvessels in the brain display BBB properties, and almost every neuron is estimated to be nourished by a distinct capillary vessel (Pardridge, 2005). When regulating its own activities, the mature BBB receives support from at least three different cell types: (1) pericytes which share the same basement membrane with endothelial cells; (2) astrocytes which envelope 99% of the abluminal face of endothelial cells; and (3) neurons (Guo and Lo, 2009; Correale and Villa, 2009). Nevertheless, under normal conditions, BBB function is regulated primarily by capillary endothelial cells (Fisher, 2009; Abbott *et al*, 2010).

In brain tissue, the barrier-type endothelial cells have a continuous basal membrane and do not exhibit fenestrations. These cells contain many mitochondria, but harbor very few caveola (pinocytotic vesicles) in their luminal surfaces. Tight junctions (TJs) between adjacent brain capillary endothelial cells possess occludin and claudin proteins that serve to preserve junctional integrity. Meanwhile, zonula occludens (ZO)-1 and 2, cingulin, cadherin, cathenin, vinculin and actin constitute accessory proteins which aid the assembly of TJs.

Passive diffusion across the BBB mainly depends on the lipid-solubility and molecular weight of molecules. Lipophilic substances with molecular weights less than 400-600 Da can pass readily into the brain tissue by passive diffusion. In normally functioning BBB, oxygen, carbon dioxide, nicotine, ethanol, lipid-soluble substances such as heroin and amphiphilic drugs (containing both hydrophobic and hydrophilic moieties) are carried by this route. Besides, a number of molecules are transported across the

BBB by other mechanisms including carrier- and receptor-mediated transport, adsorptive-mediated endocytosis and fluid phase-mediated endocytosis (Loscher and Potschka, 2005; Pardridge, 2007). However, many pathological conditions alter the functional and structural characteristics of the BBB impairing the maintenance of neural homeostasis.

Magnesium Physiology

Magnesium ion (Mg^{2+}), the most abundant divalent cation in living cells, exists not only in the intracellular compartment but also in circulation and cerebrospinal fluid (CSF). Serum Mg^{2+} concentration normally ranges between 1.7-2.3 mEq/L in humans and may decrease during several pathological conditions (Romani and Scarpa, 2000; Musso, 2009). Cell membranes have a particularly low permeability to Mg^{2+} and hence the ion moves slowly between intracellular and interstitial compartments. In physiological conditions, Mg^{2+} concentration within the cell is maintained in a relatively narrow range between 0.5 and 1 mM (Dai and Quamme, 1991; Romani and Scarpa, 2000). Mg^{2+} acts as a regulatory cation at the systemic and cellular levels, and participates in almost all anabolic and catabolic processes in the body. It plays a fundamental role in a wide range of cellular events, biochemical reactions and physiological functions, activating over 325 enzyme systems, including those involved in ATP synthesis, carbohydrate metabolism, K^+ and Ca^{2+} transport, cell proliferation and membrane stability and function (Grubbs and Maguire, 1987; Saris *et al*, 2000; Wolf and Trapani, 2008; Barbagallo and Dominguez, 2010).

During normal physiological processes, Mg^{2+} works as a voltage dependent antagonist and a noncompetitive inhibitor of the N-methyl-D-aspartic acid (NMDA) receptors and ion channels in the brain. Although pharmacokinetic and pharmacodynamic studies in rats have shown Mg^{2+} entry into the brain upon systemic treatment (Hallak *et al*, 1992; Hoane, 2007), no concomitant rise of Mg^{2+} in CSF was noted following parenteral administration in humans with brain insults (McKee *et al*, 2005).

A reduction of Mg^{2+} level within the cell in pathological states can be considered as an injury factor in the brain and may lead to serious biological and metabolic dysfunctions. Decline in intracellular free Mg^{2+} concentration reduces ATP synthesis and utilization in the maintenance of ion gradients via Na^+-K^+ ATPase (Grubbs and Maguire, 1987). Also, the reduction in Mg^{2+} concentration within the cell results in an impairment of membrane stability by promoting free radical production (Ebel and Gunther, 1980; Bara and Guiet-Bara, 1984). Among the other events associated with Mg^{2+} deficiency in brain are opening of Ca^{2+} channels, cellular entry of Ca^{2+}, release of certain neurotransmitters, activation of NMDA receptors, membrane oxidation and activation of nuclear factor-kappa B ($NF_{K}B$) (Weglicki *et al*, 1994; Altura *et al*, 2003; Billard, 2006; Rayssiguier *et al*, 2010). On the other hand, beneficial effects of magnesium supplementation have been shown in experimental models and a variety of mechanistic pathways have been put forward including decrease in intracellular Ca^{2+} concentration, increase in antioxidant capacity and induction of endothelial cell proliferation (Kaya *et al*, 2001 and 2004; Esen *et al*, 2005; Euser *et al*, 2008; Wolf *et al*, 2008 and 2009).

Brain edema and magnesium

Two major types of brain edema, termed cytotoxic and vasogenic, were described by Klatzo in the late 1960s and later two more types were added to the classification (Klatzo, 1967; Marmarou, 2004; Nag *et al*, 2009). Cytotoxic brain edema is characterized by sustained intracellular water accumulation, causing cellular injury in the absence of BBB damage and involves mainly astrocytes. On the other hand, vasogenic edema results in extracellular water accumulation in brain parenchyma through BBB disruption. The other types are interstitial edema observed in patients with hydrocephalus and osmotic edema caused by imbalances of osmotic active substances, promoting water influx into cells.

Energy depletion followed by a failure of the Na^+-K^+ ATPase plays a major role in the pathogenesis of cytotoxic brain edema and increased uptake of Na^+ into the cell cannot be equilibrated by the defective pump. Under certain pathological conditions, such as traumatic brain injury (TBI), cerebral ischemia and acute hypertension, the brain edema, which is initially cytotoxic, acquires a vasogenic character in the following stages. Besides, brain edema caused by trauma has been proposed to be mainly vasogenic due to the opening of TJs in BBB (Unterberg *et al*, 2004). Magnesium supplementation has been reported to decrease regional brain tissue water content and attenuate brain edema formation after experimental TBI (Okiyama *et al*, 1995; Feldman *et al*, 1996). In addition, magnesium treatment protects the blood-spinal cord barrier, improves clinical recovery, and preserves normal spinal cord ultrastructure in experimental spinal cord injury in rats (Kaptanoglu *et al*, 2003).

Aquaporin (AQP)-4, a bidirectional transmembrane water channel expressed mainly in astrocytes and to a lesser extent in barrier type of endothelial cells and pial membranes, may play a crucial role in the pathogenesis of cytotoxic and vasogenic brain edema and aggravation/resolution of ischemic and traumatic brain edema (Amiry-Moghaddam *et al*, 2003; Zador *et al*, 2009). Experimental studies focusing on the treatment of brain edema showed beneficial effects of magnesium administered in combination with various pharmacological drugs in animal models (Royo *et al*, 2003; Sen and Gulati, 2010). Upregulation of AQP-4 in brain injury leads to an increase in brain water content, resulting in brain edema (Taniguchi *et al*, 2000; Papadopoulos and Verkman, 2005) and treatment with magnesium causes the down-regulation of AQP-4 (Ghabriel *et al*, 2006) and thereby attenuates brain edema (Okiyama *et al*, 1995).

It is reported that Mg^{2+} exerts neuroprotective effects in anoxic insult through improving the recovery of synaptic transmission and blocking the loss of protein kinase C (PKC) (Libien *et al*, 2005). These data are mechanistically consistent with the observations that the treatment of the astrocytes with a PKC activator caused a rapid decrease in AQP-4 mRNA and this effect was inhibited by a specific PKC inhibitor (Nakahama *et al*, 1999). Among the other mechanisms put forward for the beneficial effects of Mg^{2+} in decreasing brain edema are restriction of the opening of paracellular pathway through Ca^{2+} antagonism, alleviation of the oxidative stress and prevention of hypertensive encephalopathy through reduction in cerebral perfusion pressure (Belfort *et al*, 2008; Euser and Cipolla 2009). Mg^{2+} has also been shown to reduce brain edema and protect brain morphology in experimental cold-injury by inhibition of lipid peroxidation (Turkoglu *et al*, 2008).

Blood-brain barrier and magnesium

Mg^{2+} is slowly transported across the BBB to brain by transporters and exchangers located in endothelial cell membranes, including Na^+/Mg^{2+} exchanger, Mg^{2+}/Ca^{2+} exchanger and cation channels. Following systemic administration, regional increase of Mg^{2+} has been detected in the cerebral cortex and hippocampus in rats with intact BBB (Hallak *et al*, 1992; Touyz, 2008). In both physiological and pathological conditions, Mg^{2+} can directly influence the BBB properties. Low Mg^{2+} concentration in circulation is associated with increase in endothelial permeability, decrease in vasodilator capacity and increase in the production of vasoconstrictor substances, cytokines and oxidative products (Touyz, 2003; Maier *et al*, 2004). In pathological conditions with BBB impairment, Mg^{2+} passes into the extracellular compartment of brain in significantly higher concentrations and plays an important role in the pathophysiological processes that follow BBB disruption. An elevation in free Mg^{2+} concentration in capillary endothelial cells increases the proliferation of endothelial cells, recovers the cell's ability to generate and utilize ATP for cellular repair mechanisms and improves BBB integrity disrupted under a variety of insults. In addition to the stimulatory effects of Mg^{2+} on endothelial cell migration and proliferation, the observations that high Mg^{2+} concentration facilitates the re-endothelialization of vascular injuries may also provide new insights into the role of Mg^{2+} in angiogenesis (Maier *et al*, 2004).

A decrease in Mg^{2+} level in the microcirculation of the cortical structures causes a rapid and progressive damage to microvessels, leading to focal hemorrhages and brain edema (Altura *et al*, 1991). Increasing brain bioavailability of parenterally administered magnesium by artificial BBB disruption has been considered as a necessary step in assessing the therapeutic benefits of magnesium supplementation after TBI (Sen and Gulati, 2010). Magnesium therapy has been shown to be effective in a variety of animal models of experimental BBB disruption. Accumulated data indicate that magnesium administration improves functional outcome following BBB disruption and decreases brain edema (Okiyama *et al*, 1995; Feldman *et al*, 1996; Kaya *et al*, 2004; Esen *et al*, 2005; Euser *et al*, 2008). Treatment with magnesium and MK-801 (dizocilpine), a noncompetitive NMDA receptor antagonist, alone and in combination can reduce brain edema development and help to restore BBB permeability after experimental diffuse brain injury (Feng *et al*, 2004; Imer *et al*, 2009).

One of the major mechanisms responsible for the pharmacological action of Mg^{2+} is blockage of NMDA or alpha-amino-3-hydroxy-5-methyl isoxazole-4-proprionic acid (AMPA) channels/ receptors in cerebral vascular system as well as brain parenchyma (Huang *et al,* 1994). The observations that blockade of NMDA or AMPA receptors could attenuate the BBB disruption in focal cerebral ischemia suggest that ionotropic glutamate receptors are involved, at least partly, in BBB disruption (Liu *et al*, 2010). Magnesium can modulate hypoxic-ischemic events in the cerebral cortex by blocking the action of local putative excitatory amino acid neurotransmitter and consequently, high extracellular Mg^{2+} has been shown to be effective in blocking the pathophysiological mechanisms of rupture and spasm in the brain microvasculature (Huang *et al*, 1994; Chaon *et al*, 2006). Other possible mechanisms of action of Mg^{2+} in regulating vascular function involve its antioxidant, anti-inflammatory, and growth regulatory properties via which burden of oxidative stress and inflammation in the endothelial cells of microvessels are attenuated (Weglicki *et al*, 1996; Mazur *et al*, 2007). In addition, treatment of human endothelial cells with magnesium has induced reduction of cellular pro-oxidant levels and diminished the release of pro-inflammatory cytokines (Wolf *et al*, 2008).

Although the effects of magnesium on BBB characteristics and the formation of brain edema in various pathophysiological conditions has not been thoroughly elucidated, the studies mentioned above suggest that magnesium provides protective effects on BBB integrity and reduces brain edema by more than one mechanism (Fig. 1). Yet, further studies are still needed to assess more accurately the role of magnesium in the BBB response to various insults in humans and animals.

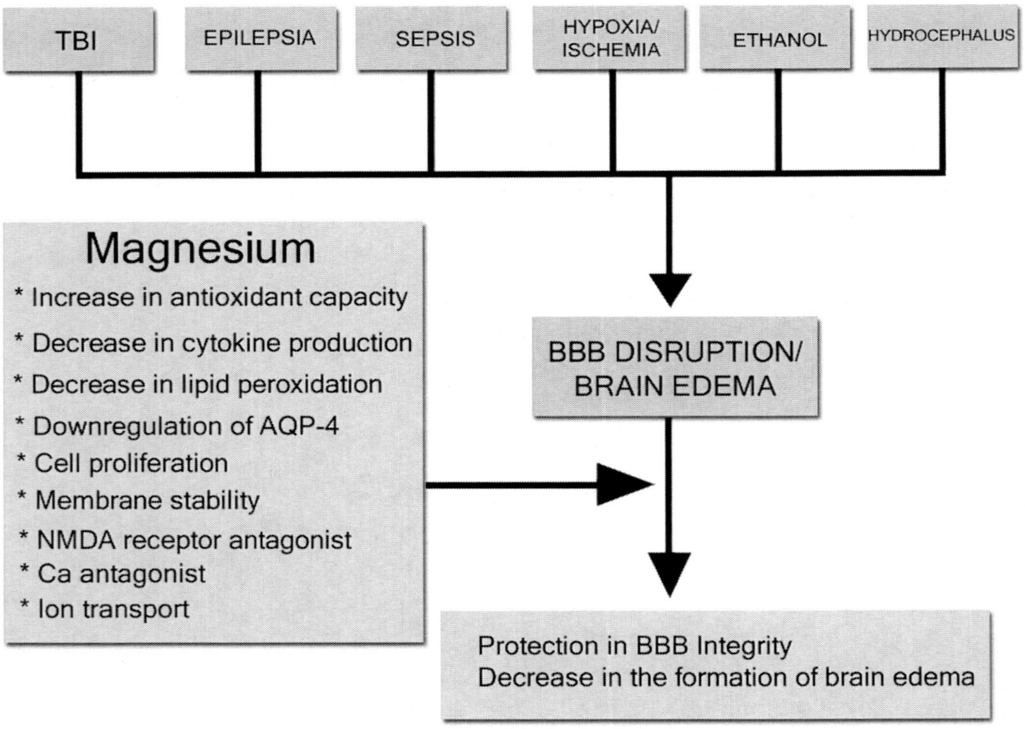

Figure 1. Effects of magnesium on BBB integrity.

Blood-brain barrier, magnesium and traumatic brain injury

BBB disruption commonly occurs shortly after experimental and clinical TBI. Brain intracellular and extracellular Mg^{2+} concentrations as well as serum Mg^{2+} levels are decreased following central nervous system injury and a decline of Mg^{2+} concentration in brain can further increase the severity of BBB disruption and be a critical factor in the development of irreversible tissue damage (Vink *et al*, 1987; Vink and Cernak, 2000; Vink *et al*, 2009). Reduction in brain intracellular free Mg^{2+} is also associated with brain intracellular acidosis and a concomitant reduction of brain energy stores (Vink *et al*, 1988; Altura *et al*, 1995).

Magnesium salts, such as magnesium sulphate ($MgSO_4$) or magnesium chloride were shown to penetrate the BBB and cause enhancement of brain intracellular free Mg^{2+} concentration following TBI (Heath and Vink, 1999). Accumulated data from animal models indicate that administration of magnesium salts into the circulation or extracellular brain compartments can provide an effective therapy for TBI (Vink and Cernak, 2000; Saatman *et al*, 2001; Hoane, 2007) by improving BBB integrity and decreasing brain edema (Esen *et al*, 2003). In contrast to the animal studies mentioned above, McKee and colleagues (McKee *et al*, 2005) described the functional characteristics of the BBB in patients with TBI by using $MgSO_4$ infusions initiated at an average of 5 days after injury. The authors showed that the increased serum Mg^{2+} concentrations yielded only a marginal increase of total and ionized Mg^{2+} in CSF and they concluded that the regulation of magnesium by the constituents of the BBB remains largely intact following brain injuries. Meanwhile, in a double-blinded trial conducted to check the validity of animal data in humans and to explore, whether magnesium infusion initiated within 8 hours of major head injury and continued for 5 days would decrease mortality and improve the functional outcome in head-injured patients, it is reported that there was no clinical suggestion of a beneficial effect of the magnesium regimen in these patients (Temkin *et al*, 2007).

Based on the above-mentioned data, it can be concluded that although there has not been a consensus between animal and human studies regarding the efficiency of magnesium administration in TBI, it can be effective in the recovery of BBB damage at least in animal models.

Blood-brain barrier, magnesium and seizures

Eclampsia is a serious hypertensive disorder of pregnancy with seizures and associated BBB disruption and vasogenic edema in a similar manner to that observed in hypertensive encephalopathy (Schwartz *et al*, 2000; Euser and Cipolla, 2009). In animal models, magnesium treatment has been shown to contribute to the protection of the BBB during eclampsia, to decrease the increased BBB permeability and to prevent the development of brain edema in certain experimental settings, such as acute hypertension and hypoglycemia-induced seizures (Kaya *et al*, 2001 and 2004; Euser *et al*, 2008). The above mentioned beneficial effects of magnesium on BBB integrity may be related to its ability to scavenge free radicals. The antioxidant action of magnesium has been reported in two recent studies (Ariza *et al*, 2005; Turkoglu *et al*, 2008), suggesting that it could protect against free radical surge associated with epileptic seizures. However, the exact mechanism/s of action of magnesium treatment in the improvement of BBB integrity in eclampsia still remains to be elucidated.

Blood-brain barrier, magnesium and sepsis

Magnesium supplementation is one of the experimental methods and pharmacological approaches developed for the treatment of BBB disruption and brain edema caused by septic encephalopathy. The impairment of BBB integrity during sepsis has been shown by several studies, and magnesium administration in the early stages of sepsis reduced BBB permeability and brain edema (Papadopoulos *et al*, 2005; Esen *et al*, 2005). Magnesium deficiency leads to an elevation in plasma inflammatory cytokines and excessive production of free radicals and aggravates endotoxic shock (Weglicki *et al*, 1994; Matsui *et al*, 2007). Treatment with magnesium decreases the concentration of inflammatory cytokines and free radicals and increases antioxidant capacity and survival rate in rats (Salem *et al*, 1995). Finally, alterations in endothelial cells, which are protagonists in the vascular changes during inflammation, are reversible upon magnesium supplementation (Mazur *et al*, 2007). Although the above mentioned studies suggest that magnesium is involved in the protection of the BBB and brain edema in sepsis, the literature data is quite limited at present and additional studies are needed to explain the patho-physiologic mechanisms involved in this protection.

Blood-brain barrier, magnesium and brain hypoxia/ischemia

Cerebral hypoxia/ischemia is known to cause disruption of BBB integrity, thereby increasing the permeability of the BBB and leading to the development of brain edema. Extracellular Mg^{2+} concentration has been shown to be significantly decreased to approximately 60% of basal values in the ipsilateral cortex in hypoxia-ischemia (Lee *et al*, 2002). Meanwhile, magnesium deficient rats are more susceptible to cerebral hypoxia/ ischemia than rats fed with a normal or high magnesium diet (Demougeot *et al*, 2004). Magnesium administration significantly attenuates the hypoxia-induced increase in reactive oxygen species and contributes to the repair of the disrupted BBB in hypoxia/ischemia (Ravishankar *et al*, 2001; Goñi-de-Cerio *et al*, 2009). The protection of the BBB by magnesium in hypoxic conditions could be multifactorial and in addition to the above mentioned effects may involve other factors such as decrease in the production of cytokines, increase in antioxidative products and blockade of NMDA or AMPA channels/ receptors. There is at present only limited knowledge about the role of magnesium on BBB integrity and brain edema in hypoxia/ischemia and future research is needed to determine the possible mechanisms of magnesium supplementation in improving the functions of BBB.

Blood-brain barrier, magnesium and ethanol

Acute and chronic ethanol treatment gives rise to significant increases in BBB permeability to a variety of molecules which do not normally cross BBB. Increase in free radical concentration in ethanol-treated endothelial cells leads to phosphorylation of TJ proteins, activation of paracellular pathway and thus disruption of BBB (Haorah *et al*, 2005). A number of studies have provided evidence for the alterations in serum Mg^{2+} levels in acute and chronic ethanol treatments. A single dose of ethanol (2 g/kg) injected to mice significantly decreased total Mg^{2+} concentration in serum (Papierkowski *et al*, 1998). Furthermore, acute or chronic alcohol consumption impairs Mg^{2+} transport and homeostasis at the capillary level in the brain (Romani, 2008). However, little is known about whether any improvement in BBB integrity can be achieved by magnesium treatment in acute or chronic ethanol intake. Therefore, this lack of basic knowledge compounds the difficulty we face when interpreting the importance of efforts of increasing serum Mg^{2+} levels under these conditions.

Blood-brain barrier, magnesium and hydrocephalus

Human and animal studies have indicated that hydrocephalus leads to disruption of BBB. In a study involving a total of 21 patients with normal-pressure hydrocephalus, a slight plasma-like protein pattern has been demonstrated in CSF in 38% of the patients prior to surgical intervention indicating BBB dysfunction (Wikkelsø and Blomstrand, 1982). There is only one study in the current literature which evaluates the effects of magnesium in hydrocephalus and a mild protection against brain damage has been shown by $MgSO_4$ therapy in a rat model of childhood-onset hydrocephalus (Khan *et al*, 2003). Further studies are necessary to increase our understanding of the effects of deficiency or supplementation of magnesium on the functional and structural characteristics of BBB in hydrocephalus by both animal and human studies.

Conclusion

It is clear from the discussion above that magnesium plays a variety of essential roles within the cell by modulating the activity of more than 325 enzymes as a cofactor. These enzymes are important for the survival of various cell types including endothelial cells of BBB. Meanwhile, magnesium deficiency leads to or worsens a variety of central nervous system pathologies by increasing inflammatory cytokines and reactive oxygen species and disturbing the activity of transporters in neurons, astrocytes, pericytes and capillary endothelial cells which together constitute the neurovascular unit of the brain. Besides, the alterations in the Mg^{2+} concentration in intra- and extracellular fluids are associated with development or aggravation of BBB disruption and brain edema in various clinical disorders and experimental settings. On the other hand, magnesium supplementation can play multiple roles in protecting BBB integrity and improving brain edema. However, owing to the availability of limited knowledge, it is hard to come to a full understanding of the highly specific actions of magnesium on BBB integrity and brain edema in the course of a variety of pathophysiologies involving the BBB. For this reason, research in this field should continue in order to provide a thorough explanation of the impact of magnesium on BBB, brain edema and related pathologies.

References

Abbott NJ, Patabendige AA, Dolman DE, Yusof SR, Begley DJ (2010) Structure and function of the blood-brain barrier. *Neurobiol Dis* 37:13-25.

Altura BM, Gebrewold A, Huang QF, Altura BT (1991) Deficits in brain-CSF magnesium result in cerebrovasospasm and rupture of cerebral microvessels: Possible relation to stroke. *Clin Res* 39:394A.

Altura BM, Gebrewold A, Altura BT, Gupta RK (1995) Role of brain [Mg2+]i in alcohol-induced hemorrhagic stroke in a rat model: a 31P-NMR in vivo study. *Alcohol* 12(2):131-6.

Altura BM, Gebrewold A, Zhang A, Altura BT (2003) Low extracellular magnesium ions induce lipid peroxidation and activation of nuclear factor-kappa B in canine cerebral vascular smooth muscle: possible relation to traumatic brain injury and strokes. *Neurosci Lett* 341:189-92.

Amiry-Moghaddam M, Otsuka T, Hurn PD, Traystman RJ, Haug FM, Froehner SC, Adams ME, Neely JD, Agre P, Ottersen OP, Bhardwaj A (2003) An alpha-syntrophin-dependent pool of AQP4 in astroglial end-feet confers bidirectional water flow between blood and brain. *Proc Natl Acad Sci USA* 100:2106–11.

Ariza AC, Bobadilla N, Fernandez C, Munoz-Fuentes RM, Larrea F, Halhali A (2005) Effects of magnesium sulfate on lipid peroxidation and blood pressure regulators in pre-eclampsia. *Clin Biochem* 38:128–33.

Bara M, Guiet-Bara A (1984) Potassium, magnesium and membranes. *Magnesium* 3:212-25.

Barbagallo M, Dominguez LJ (2010) Magnesium and aging. *Curr Pharm Des* 16:832-39.

Billard JM (2006) Ageing, hippocampal synaptic activity and magnesium. *Magnes Res* 19:199-215.

Belfort M, Allred J, Dildy G (2008) Magnesium sulfate decreases cerebral perfusion pressure in preeclampsia. *Hypertens Pregnancy* 27:315–27.

Cardoso FL, Brites D, Brito MA (2010) Looking at the blood-brain barrier: molecular anatomy and possible investigation approaches. *Brain Res Rev* 64: 328-63.

Chaon A, Lisott E, Eblen-Zajjur A (2006) Magnesium sulphate reduces cell volume in physiological conditions but not in the cytotoxic oedema during global brain ischemia. *Brain Injury* 20:1087–91.

Correale J, Villa A (2009) Cellular Elements of the Blood-Brain Barrier. *Neurochem Res* 34:2067–77.

Dai LJ, Quamme G A (1991) Intracellular Mg2+ and magnesium depletion in isolated renal thick ascending limb cells. *J Clin Invest* 88: 1255-64.

Demougeot C, Bobillier-Chaumont S, Mossiat C, Marie C, Berthelot A (2004) Effect of diets with different magnesium content in ischemic stroke rats. *Neurosci Lett* 362:17-20.

Ebel H, Gunther T (1980) Magnesium metabolism: a review. *J Clin Chem Clin Biochem* 18:257–70.

Esen F, Erdem T, Aktan D, Kalaycı R, Cakar N, Kaya M, Telci L (2003) Effects of magnesium administration on brain edema and blood brain barrier breakdown after experimental traumatic brain injury in rats. *J Neurosurg Anesthesiol* 15:119-25.

Esen F, Erdem T, Aktan D, Orhan M, Kaya M, Eraksoy H, Cakar N, Telci L (2005) Effect of magnesium sulfate administration on blood-brain barrier in a rat model of intraperitoneal sepsis: A randomized controlled experimental study. *Critical Care* 9:R18–R23.

Euser AG, Bullinger L, Cipolla MJ (2008) Magnesium sulphate treatment decreases blood brain barrier permeability during acute hypertension in pregnant rats. *Exp Physiol* 93:254–61.

Euser AG, Cipolla MJ (2009) Magnesium Sulfate for the Treatment of Eclampsia. *Stroke* 40:1169-75.

Feldman Z, Gurevitch B, Artru AA, Oppenheim A, Shohami E, Reichenthal E, Shapira Y (1996) Effect of magnesium given 1 hour after head trauma on brain edema and neurological outcome. *J Neurosurg* 85:131–7.

Feng DF, Zhu ZA, Lu YC (2004) Effect of magnesium on traumatic brain edema in rats. *Chin J Traumatol* 7:148–52.

Fisher M (2009) Pericyte signaling in the neurovascular unit. *Stroke* 40:S13–S15.

Ghabriel MN, Thomas A, Vink R (2006) Magnesium restores altered aquaporin-4 immunoreactivity following traumatic brain injury to a pre-injury state. *Acta Neurochir Suppl* 96:402–6.

Goñi-de-Cerio F, Alvarez A, Alvarez FJ, Rey-Santano MC, Alonso-Alconada D, Mielgo VE, Gastiasoro E, Hilario E (2009) MgSO4 treatment preserves the ischemia-induced reduction in S-100 protein without modification of the expression of endothelial tight junction molecules. *Histol Histopathol* 24(9):1129-38.

Grubbs RD, Maguire ME (1987) Magnesium as a regulatory cation: criteria and evaluation. *Magnes* 6:113-27.

Guo S, Lo EH (2009) Dysfunctional cell-cell signaling in the neurovascular unit as a paradigm for central nervous system disease. *Stroke* 40(3):S4-7.

Hallak M, Berman RF, Irtenkauf SM, Evans MI, Cotton DB (1992) Peripheral magnesium sulfate enters the brain and increases the threshold for hippocampal seizures in rats. *Am J Obstet Gynecol* 167:1605–10.

Haorah J, Knipe B, Leibhart J, Ghorpade A, Persidsky Y (2005) Alcohol-induced oxidative stress in brain endothelial cells causes blood-brain barrier dysfunction. *J Leukoc Biol* 78(6):1223-32.

Heath DL, Vink R (1999) Improved motor outcome in response to magnesium therapy received up to 24 hours after traumatic diffuse axonal brain injury. *J Neurosurg* 90:504-9.

Hoane MR (2007) Assessment of cognitive function following magnesium therapy in the traumatically injured brain. *Magnes Res* 20:229–36.

Huang Q F, Gebrewold A, Zhang A, Altura BT, Altura BM (1994) Role of excitatory amino acids in regulation of rat pial microvasculature. *Am J Physiol Regul Integr Comp Physiol* 266:R158–R163.

Imer M, Omay B, Uzunkol A, Erdem T, Sabanci PA, Karasu A, Albayrak SB, Sencer A, Hepgul K, Kaya M (2009) Effect of magnesium, MK-801 and combination of magnesium and MK-801 on blood-brain barrier permeability and brain edema after experimental traumatic diffuse brain injury. *Neurol Res* 31:977-81.

Kaptanoglu E, Beskonakli E, Okutan O, Selcuk Surucu H, Taskin Y (2003) Effect of magnesium sulphate in experimental spinal cord injury: evaluation and ultrastructural findings and early clinical results. *J Clin Neurosci* 10:329–34.

Kaya M, Küçük M, Bulut Kalayci R, Cimen V, Gürses C, Elmas I, Arican N (2001) Magnesium sulfate attenuates increased blood–brain barrier permeability during insulin-induced hypoglycemia in rats. *Can J Physiol Pharmacol* 79:793-8.

Kaya M, Gulturk S, Elmas I, Arican N, Kocyildiz ZC, Kucuk M, Yorulmaz H, Sivas A. (2004) The effects of magnesium sulfate on blood-brain barrier disruption caused by intracarotid injection of hyperosmolar mannitol in rats. *Life Sci* 76:201–12.

Khan OH, Enno T, Del Bigio MR (2003) Magnesium sulfate therapy is of mild benefit to young rats with kaolin-induced hydrocephalus. *Pediatr Res* 53:970-6.

Klatzo I (1967) Presidental address: neuropathological aspects of brain edema. *J Neuropathol Exp Neurol* 26:1–14.

Lee MS, Wu YS, Yang DY, Lee JB, Cheng FC (2002) Significantly decreased extracellular magnesium in brains of gerbils subjected to cerebral ischemia. *Clin Chim Acta* 318:121-5.

Libien J, Sacktor TC, Kass IS (2005) Magnesium blocks the loss of protein kinase C, leads to a transient translocation of PKC(alpha) and PKC (epsilon), and improves recovery after anoxia in rat hippocampal slices. *Brain Res Mol Brain Res* 136:104-11.

Liu X, Hunter C, Weiss HR, Chi OZ (2010) Effects of blockade of ionotropic glutamate receptors on blood-brain barrier disruption in focal cerebral ischemia. *Neurol Sci* 31:699-703.

Löscher W, Potschka H (2005) Blood-brain barrier active efflux transporters: ATP-binding cassette gene family. *NeuroRx* 2:86-98.

Maier JA, Bernardini D, Rayssiguier Y, Mazur A (2004) High concentrations of magnesiummodulate vascular endothelial cell behaviour in vitro. *Biochim Biophys Acta* 1689:6-12.

Marmarou A (2004) The pathophysiology of brain edema and elevated intracranial pressure. *Cleveland Clin J Med* 71:S6–8.

Matsui T, Kobayashi H, Hirai S, Kawachi H, Yano H (2007) Magnesium deficiency stimulated mRNA expression of tumor necrosis factor-a in skeletal muscle of rats. *Nutrition Research* 27: 66–8.

Mazur A, Maier JA, Rock E, Gueux E, Nowacki W, Rayssiguier Y (2007) Magnesium and the inflammatory response: potential physiopathological implications. *Arch Biochem Biophys* 458:48–56.

McKee JA, Brewer RP, Macy GE, Phillips-Bute B, Campbell KA, Borel CO, Reynolds JD, Warner DS (2005) Analysis of the brain bioavailability of peripherally administered magnesium sulfate: a study in humans with acute brain injury undergoing prolonged induced hypermagnesemia. *Crit Care Med* 33:661–6.

Musso CG (2009) Magnesium metabolism in health and disease. *Int Urol Nephrol* 41:357-62.

Nag S, Manias JL, Stewart DJ (2009) Pathology and new players in the pathogenesis of brain edema. *Acta Neuropathol* 118(2):197-217.

Nakahama K, Nagano M, Fujioka A, Shinoda K, Sasaki H (1999) Effect of TPA on aquaporin 4 mRNA expression in cultured rat astrocytes. *Glia* 25:240-6.

Okiyama K, Smith DH, Gennarelli TA, Simon RP, Leach M, McIntosh TK. (1995) The sodium channel blocker and glutamate release inhibitor BW1003C87 and magnesium attenuate regional cerebral edema following experimental brain injury in the rat. *J Neurochem* 64:802–9.

Papadopoulos MC, Verkman AS (2005) Aquaporin-4 gene disruption in mice reduces brain swelling and mortality in pneumococcal meningitis. *J Biol Chem* 280:13906–12.

Papierkowski A, Pasternak K (1998) The effect of a single dose of morphine and ethanol on magnesium level in blood serum and tissues in mice. *Magnes Res* 11:85-9.

Pardridge WM (2005) Molecular biology of the blood-brain-barrier. *Mol Biotechnol* 30:57-70.

Pardridge WM (2007) Blood-brain-barrier delivery. *Drug Discov Today* 12:54–61.

Rayssiguier Y, Libako P, Nowacki W, Rock E (2010) Magnesium deficiency and metabolic syndrome: stress and inflammation may reflect calcium activation. *Magnes Res* 23(2):73-80.

Ravishankar S, Ashraf QM, Fritz K, Mishra OP, Delivoria-Papadopoulos M (2001) Expression of Bax and Bcl-2 proteins during hypoxia in cerebral cortical neuronal nuclei of newborn piglets: effect of administration of magnesium sulfate. *Brain Res* 901:23-9.

Romani AM (2008) Magnesium homeostasis and alcohol consumption. *Magnes Res* 21:197-204.

Romani AM, Scarpa A (2000) Regulation of cellular magnesium. *Frontiers in Bioscience* 5:720-34.

Royo NC, Shimizu S, Schouten JW, Stover JF, McIntosh TK (2003) Pharmacology of traumatic brain injury. *Curr Opin Pharmacol* 3:27–32.

Saatman KE, Bareyre FM, Grady MS, McIntosh TK (2001) Acute cytoskeletal alterations and cell death induced by experimental brain injury are attenuated by magnesium treatment and exacerbated by magnesium deficiency. *J Neuropathol Exp Neurol* 60:183–94.

Salem M, Kasinski N, Munoz R, Chernow B (1995) Progressive magnesium deficiency increases mortality from endotoxin challenge: protective effects of acute magnesium replacement therapy. *Crit Care Med* 23:108-18.

Saris NL, Mervaala E, Karppanen H, Khawaja JA, Lewenstam A (2000) Magnesium: an update on physiological, clinical and analytical aspects. *Clin Chim Acta* 294:1–26.

Schwartz RB, Feske SK, Polak JF, DeGirolami U, Iaia A, Beckner KM, Bravo SM, Klufas RA, Chai RY, Repke JT (2000) Preeclampsia-eclampsia: Clinical and neuroradiographic correlates and insights into the pathogenesis of hypertensive encephalopathy. *Radiology* 217:371–6.

Sen AP, Gulati A (2010) Use of magnesium in traumatic brain injury. *Neurotherapeutics* 7:91-9.

Taniguchi M, Yamashita T, Kumura E, Tamatani M, Kobayashi A, Yokawa T, Maruno M, Kato A, Ohnishi T, Kohmura E, Tohyama M, Yoshimine T (2000) Induction of aquaporin-4 water channel mRNA after focal cerebral ischemia in rat. *Mol Brain Res* 78:131–7.

Temkin NR, Anderson GD, Winn HR, Ellenbogen RG, Britz GW, Schuster J, Lucas T, Newell DW, Mansfield PN, Machamer JE, Barber J, Dikmen SS (2007) Magnesium sulfate for neuroprotection after traumatic brain injury: a randomised controlled trial. *Lancet Neurol* 6:29–38.

Touyz RM (2003) Role of magnesium in the pathogenesis of hypertension. *Mol Aspects Med* 24:107-36.

Touyz RM (2008) Transient receptor potential melastatin 6 and 7 channels, magnesium transport, and vascular biology: implications in hypertension. *Am J Physiol Heart Circ Physiol* 294:H1103-8.

Turkoglu OF, Eroglu H, Okutan O, Tun MK, Bodur E, Sargon MF, Oner L, Beskonakli E (2008) A comparative study of treatment for brain edema Magnesium sulphate versus dexamethasone sodium phosphate. *J Clin Neurosci* 15:60–5.

Unterberg AW, Stover J, Kress B, Kiening KL (2004) Edema and brain trauma. *Neuroscience* 129:1021-9.

Vink R, McIntosh T K, Demediuk P, Faden AI (1987) Decrease in total and free magnesium concentration following traumatic brain injury in rats. *Biochem Biophys Res Commun* 149:594-9.

Vink R, McIntosh TK, Demediuk P, Weiner MW, Faden AI (1988) Decline in intracellular free Mg^{2+} is associated with irreversible tissue injury after brain trauma. *J Biol Chem* 263(2):757-61.

Vink R, Cernak I (2000) Regulation of intracellular free magnesium central nervous system injury. *Front Biosci* 1:656–65.

Vink R, Cook NL, van den Heuvel C (2009) Magnesium in acute and chronic brain injury: an update. *Magnes Res* 22:158S-162S.

Weglicki WB, Phillips TM, Mak IT, Cassidy MM, Dickens BF, Stafford R, Kramer JH (1994) Cytokines, neuropeptides, and reperfusion injury during magnesium deficiency. *Ann N Y Acad Sci* 723:246-57.

Weglicki WB, Mak, IT, Kramer JH, Dickens BF, Cassidy MM, Stafford RE, Phillips TM (1996) Role of free radicals and substance P in magnesium deficiency. *Cardiovasc Res* 31: 677–82.

Wikkelsø C, Blomstrand C (1982) Cerebrospinal fluid proteins and cells in normal-pressure hydrocephalus. *J Neurol* 228:171-80.

Wolf FI, Trapani V, Simonacci M, Ferré S, Maier JAM (2008) Magnesium deficiency and endothelial dysfunction: is oxidative stress involved? *Magnes Res* 21:58–64.

Wolf FI, Trapani V (2008) Cell (patho) physiology of magnesium. *Clin Sci* 114: 27–35.

Wolf FI, Trapani V, Simonacci M, Boninsegna A, Mazur A, Maier JA (2009) Magnesium deficiency affects mammary epithelial cell proliferation: involvement of oxidative stress. *Nutr Cancer* 61(1):131-6.

Zador Z, Stiver S, Wang V, Manley GT (2009) Role of aquaporin-4 in cerebral edema and stroke. In: *Aquaporins- Handbook of experimental pharmacology* 190 (Beitz E eds), Springer, Heidelberg, 159-70.

Magnesium and hearing loss

Isabelle Sendowski,[1,✉] *Xavier Holy,*[2] *Florent Raffin*[1] *and Yves Cazals*[3]

[1] Institut de Recherche Biomédicale des Armées, Antenne de la Tronche, La Tronche, France.
[2] Institut de Recherche Biomédicale des Armées, Antenne de Brétigny, Brétigny-sur-Orge, France.
[3] UMR6231, Université Paul Cézanne, Marseille, France.
✉ Isendowski@crssa.net

Abstract

Hearing loss is a major public health problem with a large number of causes. Among them, noise-induced hearing loss, drug ototoxicity and sudden sensorineural hearing loss have been proven to result in part from metabolic disorders. Metabolic disorders have multiple origins such as: ionic, ischemic, excitotoxic and production of cochlear free radicals causing cell death, via necrosis or apoptosis. The efficacy of magnesium, administered either to prevent or to treat hearing damages has been demonstrated in several studies in animals and in humans, particularly in noise-induced hearing loss. The exact mechanism by which Mg^{2+} acts is not fully known. Different hypotheses exist including calcium antagonism, vasodilatation, antioxidant and anti-NMDA properties. Because it is a relatively safe and well-known treatment, magnesium therapy, alone or in association, could be of a great interest to improve auditory recovery.

Introduction

According to the World Health Organization, 278 million people worldwide have moderate to profound hearing loss in both ears. Besides pathologies of unknown origin such as sudden hearing loss and Meniere's disease, hearing loss has so many known causes, it would be arduous to list them all. Briefly, it can be due to the aging process, exposure to loud noise, certain medications, infections, head or ear trauma, congenital or hereditary factors, diseases, as well as a number of other causes. In noise-induced hearing loss (NIHL), sudden sensorineural hearing loss (SSHL) or iatrogenic hearing loss (ototoxicity), sensory cell death involves metabolic processes. So, pharmacological intervention to prevent or ameliorate the evolution of these hearing impairments, as well as susceptibility factors, have been studied for few years in animal models or in humans. Among them, magnesium seems to play an important role. Magnesium therapy is well documented because it is usually prescribed in other pathologies. Its side effects and contraindications are few and it is cheap. Magnesium, that crosses easily the hemato-cochlear barrier, presents neuroprotective and vasodilatory effects, and is able to limit cochlear damage. These observations have led to many investigations, the aim of them being to evaluate the pertinence of magnesium administration in prevention or treatment in such a hearing impairment. This article also presents some arguments that emphasize the interest of magnesium therapy in some forms of hearing loss.

How can we hear?

Sound waves are transmitted via the bones of the middle ear to the fluid environment of the inner ear, where the sensory organ is in the cochlea. The human cochlea is a coiled tube 30-35 mm long containing three parallel chambers (Figure 1A): the scala vestibuli and scala tympani, which contain perilymph, and the scala media, which contains endolymph. Conversely to perilymph, which is similar to cerebrospinal fluid, endolymph contains a large amount of potassium (154 mM) maintained by the cells of the stria vascularis. The organ of Corti (Figure 1B) is composed of supporting cells and hair cells. Of all the sensory organs, the organ of Corti functions with the smallest number of sensory receptor cells. The human cochlea only contains about 15,000 hair cells, including approximately 3,000 inner hair cells (IHCs) and 12,000 outer hair cells (OHCs). The IHCs form one row (Figure 2A) and are the primary sensory receptors. OHCs are organized into three (and sometimes four) rows along the

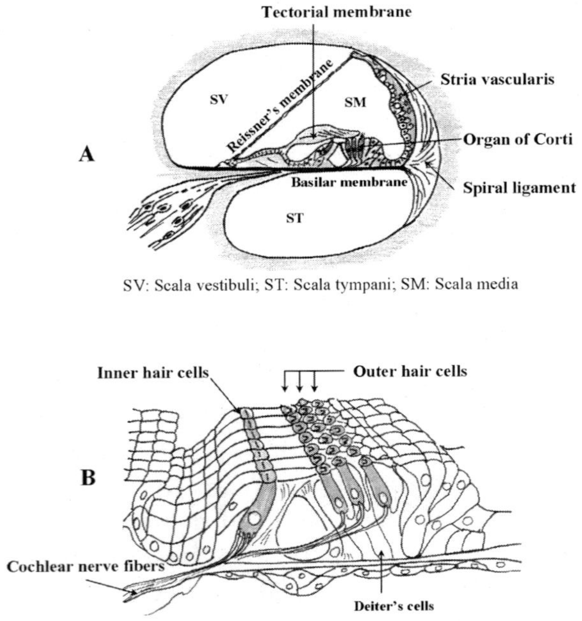

Figure 1. Schematic representation of the inner ear. A: section of the cochlea; B: organ of Corti.

outer edge of the organ of Corti. The longer stereocilia of the OHCs are connected to the tectorial membrane.

In the hearing process, the sound reaches the inner ear and the basilar membrane supporting hair cells is displaced. When the hair bundle is deflected, transduction channels are opened and K^+ enters the hair cells. The depolarisation evoked by this transduction current activates voltage-gated Ca^{2+}channels and Ca^{2+}influx. In IHCs, increased intracellular Ca^{2+} causes mobilization of synaptic vesicles and exocytotic release of glutamate at the base of the hair cells. Glutamate release modulates the activity of the auditory nerve fibers by activating specific receptors, among them the glutamate ionotropic receptors (AMPA, NMDA and Kaïnate) and the metabotropic receptors. The OHCs respond quite differently to changes in membrane potential. Their membranes include a protein (prestin), which alters their conformation with the membrane potential and forces cell length changes at acoustic frequencies. This mechanism is thought to amplify and tune the mechanical responses of the basilar membrane. This sensory system is so efficient that, near auditory threshold, a sound vibration of less than 0.1 nanometer is detected corresponding to a stereocilia displacement 10,000 times lower than its diameter (about one micrometer). However, exposure to loud noise can weaken the system.

Magnesium and noise-induced hearing loss (NIHL)

Excessive noise is the predominant cause of permanent sensorineural hearing loss. Reports from WHO state (WHO 2004) "Worldwide, 16% of the disabling hearing loss in adults is attributed to occupational noise, ranging from 7% to 21% in the various subregions". At least 30 million people in the United States encounter hazardous levels of noise at work, particularly in jobs such as construction, mining, agriculture, manufacturing, transportation, and in the military. The incidence of NIHL continues to grow, moreover, partly due to the growing popularity of portable music players with highly efficient headphones (Zhao *et al*, 2010). The hearing loss can be caused by a single exposure to very loud sounds (impulse noise) or by repeated exposure to louder sounds over an extended period. It may be temporary (temporary threshold shifts, TTS) or permanent (permanent threshold shifts, PTS). It is frequently associated with tinnitus.

The damage mechanisms are of dual origin, mechanical and metabolic. Mechanical damages are developed immediately when the movements of the basilar membrane are excessive, thus inducing detachment of the hairs of the tectorial membrane, disconnection of the interciliary bridges (Figure 2D), or even rupture of membranes. Modern research has provided new insights into the biological mechanisms of NIHL such as: free radicals production (oxidative stress), glutamatergic excitotoxicity, ionic and ischemic disorders. They are responsible for a delayed hair cell death by necrosis and apoptosis.

Oxidative stress

It has been demonstrated that an increase of reactive oxygen and nitrogen species (ROS and RNS, respectively) is involved in noise trauma (see Henderson *et al*, 2006 for review). The superoxide radical anion, nitric oxide (NO) and its redox-related forms, in conjunction with an imbalance of antioxidant defences, have been demonstrated to play a significant role in NIHL as they largely participate in cellular mechanisms that underlie hair cell death. ROS ototoxicity is believed to be associated with deleterious cellular

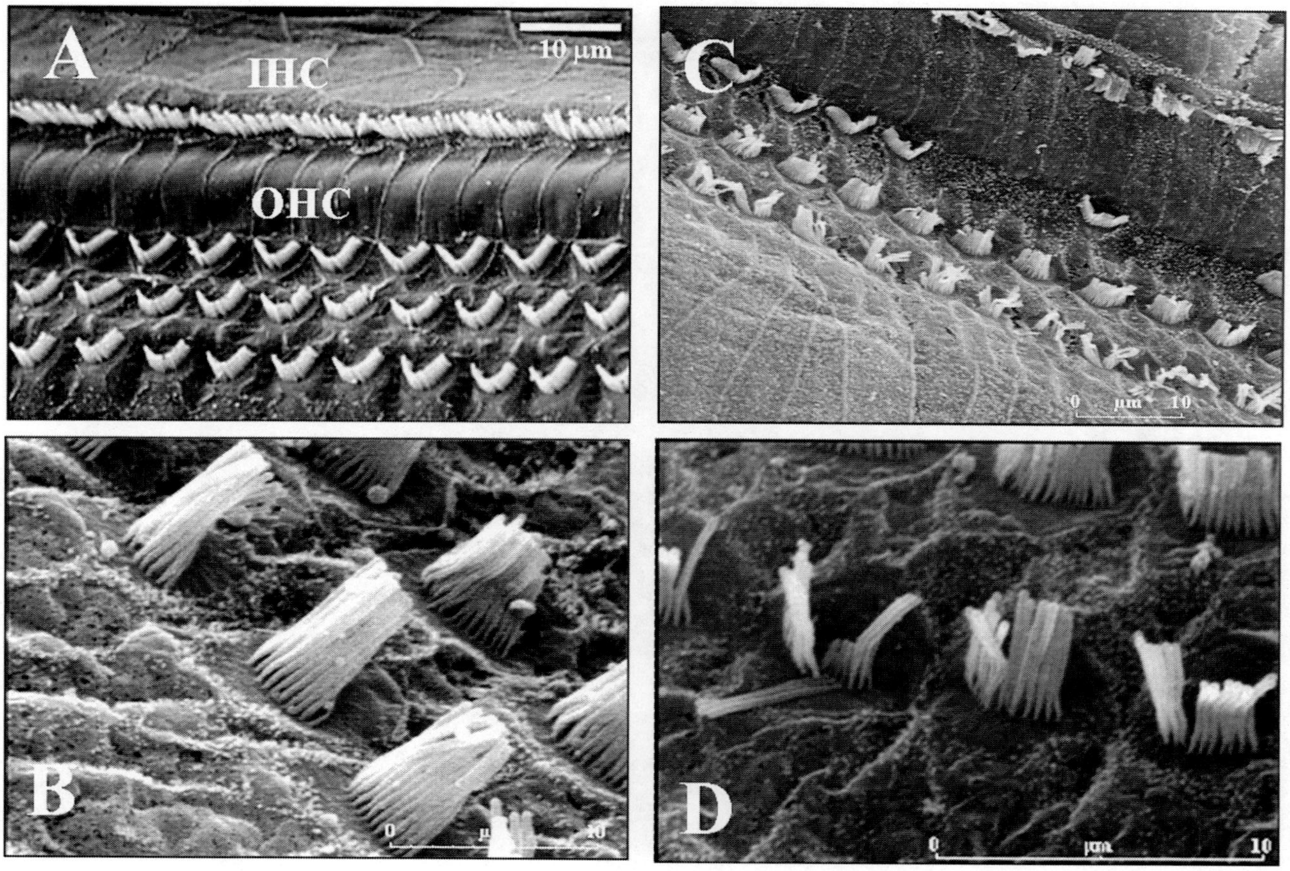

Figure 2. A,B: normal aspect of the hair cells and their stereocilia, observed with scanning electron microscopy. C and D: Organ of Corti after traumatizing noise exposure: OHCs are partially missing (C). The stereocilia of hair cells are abnormally bent with broken interciliary bridges (D).

effects at multiple sites including lipid peroxidation, DNA strand breaks, alterations in carbohydrate and protein structures and trigger cell death gens expression, leading to necrosis or apoptosis. Oxidants are also initiators in intracellular cell death signalling pathways that may lead to apoptosis. The noise-induced ROS formation may occur with a delay of 7-10 days following exposure to noise (Yamashita *et al*, 2004).

Excitotoxicity

Excitotoxicity is a phenomenon of biochemical events, triggered by the interaction of excitatory amino acids with ion channel-bound receptor complexes that can lead to cell death. During high-level noise exposure, the IHCs are highly active, leading to the release of large amounts of glutamate into the synapses with the auditory fibers. The levels of glutamate in the synapses can overstimulate the glutamate receptors, especially the NMDA receptors that involve high intracellular Ca2 + levels. The increase in cytosolic Ca^{2+}concentration is not only caused by an influx of extracellular Ca^{2+}, but also by the release of calcium ions from intracellular stores such as the endoplasmic reticulum or mitochondria. Dendritic swelling and vacuolization are a result of excessive postsynaptic ion influx into the VIIIth nerve terminals at the inner hair cell synapse (Pujol *et al*, 1990).

Ionic disorders

High-level noise stimulation involves a massive entrance of potassium through the apical channels of the stereocilia. Moreover, mechanical damage with ruptures of the membranes lining the endolymphatic spaces could involve an excessive influx of K^+. This increased K^+ concentration may be toxic for the hair cells (Zenner, 1986). The consecutive increase of intracellular Ca^{2+} overactivates a series of enzymes including phospholipases, proteases, endonucleases. The results are membrane breakdown, depolymerization of microtubules and disruption of protein synthesis.

Ischemic process

Unlike most tissues in which increased metabolism increases blood flow to provide additional oxygen to stressed cells, the cochlea shows reduced blood vessel diameter and red blood cell velocity (Quirk and Seidman, 1995) and decreased blood flow (Thorne and Nuttal, 1987) post-noise. This noise-induced vasoconstriction is a direct consequence of noise-induced formation of 8-isoprostane-F_{2a}, a vaso-active by-product of free radicals (Miller *et al*, 2003). Cochlear ischemia is aggravated in animals with low Mg^{2+} content (Scheibe *et al*, 2000a).

These different mechanisms can lead to cell death which may be more or less rapid, due to necrosis or apoptosis (Yang *et al*, 2004). Recent studies have revealed that these two types of cell death exist following exposure to intense noise and that apoptosis appears extremely rapidly after the noise stress. Apoptosis has been shown to be the primary cell death pathway in the first day following noise exposure (Hu *et al*, 2002; 2006).

Contrary to birds or reptiles, mammal's auditory hair cells do not regenerate if they are destroyed. Thus these new metabolic insights bring hope for possible prevention or treatment to limit oxidative stress, ischemia and the apoptosis cascade. A large number of treatments have been tested these last years (see Le Prell *et al*, 2007a; Shibata and Raphael, 2010 for reviews). Among them, magnesium has aroused some interest.

For the last few years, researchers and clinicians demonstrated the influence of magnesium in the susceptibility to recover following acoustic trauma: NIHL of guinea pigs was found to increase with decreasing Mg^{2+} content of the drinking water while the Mg^{2+} content of the food was low and constant. In Mg-deficient guinea pigs, the hearing threshold shift after 10 days of continuous noise exposure was negatively correlated to the Mg^{2+} content of the perilymph (Ising *et al*, 1982). Coherent results were obtained in rats (Joachims *et al*, 1983). Similarly, electrocochleographic measurements of the auditory threshold shifts induced by impulses noises (Devrière *et al*, 1991) showed that Mg-deficient animals are slightly more susceptible to this type of noise. This susceptibility is less pronounced than after a long duration exposure to a continuous noise, as observed in the previous experiments. After exposure to continuous noise, up to 75 % of the variance of PTS in guinea pigs could be explained by the level of perilymph Mg^{2+} (Vorman and Günther, 1993). The increased susceptibility to NIHL with Mg^{2+} deficit has not only been demonstrated in animal experiments: in a retrospective study in humans, subjective thresholds across frequencies of 3, 4 and 5 kHz were found to be negatively correlated to serum magnesium (Joachims *et al*, 1987). This finding was the first indication that magnesium status in humans may be one of the factors determining variations in sensitivity to noise-induced hearing loss. Günther et al (1989) reported that NIHL observed in 24 air force pilots was negatively correlated to serum Mg^{2+} concentration. However, Walden et al (2000) exploring the susceptibility of soldiers to NIHL failed to demonstrate any correlation between audiometric index and body magnesium.

Because Mg^{2+} deficiency increases the susceptibility to NIHL, several studies have been conducted in animals or in humans to point out the possible interest of a prophylactic efficacy of magnesium. Joachims et al (1983) observed that guinea pigs with physiologically high Mg^{2+}levels, exposed to a single shot impulse or a series of impulses had significantly smaller threshold increases as compared to physiologically low Mg^{2+} animals. Scheibe et al (2000b) showed that oral magnesium supplementation significantly reduces TTS and PTS in guinea pigs subjected to a series of impulsions. The mean PTS was found to correlate negatively with the total Mg^{2+} concentration of perilymph and plasma. Conversely, they did not observe any significant effect on PTS following exposure to a gunshot noise. More recently, Attias et al (2003) explored the activity of the outer hair cells in guinea pig by mean of otoacoustic emission, after impulse noise exposure. The thresholds were less significantly affected by noise exposure and the audition recovery was faster in the animals supplemented in Mg^{2+}. In humans, preventive administration of magnesium has been also shown to be effective on hearing loss related to noise. Attias et al (1994) tested the prophylactic effect of magnesium in human subjects exposed to hazardous noise. The study was carried out on 300 young, normal-hearing recruits who underwent 2 months of basic military training. This training included repeated exposures to high levels of impulse noises while using ear plugs. The subjects received daily an additional drink containing either 167 mg magnesium aspartate or a placebo. The NIHL was significantly more frequent and more severe in the placebo group (28.5 %) than in the magnesium group (11.2 %). Moreover, the severity of the NIHL was negatively correlated to the magnesium content of red and mononuclear cells. This prophylactic effect in humans was confirmed by Attias et al (2004) for temporary threshold shifts. Subjects were exposed to a traumatizing noise during 10 min in order to produce TTS without PTS. Compared to a placebo, the preventive oral intake of magnesium (122 mg Mg^{2+} aspartate during 10 days) provided significant protection against TTS. A negative correlation between the blood magnesium levels and the TTS was also noted.

Whilst magnesium is well known as a preventive treatment for sound trauma, it may also be useful therapeutically: in animals submitted to a series of sound impulses, the administration of magnesium by the systemic route significantly reduced hearing loss after 7 days (Scheibe *et al*, 2001; 2002). This treatment was more effective if it was quickly instigated. Threshold shift reduction 7 days after acoustic trauma in guinea pigs was confirmed using distorsion product otoacoustic emissions (DPOAE: a non invasive technique to test OHC function; Haupt *et al*, 2003). In another study (Sendowski *et al*, 2006) it has been shown that a 7-day post-trauma magnesium treatment reduced auditory threshold shift measured seven days after gunshot noise exposure. However, this improvement was temporary, suggesting that it could be potentially beneficial to prolong magnesium administration. This hypothesis has been confirmed thereafter (Abaamrane *et al*, 2009): the study compared 4 post-NIHL treatments: a 7-day or 1-month magnesium treatment, conventional therapy with methylprednisolone or a placebo. It was demonstrated that 3 months after an impulse noise trauma, the 1-month Mg treatment preserved more hair cells from death (Figure 3), but this preservation was found to be partial. These observations suggest that post-NIHL treatments can be improved if continued beyond the period of one week.

Another track of research concerns combination of different therapies including magnesium. Treatment with a combination of vitamins A, C, E and magnesium, initiated 1 hour before noise exposure, produced a compelling reduction in NIHL and cell death, while effects of either the antioxidant agents (vitamin A, C, or E) or magnesium were small and not statistically reliable (Le Prell *et al*, 2007b). Thus, the combination of magnesium with other agents could also present a great interest, and suggest that they act at different and complementary levels of the cellular death process.

Magnesium and ototoxicity

Various pharmaceuticals are known to impair the auditory system. The best-known substances are the aminoglycoside antibiotics and cisplatin. Both cause high frequency sensorineural hearing loss, which is usually permanent and associated with loss of outer hair cells in the basal turn of the cochlea. Aminoglycoside antibiotics (such as gentamicin, neomycin and kanamycin) are used to treat bacteria not responsive to conventional antibiotics. Their clinical use is limited by toxic side effects that include cochlear toxicity, vestibular toxicity and nephrotoxicity. Aminoglycoside antibiotics possibly cause formation of free radicals by forming complexes with iron, which is vital for normal mitochondrial function. Free radicals can rapidly react with cell constituents, including cell membranes and DNA. The resulting oxidative stress can trigger apoptotic cell death. The intrinsic apoptosis pathway is the major pathway induced by aminoglycosides in the cochlea (Rybak and Withworth, 2005).

Vormann and Günther (1991) demonstrated that Mg deficiency in growing rats aggravated the ototoxic effects of the aminoglycoside antibiotic gentamicin. Administration of gentamicin to Mg^{2+} deficient pregnant rats from day 16-20 of gestation produced hearing threshold shifts in the maternal rats as well in their offspring (Vormann and Günther 1991). Theses data suggest that Mg^{2+} deficiency is a relevant predisposing risk factor for the development of

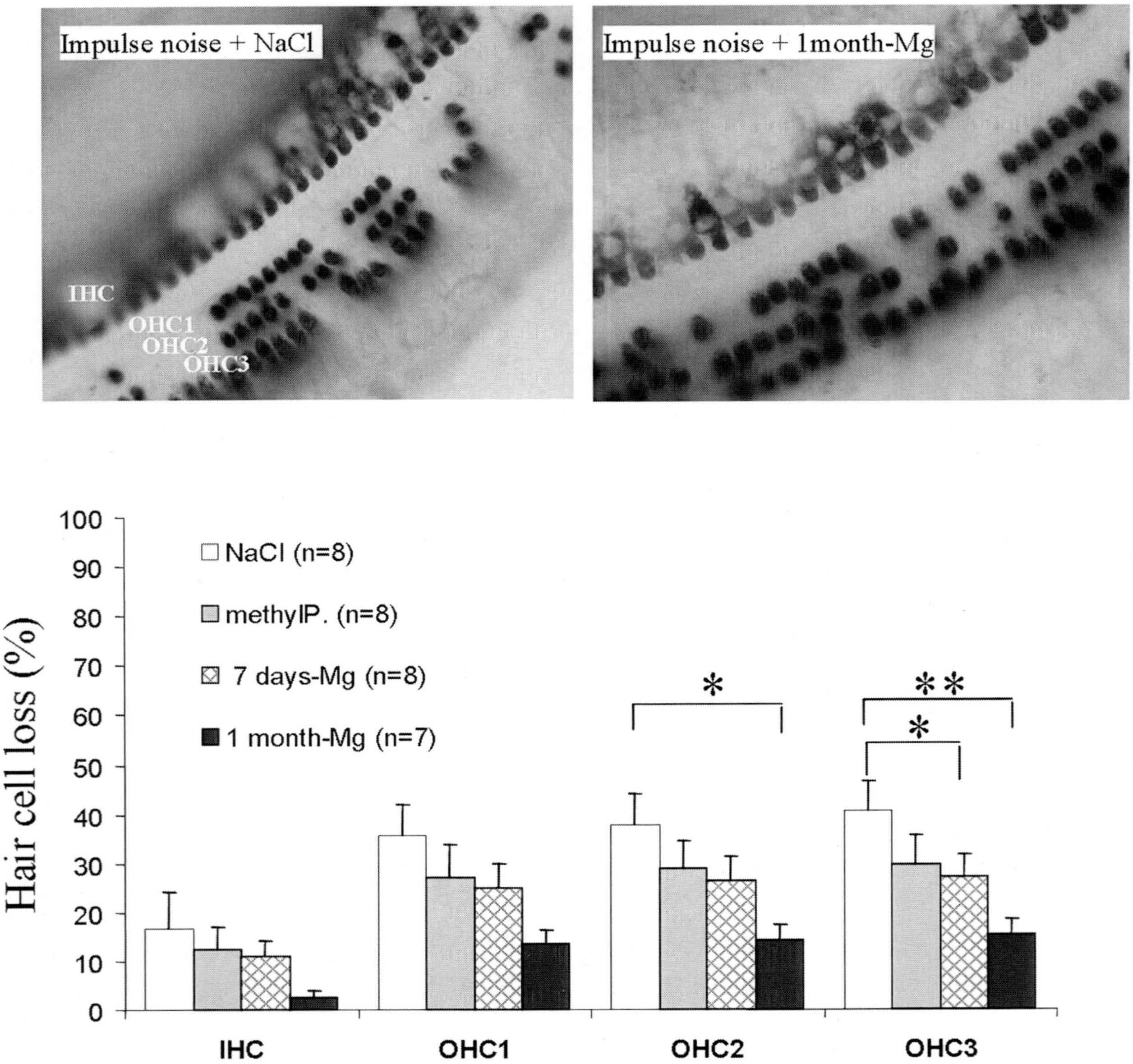

Figure 3. Global hair cells losses in guinea pigs, 3 months after an impulse noise exposure, for 4 treatments groups: placebo (NaCl), a 7-day or 1-month magnesium treatment, and conventional therapy with methylprednisolone. (* $P<0.05$; ** $P<0.01$) (after Abaamrane *et al*, 2009).

ototoxicity induced by some pharmaceuticals. Recently, it has been shown, in the zebrafish model, that extracellular magnesium or calcium ions modulated hair cell death from neomycin and gentamycin, but exerted their protective effects through different mechanisms (Coffin *et al*, 2009). In mammals, preliminary injection of magnesium solution by means of electrophoresis reduced the ototoxic effect of the kanamicin (Spasov *et al*, 1999).

Other well-known ototoxic treatments are platinum compounds. Cisplatin is a frequently used chemotherapeutic agent in the treatment of many types of neoplasias, especially of the head and neck (Rybak and Withworth, 2005). The mechanism of antineoplastic action is associated with the selective and persistent inhibition of the deoxyribonucleic acid synthesis (Williams and Whitehouse, 1979). Its side effects include ototoxicity, kidney toxicity, medullar suppression and gastrointestinal disorders. The nephrotoxic effect of cisplatin is a severe damage in the renal proximal cells within the thick ascending loop of Henle manifested by hypomagnesemia. These types of toxicity can impact treatment, as they reduce the chemotherapy dosage, frequency and duration for many patients. Some audiometric studies have reported elevated hearing threshold in 75-100% of patients treated with cisplatin (McKeage, 1995).

The auditory lesions seem to result from free radical-induced damage to many tissues (Kopke *et al*, 1997; Rybak *et al*, 1995; Dehne *et al*, 2001). Oxygen reactive species are generated in the cochlea after exposure to cisplatin (Clerici and Yang, 1996) and that such oxidative stress can cause cochlear cell death by apoptosis secondary to the activation of caspase-3 (Garcia-Berrocal *et al*, 2007; De Freitas *et al*, 2009). Inner ear cell apoptosis can be triggered by the formation of complexes between cisplatin and the DNA of the damaged cell, preventing the progression of the cell cycle. Cevette et al (2000) observed a significant increase in otoacoustic emission amplitude (which provides frequency-specific information about OHC function) in two patients undergoing cisplatin treatment supplemented with magnesium. The authors of this study concluded that Mg^{2+} might be a promising agent against cisplatin ototoxicity. However, the study of Sahin et al (2006) showed that a Mg^{2+}-rich diet can prevent the severe hypomagnesemia that cisplatin causes in guinea pigs, but failed to prove any protection against its ototoxic effect.

Magnesium and sudden sensorineural hearing loss.

The US National Institute for Deafness and Communication Disorders defines SSHL as the idiopathic loss of hearing of at least 30 dB over at least 3 contiguous test frequencies occurring within 3 days. Estimates of the overall incidence of SSHL range from 5 to 20 per 100 000 persons per year (Conlin and Parnes, 2007). Many etiologic causes of SSHL have been proposed, but many remain unconfirmed. In the majority of patients (71%), the aetiology remains idiopathic. A wide range of disorders might lead to the development of SSHL. The theorized major causative factors can be broken down into several categories: 1) viral infection (13 %); 2) vascular impairment; 3) immune-mediated mechanisms; 4) inner ear abnormality; and 5) CNS abnormalities, including tumors, trauma, hemorrhage, infarction and other pathologies (Chau *et al*, 2010). The lack of understanding of the mechanism of SSHL has rendered the development of a specific treatment difficult, and currently, empirical guidelines are used. Because of the spontaneous recovery rates of 32 % to 70 % (Colin and Parnes, 2010), some otolaryngologists choose not to treat SSHL. However the most common approach to treatment of SSHL is with systemic steroids in moderate doses. Nageris et al (2004) evaluated the efficiency of two treatments after SSHL in humans: the first one consisted in the association corsticosteroid and magnesium and the second one (control) in corticosteroid and placebo. They observed that more patients treated with magnesium experienced hearing improvement, and at a larger magnitude, than control subjects. Gordin and colleagues (2002) reported a significantly greater recovery rate among patients treated with magnesium and carbogen vs patients treated with carbogen alone.

How does magnesium therapy work?

Magnesium plays an essential role in the regulation of most cellular functions. However, it is recognized that magnesium status in humans is often deficient. In the recent French study SU.VI.MAX (The "supplementation en vitamines et mineraux antioxidants" study) concerning 5,448 subjects, it has been shown that 77 % of women and 72 % of men had dietary magnesium intakes lower than recommended dietary allowances (Galan *et al*, 1997). The deficiency is increased by chronic stress, loud noise exposure or chemotherapy with platinum compounds (Galland, 1991; Mocci *et al*, 2001, Sahin *et al*, 2006). Scheibe et al (1999) were the first to study in the same animal the correlation between the plasma, perilymph and cerebrospinal magnesium contents. Contrary to the blood brain barrier, the blood perilymph barrier is not able to concentrate Mg^{2+} taken up from plasma. Also, the perilymph Mg^{2+} concentration correlates well with the plasma level, and a Mg^{2+} deficiency affects perilymph content.

The exact manner by which Mg^{2+} affects the susceptibility to hearing loss is still unknown, but several mechanisms could be evoked. By its nature, magnesium is a **calcium antagonist** and therefore blocks the excessive release of calcium, both in the hair cells and in the cochlear vasculature, limiting cell energy depletion and inducing the vasodilatation of arterioles. Through these mechanisms, magnesium could limit ischemia induced by acoustic trauma. Haupt and Scheibe (2002) demonstrated that cochlear blood flow as well as perilymphatic pO_2 levels were significantly increased in noise-traumatized animals that received magnesium supplements. Not only does magnesium combat ischemia, but it is also thought to prevent cell damage caused by hypoxia: Konig *et al* (2003) noted a protective effect of magnesium on hypoxia-induced hair cell loss in vitro. In other models high magnesium concentration has been showed to attenuate the hypoxia/ischemia-induced disruption of mitochondrial membrane potential, a critical event in triggering cell death (Sharikabad *et al*, 2001). This mechanism is supported by the observation that an increase in the extracellular magnesium concentration led to a decrease in hypoxia induced apoptosis by maintaining the normal ratio of Bax to Bcl-2 proteins involved in determining the survival of cells or their death (Ravishankar, 2001).

Another potential mechanism explaining the Mg^{2+} efficiency in NIHL or in drug ototoxicity, involves **free radical production**. Two mechanisms have been suggested (Garcia *et al*, 1998): It may directly inhibit free radical production or it may facilitate scavenging of free radicals. Afanas'ev et al (1995) showed that Mg^{2+} inhibits reduced NADP oxidase, an enzyme that produces superoxide radical. However, despite the protective effect of magnesium against oxidative stress, as demonstrated in different models (Sharikabad *et al*. 2001, Bede *et al*., 2008) no data are currently available about the cochlea.

Lastly, Mg^{2+} could act on **glutamate excitotoxicity,** specially in NIHL. Magnesium apparently enhances the survival capability of the cochlear afferents, reducing the effect of glutamate-induced inner hair cell damage (Ehrenberger and Felix, 1995). Magnesium is able to modulate the opening of Na^{+}/Ca^{++} channels of the NMDA receptors (Mayer *et al*, 1984). The blockage of the NMDA receptors by Mg^{2+} is voltage-dependent, but extracellular Mg^{2+} behaves as a non-competitive NMDA antagonist, without the side effects presented by the other non-competitive NMDA antagonists. In the hearing process, if Mg^{2+} is low, an excess of Ca^{2+} could enter hair cells. In turn, more glutamate would then be produced in response to this Ca^{2+} influx. Increased glutamate would also greatly increase the activity of the NMDA receptor, which is also operating with low magnesium. With the double insult of high glutamate and low Mg^{2+}, a flood of Ca^{2+} could go through the NMDA channels into the nerve cell, and the energetic system could be compromised.

Conclusion

Hearing loss is a significant clinical issue. We now know many of the molecular pathways leading to apoptotic cell death that are triggered by noise and other environmentally mediated trauma such as aminoglycoside antibiotics and chemo-therapeutics. There is increasing evidence for their similarity, since free radical formation and apoptotic cascades have been implicated in all. Interventions can be directed at preventing initial ROS formation, maintaining cochlear blood flow or blocking apoptosis. A large number of therapeutics including magnesium have been tested. Magnesium, by its neuroprotective and vasodilatory effects, has the potency to prevent as well as to limit hearing loss, particularly after noise exposure or sudden sensorineural hearing loss. Magnesium therapy with recommended dosage appears to be safe with few contraindications (severe renal failure). In contrast to other therapeutic agents (like corticosteroids), it easily crosses the perilymph blood barrier and reaches the organ of Corti. The majority of studies have shown that magnesium is partly effective. Using magnesium in combination with other agents could improve the recovery after hearing loss.

References

Abaamrane L, Raffin F, Gal M, Avan P, Sendowski I (2009) Long-term administration of magnesium after acoustic trauma caused by gunshot noise in guinea pigs. *Hear Res* 247:137-45.

Afanas'ev I, Suslova T, Cheremisina Z, Abramova N, Korkina L (1995) Study of antioxidant properties of metal aspartates. *Analyst* 120:859-62.

Attias J, Bresloff I, Haupt H, Scheibe F, Ising H (2003) Preventing noise induced otoacoustic emission loss by increasing magnesium (Mg2+) intake in guinea pigs. *J Basic Clin Physiol Pharmacol* 14:119-36.

Attias J, Sapir S, Bresloff I, Reshef-Haran I, Ising H (2004) Reduction in noise-induced temporary threshold shift in humans following oral magnesium intake. *Clin Otolaryngol* 29: 635-41.

Attias J, Weisz G, Almog S, Shahar A, Wiener M, Joachims Z, Netzer A, Ising H (1994) Oral magnesium intake reduces permanent hearing loss induced by noise exposure. *Am J Otol* 15:26-32.

Bede O, Ngy D, Suranyi A, Horvath I, Szlavik M, Gyurkovits K (2008) Effects of magnesium supplementation on the glutathione redox system in atopic asthmatic children. *Inflamm Res* 57:279-86.

Cevette MJ, Drew D, Webb TM, Marion MS (2000) Cisplatin ototoxicity, incresed DPOAE amplitudes, and magnesium deficiency. Distorsion product otoacoustic emissions. *J Am Acad Audiol* 11:323-29.

Chau J, Lin J, Atashband S, Irvine R, Westerberg B (2010) Systematic review of the evidence fort he etiology of adult sudden sensorineural hearing loss. *Laryngoscope* 120:1011-21.

Clerici W, Yang L (1996) Direct effects of intraperilymphatic reactive oxygen species generation on cochlear function. *Hear Res* 101:14-22.

Coffin AB, Reinhart KE, Owens KN, Raible DW, Rubel EW (2009) Extracellular divalent cations modulate aminoglycoside-induced hair cell death in the zebrafish lateral line. *Hear Res* 253:42-51.

Conlin E, Parnes L (2007) Treatment of sudden sensorineural hearing loss: A systematic review. *Arch Otolaryngol Head Neck Surg* 133:573-81.

De Freitas MR, Figueiredo AA, Brito GA, Leitao RF, Carvalho JV, Gomes RM, Ribeiro A (2009) The role of apoptosis in cisplatin-induced ototoxicity in rats. *Braz J Otolaryngol* 75:745-52.

Dehne N, Lautermann J, Petrat F, Rauen U, De Groot H (2001) Cisplatin Ototoxicity: involvement of iron and enhanced formation of superoxide anion radicals. *Toxicol Appl Pharmacol* 174:27-34.

Devrière F, Ising H, Dancer A (1991) Déficits auditifs provoqués par l'exposition à des bruits impulsionnels chez des cobayes carencés ou enrichis en magnésium. *J Acoustique* 4:363-66.

Ehrenberger K, Felix D (1995) Receptor pharmacological models for inner ear therapies with emphasis on glutamate receptors: a survey. *Acta Otolaryngol (Stockh)* 115:236-40.

Galan P, Preziosi P, Durlach V, Valeix P, Ribas L, Bouzid D, Favier A, Hercberg S (1997) Dietary magnesium intake in a French adult population. *Magnes Res* 10:321-28.

Galland L (1991) Magnesium, stress and neuropsychiatric disorders. *Magnes Trace Elem* 10:287-301.

Garcia L, Dejong S, Martin S, Smith R, Buettner G, Kerber R (1998) Magnesium reduces free radicals in an in vivo coronary occlusion-reperfusion model. *J Am Coll Cardiol* 32:536-39.

García-Berrocal JR, Nevado J, Ramírez-Camacho R, Sanz R, González-García JA, Sánchez-Rodríguez C, Cantos B, España P, Verdaguer JM, Trinidad Cabezas A (2007) The anticancer drug cisplatin induces an intrinsic apoptotic pathway inside the inner ear. *Br J Pharmacol* 152:1012-20.

Gordin A, Goldenberg D, Golz A, Netzer A, Joachims H (2002) Magnesium: a new therapy for idiopathic sudden sensorineural hearing loss. *Otol Neurotol* 23:447-51.

Günther T, Ising H, Joachims Z (1989) Biochemical mechanisms affecting susceptibility to noise-induced hearing loss. *Am J Otol* 10:36-41.

Haupt H, Scheibe F (2002) Preventive magnesium supplement protects the inner ear against noise-induced impairment of blood flow and oxygenation in the guinea pig. *Magnes Res* 15:17-25.

Haupt H, Scheibe F, Mazurek B (2003) Therapeutic efficacy of magnesium in acoustic trauma in the guinea pig. *Otorhinolaryngol Relat Spec* 65:134-39.

Henderson D, Bielefeld EC, Harris KC, Hu BH (2006) The role of oxidative stress in noise-induced hearing loss. *Ear and Hearing* 27:1-19.

Hu BH, Henderson D, Nicotera T (2006) Extremely rapid induction of outer hair cell apoptosis in the chinchilla cochlea following exposure to impulse noise. *Hear Res* 211:16-25.

Hu BH, Henderson D, Nicotera TM (2002) Involvement of apoptosis in progression of cochlear lesion following exposure to intense noise. *Hear Res* 166:62-71.

Ising H, Handrock M, Gunther T, Fischer R, Dombrowski M (1982) Increased noise trauma in guinea pigs through magnesium deficiency. *Arch Otorhinolaryngol* 236:139-46.

Joachims Z, Babisch W, Ising H, Guenther T, Handrock M (1983) Dependence of noise-induced hearing loss upon perilymph magnesium concentration. *J Acoust Soc Am* 74:104-8.

Joachims Z, Ising H, Gunther T (1987) Noise-induced hearing loss in humans as a function of serum Mg concentration. *Magnes Bull* 9:130-1.

Konig O, Winter E, Fuchs J, Haupt H, Mazurek B, Weber N, Gross J (2003) Protective effect of magnesium and MK 801 on hypoxia-induced hair cell loss in new-born rat cochlea. *Magnes Res* 16:98-105.

Kopke RD, Liu W, Gabaizadeh R, Jacono A, Feghali J, Spray D (1997) Use of organotypic cultures of Corti's organ to study the protective effects of antioxidant molecules on cisplatin-induced damage of auditory hair cells. *Am J Otolaryngol* 18:559-71.

Le Prell CG, Hughes LF, Miller JM. (2007b) Free radical scavengers vitamins A, C, and E plus magnesium reduce noise trauma. *Free Radic Biol Med* 42(9):1454-63.

Le Prell CG, Yamashita D, Minami SB, Yamasoba T, Miller JM (2007a) Mechanisms of noise-induced hearing loss indicate multiple methods of prevention. *Hear Res* 226:22-43.

Mayer ML, Westbrook GL, Guthrie P (1984) Voltage dependent block by magnesium of NMDA response in spinal cord neurons. *Nature* 309:261-263.

McKeage MJ (1995) Comparative adverse effects of platinium drugs. Drug Safety 13:228-244.

Miller JM, Brown JN, Schacht J (2003) 8-iso-prostagladin F(2alpha), a product noise of exposure, reduces inner ear blood flow. *Audiol Neurootol* 8:207-21.

Mocci F, Canalis P, Tomasi PA, Casu F, Pettinato S (2001) The effect of noise on serum and urinary magnesium and catecholamines in humans. *Occup Med* 51:56-61.

Nageris B, Ulanovski D, Attias J (2004) Magnesium treatment for sudden hearing loss. *Ann Otol Laryngol* 113:672-5.

Pujol R, Puel JL, Gervais d'Aldin C, Eybalin M (1990) Physiopathology of the glutamatergic synapses in the cochlea. *Acta Oto-Laryngol* 113:330-4.

Quirk WS, Seidman MD (1995) Cochlear vascular changes in response to loud noise. *Am J Otol* 16(3):322-5.

Ravishankar S, Ashraf Q, Fritz K, Mishra O, Delivoria-Papadopoulos M (2001) Expression of Bax and Bcl-2 proteins during hypoxia in cerebral cortical neuronal nuclei of newborn piglets: effect of administration of magnesium sulphate. *Brain Res* 901:23-9.

Rybak LP, Ravi R, Somani SM (1995) Mechanism of protection by diethyldithiocarbamate against cisplatin ototoxicity: antioxidant system. *Fundam Appl Toxicol* 26(2):293-300.

Rybak LP, Withworth CA (2005) Ototoxicity: therapeutic opportunities. *Drug Discovery Today* 10:1313-21.

Sahin AA, Oysu CC, Yilmaz HB, Topak M, Kulekci M, Okar I (2006) Effect of oral magnesium supplementation on cisplatin ototoxicity. *J of Otolaryngol* 35(2):112-6.

Scheibe F, Haupt H, Ising H (1999) Total magnesium concentrations of perilymph, cerebrospinal fluid and blood in guinea pigs fed different magnesium-containing diets. *Eur Arch Otorhinolaryngol* 256:215-9.

Scheibe F, Haupt H, Ising H (2000b) Preventive effect of magnesium supplement on noise-induced hearing loss in the guinea pig. *Eur Arch Otorhinolaryngol* 257:10-6.

Scheibe F, Haupt H, Vlastos GA (2000a) Preventive magnesium supplement reduces ischemia-induced hearing loss and blood viscosity in the guinea pig. *Eur Arch Otorhinolaryngol* 257:355-61.

Scheibe F, Haupt H, Ising H, Cherny L (2002) Therapeutic effect of parenteral magnesium on noise-induced hearing loss in guinea pig. *Magnes Res* 15:27-36.

Scheibe F, Haupt H, Mazurek B, Konig O (2001) Therapeutic effect of magnesium on noise-induced hearing loss. *Noise & Health* 3:79-84.

Sendowski I, Raffin F, Braillon-Cros A (2006) Therapeutic efficacy of Magnesium after acoustic trauma caused by gunshot noise in guinea pigs. *Acta Oto-Laryngol* 126:122-9.

Sharikabad M, Ostbye K, Lyberg T, Brors O (2001) Effect of extracellular Mg2+ on ROS and Ca2+ accumulation during reoxygenation of rat cardiomyocytes. *Am J Phyiol Heart Circ Physiol* 280:H344-H353.

Shibata SB, Raphael Y (2010) Future approaches for inner ear protection and repair. *J Commun Disord* 43:295-310.

Spasov AA, Lobzov MS, Sanzharovskaia NK, Kozhevnikova EV, Kuzubova EA (1999) The effect of polikatan on the ototoxic action of kanamycin. *Eksp Klin Farmakol* 62:65-6.

Thorne RP, Nuttal AL (1987) Laser Doppler measurements of cochlear blood flow during loud sound exposure in guinea pigs. *Hear Res* 27:1-10.

Vormann J, Günther T (1993) Influence of magnesium on drug-and noise-induced inner ear damage. Animal studies. *Schriften Ver Wasser Boden Lufthyg* 88:491-502.

Vormann J, Günther T (1991) The role of magnesium and zinc in determining vulnerability of the auditory system to salicylate and gentamicin. *Arch Compl Env Stud* 3:75-82.

Walden BE, Henselman LW, Morris ER (2000) The role of magnesium in the susceptibility of soldiers to noise-induced hearing loss. *J Acoust Soc Am* 108:453-6.

World Health Organization (2004) *Occupational noise: assessing the burden of disease from work-related hearing impairment at national and local levels.* Environmental burden of disease Series Number 9, (Geneva).

Williams CJ, Whitehouse JM (1979) Cis-paltinum: a new anticancer agent. Br Med J 23:1689-91.
Yamashita D, Jiang H, Schacht J, Miller J (2004) Delayed production of free radicals following noise exposure. *Brain Res* 1019:201-9.

Yang W, Henderson D, Hu BH, Nicotera T (2004) Quantitative analysis of apoptotic and necrotic outer hair cells after exposure to different levels of continuous noise. *Hear Res* 196:69-76.

Zenner H (1986) K+-induced motility and depolarization of cochlear hair cells. Direct evidence for a new pathophysiological mechanism in Meniere's disease. *Arch Otorhinolaryngol* 243:108-11.

Zhao F, Manchaiah VK, French D, Price SM (2010) Music exposure and hearing disorders: an overview. *Int J Audiol* 49:54-64.

The role of magnesium in pain

Hyo-Seok Na, Jung-Hee Ryu and Sang-Hwan Do✉

Department of Anesthesiology and Pain Medicine, Seoul National University Bundang Hospital, Seongnam, South Korea.
✉ shdo@snu.ac.kr

Abstract

Magnesium plays an important role in the prevention of central sensitization and in the attenuation of established pain hypersensitivity, and its main mode of action appears to involve its voltage-gated antagonist action at N-methyl-D-aspartate (NMDA) receptor. Given the putative function of the NMDA receptor in pain transduction, magnesium has been investigated in various clinical conditions associated with acute or chronic pain. The parenteral administration of magnesium, via an intravenous, intrathecal, or epidural route, may reduce pain, and anesthetic and analgesic requirements during the intra- and postoperative periods. The beneficial effects of magnesium treatment have also been demonstrated in patients suffering from neuropathic pain, such as, in those with malignancy-related neurologic symptoms, postherpetic neuralgia, diabetic neuropathy, and chemotherapy-induced peripheral neuropathy. In addition, magnesium therapy has been shown to be effective at alleviating dysmenorrhea, headaches, and acute migraine attacks. Magnesium is playing an evolving role in pain management, but a more thorough understanding of the mechanism underlying its antinociceptive action and additional clinical studies are required to clarify its role as an analgesic adjuvant.

Introduction

The research interest in NMDA receptors has led to an examination of the interactions between NMDA receptors and the induction and maintenance of central sensitization after nociceptive stimuli (Woolf and Thompson 1991). Ketamine and magnesium are representative NMDA receptor antagonists, and in particular, magnesium can regulate calcium access into cells by antagonizing the NDMA receptor (Paoletti and Neyton 2007), which has encouraged investigations on the use of magnesium as an analgesic adjuvant. Recent studies have proposed a role for NMDA receptor antagonists in the management of postoperative pain and in other acute and chronic pain conditions. This chapter describes the pharmacologic basis of pain relief by the magnesium ion, and surveys various clinical studies that have examined the antinociceptive effects of magnesium.

Mechanism of magnesium as an analgesic adjuvant

Although magnesium has no direct analgesic effect, it inhibits calcium ions entering cells by blocking NMDA receptors, which causes an antinociceptive effect. Furthermore, this antinociceptive effect is related to its prevention of central sensitization caused by peripheral tissue injury (Woolf and Thompson 1991). Central sensitization is the result of the enhancement of neuronal properties in nociceptive pathways of the central nervous system, and is triggered by repetitive nociceptive afferent inputs, which manifests as a prolonged reduction in the pain threshold. Central sensitization produces pain hypersensitivity, such as wind-up or long-term potentiation of pain, that is, it causes pain even when peripheral stimuli are not intense and continues to cause pain after initiating stimuli have disappeared (Latremoliere and Woolf 2009; Woolf 1983; Woolf and Salter 2000).

Increased intracellular calcium levels seem to play a major role in the initiation of central sensitization (Pockett 1995; Woolf and Chong 1993), and the build-up of intracellular calcium is associated with various receptors on postsynaptic neurons of the spinal dorsal horn, such as, NMDA, α-amino-3-hydroxy-5-methyl-4-isoxazole propionate (AMPA), kainate, and glutamate receptors (Latremoliere and Woolf 2009). Of these receptors, NMDA receptor activation has been demonstrated to be essential for initiating and maintaining central sensitization.

The NMDA receptor is a membrane ion channel expressed in the central nervous system. It is a tetramer composed of four different subunits, that is, two NR1 and two NR2 (Dingledine *et al* 1999). NMDA receptors regulate the cellular inflows of Na^+ and Ca^{2+}, and the outflow of K^+. This voltage-dependent ion channel is blocked non-competitively in the resting state by the magnesium ion and by ketamine (phencyclidine site blockade), MK-801, memantine, and others (Felsby *et al,* 1996; Paoletti and Neyton 2007) (Fig. 1). On the other hand, the NMDA receptor channel is opened by the membrane depolarization induced by the sustained release of glutamate and neuropeptides, which include substance P and calcitonin gene-related peptide (CGRP) (Baranauskas and Nistri 1998; Mayer *et al,* 1984).

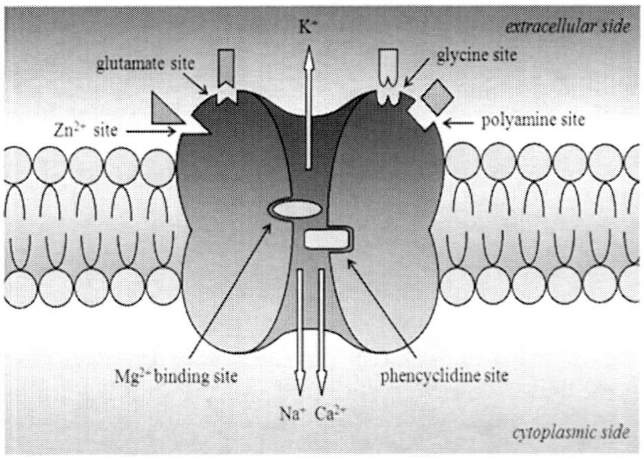

Figure 1. Scheme of the NMDA receptor and its ligand binding sites. The NMDA receptor is composed of four subunits (two NR1 and two NR2). In the extracellular region, there are agonist-binding sites for glutamate and glycine, co-agonists for the efficient opening of the ion channel. The ion channel includes the binding sites for the pore block, one of which is for the Mg^{2+} and the other is for the ketamine, MK-801, memantine, and so on.

Extracellular magnesium blocks the NMDA receptor in a voltage-dependent manner (Mayer *et al,* 1984), and thus, can prevent the establishment of central sensitization and abolish existing hypersensitivity. Other noncompetitive or competitive NMDA receptor antagonists, such as MK801 and D-CPP, also prevent and reverse the hyperexcitability of neurons produced by nociceptive afferent inputs (Ma and Woolf 1995; Woolf and Thompson 1991).

Perioperative pain

Many authors have investigated the adjuvant role of magnesium in the context of intra- and post-operative analgesia. Magnesium has been shown to be effective for treating intra- and post-operative pain and for blunting autonomic, somatic, and endocrine reflexes to noxious stimuli (Kara *et al,* 2002; Koinig *et al,* 1998; Levaux *et al,* 2003). Usually, magnesium is administered as an i.v. bolus of magnesium sulfate 30-50 mg/ kg as a loading dose, and maintained at 6-20 mg/kg/h by continuous infusion until the end of surgery (Koinig *et al,* 1998; Ryu *et al,* 2008; Ryu *et al,* 2009; Wilder-Smith *et al,* 1997) or for 4 hours after the initial bolus (Seyhan *et al,* 2006).

Tramer et al (Tramer *et al,* 1996) conducted the first, prospective, randomized study on the effect of magnesium on analgesic requirements, pain, comfort, and quality of sleep during the immediate postoperative period. They showed that magnesium sulfate reduces analgesic requirements and discomfort, and improves quality of sleep during the postoperative period and that it does not cause any adverse effect at 48 h after surgery. Oguzhan et al (Oguzhan *et al,* 2008) studied the effect of a magnesium sulfate infusion on postoperative requirements for opioids, intraoperative muscle relaxant, inhalational anesthetic consumption, and post-operative pain during and after lumbar disc surgery. Their results suggested that intra-operative magnesium administration significantly reduced intraoperative muscle relaxant and opioid requirements, and also reduced postoperative pain and opioid use.

When used during a variety of surgeries, magnesium was also found to reduce the need for intraoperative anesthetics and muscle relaxants and to reduce the amount of morphine required to treat postoperative pain. Ryu et al (Ryu *et al,* 2009) compared remifentanil and magnesium during middle ear surgery in terms of postoperative pain and other complications. In this study, magnesium or remifentanil combined with sevoflurane provided adequate hypotensive anesthesia, but patients in the magnesium group experienced a more comfortable postoperative course with better analgesia, less shivering, and less postoperative nausea and vomiting (PONV). Furthermore, the amount of sevoflurane required to maintain surgical anesthesia was significantly lower in the magnesium group than in the remifentanil group (Ryu *et al,* 2009).

The use of magnesium as an analgesic adjunct has also found to be beneficial in patients on total intravenous anesthesia (TIVA). Significant reductions in intraoperative propofol, atracurium, and postoperative morphine consumptions were observed in patients undergoing gynecological surgery (Seyhan *et al,* 2006). In another study on gynecologic patients receiving TIVA, post-operative pain scores, cumulative analgesic consumption, and shivering incidents were significantly lower in patients treated with magnesium, to the extent that the authors concluded magnesium sulfate during TIVA improved the quality of postoperative analgesia (Ryu *et al,* 2008). Furthermore, Choi et al (Choi *et al,* 2002) found that intravenous magnesium sulfate reduced propofol infusion requirements during the maintenance of propofol-nitrous oxide anesthesia in patients undergoing total abdominal hysterectomy.

The usefulness of adjunctive magnesium for postoperative pain control has also been examined in the context of regional anesthesia. Recent studies have suggested that magnesium may play a beneficial role in spinal anesthesia. For example, magnesium was found to prevent the induction of central sensitization by peripheral nociceptive stimulation at a spinal site of action by blocking NMDA receptors in a voltage-dependent fashion (Woolf and Thompson 1991). Utilizing the same mechanism, the addition of small doses of magnesium sulfate to local anesthetics for spinal anesthesia enhances the duration of anesthesia and reduced postoperative analgesic requirements and the incidence of side effects of high doses of local anesthetics and opioids. In animal studies, the intrathecal co-administration of magnesium sulfate during spinal anesthesia was found to significantly potentiate morphine analgesia in normal rats and in a surgical model of mechanical allodynia (Kroin *et al,* 2000). In other experimental model, intrathecal magnesium sulfate produced a state of spinal anesthesia and general sedation in rats that lasted for around 1 h, and at 6 h post-injection animals recovered and showed no evidence of neurotoxicity (Bahar *et al,* 1996). Clinical studies have also shown that intrathecal magnesium sulfate added to fentanyl prolongs analgesia without increasing side effects during labor analgesia (Buvanendran *et al,* 2002; Ozalevli *et al,* 2005). Furthermore, the i.v. infusion of magnesium sulfate during spinal anesthesia was found to improve postoperative analgesia and reduce the cumulative consumption of analgesics after total hip replacement arthroplasty (Hwang *et al,* 2010). Postoperative adjunctive i.v. magnesium infusion was also found to increase time to analgesic need and to reduce total analgesia consumption after spinal anesthesia (Apan *et al,* 2004).

Comparatively little is known of the effect of epidural magnesium sulfate, whereas intrathecal magnesium sulfate has been investigated on many occasions. Caudal epidural anesthesia with lidocaine plus magnesium sulfate was found to produce analgesia of longer duration than lidocaine plus distilled water in cattle (Dehghani and Bigham 2009). Arcioni et al (2007) compared intrathecal, epidural, combined intrathecal and epidural magnesium sulfate and spinal anesthesia alone (controls) in patients undergoing orthopedic surgery to investigate whether intrathecal and/or epidural magnesium sulfate could reduce postoperative analgesic requirements. The results obtained suggested that combined intrathecal and epidural magnesium sulfate significantly reduced postoperative analgesic requirements (Arcioni *et al,* 2007).

However, not all investigations have reported postoperative analgesic effects for magnesium sulfate. For example, perioperative i.v. magnesium infusion was not found to reduce postoperative pain or analgesic consumption in patients undergoing abdominal hysterectomy (Ko *et al,* 2001) or cesarean delivery (Paech *et al,* 2006). Furthermore, in a recent report issued by Tramer and Glynn (2007) pretreatment with magnesium sulfate was found to have no effect on postoperative pain or analgesic requirements over the first three postoperative days in patients undergoing ambulatory ilioinguinal hernia repair or varicose vein surgery. However, in this study, a single dose (4 g) of intravenous magnesium sulfate was used instead of a loading dose plus continuous infusion.

Although some debate exists concerning the role of magnesium sulfate as an analgesic adjuvant, the consensus is that magnesium sulfate acts to support a neuromuscular blockade. Magnesium acts as a calcium channel blocker at presynaptic nerve terminals and reduces acetylcholine release at the motor endplate (Fisher 1999). This diminishes muscle fiber excitability and reduces end plate potential amplitudes, which leads to the potentiation of a neuromuscular blockade by nondepolarizing neuromuscular blockers (Fisher 1999). Some authors have focused on the direct effect of magnesium on neuromuscular blockade (Fuchs-Buder *et al,* 1995; Fuchs-Buder and Tassonyi 1996; Kussman *et al,* 1997; Ross and Baker 1996; Telci *et al,* 2002), whereas others concluded that a perioperative adjuvant magnesium infusion enhances neuromuscular blockade (Lee and Kwon 2009; Oguzhan *et al,* 2008; Ryu *et al,* 2008; Ryu *et al,* 2009; Seyhan *et al,* 2006).

Controlled hypotension is sometimes required during surgery to maintain a bloodless operative field, and investigations on perioperative magnesium infusion for the control of hypotension during middle ear surgery decreased the incidences of postoperative nausea and vomiting (PONV) (Ryu *et al,* 2008; Ryu *et al,* 2009), which could have been due to lower sevoflurane consumption (Apfel *et al,* 2002; Ryu *et al,* 2009) rather than any antiemetic effect of the magnesium. Nevertheless, since PONV is one of the most common and distressing complications after surgery, this effect is interesting, because it could be used to benefit, for example patients undergoing ambulatory surgery. Perioperative i.v. magnesium infusion has another advantageous effect, in that it decreases the incidence of shivering by up to 70-90% (Ryu *et al,* 2008; Ryu *et al,* 2009; Tramer and Glynn 2007). Shivering is one of the leading causes of postoperative discomfort (Alfonsi 2001), and increases oxygen consumption (Alfonsi 2001). Thus, the prevention of shivering is one of the most obvious benefits of magnesium sulfate administration in surgical patients.

When mixed with local anesthetic, magnesium may also show beneficial effects in intravenous regional anesthesia. In one study, magnesium was added to lidocaine for intravenous regional anesthesia, and was found to improve quality of anesthesia and analgesia, specifically, sensory and motor block onset times were shorter and postoperative analgesia was better with magnesium (Turan *et al,* 2005). However, in this previous study, recovery after intravenous regional anesthesia was prolonged in the magnesium group (Turan *et al,* 2005). In contrast, i.v. magnesium infusion during general anesthesia has not been found to delay recovery from anesthesia in most investigations (Lee and Kwon 2009; Ozcan *et al,* 2007; Ryu *et al,* 2008). Another consideration during magnesium administration is that magnesium may cause cardiovascular depression by acting as a calcium channel blocker. The consequent inhibition of catecholamine release lowers plasma epinephrine and norepinephrine concentrations after endotracheal intubation, and therefore reduces hypertensive responses during anesthesia induction (James *et al,* 1989). Accordingly, magnesium should be used with caution in hypovolemic patients and in those with limited cardiac capacity.

Other pain conditions

Numerous clinical studies have found that magnesium has beneficial effects in patients suffering from neuropathic pain, dysmenorrhea, tension headache, acute migraine attack, and others. These effects are considered to be due to blockage of the NMDA receptor, attenuation of central sensitization, and its muscle relaxing effect.

Neuropathic pain

Neuropathic pain is caused by damage to or by the dysfunction of a component of the peripheral or central nervous system (Backonja 2003). Thus, the causes of neuropathic pain are various and include spinal cord injury, multiple sclerosis, diabetic neuropathy, radiation injury, complications of chemotherapy, a malignancy-related neurologic symptom, amongst others. Its common features include burning, a cold sensation, numbness, itching, and a shooting or abnormal sensation called dysesthesia in a continuous or episodic manner. The mechanism responsible for neuropathic pain remains unknown, but peripheral or central sensitization is a prime candidate (Bridges *et al,* 2001; Ossipov *et al,* 2000). Neuropathic pain is extremely difficult to treat, and is only partially relieved in some 40-60% of patients. Favored pharmacologic treatments are antidepressants, anticonvulsants, opioids, and NMDA receptor antagonists (O'Connor and Dworkin 2009). Magnesium has been shown to have beneficial effects on neuropathic pain in some clinical and animal studies. When magnesium sulfate (bolus doses of 500 mg or 1 g) was given intravenously to patients with uncontrolled neuropathic pain due to cancer infiltration, pain intensity and pain relief scores improved (Crosby *et al,* 2000). In another study, magnesium chloride (bolus 0.16 mmol/kg over 10 minutes followed by continuous infusion at 0.16 mmol/kg/h) reduced protracted pain and regions of allodynia in patients suffering from peripheral neuropathic pain (Felsby *et al,* 1996). In addition, in an animal model of neuropathic pain induced hyperalgesia subsided after intraperitoneal magnesium therapy (total 150 or 200 mg/kg for 5 days) (Begon *et al,* 2000).

Postherpetic neuralgia

Postherpetic neuralgia (PHN), a type of neuropathic pain, is characterized by chronic persistent pain after an acute herpes zoster attack (Rowbotham and Petersen 2001). Typically, PHN causes a burning, aching, sharp, and lancinating pain that occurs in a continuous or paroxysmal pattern, and is often accompanied by hyperalgesia and allodynia. Brill et al (Brill *et al,* 2002) showed that magnesium can relieve hyperalgesia and allodynia in PHN. When they administered i.v. magnesium sulfate at 30 mg/kg over 30 min to patients with intractable PHN, pain was either relieved completely or diminished (Brill *et al,* 2002).

Diabetic neuropathy

Diabetes mellitus is the most common etiologic factor of peripheral neuropathy, and diabetic neuropathy is often expressed as numbness, a tingling sensation, and hypersensitivity to pain. These symptoms are limited to the fingers and toes during early disease, and then spread to the proximal extremities to produce a characteristic glove and stocking pattern (Head 2006). Conventional treatments include antidepressants, anticonvulsants, lidocaine patches, opioid or non-opioids analgesics, and various alternative treatments (Head 2006). Recently, dietary magnesium supplementation has been at the focus of attention, and oral doses of magnesium sulfate have been found to be effective at reducing thermal pain thresholds in rats. However, appropriate treatment dosages and durations have not been established (Hasanein *et al,* 2006). De Leeuw et al also demonstrated that long-term magnesium supplementation (300 mg daily for 5 years) can favorably influence the progression of diabetic polyneuropathy (De Leeuw *et al,* 2004).

Chemotherapy-induced peripheral neuropathy

CIPN is one of the most common side effects in cancer patients administered many chemo-therapeutic agents, such as cisplatin, 5-fluorouracil, vinca alkaloids, taxoids, and etoposide (Head 2006; Hildebrand 2006; Wolf *et al,* 2008). The symptoms and signs of CIPN may resolve completely or partially, but are sometimes irreversible (Kannarkat *et al,* 2007). Because the pathophysiology of CIPN has not been fully elucidated, various agents have been used to prevent or treat CIPN. Recently, it was reported that a Ca^{2+}/Mg^{2+} infusion before and after oxaliplatin could prevent the development of CIPN (Gamelin *et al,* 2004), but the overall benefit of this is uncertain because of the different treatment efficacies of oxaliplatin and Ca^{2+}/Mg^{2+} infusion combinations (Hochster *et al,* 2007). Furthermore, oxaliplatin metabolites are chelated by calcium and magnesium, and this could explain the observed neuroprotective effect. However, Bujalska *et al.* found that pretreatment with magnesium (30 mg/kg, i.p.) enhanced the analgesic effects of opioids in a vincristine-induced neuropathy model, and re-emphasized the antagonistic effect that magnesium has on NMDA receptors (Bujalska *et al,* 2009).

Dysmenorrhea

Dysmenorrhea refers to a gynecological medical complaint characterized by severe uterine cramps associated with menstruation. Dysmenorrhea may precede or co-occur with menstruation, and causes a dull, nauseating, colicky to sharp or cramping pain. The overproduction of uterine prostaglandins or vasopressin, which stimulates myometrial contraction of the uterus, has been identified as a potential contributory factor (Stromberg *et al,* 1984; Woolf and Chong 1993). When dysmenorrhea is severe enough to restrict daily activities, nonsteroidal anti-inflammatory drugs or oral contraceptive pills are required to reduce uterine contraction, and thus, relieve the pain (Harel 2008). The benefits and safety of magnesium for the treatment of primary dysmenorrhea have also been reviewed (Bettendorf *et al,* 2008; Proctor and Murphy 2001), but more research is required to verify its efficacy. Briefly, oral magnesium on the day before menstruation and during the first and second days of the menstrual cycle for six consecutive cycles, was found to have a therapeutic effect on dysmenorrhea (Fontana-Klaiber and Hogg 1990). However, the optimum treatment regimen has yet to be established and the mechanism responsible has not been determined. Nevertheless, it has been hypothesized, that magnesium inhibits the biosynthesis of PGF2-α, which alleviates myometrial contraction and muscle relaxation by competing with calcium for entry into myometrial cells through voltage-gated channels (Seifert *et al,* 1989; Zahradnik and Breckwoldt 1988).

Tension headache

Tension headaches are characterized by a diffuse, gradual, and pressure-like aching pain bilaterally over the top sides of the cranium (Altura and Altura 2001). Its prevalence has been reported to range from around 10% to nearly 90% (Rasmussen *et al,* 1991; Robbins and Lipton 2010; Russell *et al,* 2006). Although the exact etiology of tension headaches is unknown, several pathophysiologies have been suggested, such as, muscle tension (Jensen and Rasmussen 1996; Langemark and Olesen 1987), increased myofascial pain sensitivity (Pfaffenrath *et al,* 1998), platelet aggregation (Mishima *et al,* 1997), and others. Furthermore, in one study, it was shown that the magnesium ion levels of platelets were lower in patients with a tension headache (Mishima *et al,* 1997), and that magnesium supplementation appeared to ameliorate headaches, including the tension headaches (Mauskop *et al,* 1996; Thomas *et al,* 1994).

Conclusion

The postoperative analgesic adjuvant role of magnesium and its use as an analgesic therapy for the treatment of acute or chronic pain have been suggested for decades. Its antinociceptive effect has been suggested to be due to the blocking of NMDA receptors, and thus, the prevention of central sensitization. More consistent and convincing evidence is required before magnesium can be viewed as an effective adjuvant pain treatment.

References

Alfonsi P (2001) Postanaesthetic shivering: epidemiology, pathophysiology, and approaches to prevention and management. *Drugs* 61:2193-205.

Altura BM, Altura BT (2001) Tension headaches and muscle tension: is there a role for magnesium? *Med Hypotheses* 57:705-13.

Apan A, Buyukkocak U, Ozcan S, Sari E, Basar H (2004) Postoperative magnesium sulphate infusion reduces analgesic requirements in spinal anaesthesia. *Eur J Anaesthesiol* 21:766-9.

Apfel CC, Kranke P, Katz MH, Goepfert C, Papenfuss T, Rauch S, Heineck R, Greim CA, Roewer N (2002) Volatile anaesthetics may be the main cause of early but not delayed postoperative vomiting: a randomized controlled trial of factorial design. *Br J Anaesth* 88:659-68.

Arcioni R, Palmisani S, Tigano S, Santorsola C, Sauli V, Romano S, Mercieri M, Masciangelo R, De Blasi RA, Pinto G (2007) Combined intrathecal and epidural magnesium sulfate supplementation of spinal anesthesia to reduce post-operative analgesic requirements: a prospective, randomized, double-blind, controlled trial in patients undergoing major orthopedic surgery. *Acta Anaesthesiol Scand* 51:482-9.

Backonja MM (2003) Defining neuropathic pain. *Anesth Analg* 97:785-90.

Bahar M, Chanimov M, Grinspun E, Koifman I, Cohen ML (1996) Spinal anaesthesia induced by intrathecal magnesium sulphate. *Anaesthesia* 51:627-33.

Baranauskas G, Nistri A (1998) Sensitization of pain pathways in the spinal cord: cellular mechanisms. *Prog Neurobiol* 54:349-65.

Begon S, Pickering G, Eschalier A, Dubray C (2000) Magnesium and MK-801 have a similar effect in two experimental models of neuropathic pain. *Brain Res* 887:436-9.

Bettendorf B, Shay S, Tu F (2008) Dysmenorrhea: contemporary perspectives. *Obstet Gynecol Surv* 63:597-603.

Bridges D, Thompson SW, Rice AS (2001) Mechanisms of neuropathic pain. *Br J Anaesth* 87:12-26.

Brill S, Sedgwick PM, Hamann W, Di Vadi PP (2002) Efficacy of intravenous magnesium in neuropathic pain. *Br J Anaesth* 89:711-4.

Bujalska M, Makulska-Nowak H, Gumulka SW (2009) Magnesium ions and opioid agonists in vincristine-induced neuropathy. *Pharmacol Rep* 61:1096-104.

Buvanendran A, McCarthy RJ, Kroin JS, Leong W, Perry P, Tuman KJ (2002) Intrathecal magnesium prolongs fentanyl analgesia: a prospective, randomized, controlled trial. *Anesth Analg* 95:661-6, table of contents.

Choi JC, Yoon KB, Um DJ, Kim C, Kim JS, Lee SG (2002) Intravenous magnesium sulfate administration reduces propofol infusion requirements during maintenance of propofol-N2O anesthesia: part I: comparing propofol requirements according to hemodynamic responses: part II: comparing bispectral index in control and magnesium groups. *Anesthesiology* 97:1137-41.

Crosby V, Wilcock A, Corcoran R (2000) The safety and efficacy of a single dose (500 mg or 1 g) of intravenous magnesium sulfate in neuropathic pain poorly responsive to strong opioid analgesics in patients with cancer. *J Pain Symptom Manage* 19:35-9.

De Leeuw I, Engelen W, De Block C, Van Gaal L (2004) Long term magnesium supplementation influences favourably the natural evolution of neuropathy in Mg-depleted type 1 diabetic patients (T1dm). *Magnes Res* 17:109-14.

Dehghani SN, Bigham AS (2009) Comparison of caudal epidural anesthesia by use of lidocaine versus a lidocaine-magnesium sulfate combination in cattle. *Am J Vet Res* 70:194-7.

Dingledine R, Borges K, Bowie D, Traynelis SF (1999) The glutamate receptor ion channels. *Pharmacol Rev* 51:7-61.

Felsby S, Nielsen J, Arendt-Nielsen L, Jensen TS (1996) NMDA receptor blockade in chronic neuropathic pain: a comparison of ketamine and magnesium chloride. *Pain* 64:283-91.

Fisher DM (1999) Clinical pharmacology of neuromuscular blocking agents. *Am J Health Syst Pharm* 56:S4-9.

Fontana-Klaiber H, Hogg B (1990) Therapeutic effects of magnesium in dysmenorrhea. *Schweiz Rundsch Med Prax* 79:491-4.

Fuchs-Buder T, Wilder-Smith OH, Borgeat A, Tassonyi E (1995) Interaction of magnesium sulphate with vecuronium-induced neuromuscular block. *Br J Anaesth* 74:405-9.

Fuchs-Buder T, Tassonyi E (1996) Magnesium sulphate enhances residual neuromuscular block induced by vecuronium. *Br J Anaesth* 76:565-6.

Gamelin L, Boisdron-Celle M, Delva R, Guerin-Meyer V, Ifrah N, Morel A, Gamelin E (2004) Prevention of oxaliplatin-related neurotoxicity by calcium and magnesium infusions: a retrospective study of 161 patients receiving oxaliplatin combined with 5-Fluorouracil and leucovorin for advanced colorectal cancer. *Clin Cancer Res* 10:4055-61.

Harel Z (2008) Dysmenorrhea in adolescents and young adults: from pathophysiology to pharmacological treatments and management strategies. *Expert Opin Pharmacother* 9:2661-72.

Hasanein P, Parviz M, Keshavarz M, Javanmardi K, Mansoori M, Soltani N (2006) Oral magnesium administration prevents thermal hyperalgesia induced by diabetes in rats. *Diabetes Res Clin Pract* 73:17-22.

Head KA (2006) Peripheral neuropathy: pathogenic mechanisms and alternative therapies. *Altern Med Rev* 11:294-329.

Hildebrand J (2006) Neurological complications of cancer chemotherapy. *Curr Opin Oncol* 18:321-4.

Hochster HS, Grothey A, Childs BH (2007) Use of calcium and magnesium salts to reduce oxaliplatin-related neurotoxicity. *J Clin Oncol* 25:4028-9.

Hwang JY, Na HS, Jeon YT, Ro YJ, Kim CS, Do SH (2010) I.V. infusion of magnesium sulphate during spinal anaesthesia improves postoperative analgesia. *Br J Anaesth* 104:89-93.

James MF, Beer RE, Esser JD (1989) Intravenous magnesium sulfate inhibits catecholamine release associated with tracheal intubation. *Anesth Analg* 68:772-6.

Jensen R, Rasmussen BK (1996) Muscular disorders in tension-type headache. *Cephalalgia* 16:97-103.

Kannarkat G, Lasher EE, Schiff D (2007) Neurologic complications of chemotherapy agents. *Curr Opin Neurol* 20:719-25.

Kara H, Sahin N, Ulusan V, Aydogdu T (2002) Magnesium infusion reduces perioperative pain. *Eur J Anaesthesiol* 19:52-6.

Ko SH, Lim HR, Kim DC, Han YJ, Choe H, Song HS (2001) Magnesium sulfate does not reduce postoperative analgesic requirements. *Anesthesiology* 95:640-6.

Koinig H, Wallner T, Marhofer P, Andel H, Horauf K, Mayer N (1998) Magnesium sulfate reduces intra- and postoperative analgesic requirements. *Anesth Analg* 87:206-10.

Kroin JS, McCarthy RJ, Von Roenn N, Schwab B, Tuman KJ, Ivankovich AD (2000) Magnesium sulfate potentiates morphine antinociception at the spinal level. *Anesth Analg* 90:913-7.

Kussman B, Shorten G, Uppington J, Comunale ME (1997) Administration of magnesium sulphate before rocuronium: effects on speed of onset and duration of neuromuscular block. *Br J Anaesth* 79:122-4.

Langemark M, Olesen J (1987) Pericranial tenderness in tension headache. A blind, controlled study. *Cephalalgia* 7:249-55.

Latremoliere A, Woolf CJ (2009) Central sensitization: a generator of pain hypersensitivity by central neural plasticity. *J Pain* 10:895-926.

Lee DH, Kwon IC (2009) Magnesium sulphate has beneficial effects as an adjuvant during general anaesthesia for Caesarean section. *Br J Anaesth* 103:861-6.

Levaux C, Bonhomme V, Dewandre PY, Brichant JF, Hans P (2003) Effect of intra-operative magnesium sulphate on pain relief and patient comfort after major lumbar orthopaedic surgery. *Anaesthesia* 58:131-5.

Ma QP, Woolf CJ (1995) Noxious stimuli induce an N-methyl-D-aspartate receptor-dependent hypersensitivity of the flexion withdrawal reflex to touch: implications for the treatment of mechanical allodynia. *Pain* 61:383-90.

Mauskop A, Altura BT, Cracco RQ, Altura BM (1996) Intravenous magnesium sulfate rapidly alleviates headaches of various types. *Headache* 36:154-60.

Mayer ML, Westbrook GL, Guthrie PB (1984) Voltage-dependent block by Mg2+ of NMDA responses in spinal cord neurones. *Nature* 309:261-3.

Mishima K, Takeshima T, Shimomura T, Okada H, Kitano A, Takahashi K, Nakashima K (1997) Platelet ionized magnesium, cyclic AMP, and cyclic GMP levels in migraine and tension-type headache. *Headache* 37:561-4.

O'Connor AB, Dworkin RH (2009) Treatment of neuropathic pain: an overview of recent guidelines. *Am J Med* 122:S22-32.

Oguzhan N, Gunday I, Turan A (2008) Effect of magnesium sulfate infusion on sevoflurane consumption, hemodynamics, and perioperative opioid consumption in lumbar disc surgery. *J Opioid Manag* 4:105-10.

Ossipov MH, Lai J, Malan TP, Jr., Porreca F (2000) Spinal and supraspinal mechanisms of neuropathic pain. *Ann N Y Acad Sci* 909:12-24.

Ozalevli M, Cetin TO, Unlugenc H, Guler T, Isik G (2005) The effect of adding intrathecal magnesium sulphate to bupivacaine-fentanyl spinal anaesthesia. *Acta Anaesthesiol Scand* 49:1514-9.

Ozcan PE, Tugrul S, Senturk NM, Uludag E, Cakar N, Telci L, Esen F (2007) Role of magnesium sulfate in postoperative pain management for patients undergoing thoracotomy. *J Cardiothorac Vasc Anesth* 21:827-31.

Paech MJ, Magann EF, Doherty DA, Verity LJ, Newnham JP (2006) Does magnesium sulfate reduce the short- and long-term requirements for pain relief after caesarean delivery? A double-blind placebo-controlled trial. *Am J Obstet Gynecol* 194:1596-602; discussion 602-3.

Paoletti P, Neyton J (2007) NMDA receptor subunits: function and pharmacology. *Curr Opin Pharmacol* 7:39-47.

Pfaffenrath V, Brune K, Diener HC, Gerber WD, Gobel H (1998) The treatment of tension type headache. *Headache* 38:725-6.

Pockett S (1995) Spinal cord synaptic plasticity and chronic pain. *Anesth Analg* 80:173-9.

Proctor ML, Murphy PA (2001) Herbal and dietary therapies for primary and secondary dysmenorrhoea. *Cochrane Database Syst Rev*:CD002124.

Rasmussen BK, Jensen R, Schroll M, Olesen J (1991) Epidemiology of headache in a general population--a prevalence study. *J Clin Epidemiol* 44:1147-57.

Robbins MS, Lipton RB (2010) The epidemiology of primary headache disorders. *Semin Neurol* 30:107-19.

Ross RM, Baker T (1996) An effect of magnesium on neuromuscular function in parturients. *J Clin Anesth* 8:202-4.

Rowbotham MC, Petersen KL (2001) Zoster-associated pain and neural dysfunction. *Pain* 93:1-5.

Russell MB, Levi N, Saltyte-Benth J, Fenger K (2006) Tension-type headache in adolescents and adults: a population based study of 33,764 twins. *Eur J Epidemiol* 21:153-60.

Ryu JH, Kang MH, Park KS, Do SH (2008) Effects of magnesium sulphate on intraoperative anaesthetic requirements and postoperative analgesia in gynaecology patients receiving total intravenous anaesthesia. *Br J Anaesth* 100:397-403.

Ryu JH, Sohn IS, Do SH (2009) Controlled hypotension for middle ear surgery: a comparison between remifentanil and magnesium sulphate. *Br J Anaesth* 103:490-5.

Seifert B, Wagler P, Dartsch S, Schmidt U, Nieder J (1989) Magnesium--a new therapeutic alternative in primary dysmenorrhea. *Zentralbl Gynakol* 111:755-60.

Seyhan TO, Tugrul M, Sungur MO, Kayacan S, Telci L, Pembeci K, Akpir K (2006) Effects of three different dose regimens of magnesium on propofol requirements, haemodynamic variables and postoperative pain relief in gynaecological surgery. *Br J Anaesth* 96:247-52.

Stromberg P, Akerlund M, Forsling ML, Granstrom E, Kindahl H (1984) Vasopressin and prostaglandins in premenstrual pain and primary dysmenorrhea. *Acta Obstet Gynecol Scand* 63:533-8.

Telci L, Esen F, Akcora D, Erden T, Canbolat AT, Akpir K (2002) Evaluation of effects of magnesium sulphate in reducing intraoperative anaesthetic requirements. *Br J Anaesth* 89:594-8.

Thomas J, Tomb E, Thomas E, Faure G (1994) Migraine treatment by oral magnesium intake and correction of the irritation of buccofacial and cervical muscles as a side effect of mandibular imbalance. *Magnes Res* 7:123-7.

Tramer MR, Schneider J, Marti RA, Rifat K (1996) Role of magnesium sulfate in postoperative analgesia. *Anesthesiology* 84:340-7.

Tramer MR, Glynn CJ (2007) An evaluation of a single dose of magnesium to supplement analgesia after ambulatory surgery: randomized controlled trial. *Anesth Analg* 104:1374-9, table of contents.

Turan A, Memis D, Karamanlioglu B, Guler T, Pamukcu Z (2005) Intravenous regional anesthesia using lidocaine and magnesium. *Anesth Analg* 100:1189-92.

Wilder-Smith CH, Knopfli R, Wilder-Smith OH (1997) Perioperative magnesium infusion and postoperative pain. *Acta Anaesthesiol Scand* 41:1023-7.

Wolf S, Barton D, Kottschade L, Grothey A, Loprinzi C (2008) Chemotherapy-induced peripheral neuropathy: prevention and treatment strategies. *Eur J Cancer* 44:1507-15.

Woolf CJ (1983) Evidence for a central component of post-injury pain hypersensitivity. *Nature* 306:686-8.

Woolf CJ, Thompson SW (1991) The induction and maintenance of central sensitization is dependent on N-methyl-D-aspartic acid receptor activation; implications for the treatment of post-injury pain hypersensitivity states. *Pain* 44:293-9.

Woolf CJ, Chong MS (1993) Preemptive analgesia--treating postoperative pain by preventing the establishment of central sensitization. *Anesth Analg* 77:362-79.

Woolf CJ, Salter MW (2000) Neuronal plasticity: increasing the gain in pain. *Science* 288:1765-9.

Zahradnik HP, Breckwoldt M (1988) Drug therapy of dysmenorrhea. *Gynakologe* 21:58-62.

The role of magnesium in CNS injury

Naomi L. Cook, Frances Corrigan and Corinna van den Heuvel ✉

Discipline of Anatomy and Pathology & Adelaide Centre for Neuroscience Research, School of Medical Sciences, The University of Adelaide, Adelaide, South Australia 5005, Australia.
✉ corinna.vandenheuvel@adelaide.edu.au

Abstract

Traumatic injury to the central nervous system (CNS) is a leading cause of morbidity and mortality, and represents a significant public health issue. Despite intensive research, no effective neuroprotective therapy exists, and survivors of CNS injury, including traumatic brain injury (TBI) and spinal cord injury (SCI), can be left with severe disabilities that require long-term rehabilitation. Much of the damage that occurs after TBI and SCI develops over time with the primary injury initiating a secondary injury cascade made up of deleterious biochemical and pathophysiological reactions. This delayed development of secondary injury provides a vital opportunity for therapeutic intervention and considerable effort is currently being directed toward identifying these injury factors and developing interventions that may potentially prevent their actions. Magnesium (Mg^{2+}) decline has been identified as playing a key role in the secondary injury process, in part because of its central role in the regulation of a large number of known injury factors and that its decline is associated with the development of motor and cognitive deficits. Mg^{2+} administration has been extensively investigated both preclinically in TBI and SCI and clinically as a neuroprotectant in TBI with varied success. This chapter focuses on the role of Mg^{2+} in TBI and SCI pathophysiology, with particular emphasis on Mg^{2+} as a potential therapeutic agent.

Introduction

A decline in Mg^{2+} following TBI was first identified using *in vivo* magnetic resonance spectroscopy (Vink *et al*, 1988) and further declines have subsequently been reported by numerous laboratories following a variety of insults to the CNS including TBI, SCI, stroke and drug intoxication. It has been observed that a traumatic insult to the CNS results in a decrease in the intracellular free Mg^{2+} concentration of between 40 and 60%, while the total tissue Mg^{2+} falls by between 10-15%. This Mg^{2+} decline is confined to the site of injury and the decrease is associated with the development of neurological dysfunction. Treatment with Mg^{2+} has been shown to attenuate the neurological changes experimentally following TBI and SCI, however, clinical studies of Mg^{2+} as a neuroprotective agent show conflicting results (Dhandapani *et al*, 2008; Temkin *et al*, 2007).

Traumatic CNS injury

Injuries to the CNS are a significant problem, with TBI the leading cause of death and disability in people under the age of 40 years (Fleminger and Ponsford, 2005). In the USA, approximately 1.5 million people are affected by TBI annually. Of these, 230,000 people are hospitalized and survive, 80,000 people develop a TBI-related disability, and 50,000 people die (Pitkänen *et al*, 2005). In addition, SCI affects around 200,000 people in the USA with 10,000 new cases each year (Anonymous, 2008; Buechner *et al*, 2000) with the cost of caring for patients with SCI in the US estimated to be $9.73 billion (Weaver *et al*, 2000). Since no effective treatment is available, survivors of TBI and SCI may be left with debilitating neurological deficits that confer social, financial and emotional burdens and adversely affect their quality of life.

The neurological damage resulting from traumatic injuries to the CNS is due to both direct, immediate biomechanical processes (the primary injury) and indirect, delayed (secondary) injury mechanisms (Morales *et al*, 2005) and the neuronal death in TBI and SCI is likely to involve both necrotic and apoptotic pathways (Liou *et al*, 2003). The primary event is irreversible and in TBI comprises contusions, lacerations, tissue shearing and stretching of nerve fibers (Gentile and

McIntosh, 1993), whereas the most common primary injuries to the spinal cord result from fracture/dislocation or crush injury to the vertebral column. In contrast, secondary injury consists of a series of complex biochemical changes that are triggered by the primary event and evolve over the minutes to days and even months after the insult (Vink and Van Den Heuvel, 2010). A number of secondary injury factors have been identified, including disruption to the blood-brain barrier (BBB), edema, ischemia, hypertension, inflammation, excito-toxicity, oxidative stress and Mg^{2+} decline, all of which can be deleterious to neuronal cells (Barone and Kilgore, 2006; Cormio *et al,* 1997; Gentile and McIntosh 1993; Golding, 2002).

Secondary injury factors

As stated above, secondary injury involves series of complex biochemical changes that are triggered by the primary event and may continue for days to weeks after the insult (Roth and Farls 2000). To provide an example of the secondary injury cascade, shearing of nerve fibers at the time of insult results in massive ion fluxes across cell membranes, loss of membrane potential and rapid release of neurotransmitters from damaged neurons. This may result in excitotoxicity, which can evoke an inflammatory response, thereby stimulating further processes (such as the changes described above), eventually leading to cell death (Vink and Van Den Heuvel, 2004). Secondary injury is associated with significant morbidity and mortality following traumatic CNS injury (Gentile and McIntosh, 1993), but given that it manifests over time, this provides an opportunity to administer a pharmacological agent to impede or prevent further injury and thus improve outcome. Several injury processes relevant to traumatic CNS injury will now be discussed including diffuse axonal injury (DAI), edema, oxidative stress, mitochondrial dysfunction, inflammation and lastly significant discussion will be given to magnesium decline.

Diffuse Axonal Injury

DAI is a principal cause of coma following TBI, and significantly contributes to TBI-related morbidity and mortality (Li and Feng, 2009). Classically, DAI was categorized as a primary injury, whereby axons are torn and rupture at the time of insult (Adams *et al,* 1982). However, more recent evidence suggests that DAI is triggered at the time of injury by inertial forces and may evolve over a period of hours to days, progressing from focal disruptions to axons to impaired axonal transport, axolemmal swelling and, ultimately, axonal disconnection (Büki and Povlishock, 2006; Mazzeo *et al,* 2009; Stone *et al,* 2004). DAI is generally diagnosed at post-mortem by immunostaining for β-amyloid precursor protein (APP) (Gentleman *et al,* 1993), although recent imaging advances may allow its detection at an earlier stage (Li and Feng, 2009).

Edema

Cerebral edema is defined as an abnormal accumulation of fluid within the brain parenchyma, resulting in a volumetric enlarge-ment (swelling) of brain tissue (Heo *et al,* 2005). Swollen tissues may exert harmful effects by increasing pressure in surrounding tissues, leading to ischemia and additional edema (Simard *et al,* 2007). Swelling has particularly deleterious consequences in the brain, due to the fact that the volume of the intracranial cavity is fixed (Ayata and Ropper, 2002). The resulting rise in intracranial pressure (ICP) with cerebral edema formation is a potentially lethal process (Kimelberg, 1995). Indeed, cerebral edema plays an important role in the outcome of TBI victims: uncontrolled brain swelling with the accompanying rise in ICP is the leading cause of death in TBI patients (Marmarou *et al,* 2000).

Cerebral edema is classified as cytotoxic and vasogenic, depending upon whether or not BBB permeability is increased (Verlooy and Van Reempts, 2005). The BBB is composed of a monolayer of endothelial cells forming tight junctions that prevent the direct interaction of the peripheral circulation with the CNS (Palmer, 2010). Cytotoxic edema refers to the movement of water, Na^+ and Cl^- from the extracellular to the intracellular space, which results in cell swelling and predisposes cells to oncotic cell death. However, cytotoxic edema does not involve increases in BBB permeability, nor does it contribute to the actual net increase in brain water (Ayata and Ropper, 2002; Simard *et al,* 2007). Conversely, vasogenic edema is associated with the degradation of tight junctions between endothelial cells of the BBB (Heo *et al,* 2005). Consequently, the BBB becomes more permeable to macromolecules and permits the movement of fluid from capillaries to the extravascular compartment (Heo *et al,* 2005; Simard *et al,* 2007); hence vasogenic edema causes a net increase in brain water content (Ayata and Ropper 2002). In TBI, the increase in BBB permeability may occur by mechanical injury, autodestructive mediators or both (Unterberg *et al,* 2004). However, despite the potentially lethal consequences of edema in TBI, there is currently no effective therapy to prevent its formation or progression. Treatments such as mannitol, corticosteroids, barbiturates, induction of hypothermia, drainage of the cerebrospinal fluid (CSF) and surgical decompression (Ayata and Ropper, 2002; Clausen and Bullock, 2001) have had limited success in managing rises in ICP (Vink and Van Den Heuvel, 2004).

Neurogenic inflammation is a local inflammatory reaction of neurons in response to infection, toxins or trauma, which is characterized by vasodilation, plasma extravasation and edema (Black, 2002; Ro *et al,* 2005; Turner *et al,* 2006). Studies from our laboratory (Nimmo *et al,* 2004; Vink *et al,* 2003) have shown that neurogenic inflammation may be involved in the formation of vasogenic edema and the functional deficits following diffuse TBI in rats, and that the neuropeptide, substance P (SP), is a potent initiator of neurogenic inflammation. Further research from our laboratory (Donkin *et al,* 2009) has demonstrated that a SP receptor antagonist inhibits BBB breakdown and edema formation, and significantly improves long-term functional outcome and motor deficits resulting from TBI. These important results may provide a novel pharmacological treatment for TBI.

Oxidative Stress

Reactive oxygen species (ROS) comprise a range of chemical entities, including hydroxyl radicals, peroxynitrite, superoxide anions, hydrogen peroxide, nitric oxide and singlet oxygen (Chong *et al,* 2005; Ellis, 2007). ROS are highly reactive molecules, possessing one or more unpaired electrons in their outer orbits (Halliwell, 1992). While some ROS are normal by-products of cellular metabolism (Yu, 1994), their overproduction can lead to cell injury and tissue damage via reactions with proteins, lipids and nucleic acids, and cellular activation by ROS induces signaling cascades that lead to rises in intracellular Ca^{2+} concentrations (Alexandrova and Bochev, 2005; Massullo *et al,* 2006). When ROS are generated in excess of endogenous antioxidant mechanisms, the result is oxidative stress (Finkel and Holbrook, 2000).

Brain tissue is highly susceptible to damage by oxidative stress for a number of reasons. The brain has a high rate of oxygen metabolism, which increases the likelihood of excess ROS production (Chong *et al,* 2005). Furthermore, it contains high levels of polyunsaturated fatty acids, which are particularly vulnerable to damage by free radicals (Halliwell, 1992). Critically, the brain has relatively low antioxidant and repair capacities compared with other organs (Vink and Nimmo, 2009). All of these factors render brain tissue extremely sensitive to increases in ROS, and oxidative stress is indeed relevant to TBI. Studies demonstrate that the production of ROS is enhanced following TBI, and this is accompanied by an impairment of antioxidant defenses (Ansari *et al,* 2008; Lima *et al,* 2008). TBI-induced oxidative stress can lead to cytoskeletal damage, mitochondrial dysfunction and altered signal transduction, which can be deleterious to neuronal and vascular cells (Ansari *et al,* 2008; Chong *et al,* 2005).

Mitochondrial Dysfunction

Mitochondria are organelles that are present in all cells and play a critical role in regulating cellular energy production via the electron transport chain (Bayir and Kagan, 2008; Mazzeo *et al,* 2009). Consequently, it would be expected that disruption to mitochondrial function would have serious adverse consequences to cells, particularly those with a high-energy demand, such as neurons. Indeed, mitochondrial dysfunction is an important factor in TBI pathophysiology that can lead to energy depletion, free radical release and apoptosis, or programmed cell death (Vink and Nimmo, 2009). In experimental TBI, alterations in mitochondrial function have been reported within hours of injury and may persist for days (Robertson, 2004). Furthermore, in clinical TBI studies, patients with profound mitochondrial dysfunction have a poor outcome (Signoretti *et al,* 2008).

As discussed, traumatic CNS injury leads to conditions of oxidative stress. Oxidative stress directly contributes to mitochondrial dysfunction, promoting the release of cytochrome c from the inner membrane of the mitochondrion, which triggers an apoptotic cascade involving caspases and other pro-apoptotic proteins (Bayir and Kagan, 2008; Chong *et al,* 2005). Mitochondria also constitute an important intracellular source of ROS, which are produced during the synthesis of ATP (Kowaltowski *et al,* 2009). During states of electron transport chain dysregulation, as may occur following TBI, there is an increase in the production of ROS (Bayir and Kagan, 2008). Mitochondria have also been implicated in glutamate-mediated excitotoxicity, by participating in the release of glutamate, Ca^{2+} sequestration and the generation of ROS (Nicholls and Budd, 2000).

Inflammation

The inflammatory response represents another important secondary injury process of traumatic CNS injury. Injury-induced inflammation may be beneficial in the short term, by removing cellular debris or promoting regeneration, however, in excess, inflammatory responses can have severe deleterious effects that lead to neurodegeneration (Maas *et al,* 2008; Vink *et al,* 2009). Inflammation can occur within the neural tissue, where activated microglia and astrocytes release cytokines, chemokines and ROS. There is also evidence that the complement system is activated following TBI (Stahel *et al,* 1998). Furthermore, disruption to the BBB in response to brain insult is associated with the transmigration of leukocytes to the area of damage, which themselves produce cytokines (Jain 2008). Indeed, levels of the pro-inflammatory cytokines, tumor necrosis factor (TNF)-α and interleukin (IL)-1β are elevated following experimental TBI (Fan *et al,* 1995; Fan *et al,* 1996), and may act synergistically to exacerbate the neuroinflammatory response and excitotoxicity (Morganti-Kossmann *et al,* 2007). On the other hand, anti-inflammatory cytokines, such as IL-10 and transforming growth factor (TGF)-β, may exert neuroprotective effects in TBI (Knoblach and Faden, 1998) by suppressing the actions of TNF-α and IL-1β (Benveniste *et al,* 1995). Finally, IL-6 may act either to promote or inhibit inflammation in different situations, exemplifying the complexity of the neuro-inflammatory pathways associated with TBI (Morganti-Kossmann *et al,* 2007).

Mg^{2+} depletion following traumatic CNS injury

Mg^{2+} depletion has been observed both experimentally within the brain of animals and clinically in the blood of humans following traumatic CNS injuries. This depletion is an important secondary injury factor that has been associated with poor neurological outcome in both humans and experimental animals. A significant decline in serum ionized Mg^{2+} levels was measured in TBI patients, with the magnitude of Mg^{2+} decline linked to the severity of TBI (Kahraman *et al,* 2003). Similarly Mg^{2+} levels decline following experimental SCI in the acute phase, with levels significantly lower for up to 3 days following injury, before gradually returning to sham levels (Chanimov *et al,* 2006; Lemke *et al,* 1987). Like TBI, the degree of reduction is also dependent on injury severity (Lemke and Faden, 1990) suggesting a drop in Mg^{2+} levels plays a central role in the secondary injury cascade. Indeed, following TBI in rats the decrease in brain intracellular free Mg^{2+} concentration observed following injury was correlated with the development of neurological deficits (Heath and Vink, 1996; Vink *et al,* 1988). In a study investigating the consequences of Mg^{2+} deficiency prior to TBI in rats, the Mg^{2+}-deficient group was shown to have significantly greater cortical cell loss compared to the vehicle group, as well as cytoskeletal alterations in cortical and hippocampal neurons (Saatman *et al,* 2001).

Mechanisms of Mg^{2+} neuroprotection

Given the significance of Mg^{2+} decline with respect to neurological outcome following CNS injury, Mg^{2+} has been investigated as a potential neuroprotective agent for CNS injury. Mg^{2+} represents an attractive interventional therapy due to its low cost, ease of use, low risk of adverse effects and its ability to penetrate the BBB (Sacco *et al,* 2007). Furthermore, it is able to modulate many processes relevant to both TBI and SCI.

Mg^{2+} is crucial to many diverse biological processes and is an essential co-factor required for the function of numerous enzymes (Ebel and Günther, 1980). Given its vital physiological roles, a decline in Mg^{2+} concentration is likely to have an adverse effect on cellular functioning, the maintenance of membrane potential and the capacity for cells to undergo repair (Vink and Cernak, 2000). Mg^{2+} also blocks N-methyl-D-aspartate receptors (NMDAR), thereby regulating Ca^{2+} influx (Sen and Gulati, 2010), with a decline in Mg^{2+} exacerbating excitotoxicity post-injury. In the absence of injury, Mg^{2+} deficiency impairs antioxidant defenses (Blache *et al,* 2006), with Mg^{2+} inhibiting the production of reactive oxygen species (Blache *et al,* 2006), reducing lipid peroxidation (Regan *et al,* 1998; Suzer *et al,* 1999), and ultimately decreasing oxidative stress in TBI patients (Cernak *et al,* 2000). In addition Mg^{2+} has a positive effect on cerebral energy state, preserving mitochondrial membrane potential with an improvement in oxidative phosphorylation and decrease in lactic acid production when administered post-injury (Feldman *et al,* 1996; Van Den Heuvel and Vink, 2004). The acute inflammatory response is also modulated by Mg^{2+}, with neutrophil invasion reduced following SCI in animals treated with $MgSO_4$ (Gok *et al,* 2007). This correlates with studies that show that Mg^{2+} deficiency evokes an inflammatory response (Malpuech-Brugère *et al,* 2000), including the release of pro-inflammatory cytokines and SP (Mazur *et al,* 2006).

Mg^{2+} and Substance P

Within one week of Mg^{2+} deficiency, plasma SP concentration was elevated (Weglicki and Phillips 1992) and this was associated with the development of neurogenic inflammation (Weglicki *et al,* 1994). This is relevant to TBI, as SP expression increases following experimental TBI (Donkin *et al,* 2009), with administration of SP receptor antagonists increasing levels of free Mg^{2+} in the brain, indicating that the decline in Mg^{2+} could be mediated, in part, by elevations in SP (Vink *et al,* 2004).

SP has a number of neuroinflammatory roles, including stimulating the release of histamine and serotonin (5HT) from mast cells, which can compromise the BBB along with nitric oxide (NO) and bradykinin. It is also a potent initiator of neurogenic inflammation (vasodilation, plasma protein extravasation and edema) (Harrison and Geppetti, 2001) with the resulting disruption to the BBB resulting in the entry of toxins, metal ions and inflammatory cells into the brain (see Figure 1). Furthermore, SP stimulates immune cells to release pro-inflammatory cytokines, including TNF-α and several interleukin family members (IL-1β, 1L-2 and Il-6) resulting in further inflammation (Delgado *et al,* 2003). Additionally, NK-1R activation stimulates second messenger pathways which increase Ca^{2+} entry to neurons (Suh and Hille, 2005; Yang *et al,* 2003). Since SP also activates NMDAR (Wu *et al,* 2004) Ca^{2+} influx through these channels may lead to excitotoxicity and the production of free radicals such as peroxynitrite, which can be highly toxic to cellular macromolecules (Giruouard, 2003). This Ca^{2+} influx is facilitated by low Mg^{2+} levels, as blockade of NMDAR is reduced and members of the transient receptor potential melastatin (TRPM) family may be activated allowing further Ca^{2+} entry (Schmitz *et al,* 2003). The induction of this secondary injury cascade by SP correlates with results which show increased SP is deleterious following TBI, as it is associated with the development of cerebral edema and poorer neurological outcome (Donkin *et al,* 2009). Taken together, SP release and the associated Mg^{2+} decline following TBI can result in neuro-inflammation, BBB disruption, excitotoxicity and oxidative stress, with restoring Mg^{2+} homeostasis a potential target to limit these secondary injury factors and thus cell death.

Mg^{2+} and TRPM channels

TRPM7 is one of the few mammalian Mg^{2+} transporters described to date, playing an important role in regulating Mg^{2+} entry into cells. It is ubiquitously expressed and consists of an ion channel fused to a protein kinase domain (Runnels *et al,* 2001), with the channel permeable to a number of divalent cations including Mg^{2+} (Monteilh-Zoller *et al,* 2003). Of note TRPM7 has been implicated in the anoxic death of neuronal cells (Aarts *et al,* 2003), and activation of TRPM7 during ischemia has been proposed as a key factor contributing to excitotoxicity and other deleterious processes (MacDonald *et al,* 2006). We have recently found changes in TRPM7 channel expression following experimental TBI in rats (Cook *et al,* unpublished), suggesting a role for this protein in traumatic CNS injury.

TRPM7 has been suggested to mediate cell death via a positive feedback loop whereby Ca^{2+} entry into cells as a result of injury causes the production of free radicals, which activate TRPM7, leading to further Ca^{2+} influx and

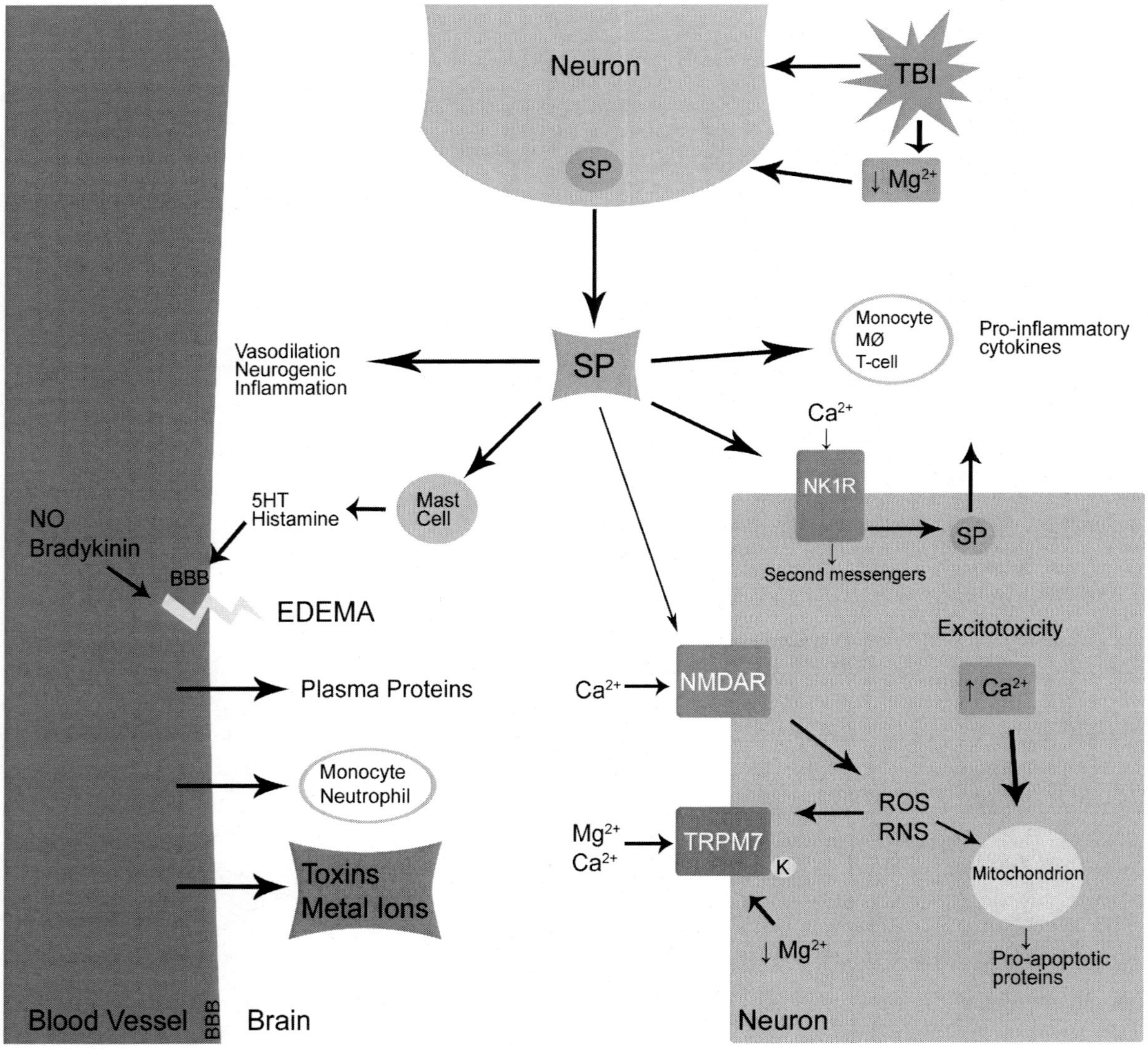

Figure 1. Potential mechanisms of neuronal damage resulting from Mg^{2+} depletion and SP release in TBI.

additional free radical production (Aarts and Tymianski, 2005). Importantly, a decline in intracellular Mg^{2+} concentration, such as that observed following TBI and SCI, can lead to the generation of reactive oxygen and nitrogen species (Altura *et al,* 2003), which could further activate TRPM7, thereby exacerbating inflammation, oxidative stress and cell death pathways (see Figure 1). Given that Mg^{2+} levels remain suppressed for several days following injury (Heath and Vink 1996), this is potentially a critical and persistent pathway leading to cell death after TBI and SCI. However, additional studies are required to determine whether TRPM7 directly mediates cell death in traumatic CNS injury, and if changes in TRPM7 expression following TBI are linked to the observed decline in Mg^{2+} levels.

Mg^{2+} administration in traumatic CNS studies

Experimental TBI Studies

A number of studies have investigated whether this attenuation of secondary injury factors by restoring Mg^{2+} homeostasis after TBI is effective in improving neurological and functional outcome. Substantial evidence from studies of experimental TBI suggests that Mg^{2+} administration may be beneficial following head injury. Mg^{2+} significantly reduced cortical cell loss (Saatman *et al,* 2001) and motor deficits (Bareyre *et al,* 1999) in injured rats compared to vehicle controls. A number of other studies have also demonstrated a neuroprotective effect of Mg^{2+} following experimental TBI (Browne *et al,* 2004; Fromm *et al,* 2004; McIntosh *et al,* 1989; Turner *et al,* 2004). Mg^{2+} treatment following TBI in rats has been shown to reduce apoptosis and the expression of p53-related (apoptosis-inducing) proteins (Lee *et al,* 2004) as well as modulating levels of Bax and Bcl-2, which are also regulators of apoptosis (Ravishankar *et al,* 2001).

Although Mg^{2+} has been shown to improve neurological outcome when administered up to 24 hours after injury (Hoane and Barth 2002), the best results have been achieved when the therapeutic window is restricted to 12 hours (Vink and Cernak 2000). Mg^{2+} decline has been shown to persist for at least 4 days after injury (Heath and Vink 1996), however, the concentration of Mg^{2+} in CNS injury has been shown never to fall below 0.2 mM (Vink *et al,* 1988). Thus, it is likely that the length of time for which free Mg^{2+} concentration is reduced, rather than the magnitude of decline, is the parameter that influences neurological outcome (Vink and Cernak 2000). In addition to the positive effect seen with respect to motor performance, Mg^{2+} also significantly improves cognitive function following TBI (reviewed in (Hoane 2007)).

Experimental SCI Studies

In experimental SCI, administration of Mg^{2+} has been found to have beneficial effects when administered to rats using both the clip compression (Ditor *et al,* 2007; Suzer *et al,* 1999) and weight drop models of SCI (Gok *et al,* 2007; Kaptanoglu *et al,* 2003a; Kaptanoglu *et al,* 2003b; Kwon *et al,* 2009) as well as when administered to rabbits following SCI (Ozdemir *et al,* 2005). The beneficial effect of Mg^{2+} include decreases in membrane damage (Kaptanoglu *et al,* 2003a; Kaptanoglu *et al,* 2003b), normalization of energy balance (Ozdemir *et al,* 2005), protection against axonal damage (Suzer *et al,* 1999), preservation of the BBB (Kaptanoglu *et al,* 2003a; Kaptanoglu *et al,* 2003b) and reduction in apoptosis as seen by a reduction in activated caspase-3 (Solaroglu *et al,* 2005). However, unlike TBI, the clinical window for administration of Mg^{2+} in SCI appears to only extend to 8 hours, with no improvement in outcome seen in animals treated at later time points (Kwon *et al,* 2009; Wiseman *et al,* 2009). In contrast, earlier treatment leads to a decrease in lesion size with an associated significant improvement in motor outcome seen early, at 24 hours following injury (Kaptanoglu *et al,* 2003a; Kaptanoglu *et al,* 2003b; Suzer *et al,* 1999), as well as later, at 4 weeks post-injury (Wiseman *et al,* 2009).

Despite this evidence supporting a potential therapeutic role of Mg^{2+} in SCI, the neuroprotective effects were only demonstrated following extremely high doses of $MgSO_4$ (600 mg/kg) and smaller doses were less effective at providing significant histological or functional benefit (Kaptanoglu *et al,* 2003a; Kaptanoglu *et al,* 2003b; Suzer *et al,* 1999). Such a bolus dose of 600 mg/kg far exceeds the 2-4 gram bolus dose given to patients with emergencies such a pre-eclampsia or cardiac arrest (Gowda and Khan, 2004; Leeman and Fontaine 2008). Given the high doses necessary to see these clinical improvements, further studies investigated whether combining Mg^{2+} with polyethylene glycol (PEG), a hydrophilic polymer used as excipient for many pharmacological agents, would reduce the dosage needed. Indeed, by treating animals with 60 mg/kg of $MgSO_4$ in a PEG formulation, lesion volume was reduced to a greater extent than seen in animals treated with $MgSO_4$ or PEG alone, with only the $MgSO_4$ in PEG leading to a significant improvement of motor outcome at 6 weeks post-injury (Kwon *et al,* 2009). Similarly with a higher dose of Mg^{2+} (300 mg/kg), only the combination of $MgSO_4$ in PEG led to a significant reduction in lesion volume, tissue sparing at the site of injury and modest BBB improvements at 6 weeks post injury (Ditor *et al,* 2007). The ability to reduce the necessary dosage for treating SCI by placing Mg^{2+} in PEG makes it more likely that a clinical translation can be made, with the dosage optimized so that beneficial effects are seen with a comparable amount of Mg^{2+} administered to that shown to be safe in patients suffering from cardiac arrest and pre-eclampsia (Kwon *et al,* 2009).

Clinical translation

Although Mg^{2+} is a multifactorial pharmacological intervention with a proven safety record in previous clinical studies, it has yet to be used clinically to treat SCI. Interestingly, experimental data suggest that the Mg^{2+} in PEG formulation is more effective than methylprednisolone, the only pharmacological treatment currently available clinically for SCI (Bracken and Holford, 2002). This formulation reduced lesion volume by 67% compared to 34% following SCI, with an associated significant improvement in motor outcome at 6 weeks post-injury in the animals treated with Mg^{2+} compared to the methyl-prednisolone group (Kwon *et al,* 2009). This is important as treatment with methylprednisolone remains controversial with only modest improvements noted in motor and sensory outcome of patients treated within 8 hours (Bracken and Holford 2002), which are offset by an increase in complications such as severe sepsis and pneumonia (Hurlbert 2006). This highlights the importance of finding new treatments for SCI, with the Mg^{2+}/PEG formulation soon poised to be translated into human SCI clinical trials (as reviewed by (Kwon *et al,* 2010).

Despite the positive results obtained using Mg^{2+} as a therapy for TBI in animal models, a recent Phase III clinical trial (Temkin *et al,* 2007) found that $MgSO_4$ given to patients for 5 days after injury was not neuroprotective and possibly even had a negative effect on outcome. Given that all patients (including the control group) received Mg^{2+} to restore depleted serum levels to normal, it is unclear whether this restoration of serum Mg^{2+} level was sufficient to confer positive effect in all patients irrespective of the treatment group. This result was in marked contrast to another clinical trial (Dhandapani *et al,* 2008) which reported that acute Mg^{2+} administration (less than 24 hours) resulted in significant improvements in neurological outcome, post-operative brain swelling and 1-month mortality. The differences in trial results could be attributed to possible limitations in central Mg^{2+} transport (McKee *et al,* 2005), and the recently described Mg^{2+} transporters from the TRPM family have been suggested to be involved in this process (Cook *et al,* 2009). However, as described in this review further investigation is warranted to elucidate the exact role of these channels in the pathophysiology of TBI and SCI.

Conclusions

Secondary injury factors involve numerous pathological processes that account for significant morbidity and mortality following traumatic CNS injury. Deficits in intracellular Mg^{2+} concentration occurring following TBI and SCI are associated with poor neurological outcome, but despite promising experimental studies, Mg^{2+} has not been proven clinically effective. While it is unlikely that targeting a single factor will significantly improve neurological outcome, Mg^{2+} may still be a useful neuroprotective agent as part of a combination treatment regime that targets multiple components of the secondary injury cascade.

Acknowledgments
Supported, in part, by the Neurosurgical Research Foundation of Australia and a National Health and Medical Research Council postgraduate research award (NLC).

References

Aarts M, Iihara K, Wei W-L, Xiong Z, -G., Arundine M, Cerwinski W, MacDonald JF, Tymianski M (2003) A key role for TRPM7 channels in anoxic neuronal death. *Cell* 115:863-77.

Aarts MM, Tymianski M (2005) TRPMs and neuronal cell death. *Pflugers Arch* 451:243-9.

Adams JH, Graham DI, Murray LS, Scott G (1982) Diffuse axonal injury due to nonmissile head injury in humans: an analysis of 45 cases. *Ann Neurol* 12:557-63.

Alexandrova ML, Bochev PG (2005) Oxidative stress during the chronic phase after stroke. *Free Rad Biol Med* 39:297-316.

Altura BM, Gebrewold A, Zhang A, Altura BT (2003) Low extracellular magnesium ions induce lipid peroxidation and activation of nuclear factor-kappa B in canine cerebral vascular smooth muscle: possible relation to traumatic brain injury and strokes. *Neurosci Lett* 341:189-92.

Anonymous (2008) Spinal cord injury Facts and figures at a glance. *J Spinal Cord Med* 31:357-8.

Ansari MA, Roberts KN, Scheff SW (2008) Oxidative stress and modification of synaptic proteins in hippocampus after traumatic brain injury. *Free Rad Biol Med* 45:443-52.

Ayata C, Ropper AH (2002) Ischaemic brain oedema. *J Clin Neurosci* 9:113-24.

Bareyre FM, Saatman KE, Helfaer MA, Sinson G, Weisser JD, Brown AL, McIntosh TK (1999) Alterations in ionized and total blood magnesium after experimental traumatic brain injury: relationship to neurobehavioral outcome and neuroprotective efficacy of magnesium chloride. *J Neurochem* 73:271-80.

Barone FC, Kilgore KS (2006) Role of inflammation and cellular stress in brain injury and central nervous system diseases. *Clin Neurosci Res* 6:329-56.

Bayir H, Kagan VE (2008) Bench-to-bedside review: mitochondrial injury, oxidative stressand apoptosis - there is nothing more practical than a good theory. *Crit Care* 12.

Benveniste EN, Tang LP, Law R, M. (1995) Differential regulation of astrocyte TNF-a expression by the cytokines TGF-b, IL-6 and IL-10. *Int J Dev Neurosci* 13:341-9.

Blache D, Devaux S, Joubert O, Loreau N, Schneider M, Durand P, Prost M, Guame V, Adrian M, Laurant P, Berthelot A (2006) Long-term magnesium-deficient diet shows relationships between blood pressure, inflammation and oxidant stress defense in aging rats. *Free Radic Biol Med* 41:277-84.

Black PH (2002) Stress and the inflammatory response: a review of neurogenic inflammation. *Brain Beh Immun* 16:622-53.

Bracken MB, Holford TR (2002) Neurological and functional status 1 year after acute spinal cord injury: estimates of functional recovery in National Acute Spinal Cord Injury Study II from results modeled in National Acute Spinal Cord Injury Study III. *J Neurosurg* 96:259-66.

Browne KD, Leoni MJ, Iwata A, Chen X-H, Smith DH (2004) Acute treatment with $MgSO_4$ attenuates long-term hippocampal tissue loss after brain trauma in the rat. *J Neurosci Res* 77:878-83.

Buechner JS, Speare MC, Fontes J (2000) Hospitalizations for spinal cord injuries, 1994-1998. *Med Health R I* 83:92-3.

Cernak I, Savic VJ, Kotur J, Prokic V, Veljovic M, Grbovic D (2000) Characterization of plasma magnesium concentration and oxidative stress following graded traumatic brain injury in humans. *J Neurotrauma* 17:53-68.

Chanimov M, Berman S, Gofman V, Weissgarten Y, Averbukh Z, Cohen ML, Vitin A, Bahar M (2006) Total cell associated electrolyte homeostasis in rat spinal cord cells following apparently irreversible injury. *Med Sci Monit* 12:BR63-7.

Chong ZZ, Li F, Maiese K (2005) Oxidative stress in the brain: novel cellular targets that govern survival during neurodegenerative disease. *Prog Neurobiol* 75:207-46.

Clausen T, Bullock R (2001) Medical treatment and neuroprotection in traumatic brain injury. *Curr Pharm Design* 7:1517-32.

Cook NL, Van Den Heuvel C, Vink R (2009) Are the transient receptor potential melastatin (TRPM) channels important in magnesium homeostasis following traumatic brain injury? *Magnes Res* 22:225-34.

Cormio M, Robertson CS, Narayan RK (1997) Secondary insults to the injured brain. *J Clin Neurosci* 4:132-48.

Delgado AV, McManus AT, Chambers JP (2003) Production of tumor necrosis factor-alpha, interleukin 1-beta, and interleukin 6 by rat leukocyte subpopulations after exposure to substance P. *Neuropeptides* 37:355-61.

Dhandapani SS, Gupta A, Vivekanandhan S, Sharma BS, Mahapatra AK (2008) Randomized controlled trial of magnesium sulphate in severe closed traumatic brain injury. *Ind J Neurotrauma* 5:27-33.

Ditor DS, John SM, Roy J, Marx JC, Kittmer C, Weaver LC (2007) Effects of polyethylene glycol and magnesium sulfate administration on clinically relevant neurological outcomes after spinal cord injury in the rat. *J Neurosci Res* 85:1458-67.

Donkin JJ, Nimmo AJ, Cernak I, Blumbergs PC, Vink R (2009) Substance P is associated with the development of brain edema and functional deficits after traumatic brain injury. *J Cereb Blood Flow Metab* 29:1388-98.

Ebel H, Günther T (1980) Magnesium metabolism: a review. *J Clin Chem Clin Biochem* 18:257-70.

Ellis EM (2007) Reactive carbonyls and oxidative stress: potential for therapeutic intervention. *Pharmacol & Therapeutics* 115:13-24.

Fan L, Young PR, Barone FC, Feuerstein GZ, Smith DH, McIntosh TK (1995) Experimental brain injury induces expression of interleukin-1b mRNA in the rat brain. *Mol Brain Res* 30:125-30.

Fan L, Young PR, Barone FC, Feuerstein GZ, Smith DH, McIntosh TK (1996) Experimental brain injury induces differential expression of tumor necrosis factor-a mRNA in the CNS. *Mol Brain Res* 36:287-91.

Feldman Z, Gurevitch B, Artru AA, Oppenheim A, Shohami E, Reichenthal E, Shapira Y (1996) Effect of magnesium given 1 hour after head trauma on brain edema and neurological outcome. *J Neurosurg* 85:131-7.

Finkel T, Holbrook NJ (2000) Oxidants, oxidative stress and the biology of ageing. *Nature* 408:239-47.

Fleminger S, Ponsford J (2005) Long term outcome after traumatic brain injury. *Br Med J* 331:1419-20.

Fromm L, Heath DL, Vink R, Nimmo AJ (2004) Magnesium attenuates post-traumatic depression/anxiety following diffuse traumatic brain injury in rats. *J Am Coll Nutr* 23:529S-33S.

Gentile NT, McIntosh TK (1993) Antagonists of excitatory amino acids and endogenous opioid peptides in the treatment of experimental central nervous system injury. *Ann Emerg Med* 22:1028-34.

Gentleman SM, Nash MJ, Sweeting CS, Graham DI, Roberts GW (1993) B-Amyloid precursor protein (B-APP) as a marker for axonal injury after head injury. *Neurosci Lett* 160:139-44.

Gok B, Okutan O, Beskonakli E, Kilinc K (2007) Effects of magnesium sulphate following spinal cord injury in rats. *Chin J Physiol* 50:93-7.

Golding EM (2002) Sequelae following traumatic brain injury: the cerebrovascular perspective. *Brain Res Rev* 38:377-88.

Gowda RM, Khan IA (2004) Magnesium in treatment of acute myocardial infarction. *Int J Cardiol* 96:467-9.

Halliwell B (1992) Reactive oxygen species and the central nervous system. *J Neurochem* 59:1609-23.

Harrison S, Geppetti P (2001) Substance P. *Int J Biochem Cell Biol* 33:555-76.

Heath DL, Vink R (1996) Traumatic brain axonal injury produces sustained decline in intracellular free magnesium concentration. *Brain Res* 738:150-3.

Heo JH, Han SW, Lee SK (2005) Free radicals as triggers of brain edema formation after stroke. *Free Rad Biol Med* 39:51-70.

Hoane MR, Barth TM (2002) The window of opportunity for administration of magnesium therapy following focal brain injury is 24 h but is task dependent in the rat. *Physiol Behav* 76:271-80.

Hoane MR (2007) Assessment of cognitive function following magnesium therapy in the traumatically injured brain. *Magnes Res* 20:229-36.

Hurlbert RJ (2006) Strategies of medical intervention in the management of acute spinal cord injury. *Spine (Phila Pa 1976)* 31:S16-21; discussion S36.

Jain KK (2008) Neuroprotection in traumatic brain injury. *Drug Discovery Today* 13:1082-9.

Kahraman S, Ozgurtas T, Kayalt H, Atabey C, Kutluay T, Timurkaynak E (2003) Monitoring of serum ionized magnesium in neurosurgical intensive care unit: preliminary results. *Clin Chim Acta* 334:211-5.

Kaptanoglu E, Beskonakli E, Okutan O, Selcuk Surucu H, Taskin Y (2003a) Effect of magnesium sulphate in experimental spinal cord injury: evaluation with ultrastructural findings and early clinical results. *J Clin Neurosci* 10:329-34.

Kaptanoglu E, Beskonakli E, Solaroglu I, Kilinc A, Taskin Y (2003b) Magnesium sulfate treatment in experimental spinal cord injury: emphasis on vascular changes and early clinical results. *Neurosurg Rev* 26:283-7.

Kimelberg HK (1995) Current concepts of brain edema. *J Neurosurg* 83:1051-9.

Knoblach SM, Faden AI (1998) Interleukin-10 improves outcome and alters proinflammatory cytokine expression after experimental traumatic brain injury. *Exp Neurol* 153:143-51.

Kowaltowski AJ, de Souza-Pinto NC, Castilho RF, Vercesi AE (2009) Mitochondria and reactive oxygen species. *Free Rad Biol Med* 47:333-43.

Kwon BK, Okon E, Hillyer J, Mann C, Baptiste D, Weaver LC, Fehlings MG, Tetzlaff W (2010) A systematic review of non-invasive pharmacologic neuroprotective treatments for acute spinal cord injury. *J Neurotrauma* 27:1-44.

Kwon BK, Roy J, Lee JH, Okon E, Zhang H, Marx JC, Kindy MS (2009) Magnesium chloride in a polyethylene glycol formulation as a neuroprotective therapy for acute spinal cord injury: preclinical refinement and optimization. *J Neurotrauma* 26:1379-93.

Lee JS, Han YM, Yoo DS, Choi SJ, Choi BH, Kim JH, Kim YH, Huh PW, Ko YJ, Rha HK, Cho KS, Kim DS (2004) A molecular basis for the efficacy of magnesium treatment following traumatic brain injury. *J Neurotrauma* 21:549-61.

Leeman L, Fontaine P (2008) Hypertensive disorders of pregnancy. *Am Fam Physician* 78:93-100.

Lemke M, Demediuk P, McIntosh TK, Vink R, Faden AI (1987) Alterations in tissue Mg++, Na+ and spinal cord edema following impact trauma in rats. *Biochem Biophys Res Commun* 147:1170-5.

Lemke M, Faden AI (1990) Edema development and ion changes in rat spinal cord after impact trauma: injury dose-response studies. *J Neurotrauma* 7:41-54.

Li X-Y, Feng D-F (2009) Diffuse axonal injury: Novel insights into detection and treatment. *J Clin Neurosci* 16:614-9.

Lima FD, Souza MA, Furian AF, Rambo LM, Ribeiro LR, Martignoni FV, Hoffmann MS, Fighera MR, Royes LFF, Oliveria MS, de Mello CF (2008) Na+,K+-ATPase activity impairment after experimental traumatic brain injury: relationship to spatial learning deficits and oxidative stress. *Behav Brain Res* 193:306-10.

Liou AKF, Clark RS, Henshall DC, Yin X-M, Chen J (2003) To die or not to die for neurons in ischemia, traumatic brain injury and epilepsy: a review on the stress-activated signaling pathways and apoptotic pathways. *Prog Neurobiol* 69:103-42.

Maas AIR, Stocchetti N, Bullock R (2008) Moderate and severe traumatic brain injury in adults. *Lancet Neurol* 7:728-41.

MacDonald JF, Xiong Z, -G., Jackson MF (2006) Paradox of Ca^{2+} signaling, cell death and stroke. *Trends Neurosci* 29:75-81.

Malpuech-Brugère C, Nowacki W, Daveau M, Gueux E, Linard C, Rock E, Lebreton J-P, Mazur A, Rayssiguier Y (2000) Inflammatory response following acute magnesium deficiency in the rat. *Biochim Biophys Acta* 1501:91-8.

Marmarou A, Fatouros PP, Barzo P, Portella G, Yoshihara M, Tsuji O, Yamamoto T, Laine F, Signoretti S, Ward JD, Bullock R, Young HF (2000) Contribution of edema and cerebral blood volume to traumatic brain swelling in head-injured patients. *J Neurosurg* 93:183-93.

Massullo P, Sumoza-Toledo A, Bhagat H, Partida-Sánchez S (2006) TRPM channels, calcium and redox sensors during innate immune responses. *Sem Cell Dev Biol* 17:654-66.

Mazur A, Maier JAM, Rock E, Gueux E, Nowacki W, Rayssiguier Y (2006) Magnesium and the inflammatory response: potential physiopathological implications. *Arch Biochem Biophys* 458:48-56.

Mazzeo AT, Beat A, Singh A, Bullock R (2009) The role of mitochondrial transition pore, and its modulation, in traumatic brain injury and delayed neurodegeneration after TBI. *Exp Neurol* 218:363-70.

McIntosh TK, Vink R, Yamakami I, Faden AI (1989) Magnesium protects against neurological deficit after brain injury. *Brain Res* 482:252-60.

McKee JA, Brewer RP, Macy GE, Borel CO, Reynolds JD, Warner DS (2005) Magnesium neuroprotection is limited in humans with acute brain injury. *Neurocrit Care* 2:342-51.

Monteilh-Zoller MK, Hermosura MC, Nadler MJS, Scharenberg AM, Penner R, Fleig A (2003) TRPM7 provides an ion channel mechanism for cellular entry of trace metal ions. *J Gen Physiol* 121:49-60.

Morales DM, Marklund N, Lebold D, Thompson HJ, Pitkänen A, Maxwell WL, Longhi L, Laurer H, Maegele M, Neugebauer E, Graham DI, Stocchetti N, McIntosh TK (2005) Experimental models of traumatic brain injury: do we really need to build a better mousetrap? *Neuroscience* 136:971-89.

Morganti-Kossmann MC, Satgunaseelan L, Bye N, Kossmann T (2007) Modulation of immune response by head injury. *Injury* 38:1392-400.

Nicholls DG, Budd SL (2000) Mitochondria and neuronal survival. *Physiol Rev* 80:315-60.

Nimmo AJ, Cernak I, Heath DL, Hu X, Bennett CJ, Vink R (2004) Neurogenic inflammation is associated with development of edema and functional deficits following traumatic brain injury in rats. *Neuropeptides* 38:40-7.

Ozdemir M, Cengiz SL, Gurbilek M, Ogun TC, Ustan ME (2005) Effects of magnesium sulphate on spinal cord tissue lactate and malondialdehyde levels after spinal cord trauma. *Magnes Res* 18:170-4.

Palmer AM (2010) The role of the blood-CNS barrier in CNS disorders and their treatment. *Neurobiol Dis* 37:3-12.

Pitkänen A, Longhi L, Marklund N, Morales DM, McIntosh TK (2005) Neurodegeneration and neuroprotective strategies after traumatic brain injury. *Drug Discov Today* 2:409-18.

Ravishankar S, Ashraf QM, Fritz K, Mishra OP, Delivoria-Papadopoulos M (2001) Expression of Bax and Bcl-2 proteins during hypoxia in cerebral cortical neuronal nuclei of newborn piglets: effect of administration of magnesium sulfate. *Brain Res* 901:23-9.

Regan RF, Jasper E, Guo Y, Panter SS (1998) The effect of magnesium on oxidative neuronal injury in vitro. *J Neurochem* 70:77-85.

Ro JY, Zhang Y, Nies M (2005) Substance P does not play a critical role in neurogenic inflammation in the rat masseter muscle. *Brain Res Rev* 1047:38-44.

Robertson CL (2004) Mitochondrial dysfunction contributes to cell death following traumatic brain injury in adult and immature animals. *J Bioenerg Biomemb* 36:363-8.

Roth P, Farls K (2000) Pathophysiology of traumatic brain injury. *Crit Care Nurs Quart* 23:14-25.

Runnels LW, Yue L, Clapham DE (2001) TRP-PLIK, a bifunctional protein with kinase and ion channel activities. *Science* 291:1043-7.

Saatman KE, Bareyre FM, Grady MS, McIntosh TK (2001) Acute cytoskeletal alterations and cell death induced by experimental brain injury are attenuated by magnesium treatment and exacerbated by magnesium deficiency. *J Neuropathol Exp Neurol* 60:183-94.

Sacco RL, Chong JY, Prabhakaran S, Elkind MSV (2007) Experimental treatments for acute ischaemic stroke. *Lancet* 369:331-41.

Schmitz C, Perraud A-L, Johnson CO, Inabe K, Smith MK, Penner R, Kurosaki T, Fleig A, Scharenberg AM (2003) Regulation of vertebrate cellular Mg^{2+} homeostasis by TRPM7. *Cell* 114:191-200.

Sen AP, Gulati A (2010) Use of magnesium in traumatic brain injury. *Neurotherapeutics* 7:91-9.

Signoretti S, Marmarou A, Aygok GA, Fatouros PP, Portella G, Bullock RM (2008) Assessment of mitochondrial impairment in traumatic brain injury using high-resolution proton magnetic resonance spectroscopy. *J Neurosurg* 108:42-52.

Simard JM, Kent TA, Chen M, Tarasov KV, Gerzanich V (2007) Brain oedema in focal ischaemia: molecular pathophysiology and theoretical implications. *Lancet Neurol* 6:258-68.

Solaroglu I, Kaptanoglu E, Okutan O, Beskonakli E, Attar A, Kilinc K (2005) Magnesium sulfate treatment decreases caspase-3 activity after experimental spinal cord injury in rats. *Surg Neurol* 64 Suppl 2:S17-21.

Stahel PF, Morganti-Kossmann MC, Kossmann T (1998) The role of the complement system in traumatic brain injury. *Brain Res Rev* 27:243-56.

Suh BC, Hille B (2005) Regulation of ion channels by phosphatidylinositol 4,5-bisphosphate. *Curr Opin Neurobiol* 15:370-8.

Suzer T, Coskun E, Islekel H, Tahta K (1999) Neuroprotective effect of magnesium on lipid peroxidation and axonal function after experimental spinal cord injury. *Spinal Cord* 37:480-4.

Temkin NR, Anderson GD, Winn HR, Ellenbogen RG, Britz GW, Schuster J, Lucas T, Newell DW, Mansfield PN, Machamer JE, Barber J, Dikmen SS (2007) Magnesium sulfate for neuroprotection after traumatic brain injury: a randomised controlled trial. *Lancet Neurol* 6:29-38.

Turner RJ, DaSilva KW, O'Connor C, Van Den Heuvel C, Vink R (2004) Magnesium gluconate offers no more protection than magnesium sulphate following diffuse traumatic brain injury in rats. *J Am Coll Nutr* 23:541S-4S.

Turner RJ, Blumbergs PC, Sims NR, Helps SC, Rodgers KM, Vink R (2006) Increased substance P immunoreactivity and edema formation following reversible ischemic stroke. *Acta Neurochir* S96:263-6.

Unterberg AW, Stover J, Kress B, Kiening KL (2004) Edema and brain trauma. *Neuroscience* 129:1021-9.

Van Den Heuvel C, Vink R (2004) The role of magnesium in traumatic brain injury. *Clin Calcium* 14:1187-92.

Verlooy J, Van Reempts J (2005) The blood-brain barrier in trauma, stroke and edema. *Int Congr Series* 1277:227-34.

Vink R, McIntosh TK, Demediuk P, Weiner MW, Faden AI (1988) Decline in intracellular free Mg^{2+} is associated with irreversible tissue injury after brain trauma. *J Biol Chem* 263:757-61.

Vink R, Cernak I (2000) Regulation of intracellular free magnesium in central nervous system injury. *Front Biosci* 5:d656-65.

Vink R, Young A, Bennett CJ, Hu X, O'Connor C, Cernak I, Nimmo AJ (2003) Neuropeptide release influences brain edema formation after diffuse traumatic brain injury. *Acta Neurochir* S86:257-60.

Vink R, Donkin JJ, Cruz MI, Nimmo AJ, Cernak I (2004) A substance P antagonist increases brain intracellular free magnesium concentration after diffuse traumatic brain injury in rats. *J Am Coll Nutr* 23:538S-40S.

Vink R, Van Den Heuvel C (2004) Recent advances in the development of multifactorial therapies for the treatment of traumatic brain injury. *Exp Opin Investig Drugs* 13:1263-74.

Vink R, Cook NL, van den Heuvel C (2009) Magnesium in acute and chronic brain injury: an update. *Magnes Res* 22:158S-62S.

Vink R, Nimmo AJ (2009) Multifunctional drugs for head injury. *Neurotherapeutics* 6:28-42.

Vink R, Van Den Heuvel C (2010) Substance P antagonists as a therapeutic approach to improving outcome following traumatic brain injury. *Neurotherapeutics* 7:74-80.

Weaver FM, Hammond MC, Guihan M, Hendricks RD (2000) Department of Veterans Affairs Quality Enhancement Research Initiative for spinal cord injury. *Med Care* 38:I82-91.

Weglicki WB, Phillips TM (1992) Pathobiology of magnesium deficiency: a cytokine/neurogenic inflammation hypothesis. *Am J Physiol Regul Integr Comp Physiol* 263:734-7.

Weglicki WB, Mak I-T, Phillips TM (1994) Blockade of cardiac inflammation in Mg^{2+} deficiency by substance P receptor inhibition. *Circ Res* 74.

Wiseman DB, Dailey AT, Lundin D, Zhou J, Lipson A, Falicov A, Shaffrey CI (2009) Magnesium efficacy in a rat spinal cord injury model. *J Neurosurg Spine* 10:308-14.

Wu ZZ, Guan BC, Li ZW, Yang Q, Liu CJ, Chen JG (2004) Sustained potentiation by substance P of NMDA-activated current in rat primary sensory neurons. *Brain Res* 1010:117-26.

Yang YL, Yao KH, Li ZW (2003) Similarities of SP-, NKA- and NKB-induced currents in rat dorsal root ganglion neurons. *Brain Res* 991:18-25.

Yu BP (1994) Cellular defenses against damage from reactive oxygen species. *Physiol Rev* 74:139-62.

The use of magnesium in experimental cerebral ischemia

Bruno P. Meloni, ✉ *Kym Campbell and Neville W. Knuckey*

Centre for Neuromuscular and Neurological Disorders, University of Western Australia, and the Australian Neuromuscular Research Institute, Department of Neurosurgery, Sir Charles Gairdner Hospital, Nedlands, WA, 6009, Australia.
✉ meloni@cyllene.uwa.edu.au

Abstract

The rationale for trialing magnesium as a neuroprotective agent following cerebral ischemia has been based both on its role in maintaining brain tissue homeostasis and on its known cellular actions that are likely to counteract damaging ischemic processes. A number of studies using animal models of cerebral ischemia, seizure, perinatal hypoxia-ischemia, subarachnoid hemorrhage and traumatic brain injury have reported positive outcomes with magnesium therapy. However, scrutiny of the animal cerebral ischemia data shows that about 46% of studies have not shown a neuroprotective effect. Furthermore, the IMAGES clinical trial found magnesium to be largely ineffective in treating strokes. In this review, we present the majority of published cerebral ischemia animal studies (focal and global) that have used magnesium as a neuroprotective therapy, and discuss the possible reasons for the inconsistent results. Our examination suggests that, in the majority of experiments, post-ischemic hypothermia has probably been a confounding factor in producing the positive outcomes. In addition, experimental design has not always been appropriate with respect to magnesium dosage, and to the time and route of magnesium administration. Moreover, data from our own laboratory indicates that magnesium is only neuroprotective when combined with post-ischemic hypothermia. Finally, additional information regarding the efficacy of magnesium as a stroke treatment will be available on completion of the FAST-Mag trial, but in the meantime the neuroprotective potential of magnesium should be explored when combined with post-ischemic hypothermia, and potentially with other agents, in cerebral ischemia models.

Introduction

More than any other organ, the brain is dependent on the aerobic metabolism of glucose for energy, making it exceedingly sensitive to ischemic disease. Inadequate supply of oxygenated blood leads to a rapidly developing energy crisis that, within minutes, results in the death of cells comprising the neurovascular unit. Restoration of blood supply, or the presence of collateral circulation, may preserve some tissue only for it to die over the hours or days that follow an ischemic event. Such delayed death may occur from one or more of a range of pathological processes; glutamate excitotoxicity, calcium dysregulation and overload, apoptosis, autophagy, inflammation, oxygen free radical generation and edema have all been implicated. Consequently, interruption of these processes presents an opportunity for therapeutic intervention to protect the damaged cells within the neurovascular unit after cerebral ischemia. Many therapies have been found to offer neuroprotection in experimental models of cerebral ischemia, magnesium among them.

Since magnesium is important in many normal cellular processes such as protein synthesis, energy metabolism, maintenance of ionic gradients and vascular smooth muscle tone, abnormalities in serum and CNS magnesium status before, during and after cerebral ischemia can be expected to have an effect on neurological outcome. Indeed, clinical and experimental studies have shown that subjects with low serum or CSF magnesium have worsened neurological outcomes following brain ischemia and trauma (Lampl *et al*, 1998; McIntosh *et al* 1988; Vink *et al*, 1988). There is also ample evidence demonstrating that there are marked changes in intracellular and extracellular free magnesium concentrations in brain tissue following ischemic and traumatic insults (Helpern *et al*, 1993; Vande Linde and Chopp, 1991; Vink *et al*, 1996; Lee *et al*, 2002). As such, maintaining normal serum magnesium concentration should be considered a part of standard supportive care in such patients. On top of that, however, the Mg^{2+} cation has properties that may specifically counteract a number of the damaging process associated with cerebral ischemia. In particular, magnesium can reduce synaptic glutamate release (Nowak *et al*, 1984), decrease calcium influx via voltage gated calcium channels (Iseri and French, 1984), stabilise mitochondria (Kowaltowski *et al*, 1998; Xu *et al*, 2002), increase cerebral blood flow (Chi *et al*, 1990) and reduce free radical production (Garcia *et al*, 1998).

For these reasons, restoration of magnesium homeostasis and exploration of the potential positive effects in the ischemic brain have prompted the investigation of magnesium as a neuroprotective agent following such disorders as traumatic brain injury (Heath and Vink, 1996; Vink *et al*, 1988), seizure (Cotton *et al*, 1993), subarachnoid hemorrhage (Van den Bergh *et al*, 2002) and cerebral ischemia (Muir, 1998). Here we overview the experimental animal studies that have to date tested magnesium as a neuroprotectant in the major animal models of cerebral ischemia, specifically focal (ischemic stroke) and global (cardiac arrest) brain ischemia models.

This review will present experimental findings from these studies, offer potential explanations for conflicting or inconsistent results and consider the future application of magnesium in cerebral ischemia.

Efficacy of magnesium treatment in models of focal cerebral ischemia

The results from 16 studies using magnesium in animal models of focal cerebral ischemia are summarized in Table 1. As can be seen in this table, there is considerable variability in study design (stroke model, animal species used, magnesium dose, route and timing of administration, outcome measures), which precludes direct comparison of outcomes. There were 5 studies using permanent focal ischemia models, 9 using transient models and single studies using an embolic and an endothelin-1 (lacunar stroke) model. As a broad summary, 10 of the 16 studies reported a neuroprotective effect for magnesium based on infarct volume reduction. Magnesium treatment in the endothelin-1 model did not reduce infarct volume, but did improve some behavioral outcomes. Thus, there is slightly better than equivocal support for the claim that magnesium has a neuroprotective effect in these models.

Magnesium in Permanent Focal Cerebral Ischemia

In the 5 studies using permanent middle cerebral artery occlusion (MCAO), 3 reported positive outcomes with magnesium treatment. Two of the studies, 1 using rats (Izumi *et al*, 1991) and 1 using mice (Roffe *et al*, 1996), were otherwise similar in their experimental procedures, yet reported contrasting results. Izumi et al (1991) observed both a neuroprotective effect and a hyperglycemia associated with administration of magnesium chloride; if the hyperglycemia was managed with insulin, there was a further reduction of infarct volume. In contrast, Roffe et al (1996) found no neuroprotection, and in fact reported that magnesium chloride treatment increased edema in the infarcted hemispheres. While increased edema was not evident in animals treated with magnesium and insulin, the combined treatment did not reduce infarct volume.

Two other studies (Lee *et al*, 1999; Chung *et al*, 2004), which were similar with respect to magnesium dose and timing of administration, but different in animal species used and route of administration, reported positive findings, while a study from our laboratory was negative (Campbell *et al*, 2008a). Among these, our study was the only trial to use a dosing regimen (IV loading dose and 24 hour infusion) similar to the IMAGES human stroke trial. Furthermore, we paid careful attention to body temperatures post-surgery to ensure that animals did not become hypothermic during the recovery period or thereafter. The possibility of post-ischemic hypothermia having confounded these experimental results, especially in the earlier animal studies, will be discussed in a later section.

It is of interest that Lee *et al* (1999) commented that, in unpublished experiments, if the intra-arterial route of magnesium administration was changed to an intravenous route, magnesium was no longer protective.

TABLE 1. Summary of animal studies using magnesium following focal cerebral ischemia

Reference	Animal model	Mg salt	Route	Magnesium dose	Time of treatment	Post-ischemic temperature monitoring	Neuroprotection/Outcome
Permanent Model							
Izumi *et al.*, 1991	pMCAO, rat	$MgCl_2$	IP	1 mmol/kg x 2	Immediately & 1h after MCAO	Measured 1.5, 4, 24 & 48h post MCAO	Yes; reduced infarct volume at 48h
Roffe *et al.*, 1996	pMCAO, mouse	$MgCl_2$	IP	1 mmol/kg x 2	Immediately & 1h after MCAO	No	No; based on infarct volume at 24h
Lee *et al.*, 1999	pMCAO, rat	$MgSO_4$	IA	0.75 mmol/kg	10min before MCAO	No	Yes; reduced infarct volume at 24h[#]
Chung *et al.*, 2004	pMCAO, gerbil	$MgSO_4$	IP	0.75 mmol/kg	10min before MCAO	No	Yes; reduced infarct volume at 24h
Campbell *et al.*, 2008a	pMCAO, rat	$MgSO_4.7H_2O$	IV	0.36 + 0.12 mmol/kg/h for 24h	2h after MCAO	Yes, actively monitored & controlled	No; based on infarct volume at 48h
Transient Model							
Marinov *et al.*, 1996	2 or 1.5h tMCAO, rat	$MgSO_4$	IA	0.25 or 0.75 mmol/kg	Immediately before MCAO	Monitored for 45min after ischemia	Yes; reduced infarct volume at 24h
Schmid-Elsaesser *et al.*, 1999	1.5h tMCAO, rat	$MgCl_2$	IV	1 mmol/kg x 2	Before MCAO & at time of reperfusion	Monitored for 1h after ischaemia & rats housed in warm cages for 8h	No; (25% reduction infarct volume at 7 days)
Kinoshita *et al.*, 2001	2h tMCAO, rat	$MgSO_4$	IV	0.21 mmol/kg over 2h	During MCAO	No	Yes; reduced infarct volume at 24h
Lin *et al.*, 2002	1h tMCAO, gerbil	$MgSO_4$	IP	0.75 mmol/kg	30min before ischaemia	No	Yes; reduced infarct volume at 24h
Westermaier *et al.*, 2003	1.5h tMCAO, rat	$MgSO_4$	IV & IA	0.75 mmol/kg	Immediately before MCAO	As for Schmid-Elsaesser *et al.*, 1999	No; (25% reduction) based on infarct volume at 7 days
Zhu *et al.*, 2004a	1. 45min tMCAO, rat	$MgSO_4.7H_2O$	IV	0.18, 0.36 or 0.72 mmol/kg	Immediately before MCAO	Monitoring & maintained for 6h	No; based on infarct volume at 24h
	2. 2h tMCAO, rat		IA	0.37 or 0.74 mmol/kg	Immediately before MCAO	No	No; based on infarct volume at 72h
Lee *et al.*, 2005	1.5h tMCAO, rat	$MgSO_4$	IA	0.75 mmol/kg	At time of reperfusion	Yes warm environment 4h post reperfusion. Less hyperthermia in Mg treated	Yes; reduced infarct volume at 72h & improve functional outcomes
Westermaier *et al.*, 2005	1.5h tMCAO, rat	$MgSO_4$	IV	0.75 or 2 x 1mmol/kg or 1 mmol/kg + 0.5 mmol/kg/h for ≈2.5h	Immediately before MCAO	As for Schmid-Elsaesser *et al.*, (1999)	Yes; based on infarct volume at 7 days. Note: 31% reduction for 0.75 mmol/kg dose was not significant
Campbell *et al.*, 2008b	45min tMCAO, rat	$MgSO_4.7H_2O$	IV	0.36 or 0.72 mmol/kg	Immediately before MCAO	No, rats mildly hypothermic for 1 - 4h post surgery	Yes; for 0.36 mmol at 24h
Other Models							
Yang *et al.*, 2000	Embolic, rat	$MgSO_4$	IV	0.75 mmol/kg	2, 6 or 8h after ischaemia	No	Yes; reduced infarct volume at 72h
Lecrux *et al.*, 2008	ET-1 injection, rat	$MgSO_4$	SC	2.5 mmol/kg + 1.66 mmol/kg x 4	30min before ET-1 injection & every h for 4h	No mentioned	No infarct reduction, but improved functional outcomes at day 3 & 10
IMAGES trial, 2004*	Human stroke	$MgSO_4$	IV	0.2 + 0.034 mmol/kg/h for 24h	Within 12h	Normal patient care	No based on neurological outcome, except in lacunar stroke patients

[#]Authors mentioned (unpublished data) that same dose administered IV was ineffective. *IMAGES trial has been included for references purposes

TABLE 2. Summary of animal studies using magnesium following global cerebral ischemia

Reference	Animal model	Mg salt	Route	Magnesium dose	Time of treatment	Post-ischemic temperature monitoring	Neuroprotection/outcome
Blair *et al*, 1989	10min: 2VO rat	$MgCl_2$	IV	5.0 mmol/kg	Immediately before ischemia	No	No; Mg exacerbated CA1 injury due to elevated plasma glucose levels
Tsuda *et al*, 1991	20min: 4VO rat	$MgCl_2$	IC: CA1 region	1 μl of 50 mM	10min before, 0, 2, 12, 24 or 48h after ischemia	No	Yes; at 10min before & 0, 2, 12, 24h after ischemia; based on CA1 injury
Okawa, 1992	18min: aorta occlusion dog	$MgSO_4$	IV	0.66 mmol/kg + 0.33 mmol/kg/h for 3h + 0.083 mmol/kg/h for 45h	Immediately after ischemia	No	Yes; based on neurological outcome
Sirin *et al*, 1998	15min: 4VO rat	$MgSO_4$	SC	5 mmol/kg	48h before ischemia	No	Yes; reduced CA1 injury & improved neurological outcomes
Milani *et al*, 1999	15min: 4VO rat	$MgCl_2$	SC	2.5 mmol/kg x 4 5.0 mmol/kg x 4 7.5 mmol/kg x 4	1, 2, 24 & 48h after ischemia for 2.5, 5 & 7.5 mmol/kg dose	First few hours after ischemia rats housed at 30°C	No; based on CA1 & subiculum injury
				5.0 mmol/kg x1	2h after ischemia for 5 mmol/kg dose		
Miles *et al*, 2001	8min: 2VO rat	$MgSO_4 . 7H_2O$	IV	0.36 mmol/kg + 0.06, 0.12, 0.24 or 0.48 mmol/kg/h for 48h	Before, 4, 8, 12 or 24h after ischemia	No	Yes; reduced CA1 injury when 0.12 mmol/kg/h infusion dose used
		$MgCl_2$		0.36 mmol/kg + 0.12 mmol/kg/h for 48h	Before or 8h after ischemia	No	Yes; before ischemia. No; at 8h after ischemia; based on CA1 injury
Zhou *et al*, 2003	10min: 2VO gerbil	$MgSO_4$	IP	16.6 mmol/kg	30min before ischemia	No	Yes; based on TUNEL staining
Zhu *et al*, 2004b	8min: 2VO rat	$MgSO_4 . 7H_2O$	IV	0.36 mmol/kg + 0.06 or 0.12 or 0.24 mmol/kg/h for 48h	Before ischemia	Maintained normothermic or self-regulated	No when animals maintained normothermic; based on CA1 injury Yes when combined with hypothermia
Zhu *et al*, 2005	8min: 2VO rat	$MgSO_4 . 7H_2O$	IV	0.36 mmol/kg + 0.12 mmol/kg/h for 48h	Immediately before or 2h after ischemia	Maintained normothermic or hypothermic	No; based on CA1 injury in normothermic rats Yes when combined with hypothermia

Magnesium in Transient Focal Cerebral Ischemia

In the 10 studies using transient focal ischemia, 6 reported positive outcomes with magnesium treatment. As in the permanent focal ischemia studies, some of the trials, while similar in key respects, reported contrasting results. For example, Marinov et al (1996) reported positive findings when either of 2 doses of magnesium sulphate (0.75 or 0.25 mmol/kg) were administered intra-arterially before 2 or 1.5 hours of MCAO in rats. In contrast, Zhu *et al* (2004a) reported negative findings in trials consisting of different doses of magnesium sulphate (0.18, 0.36, 0.72 or 0.74 mmol/kg) administered either intra-arterially or intravenously before 45 minutes or 2 hours of MCAO in rats. In a subsequent experiment from the Zhu laboratory (Campbell *et al*, 2008b), rats administered 0.36 mmol/kg magnesium intravenously before MCAO, and allowed to self-regulate their body temperatures post-ischemia, experienced up to 4 hours of mild hypothermia and had significantly reduced striatal infarct volumes.

Similarly, Lee et al (2005) observed a modest, magnesium-induced hypothermic effect in that magnesium treatment attenuated the post-ischemic hyperthermia normally observed in their focal model. When administered immediately after reperfusion, magnesium reduced infarct volumes and improved behavioral outcomes in rats. They ruled out magnesium's hypothermic effect as being responsible for the neuroprotection by inducing the same level of hypothermia in a separate group of animals, showing that these animals did not have either reduced infarct volumes or improved behavioral outcomes.

The Schmid-Elsaesser laboratory has been exploring the efficacy of magnesium following cerebral ischemia, alone and in combination with other treatments (e.g., tirilazad, hypothermia), dating back to 1999 (Schmid-Elsaesser *et al*, 1999; Zausinger *et al,* 2003ab; Westermaier *et al,* 2003; 2005). To summarize their several studies, they have shown that when magnesium is administered before, during or after MCAO it results in infarct volume reductions ranging from 25 - 42%, with reductions of >31% being statistically significant. After surgery, they routinely monitored animals' body temperatures for 1 hour after reperfusion and kept them in a warm environment for the first eight hours (though without further monitoring) to minimize the possibility of hypothermia (Robert Schmid-Elsaesser, personal communication).

Other Focal Cerebral Ischemia Models

Yang et al (2000) assessed the neuroprotective efficacy of intravenously administered magnesium at different time points following ischemia (2, 6 or 8 hours) using an embolic stroke model in rats. They found that magnesium treatment administered 2 or 6 hours, but not 8 hours, after ischemia significantly reduced infarct volumes. In addition, magnesium treatment appeared to improve animal survival and neurological outcome. While animals' body temperatures were monitored during surgical recovery, it was not reported what measures were taken to control their temperatures or to ensure they did not become hypothermic until the 72-hour trial end-point.

To assess the effects of magnesium on white matter injury associated with lacunar stroke, Lecrux et al (2008) injected the vasoconstrictive peptide endothelin-1 into the internal capsule in rats (the study was prompted by post-hoc analysis of the IMAGES stroke trial data, which revealed that magnesium provided a small, but significant benefit in lacunar stroke patients (IMAGES, 2004)). In this study, relatively high subcutaneous doses of magnesium sulphate were given, which increased magnesium serum levels nearly four fold and reduced blood pressure. The treatment did not influence infarct volumes, but motor functional impairments were reduced in magnesium treated animals when assessed at 3 and 10 days.

Efficacy of magnesium treatment in models of global (forebrain) cerebral ischemia

The results from 9 studies using magnesium in models of global cerebral ischemia are summarized in Table 2. As in the focal ischemia studies, there is considerable variability in study design and protocols. At the histological level, 4 of the studies found a neuroprotective effect, 2 studies did not, while 2 studies reported a positive outcome only when magnesium treatment was combined with post-ischemic hypothermia. One study, using an aortic occlusion model in dogs, reported improved neurological outcomes with magnesium treatment. Again, this is moderate support for the contention that magnesium is neuroprotective in these models.

In the first study, by Blair et al (1989), intravenous magnesium chloride appeared in fact to exacerbate CA1 neuronal injury. In this study, the magnesium dose was relatively high (5 mmol/kg), and was considered responsible for elevating serum glucose levels from 150 mg/dl to 220 mg/dl, and thus contributing to increased CA1 neuronal loss. When hyperglycemia was controlled by the simultaneous administration of magnesium and insulin, CA1 injury was no different to saline treated controls. As a measure to ensure the delivery of magnesium to the target tissue, Tsuda et al (1991) administered magnesium chloride (1µl; 50 mM solution) directly to the CA1 sector of the hippocampus at 10 minutes before ischemia or at 0, 2, 12, 24 or 48 hours after ischemia. A neuroprotective effect was observed in CA1 neurons at all time points except 48 hours post-ischemia. A lower dose of magnesium chloride (1 µl; 10 mM) administered at the 24 hour time point also showed a neuroprotective trend, but was not significant at the $P < 0.01$ level. Animal body temperatures were not monitored during recovery, so a potential confounding factor is that the animals might have become hypothermic during this period. The potential for hypothermia will also have been compounded since the animals were re-anaesthetized in those groups receiving magnesium post-ischemia.

While the implications of post-ischemic hypothermia will be discussed in more detail later, it should be emphasized that 3 studies (Milani *et al*, 1999; Zhu *et al*, 2004b; 2005) in which measures were taken to avoid post-ischemic hypothermia, including 2 from our laboratory, found no significant neuroprotection (CA1 neuronal survival) despite starting magnesium treatment before or early after cerebral ischemia and using multiple and continuous dosing regimens. Furthermore, in the 2 studies from our laboratory (Zhu *et al*, 2004b; 2005), when either spontaneous or controlled mild hypothermia occurred during treatment, a neuroprotective effect was observed. In the remaining studies (Okawa *et al*, 1992; Sirin *et al*, 1998; Miles *et al*, 2001; Zhou *et al*, 2003) no measures were reported to have been taken to avoid post-ischemic hypothermia, and all of these reported positive histological or behavioral outcomes.

Reasons for inconsistent results with magnesium following cerebral ischemia

On the evidence from these studies, to the question of whether magnesium is neuroprotective following cerebral ischemia, the answer must be: sometimes. A second question arises, then, as to what factor or factors determine when magnesium will be neuroprotective, and when it will not. Taking into account the differences in study design (species; ischemia model; post-surgical temperature control; dosage, route and time of magnesium administration) we propose several explanations that may reasonably account for the inconsistencies in the reported data.

Confounding effects of post-ischemic hypothermia

As previously reported (Meloni *et al*, 2006) there is reason to believe that the discrepant results found in these studies most likely can be attributed to the confounding effects of post-ischemic hypothermia. In the magnesium studies described in Tables 1 and 2, the animals were invariably maintained normothermic *during* ischemia, but in most cases there is no mention of body temperature monitoring or maintenance during recovery from surgery and in the post-ischemic period. This is crucial because it is now accepted and documented that post-surgical hypothermia commonly occurs in these models of cerebral ischemia, and it has been shown that post-ischemic hypothermia has confounded the results of previous studies (Buchan and Pulsinelli, 1990; Corbett *et al*, 1990; Welsh *et al*, 1990; Dietrich *et al*, 1995; Behringer *et al*, 2002). This is especially relevant in magnesium studies since there is also evidence that magnesium itself has hypothermia inducing properties (Zweifler *et al*, 2004; Wadhwa *et al*, 2005). Therefore, in those studies that did not actively maintain animals normothermic after ischemia, the occurrence of spontaneous hypothermia cannot be ruled out, and in fact is highly likely.

Further than that, direct evidence of the synergistic effects of mild hypothermia with magnesium has been generated from several studies in our laboratory. In an early global ischemia study (Miles *et al*, 2001) we did not monitor or control for animal body temperatures after ischemia; in this study we observed a neuroprotective effect. In subsequent studies (Zhu *et al*, 2004b; 2005), however, using the same model and magnesium treatment, but using controlled normothermic conditions after ischemia, we did not see a neuroprotective effect. Moreover, we observed that if body temperature was only monitored without being controlled, the animals did become mildly hypothermic during surgical recovery, and magnesium treatment in these animals did significantly reduce CA1 neuronal death. Note that control animals also became hypothermic to a similar degree, yet they did not show neuroprotection.

In subsequent experiments, when we compared magnesium efficacy in normothermic animals and in animals rendered mildly hypothermic (35°C) for 6 hours immediately after global ischemia, we observed that treatment with magnesium and mild hypothermia together increased CA1 neuronal survival. Importantly, no neuroprotection was observed either in normothermic animals receiving magnesium or in animals rendered hypothermic for 6 hours post-ischemia. We have also obtained similar findings with focal ischemia experiments. For example, we have demonstrated that following focal ischemia, magnesium treatment in normothermic animals does not result in reduced infarct volumes. In contrast, if magnesium treatment is combined with a period of mild hypothermia (spontaneous or controlled) reduced brain infarcts are observed (Campbell *et al*, 2008ab). In our controlled hypothermia experiments using a permanent focal model (Campbell *et al*, 2008b) we did not observe a protective effect with mild hypothermia alone.

Taken together, these experiments illustrate two important points. The first is that ischemic control animals, though they might experience some level of hypothermia, are unlikely to show any evidence of neuroprotection. The second is that the combination of magnesium and mild hypothermia does not appear to act in an additive way, but rather synergistically to unmask a neuroprotective effect. These findings highlight the necessity to maintain post-ischemic animal body temperatures in drug evaluation studies and, since in the majority of magnesium/cerebral ischemia studies this was not reported to have been done, there is reason to question the validity of the results.

Dosage, route and time of magnesium administration

It is a matter of speculation as to the degree to which magnesium dosage and route of administration is another contributing factor for the discrepant findings, in large part due to the fact that the optimal dose of magnesium remains unknown.

As a rule of thumb, early experimental and clinical studies have aimed to achieve serum concentrations of about double the baseline (i.e., to increase serum magnesium from ≈ 0.8 to ≈ 1.5 mmol/l), which seems reasonable as magnesium at this level appears to be safe and well tolerated (Muir and Lees, 1995; 1998). However, data from our laboratory indicate that magnesium doses that double baseline serum levels may be too high. For example, magnesium doses that resulted in serum magnesium levels >1.4 mmol/L (e.g., using an IV loading dose of 0.36 mmol/kg, followed by an infusion of 0.24 or 0.48 mmol/kg/h) provided no or minimal CA1 protection. On the other hand, a lower dose (0.36 mmol/kg IV, then 0.12 mmol/kg/h), which resulted in serum magnesium from 1 - 1.2 mmol/l, provided marked CA1 survival following global ischemia (note that in these experiments the animals' body temperatures were not monitored during the post-ischemia period; Miles *et al*, 2001). In addition, we have shown that the higher loading dose of 0.72 mmol/kg, when given before focal ischemia (in animals that were maintained normothermic in the 6 hour post-ischemic period), produced a trend towards *increased* infarct volume.

The time of administration will also have a marked influence on the potential neuroprotective effect of any intervention. Most of the studies here administered magnesium before or immediately after induction of cerebral ischemia; hence, increased magnesium levels were present in serum, and possibly the brain, at the time of ischemia. Post-ischemic treatments with magnesium, following both focal and global cerebral ischemia, have, however, produced positive outcomes, with treatment as late as 6 hours after focal ischemia (Yang *et al,* 2000) and 24 hours after global ischemia showing a benefit (Tsuda *et al,* 1991). Even allowing that hypothermia has likely confounded some outcomes, it is encouraging to note that delayed treatment with magnesium can be effective.

While different routes of administration (intravenous, intra-arterial, intraperitoneal, subcutaneous, intracranial) have been used to deliver magnesium, it is difficult to comment on how this may have influenced outcomes in the absence of measures such as the serum and CSF concentrations achieved. Again of particular interest is the positive study using intracranial delivery (Tsuda *et al*, 1991), which reported efficacy even at 24 hours post-ischemia. By bypassing the blood brain barrier, intracranial delivery would guarantee increased brain magnesium and thus maximize its effects.

CSF magnesium levels and magnesium salt

Only 1 cerebral ischemia study has examined the extent to which exogenously administered magnesium penetrates into either brain or CSF. This study, by Okawa et al (1992), used an IV loading dose (0.664 mmol/kg) followed by an infusion of magnesium sulphate (0.332 mmol/kg/h for 3 h, then 0.083 mmol/kg/h for 45 h) in dogs subjected to global cerebral ischemia. They showed a significant increase in CSF magnesium lasting from 20 minutes to 7 days after treatment. Interestingly, dogs not subjected to global ischemia, but treated with the same magnesium regimen, did not show significantly elevated CSF magnesium. In a study using rats not subjected to cerebral ischemia, Sjöström and Wester (1990) showed elevated brain and CSF magnesium shortly after IV administration of 2.0 mmol/kg magnesium chloride. The Okawa et al (1992) study suggests that exogenously administered magnesium may have increased access to the brain following cerebral ischemia, making it likely that in cerebral ischemia experiments magnesium has been present in the target tissue, and thus able to exert both vascular and neural effects.

Magnesium sulphate and magnesium chloride have both been used in models of cerebral ischemia, with both positive and negative results, yet no studies have directly compared their efficacy. The only study that has assessed both magnesium salts was an early global ischemia study from our laboratory (Miles *et al*, 2001). Our data appeared to favour greater efficacy for magnesium sulphate, but unfortunately the trials with the two magnesium salts were not performed concurrently, and once again there is the likelihood of post-ischemic hypothermia confounding the results. Interestingly, in our experiments animals treated with magnesium chloride did not become hyperglycaemic (unpublished observation), which is in contrast to two earlier studies (Blair *et al,* 1989; Izumi *et al,* 1991). A possible contributing factor to the hyperglycaemia reported by Blair et al (1989) and Izumi *et al* (1991) is that they found magnesium treatment was associated with hypothermia, which can reduce insulin secretion (Polderman, 2009) predisposing the animals to hyperglycaemia.

In summary, the discrepancies in the outcomes of these studies are explicable in light of several unanswered questions that still surround magnesium treatment for cerebral ischemia. On the available evidence, it seems fair to say that magnesium does indeed have neuroprotective properties when a suitable dose is given to achieve moderately increased (above normal) levels in the target tissue in conjunction with a mild degree of hypothermia.

Future use of magnesium following stroke and cerebral ischemia

As it stands, in light of the failure of the IMAGES stroke trial to find a significant treatment effect with magnesium (IMAGES, 2004), the future use of magnesium for the treatment of stroke, and possibly other forms of cerebral ischemia, will depend heavily on the outcome of the FAST-MAG Phase 3 trial (Saver *et al*, 2004, Stroke Trials Directory, 2010). This trial is currently underway, and is assessing whether field administration of magnesium within 2 hours of stroke onset improves clinical outcomes. In essence, the FAST-MAG trial will address whether the long delay to magnesium treatment in the IMAGES trial (enrolment up to 12 hours after the onset of stroke) was the principal reason for its ineffectiveness. However, based on our own assessment of magnesium under normothermic conditions, we predict that if FAST-MAG patients are maintained normothermic this trial will also show little or no benefit. As discussed, the evidence suggests that in order for magnesium to produce a positive outcome after stroke/cerebral ischemia it needs to be combined with mild hypothermia (Meloni *et al*, 2009). Fortunately, hypothermia induction may only require a reduction in body temperature of 1 - 2°C involving basic cooling measures, which may be achievable in conscious patients. It is anticipated that future cerebral ischemia experimental studies will play a vital role in assessing magnesium in combination with hypothermia, and potentially with other agents as well, with successful outcomes guiding the design of clinical trials.

Conclusion

There is evidence from several models and using a number of treatment regimens that magnesium has neuroprotective properties that can reduce brain damage and neurological deficits after cerebral ischemia. Given that hypomagnesaemia is known to occur after stroke, magnesium supplementation has a place in the normal supportive care of such patients. Beyond that, the question remains as to whether, and by how much, supplementation should aim to increase, rather than just restore, serum magnesium levels. The FAST-MAG trial may provide part of the answer, though probably without being definitive.

The rationale for trialing magnesium as a neuroprotective agent following stroke has been based on its role in maintaining normal brain functions, on its known cellular actions that are anticipated to counteract damaging ischemic processes and subsequently on positive experimental data from animal models of cerebral ischemia. However, close scrutiny of the animal data shows that about 46% of studies have not shown a neuroprotective effect, and that the majority, if not all, of the positive studies were potentially confounded by post-ischemic hypothermia. In addition, experimental design has not always been well-founded with respect to magnesium dosage, and to the time and route of magnesium administration. Moreover, recent animal studies under controlled post-ischemic conditions indicate that magnesium is only neuroprotective when combined with hypothermia. Finally, additional information regarding the efficacy of magnesium as a stroke treatment will be available on completion of the FAST-MAG trial, but in the meantime the neuroprotective potential of magnesium remains a valid subject for investigation in cerebral ischemia models, with emphasis on its combination with post-ischemic hypothermia.

Acknowledgments
The authors would like to thank William Gow for compiling the reference list.

References

Behringer W, Safar P, Kentner R, Wu X, Kagan VE, Radovsky A, Clark RSB, Kochanek PM, Subramanian M, Tyurin VA, Tyurin YY, Tisherman SA (2002) Antioxidant tempol enhances hypothermic cerebral preservation during prolonged cardiac arrest in dogs. *J Cereb Blood Flow Metab* 22:105-17.

Blair JL, Warner DS, Todd MM (1989) Effects of elevated plasma magnesium versus calcium on cerebral ischemic injury in rats. *Stroke* 20:507-12.

Buchan A, Pulsinelli WA (1990) Hypothermia but not N-methyl-D-aspartate antagonist, MK-801, attenuates neuronal damage in gerbils subjected to transient global ischemia. *J Neurosci* 10:311-16.

Campbell K, Meloni BP, Knuckey NW (2008a) Combined magnesium and mild hypothermia (35°C) treatment reduces infarct volumes after permanent middle cerebral artery occlusion in the rat at 2 and 4, but not 6 hours. *Brain Res* 1230:258-64.

Campbell K, Meloni BP, Zhu H, Knuckey NW (2008b) Magnesium treatment and spontaneous mild hypothermia after transient focal cerebral ischemia in the rat. *Brain Res Bull* 77:320-2.

Chi OZ, Pollak P, Weiss HR (1990) Effects of magnesium sulfate and nifedipine on regional cerebral blood flow during middle cerebral artery ligation in the rat. *Arch Int Pharmacodyn Ther* 304:196-205.

Chung SY, Lin JY, Lin MC, Liu HM, Wang MF, Chung FC (2004) Synergistic efficacy of magnesium sulfate and FK506 on cerebral ischemia-induced infarct volume in gerbil. *Med Sci Monit* 10:105-8.

Corbett D, Evans S, Thomas C, Wang D, Jonas AR (1990) MK-801 reduced cerebral ischemic injury by inducing hypothermia. *Brain Res* 514:300-4.

Cotton DB, Hallak M, Janusz C, Irtenkauf SM, Berman RF (1993) Central anticonvulsant effects of magnesium sulfate on N-methyl-D-aspartate-induced seizures. *Am J Obstet Gynecol* 168:974-8.

Dietrich WD, Lin B, Globus MY-T, Green EJ, Ginsberg MD, Busto R (1995) Effect of delayed MK-801 (dizocilpine) treatment with or without immediate postischemic hypothermia on chronic neuronal survival after global forebrain ischemia in rats. *J Cereb Blood Flow Metab* 15:960-8.

Garcia LA, Dejong SC, Martin SM, Smith RS, Buettner GR, Kerber RE (1998) Magnesium reduces free radicals in an in vivo coronary occlusion-reperfusion model. *J Am Coll Cardiol* 32:536-9.

Heath DL, Vink R (1996) Traumatic brain axonal injury produces sustained decline in intracellular free magnesium concentration. *Brain Res* 738:150-3.

Helpern JA, Vande Linde AMQ, Welch KMA, Levine SR, Schultz LR, Ordidge RJ Halvorson HR, Hugg JW (1993) Acute elevation and recovery of intracellular [Mg^{2+}] following human focal cerebral ischemia. *Neurology* 43:1577-81.

IMAGES (2004) Magnesium for acute stroke (Intravenous Magnesium Efficacy in Stroke trial): randomized controlled trial. Lancet 363:439-45.

Iseri LT, French JH (1984) Magnesium: nature's physiologic calcium blocker. *Am Heart J* 108:188-93.

Izumi Y, Roussel S, Pinard E, Seylaz J (1991) Reduction of infarct volume by magnesium after middle cerebral artery occlusion in rats. *J Cereb Blood Flow Metab* 11:1025-30.

Kinoshita Y, Ueyama T, Senba E, Terada T, Nakai K, Itakura T (2001) Expression of c-fos, heat shock protein 70, neurotrophins, and cyclooxygenase-2 mRNA in response to focal cerebral ischemia/reperfusion in rats and their modification by magnesium sulfate. *J Neurotrauma* 18:435-45.

Kowaltowski AJ, Naia-da-Silva ES, Castilho RF, Vercesi AE (1998) Ca^{2+}-stimulated mitochondrial reactive oxygen species generation and permeability transition are inhibited by dibucaine or Mg^{2+}. *Arch Biochem Biophys* 359:77-81.

Lampl Y, Geva D, Gilad R, Eshel Y, Ronen L, Sarova-Pinhas I (1998) Cerebrospinal fluid magnesium level as a prognostic factor in ischaemic stroke. *J Neurol* 245:584-8.

Lecrux C, McCabe C, Weir CJ, Gallagher L, Mullin J, Touzani O, Muir KW, Lees KR, Macrae IM (2008) Effects of magnesium treatment in a model of internal capsule lesion in spontaneously hypertensive rats. *Stroke* 39:448-54.

Lee EJ, Ayoub IA, Harris FB, Hassan M, Ogilvy CS, Maynard KI (1999) Mexiletine and magnesium independently, but not combined, protect against permanent focal cerebral ischemia in Wistar rats. *J Neurosci Res* 58:442-8.

Lee EJ, Lee MY, Chang GL, Chen LH, Hu YL, Chen TY, Wu TS (2005) Delayed treatment with magnesium: reduction of brain infarction and improvement of electrophysiological recovery following transient focal cerebral ischemia in rats. *J Neurosurg* 102:1085-93.

Lee M-S, Wu YS, Yang DY, Lee JB, Cheng FC (2002) Significantly decreased extracellular magnesium in brains of gerbils subjected to cerebral ischemia. *Clin Chim Acta* 318:121-5.

Lin J-Y, Chung S-Y, Lin MC, Cheng FC (2002) Effects of magnesium sulfate on energy metabolites and glutamate in the cortex during focal cerebral ischemia and reperfusion in the gerbil monitored by a dual-probe microdialysis technique. *Life Sci* 71:803-11.

Marinov MB, Harbaugh KS, Hoopes PJ, Pikus HJ, Harbaugh RE (1996) Neuroprotective effects of preischemia intraarterial magnesium sulfate in reversible focal cerebral ischemia. *J Neurosurgery* 85:117-24.

McIntosh TK, Faden AI, Yamakami I, Vink R (1988) Magnesium deficiency exacerbates and pre-treatment improves outcome following traumatic brain injury in rats: ^{31}P magnetic resonance spectroscopy and behavioral studies. *J Neurotrauma* 5:17-30.

Meloni BP, Campbell K, Zhu H, Knuckey NW (2009) In search of clinical neuroprotection after brain ischemia: the case for mild hypothermia (35°C) and magnesium. *Stroke 40*:2236-40.

Meloni BP, Zhu H, Knuckey NW (2006) Is magnesium neuroprotective following global and focal cerebral ischaemia? A review of published studies. *Magnes Res* 19:123-37.

Milani H, Lepri ER, Giordani F, Favero-Filho LA (1999) Magnesium chloride alone or in combination with diazepam fails to prevent hippocampal damage following transient forebrain ischemia. *Braz J Med Biol* Res 32:1285-93.

Miles AN, Majda BT, Meloni BP, Knuckey NW (2001) Postischemic intravenous administration of magnesium sulfate inhibits hippocampal CA1 neuronal death after transient global ischemia in rats. *Neurosurgery* 49:1443-51.

Muir KW (1998) New experimental and clinical data on the efficacy of pharmacological magnesium infusions in cerebral infarcts. *Magnes Res* 11:43-56.

Muir KW, Lees KR (1995) A randomised, double blind, placebo-controlled pilot trial of intravenous magnesium sulphate in acute stroke. *Stroke* 26:1183-8.

Muir KW, Lees KR (1998) Dose optimization of intravenous magnesium sulphate after acute stroke. *Stroke* 29:918-23.

Nowak L, Bregestovski P, Ascher P, Herbet A, Prochiantz A (1984) Magnesium gates glutamate-activated channels in mouse central neurones. *Nature* 307:462-5.

Okawa M (1992) Effects of magnesium sulfate on brain damage by complete global brain ischemia (Japanese). *Masui (Jap J Anesthesiol)* 41:341-55.

Polderman KS (2009) Mechanisms of action, physiological effects, and complications of Hypothermia. *Crit Care Med* 37 (Suppl.): S186 –S202.

Roffe C, Thomas L, Fotheringham A, Davies I (1996) The effect of magnesium on infarct size and oedema after middle cerebral artery occlusion. *Cerebrovasc Dis* 6 (Supplement 2):42 (Abstract).

Saver JL, Kidwell C, Eckstein M, Starkmam S (2004) Pre-hospital neuroprotective therapy for acute stroke: results of the field administration of stroke therapy-magnesium (FAST-MAG) pilot trial. *Stroke* 35, e106-8.

Schmid-Elsaesser R, Zausinger S, Hungerhuber E, Baethmann A, Reulen HJ (1999) Neuroprotective effects of combination therapy with tirilazad and magnesium in rats subjected to reversible focal cerebral ischemia. *Neurosurgery* 44:163-72.

Sirin BH, Coskun E, Yilik L, Ortac R, Sirin H, Tetik C (1998) Neuroprotective effects of preischemia subcutaneous magnesium sulfate in transient cerebral ischemia. *Eur J Cardiothorac Surg* 14:82-8.

Sjöström LG, Wester PO (1990) Accumulation of magnesium in rat brain after intravenously induced hypermagnesemia. *Cerebrovasc Dis* 5: 241 (Abstract).

Stroke Trials Directory (2010). www.stroke.org/.
Tsuda T, Kogure K, Nishioka K, Watanabe T (1991) Mg^{2+} administered up to twenty-four hours following reperfusion prevents ischemic damage of the CA1 neurons in the rat hippocampus. *Neuroscience* 44:335-41.

Van den Bergh WM, Zuur JK, Kamerling NA, Van Asseldonk JT, Rinkel GJ, Tulleken CA, Nicolay K (2002) Role of magnesium in the reduction of ischemic depolarisation and lesion volume after experimental subarachnoid hemorrhage. *J Neurosurg* 97:416-22.

Vande Linde AMQ, Chopp M (1991) Chronic changes in brain Mg^{2+} concentration after forebrain ischemia in the rat. *Metab Brain Dis* 6:199-206.

Vink R, Heath DL, McIntosh TK (1996) Acute and prolonged alterations in brain free magnesium following fluid percussion-induced brain trauma in rats. *J Neurochem* 66:2477-83.

Vink R, McIntosh TK, Demediuk P, Weiner MW, Faden AI (1988) Decline in intracellular free Mg^{2+} is associated with irreversible tissue injury after brain trauma. *J Biol Chem* 263:757-61.

Wadhwa A, Sengupta P, Durrani J, Akca O, Lenhardt R, Sessler DI, Doufas AG (2005) Magnesium sulphate only slightly reduces the shivering threshold in humans. *Br J Anaesth* 94:756-62.

Welsh FA, Sims RE, Harris VA (1990) Mild hypothermia prevents ischemic injury in gerbil hippocampus. *J Cereb Blood Flow Metab* 10:557-63.

Westermaier T, Hungerhuber E, Zausinger S, Baethmann A, Schmid-Elsaesser R (2003) Neuroprotective efficacy of intra-arterial and intravenous magnesium sulfate in a rat model of transient focal cerebral ischemia. *Acta Neurochir* 145:393-9.

Westermaier T, Zausinger S, Baethmann A, Schmid-Elsaesser R (2005) Dose finding of intravenous magnesium sulphate in transient focal cerebral ischemia in rats. *Acta Neurochir* 147:525-32.

Xu M, Dai W, Deng X (2002) Effects of magnesium sulfate on brain mitochondrial respiratory function in rats after experimental traumatic brain injury. *Chin J Traumatol* 5:361-4.

Yang Y, Li Q, Ahmad F, Shuaib A (2000) Survival and histological evaluation of therapeutic window of post-ischemia treatment with magnesium sulfate in embolic stroke model of rat. *Neurosci Lett* 285:119-22.

Zausinger S, Schöller K, Plesnila N, Schmid-Elsaesser R (2003a) Combination drug therapy and mild hypothermia after transient focal cerebral ischemia in rats. *Stroke* 34:2246-51

Zausinger S, Westermaier T, Plesnila N, Steiger HJ, Schmid-Elsaesser R (2003b) Neuroprotection in transient focal cerebral ischemia by combination drug therapy and mild hypothermia: comparison with customary therapeutic regimen. *Stroke* 34:1526-32.

Zhou H, Ma Y, Zhou Y, Liu Z, Wang K, Cheng G (2003) Effects of magnesium sulfate on neuron apoptosis and expression of caspase-3, bax and bcl-2 after cerebral ischemia-reperfusion injury. *Chin Med J* 116:1532-34.

Zhu H, Martin RL, Meloni BP, Oltvolgyi C, Moore S, Majda BT, Knuckey NW (2004a) Magnesium sulfate fails to reduce infarct volume following transient focal ischemia in rats. *Neurosci Res* 49:347-53.

Zhu H, Meloni BP, Bojarski C, Knuckey MW, Knuckey NW (2005) Post-ischemic modest hypothermia (35°C) combined with intravenous magnesium is more effective at reducing CA1 death than either treatment used alone following global cerebral ischemia in rats. *Exp Neurol* 193:361-8.

Zhu H, Meloni BP, Moore SR, Majda BT, Knuckey NW (2004b) Intravenous administration of magnesium is only neuroprotective following transient global ischemia when present with post-ischemic mild hypothermia. *Brain Res* 1014:53-60.

Zweifler RM, Voorhees ME, Mahmood MA, Parnell M (2004) Magnesium sulfate increases the rate of hypothermia via surface cooling and improves comfort. *Stroke* 35:2331-4.

Magnesium in subarachnoid hemorrhage

Walter M. van den Bergh✉

Department of Intensive Care, Academic Medical Center, Amsterdam, The Netherlands.
✉ w.m.vandenbergh@amc.nl

Abstract

Subarachnoid hemorrhage caused by a ruptured aneurysm accounts for only 5% of strokes, but occurs at a fairly young age and carries a worse prognosis. Delayed cerebral ischemia is an important cause of death and dependence after aneurysmal SAH. The current mainstay of preventing delayed cerebral ischemia is nimodipine and maintenance of normovolemia, but even with this strategy delayed cerebral ischemia occurs in a considerable proportion of patients. Magnesium is an inexpensive, easily available neuroprotective agent that reduces cerebral vasospasm and infarct volume after experimental subarachnoid hemorrhage. In a meta-analysis of all randomized clinical trials, magnesium shows a tendency to reduce the occurrence of delayed cerebral ischemia and poor outcome after subarachnoid hemorrhage, but the question if magnesium is advantageous in subarachnoid hemorrhage patients is still in abeyance. Currently a large phase III trial aiming for 1200 patients is being conducted that will hopefully provide definite evidence whether magnesium treatment is beneficial in subarachnoid hemorrhage patients.

Subarachnoid hemorrhage

Subarachnoid hemorrhage (SAH) caused by a ruptured aneurysm accounts for only 5% of strokes, but occurs at a fairly young age and carries a worse prognosis than other types of stroke (van Gijn *et al*, 2007). The cardinal feature is a history of unusually severe headache that started suddenly, but patients frequent deteriorate into unconsciousness shortly after onset. On admission two-thirds of all patients have depressed consciousness, of whom half are in coma (Brilstra *et al*, 2000) The school of Hippocrates already described the clinical picture of a subarachnoid hemorrhage; " When persons in good health are suddenly seized with pains in the head, and straightway are laid down speechless, and breathe with stertor, they die in seven days, unless fever comes on" (Hippocrates *et al*, 1527; Clarke, 1963). Attila the Hun is suspected to had a subarachnoid hemorrhage as he died suddenly during sexual intercourse after severe headache (Babinski, 1893).

The incidence of SAH in most populations is 6-7 per 100000 person-years (Linn *et al*, 1996) About one in eight patients die before reaching the hospital. The in-hospital case fatality is about one-third (Nieuwkamp *et al*, 2009). Of patients who survive the SAH approximately one-third remain dependent. Because of the young age SAH occurs and its poor prognosis, the loss of productive life years from SAH is as large as that from ischemic stroke, the most frequent subtype of stroke.

The presence of an aneurysm was first demonstrated by an angiograph of the carotid artery by Moniz (Moniz, 1933) in 1933, 6 years after he had introduced this technique (Moniz, 1927) Aneurysms arise at sites of arterial branching, usually at the base of the brain, either on the circle of Willis itself or at a nearby branching point. Most intracranial aneurysms will never rupture. Risk factors for subarachnoid hemorrhage are hypertension, smoking, and excessive alcohol intake, all of which more-or-less double the risk (Feigin *et al*, 2005).

Diagnosis is made by CT brain scanning. Recurrent bleeding is the most imminent danger; a first aim is therefore occlusion of the aneurysm. Endovascular obliteration by means of platinum spirals (coiling) is the preferred mode of treatment, but some patients require a direct neurosurgical approach (clipping) (Molyneux *et al*, 2002).

Delayed cerebral ischemia

For those patients who survive the first 24 hours after the hemorrhage, delayed cerebral ischemia (DCI) is consistently the leading cause of death and disability, adversely affecting more than one in five of all patients who have suffered SAH and survived (Dorsch, 1995; Roos *et al*, 2000).

Unlike thrombo-embolic stroke, cerebral ischemia after subarachnoid hemorrhage has a gradual onset and often involves more than the territory of a single cerebral artery or one of its branches. The clinical manifestations evolve gradually, over several hours, and consist of hemispheric focal deficits, a reduction in the level of consciousness, or both. It is mainly a diagnosis of exclusion, when clinical deterioration occurs and hydrocephalus, recurrent bleeding, hypoxia, and metabolic abnormalities have been ruled out. The peak frequency of cerebral ischemia is from 5 to 14 days after subarachnoid hemorrhage. The time course for delayed cerebral ischemia parallels that of angiographic vasospasm, but arterial narrowing – a complex process in itself – is neither a necessary nor a sufficient condition; although about 70% of patients may develop arterial narrowing, only 20-30% will manifest neurological deficits (Weir *et al*, 1999; Rabinstein *et al*, 2004).

Nimodipine is a dihydropyridine calcium channel blocker that selectively blocks the voltage-dependent L-type calcium channel. Nimodipine is accepted as beneficial in preventing DCI and subsequent poor outcome when given orally 6 times 60 mg. for 21 days after the hemorrhage (Dorhout Mees *et al*, 2007b). The initial thought was that nimodipine could prevent or ameliorate cerebral vasospasm, but nimodipine does not influence large vessel diameter and its pivotal method of action must be explained otherwise.

Cerebral vasospasm, although often used as a synonym, apparently is a too simplistic explanation for delayed cerebral ischemia. Research, however, has focused on the mechanisms involved in the development of cerebral vasospasm as a mean by which cerebral ischemia can be prevented. The precise underlying pathogenic mechanisms remain obscure, but it seems that endothelial mechanisms provide the most prominent contribution to this process and there is growing evidence that the constituents of a subarachnoid blood clot, especially oxyhemoglobin, a product of hemoglobin breakdown, seem to be the principle initiating factor (Pluta *et al*, 1998; Dumont *et al*, 2003; Kolias *et al*, 2009).

The current mainstay of preventing and treat DCI include neuroprotection with nimodipine and maintenance of normovolemia, but even with this strategy DCI still occurs in up to 30% of patients and improvement in clinical outcome has been modest (Hop *et al*, 1997; Brilstra *et al*, 2000; Roos *et al*, 2000; Dorhout Mees *et al*, 2008). Reducing the consequences of ischemia through neuroprotection may therefore improve outcome after SAH. DCI after subarachnoid hemorrhage is a unique pathophysiological process because the timing and development of potential cerebral ischemia can be predicted; the interval of 4 days or more between the bleeding and the onset of ischemia provides an opportunity for preventive treatment.

Magnesium and cerebral ischemia, opportunities and concerns

Magnesium is a popular drug for acute treatment of ischemia because of its ease of use, low cost, and favorable side-effect profile. In several experimental models of cerebral ischemia a significant neuroprotective effect of magnesium is demonstrated, with reported infarct reduction of 25 to 61% (Izumi *et al*, 1991; Marinov *et al*, 1996; Muir, 1998). Putative modes of action include inhibition of the presynaptic release of the excitatory amino acid glutamate, and blockade of the postsynaptic NMDA glutamate receptor and voltage dependent calcium channels (van den Bergh *et al*, 2004b). Magnesium reduces the production of endothelin and completely attenuates the vasoconstrictive effect of endothelin, possibly by inhibiting calcium channels mediated smooth-muscle contraction (Kemp *et al*, 1999; Berthon *et al*, 2003). Furthermore, magnesium increases cardiac contractility, which may improve cerebral perfusion in dysautoregulated brain tissue.

However, acute ischemic stroke has not the quality of cerebral vasospasm associated DCI in subarachnoid hemorrhage that occurs mostly more than 4 days after the initial bleeding, allowing the administration of a treatment before ischemia develops. Delayed treatment might explain why magnesium was ineffective in ischemic stroke in the IMAGES study (Muir *et al*, 2004). Again a precedent exists for nimodipine, which was ineffective when tested in ischemic stroke. A study of acute administration of magnesium in stroke (FAST-MAG) is underway (Saver *et al*, 2004).

Another concern about the suitability of magnesium to protect the ischemic brain is that regulation of cerebrospinal fluid magnesium is largely maintained following acute brain injury and limits the brain bioavailability of magnesium sulfate. Current dose regimens may only marginally increase concentrations of magnesium in CSF (McKee *et al*, 2005) in brain-injured humans this modest increase occurs in the range of 10 to 19%. However, experimental evidence suggests that this modest elevation may be sufficient for neuroprotection. In a study using ^{31}P-MR spectroscopy (MRS) to investigate intracellular brain free magnesium 37 patients with good-grade aneurysmal SAH patients randomized for magnesium therapy were compared (Wong *et al*, 2009). Magnesium treatment after aneurysmal SAH produced a small (+13%; mean difference 0.018 ± 0.007 mM), but significant elevation of intracellular free magnesium. In a RCT were magnesium therapy was compared with nimodipine, CSF magnesium concentration was non statistically significant higher in the magnesium group; 1.19 ± 0.20 vs. 1.14 ± 0.21 (p= 0.26) (Schmid-Elsaesser *et al*, 2006).

The negative effect of magnesium on blood pressure may also have an impact on results. Currently vasopressors after often used to prevent hypotension in SAH patients and DCI is often treated with induced hypertension with the aim to increase cerebral perfusion. However, the lowering effect of magnesium on blood pressure is limited and far less than that of nimodipine.

Finally, there is a dose related association between magnesium sulfate administration and hypocalcaemia, but symptomatic hypocalcaemia is rare and it does not result in an increased risk of poor outcome (van den Bergh *et al*, 2008b). There is no base for routine suppletion of calcium in patients with hypocalcaemia when treated with magnesium. Of course suppletion might be considered in individual patients to prevent isolated clinical symptoms of hypocalcaemia such as muscle weakness or cardiac arrhythmias.

Hypomagnesemia in subarachnoid hemorrhage

In observational clinical studies the vast majority of SAH patients develop hypomagnesaemia at some time within three weeks after the hemorrhage (Warren *et al*, 1993; van den Bergh *et al*, 2003). Low magnesium serum levels are frequently present at admission and are thus most likely caused by intracellular shift of magnesium ions. Intracellular Mg^{2+} levels are indeed increased in SAH. However, 90% of the intracellular Mg^{2+} is complexed with ATP, and the increase of intracellular Mg^{2+} during ischemia may also be the result of the release of Mg^{2+} from this complex. ATP binds with Mg^{2+} with an associate constant of 4, while binding affinity with ADP is about 2 times smaller. The cytosolic and mitochondrial Mg^{2+} concentration will increase in cells with a poor energy state and less ATP (Jung *et al*, 1990; Saris *et al*, 2000; Wong *et al*, 2009). The increase of intracellular Mg^{2+} is even less than might be expected from ATP utilization. Probably because of a disappearance of Mg^{2+} by binding to other cell components. Hypomagnesaemia that developed later on in the course might also be caused by renal loss as very often is the case in critically ill patients.

The diminished availability and subsequent decreased extracellular Mg^{2+} after SAH results in significantly increased intracellular free Ca^{2+} in cerebral vascular muscle cells. This may cause cerebral microvascular constriction, followed by a proinflammatory response, inducing vascular smooth muscle, endothelial and neuronal cell damage (Barbour *et al*, 2002). Furthermore, hypomagnesaemia results in a reduced endothelial NO release by which means hypomagnesaemia can induce vasoconstriction (Pearson *et al*, 1998; Shechter 2000). All the above gives rise to the concept of a causal relation between the decreased availability of magnesium and the development of vasospasm associated DCI. When testing this hypothesis in 107 prospectively studied consecutive patients, we found that hypomagnesaemia during day 4 and 10 after the hemorrhage increased the risk for DCI three folded (van den Bergh *et al*, 2003).

Apart from DCI, in a study in 62 patients more than one-third had hypomagnesaemia at admission which was independent related to cardiac dysrhythmias, especially a long PR interval and a shorter QTc interval (van den Bergh *et al*, 2004a). This link with cardiac complications might be another reason why hypomagnesaemia may be related to poor outcome (van der Bilt *et al*, 2009).

Magnesium treatment in subarachnoid hemorrhage

Animal studies

Magnesium has a vasorelaxing effect in oxyhemoglobin-induced vasospasm and it ameliorates cerebral vasospasm in experimental SAH, (Miura, 1988; Ram *et al*, 1991; Pyne *et al*, 2001) although no effect of magnesium sulfate on the angiographic diameter of large cerebral vessels in a monkey model of SAH could be noted (Macdonald *et al*, 2004). Neither does magnesium infusion decrease middle cerebral artery blood flow velocities in patients with DCI [*unpublished data*].

Magnesium induces a dose-dependent vasodilatation, reduces cerebrovascular tone, increases CBF and protects the metabolism (Seelig *et al*, 1983; Altura and Altura 1984; Torregrosa *et al*, 1994) However, in a human study in 6 patients magnesium sulfate infusion did not increase cerebral blood volume and cerebral blood flow compared with pre-treatment levels or compared with 6 control patients (Wong *et al*, 2010a).

We have demonstrated in an experimental model that the duration of ischemic depolarization's after SAH is substantially reduced after pre-treatment with magnesium sulfate (van den Bergh *et al*, 2002). Magnesium also postpones anoxic depolarization (van der Hel *et al*, 1998). This maintenance of the membrane potential may at least partly explain the neuroprotective properties of magnesium in SAH. We have shown in a rat model of SAH that pre-treatment with magnesium sulfate reduces acute cerebral lesion volume with more than 60% (van den Bergh *et al*, 2002).

Large randomized controlled trials

In 2005 the "Magnesium and Acetylsalicylic acid in Subarachnoid Hemorrhage" (MASH-I) trial was published, in which 283 patients between November 2000 and January 2004 were randomized to placebo or a continuous infusion of 64 mmol/l/day of magnesium sulfate starting within 4 days of SAH and continuing 14 days after occlusion of the aneurysm (van den Bergh *et al*, 2005). The results showed a trend towards less cerebral ischemia in patients allocated to magnesium and improved overall outcome, with a 35% reduction in DCI (RR 0.65; 95% CI 0.40–1.05) and a 23% reduction in poor outcomes (RR 0.77; 0.54–1.09). The mean magnesium level during treatment was 1.47 ± 0.32 mmol/L, side effects were mild and sparse (van Norden *et al*, 2005). A post-hoc analysis suggests that the treatment effect of magnesium is larger after endovascular occlusion than after neurosurgical clipping, which underlines the conclusion that further trials are not at risk to be underpowered if the proportion of endovascular treated patients increases (van den Bergh *et al*, 2009).

In 2010 the results of the Intravenous Magnesium Sulfate in Aneurysmal Subarachnoid Hemorrhage (IMASH) trial were published (Wong *et al*, 2010b). IMASH was a phase III randomized, clinical international multicentre trial that evaluate the effect of magnesium sulfate on the clinical outcome of 327 patients with aneurysmal SAH, of which 90% were recruited in Hong Kong and China and the remaining 10% in Australia from 2002 to 2008. After randomization 20 mmol of magnesium sulfate was given over 30 minutes, followed by infusion of 80 mmol/day or equivalent volume of saline within 48 h after onset of symptom and continued for up to 14 days from the day of hemorrhage. Mean time from ictus to start of study drug infusion was 32 +/- 15 SD hours. More than 90% of the patients completed at least 10 days of study drug infusion. The randomization was single-blind; the study aims for a plasma magnesium concentration in the treatment group of twice the serum baseline level but below 2.5 mmol/L. Average serum magnesium concentrations in the treatment group were 1.67 ± 0.27 mmol/L compared with 0.91 ± 0.16 mmol/L in controls.

The proportion of patients with a 6-month favorable outcome, defined as an extended Glasgow Outcome Scale 5 to 8, were similar for both treatment groups (OR 1.0; 95% CI 0.7-1.6). Also in the secondary outcome analyses, which includes incidence of clinical vasospasm, Barthel Index, modified Rankin score, modified National Institute of Health Stroke Score, and MCA velocities as measured by transcranial Doppler, there were no significant differences between the 2 groups.

Although the study was underpowered, the results do not support a significant clinical benefit of magnesium therapy in SAH. Possible explanations for the differences in results between MASH-1 and IMASH are the assumed predominant Asian origin of recruited patients and the time window of administration; too late or too short. In the MASH-1 study the median start of treatment was 28 hours, and it was continued for at least 2 weeks. On the other hand, the achieved serum magnesium concentration might have been too high, as in the treatment group higher magnesium concentrations were associated with a worse outcome (Wong *et al*, 2010c). Furthermore, the average serum magnesium concentration of 0.91 ± 0.16 mmol/L in the control group was quit high and could have diluted the results.

Is there an optimal serum magnesium concentration for neuroprotection?

In animal models of stroke, evidence was found for a dose–response effect, with optimal serum magnesium concentrations of approximately 1.40 to 1.50 mmol/l (Marinov *et al*, 1996; Yang *et al*, 2000; Miles *et al*, 2001).

The mean serum magnesium level of 1.47 mmol/L achieved in the MASH-1 study was close to the proposed optimal serum magnesium level for achieving maximal neuroprotection. In a sub-study performed in patients with a serum magnesium concentration ≥ 1.10 mmol/L we found no linear relationship between serum magnesium levels and risk reduction for DCI (Dorhout Mees *et al*, 2007a). Magnesium sulfate therapy results in a stable risk reduction of DCI over a broad range of achieved serum magnesium concentrations, and strict titration of the dosage therefore does not seem necessary, although concentrations below 1.28 mmol/l could decrease the effect on DCI. In contrast, no such relationship was observed for poor outcome; risks tended to be higher in patients with magnesium concentrations above the 75th percentile (1.62 mmol/L) with an OR for poor outcome of 4.9 (95% CI 1.2 to 19.7) in patients with a serum concentration above 1.62 mmol/L compared to the lowest quartile (1.10-1.28 mmol/L).

The aim of the IMASH study to achieve a plasma magnesium concentration of twice the serum baseline level resulted in an average serum magnesium concentration in the treatment group of 1.67 +/- 0.27 mmol/L, which might have had a negative effect on clinical outcome. Of course an optimal neuroprotective concentration of serum magnesium can only be validated if current large trials show that magnesium therapy is effective.

Systematic review and meta-analysis

We assessed in a systematic review whether magnesium decreases the occurrence of secondary ischemia and poor outcome after aneurysmal subarachnoid hemorrhage. We sought to identify all unconfounded clinical controlled trials with magnesium in patients with aneurysmal SAH. Trials were identified in the Stroke Group Trials Register of the Cochrane Library, PUBMED and MEDLINE. Outcome measures were DCI and poor outcome. An estimate of the treatment effect across trials was calculated with the Mantel-Haenszel method according to the intention-to-treat principle.

Between 2002 and 2010 four non-randomized and eight randomized controlled trials on magnesium were published, all but one compared magnesium therapy with placebo in addition to nimodipine. The exception was a small RCT in 104 patients that found similar outcomes in patients treated with nimodipine versus patients treated with magnesium (Schmid-Elsaesser *et al*, 2006). When the four non-randomized studies are combined, 118 patients with magnesium therapy were compared with a historical control group of 138 patients (Chia *et al*, 2002; Prevedello *et al*, 2006; Stippler *et al*, 2006; Friedlich *et al*, 2009). When the results are pooled it all boils down to the conclusion that a trend towards less symptomatic vasospasm was found in favor of the treatment group and, if provided, a positive effect with a less extent on outcome.

Table 1: Characteristics and results of randomized control trials of magnesium in aneurysmal subarachnoid hemorrhage.

Year **Author** ***Journal***	**Start**	**Duration**	**Bolus (mmol)**	**Infusion**	**Target** $[Mg]_s$ **(mmol/L)**	**Sample size (Mg/controls) Total**	**DCI** **RR [95%CI]**	**Poor outcome** **RR [95%CI]**
2002 Veyna *J Neurosurg*	< 3 days	10 days	25 / 30min	144 mmol/d	1.6-2.3	(20/20) 40	0.96 [0.36-2.58	0.70 [0.32-1.52
2005 Van den Bergh *Stroke*	< 4 days	14 days after occlusion aneurysma	no	64 mmol/d	1.0-2.0	(139/144) 283	0.65 [0.40-1.05]	0.77 [0.54-1.09]
2006 Wong *Neurosurg Anesthesiol*	< 2 days	14 days	20 / 30min	80 mmol/d	2x baseline but < 2.5	(30/30) 60	0.54 [0.25-1.16]	0.71 [0.38-1.35
2006 Schmid-Elsaesser *Neurosurgery*	< 4 days	7-21 days or TCD < 120 cm/s	0.4 mmol/kg	1.2 mmol/kg	2x baseline	(53/51) 104	no differences vs. nimodipine	no differences vs. nimodipine
2008 Muroi *Surg Neurol*	< 3 days	12 days	16 / 15min	64 mmol/d, adjusted every 12 h	2x baseline	(31/27) 58	0.87 [0.24-3.15]	0.68 [0.38-1.25]
2009 Akdemir *Neurosurg Q*	< 3 days	10 days after occlusion aneurysma	20 / 30min	64 mmol/d, adjusted daily	1.0-2.0	(40/43) 83	TCD values only	1.43 [0.68-3.03]
2010 Westermaier *Crit Care Med*	< 4 days	10 days	16 / 30min	8 mmol/h, adjusted every 8 hours	2.0-2.5	(54/53) 107	0.44 [0.25-0.77]	0.75 [0.48-1.18]
2010 Wong *Stroke*	< 2 days	14 days	20 / 30min	80 mmol/d	2x baseline but < 2.5	(169/158) 327	1.35 [0.89-2.06]	0.98 [0.74-1.31]

Seven trials totaling 954 patients were eligible for the meta-analyses [Table 1] (Veyna *et al*, 2002; van den Bergh *et al*, 2005; Wong *et al*, 2006; Muroi *et al*, 2008; Westermaier *et al*, 2010; Akdemir *et al*, 2010; Wong *et al*, 2010b). All used magnesium sulfate in addition to nimodipine. The overall relative risk for DCI was 0.86 (95% CI 0.67-1.11) (Figure 1), and for poor outcome 0.89 (95% CI 0.78-1.02) (Figure 2).

Headache

In patients with SAH, headache typically is severe, usually lasts for 1 to 2 weeks and often requires treatment with opioids. Opioids, however, have a wide range of potential side effects, which may have a negative effect on patient comfort and functional outcome. Blocking of the NMDA receptor is thought to be involved in pain modulation by preventing the induction of central pain sensitization. Several studies have reported that magnesium reduces perioperative pain or analgesic requirements. Headache relief would be an important additional effect of magnesium because this would reduce the need of opioids with their potentially harmful side effects. In a sub-study of the MASH-1 trial we found that magnesium treatment was associated with less severe headache and less frequent use of opioids (Dorhout Mees *et al*, 2010). These data imply that intravenous magnesium therapy, besides a supposed beneficial effect on outcome, also provides pain relief for SAH patients.

On-going phase 3 clinical controlled trials

There is currently one on-going phase 3 clinical controlled trial evaluating the effect of magnesium in SAH; the Magnesium in Aneurysmal Subarachnoid Hemorrhage (MASH-II) study is a phase III randomized, clinical international multicentre trial that studies the effect of magnesium sulfate after aneurysmal SAH [ISRCTN68742385] (van der Bilt *et al*, 2009). Study medication (magnesium sulfate 64 mmol/day or placebo) is given via continuous infusion within 4 days and until 20 days after the hemorrhage. Outcome is determined with the

Figure 1. Studies with magnesium in addition to nimodipine – effect on delayed cerebral ischemia.

Study or Subgroup	Treatment Events	Treatment Total	Control Events	Control Total	Weight	Risk Ratio M-H, Fixed, 95% CI
van den Bergh 2005	22	139	35	144	33.6%	0.65 [0.40, 1.05]
Veyna 2002	6	20	5	16	5.4%	0.96 [0.36, 2.58]
Wong 2006	7	30	13	30	12.7%	0.54 [0.25, 1.16]
Muroi 2008	4	31	4	27	4.2%	0.87 [0.24, 3.15]
Wong 2010	42	169	29	158	29.3%	1.35 [0.89, 2.06]
Westermaier 2010	9	54	15	53	14.8%	0.59 [0.28, 1.23]
Total (95% CI)		**443**		**428**	**100.0%**	**0.86 [0.67, 1.11]**
Total events	90		101			

Heterogeneity: Chi² = 8.27, df = 5 (P = 0.14); I² = 40%
Test for overall effect: Z = 1.18 (P = 0.24)

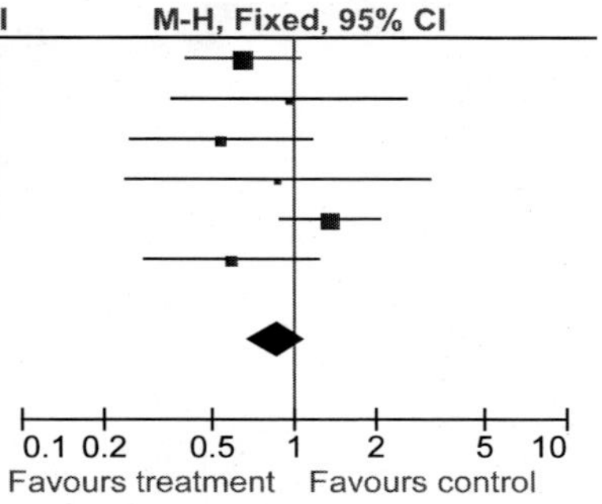

Figure 2. Studies with magnesium in addition to nimodipine – effect on poor outcome.

Study or Subgroup	Treatment Events	Treatment Total	Control Events	Control Total	Weight	Risk Ratio M-H, Fixed, 95% CI
Akdemir 2009	12	40	9	43	3.8%	1.43 [0.68, 3.03]
Muroi 2008	11	31	14	27	6.6%	0.68 [0.38, 1.24]
van den Bergh 2005	38	139	51	144	22.1%	0.77 [0.54, 1.09]
Veyna 2002	7	20	8	16	3.9%	0.70 [0.32, 1.52]
Westermaier 2010	20	54	26	53	11.6%	0.75 [0.48, 1.18]
Wong 2006	10	30	14	30	6.2%	0.71 [0.38, 1.35]
Wong 2010	108	169	100	158	45.7%	1.01 [0.86, 1.19]
Total (95% CI)		**483**		**471**	**100.0%**	**0.89 [0.78, 1.02]**
Total events	206		222			

Heterogeneity: Chi² = 6.54, df = 6 (P = 0.37); I² = 8%
Test for overall effect: Z = 1.66 (P = 0.10)

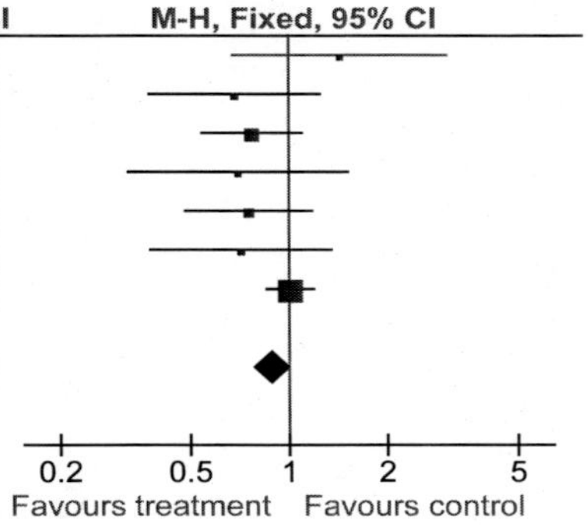

modified Rankin scale three months after the hemorrhage. Analysis will be according to the intention-to-treat principle. So far, in August 2010 over 1000 patients have been included in 6 Dutch, 1 UK, and 1 Chilean hospital. Based on the results of the MASH-1 study sample size calculations indicate that 1200 patients are needed to give a statistically significant result (with $\alpha = 5\%$ and a power of 80%). We aim to include these patients before the end of 2011. A first interim analysis was performed after 300 patients and the second and last interim analysis was performed after recruitment and follow-up of 750 patients. At both interim analyses the Data Monitoring Committee gave a unanimous advice to continue the study.

Conclusion

In conclusion, magnesium is a promising agent to prevent the occurrence of delayed cerebral ischemia and to improve outcome in patients with SAH. Hence, at present, the evidence is insufficient and larger randomized controlled trials are needed to determine the safety and efficacy of magnesium sulfate infusion before it can be recommended for patients with aneurysmal SAH. Currently a large phase III trial is being conducted that will hopefully provide definite evidence whether magnesium treatment is beneficial in SAH patients.

In the meantime, it is probably wise to maintain serum magnesium in the high-normal range, e.g. 0.8-1.0 mmol/l, after SAH to prevent the hypomagnesaemia associated neurological and cardiac complications. Magnesium therapy can be considered as a safe alternative for morphine in the treatment of headache. In case magnesium therapy is considered as a remedy to improve outcome, target serum magnesium levels are probably around 1.4 mmol/l and better not exceed 1.6 mmol/l.

Acknowledgements

The Netherlands Heart Foundation (grants 99.107 and 2005B016) and the Dutch Brain Foundation (grants *8F00(2).26 and 15F07(2)* are gratefully acknowledged for their financial support for some of the studied mentioned in this overview. Drs. Sanne Dorhout Mees is gratefully acknowledged for her assistance with the meta-analysis.

References

Akdemir H, Kulaksizoglu EO, Tucer B, Menku A, Postalci L, Gunaldi O (2010) Magnesium sulfate therapy for cerebral vasospasm after aneurysmal subarachnoid hemorrhage. *Neurosurg Q* 19:35-39.

Altura BT, Altura BM (1984) Interactions of Mg and K on cerebral vessels--aspects in view of stroke. Review of present status and new findings. *Magnesium* 3:195-211.

Babinski J (1893) Contractures organique et hystérique. *Bull Soc méd Hôp* 3:327-343.

Barbour RL, Gebrewold A, Altura BT, Altura BM (2002) Optical spectroscopy and prevention of deleterious cerebral vascular effects of ethanol by magnesium ions. *Eur J Pharmacol* 447:79-86.

Berthon N, Laurant P, Fellmann D, Berthelot A (2003) Effect of magnesium on mRNA expression and production of endothelin-1 in DOCA-salt hypertensive rats. *J Cardiovasc Pharmacol* 42:24-31.

Brilstra EH, Rinkel GJ, Algra A, van Gijn J (2000) Rebleeding, secondary ischemia, and timing of operation in patients with subarachnoid hemorrhage. *Neurology* 55:1656-1660.

Chia RY, Hughes RS, Morgan MK (2002) Magnesium: a useful adjunct in the prevention of cerebral vasospasm following aneurysmal subarachnoid haemorrhage. *J Clin Neurosci* 9:279-281.

Clarke E (1963) Apoplexy in Hippocratic writings. *Bull Hist Med* 37:301.

Dorhout Mees SM, Bertens D, van der Worp HB, Rinkel GJ, van den Bergh WM (2010) Magnesium and headache after aneurysmal subarachnoid haemorrhage. *J Neurol Neurosurg Psychiatry* 81:490-493.

Dorhout Mees SM, Rinkel GJ, Feigin VL, Algra A, van den Bergh WM, Vermeulen M, van Gijn J (2008) Calcium Antagonists for Aneurysmal Subarachnoid Hemorrhage. *Stroke* [Epub ahead of print].

Dorhout Mees SM, van den Bergh WM, Algra A, Rinkel GJ (2007a) Achieved serum magnesium concentrations and occurrence of delayed cerebral ischaemia and poor outcome in aneurysmal subarachnoid haemorrhage. *J Neurol Neurosurg Psychiatry* 78:729-731.

Dorhout Mees SM, van den Bergh WM, Algra A, Rinkel GJ (2007b) Antiplatelet therapy for aneurysmal subarachnoid haemorrhage. *Cochrane Database Syst Rev*CD006184.

Dorsch NW (1995) Cerebral arterial spasm--a clinical review. *Br J Neurosurg* 9:403-412.

Dumont AS, Dumont RJ, Chow MM, Lin CL, Calisaneller T, Ley KF, Kassell NF, Lee KS (2003) Cerebral vasospasm after subarachnoid hemorrhage: putative role of inflammation. *Neurosurgery* 53:123-133.

Feigin VL, Rinkel GJ, Lawes CM, Algra A, Bennett DA, van GJ, Anderson CS (2005) Risk factors for subarachnoid hemorrhage: an updated systematic review of epidemiological studies. *Stroke* 36:2773-2780.

Friedlich D, Agner C, Boulos AS, Mesfin F, Feustel P, Bernardini GL, Popp AJ (2009) Retrospective analysis of parenteral magnesium sulfate administration in decreased incidence of clinical and neuroradiological cerebral vasospasm: a single center experience. *Neurol Res* 31:621-625.

Hippocrates:, Leonicenus N, Laurentianus L (1527) *(trans.) Aphorismi, cum Galeni Commentariis; Praedictiones, cum Galeni Commentariis*, Paris: Simon Sylvius.

Hop JW, Rinkel GJ, Algra A, van Gijn J (1997) Case-fatality rates and functional outcome after subarachnoid hemorrhage: a systematic review. *Stroke* 28:660-664.

Izumi Y, Roussel S, Pinard E, Seylaz J (1991) Reduction of infarct volume by magnesium after middle cerebral artery occlusion in rats. *J Cereb Blood Flow Metab* 11:1025-1030.

Jung DW, Apel L, Brierley GP (1990) Matrix free Mg2+ changes with metabolic state in isolated heart mitochondria. *Biochemistry* 29:4121-4128.

Kemp PA, Gardiner SM, March JE, Rubin PC, Bennett T (1999) Assessment of the effects of endothelin-1 and magnesium sulphate on regional blood flows in conscious rats, by the coloured microsphere reference technique. *Br J Pharmacol* 126:621-626.

Kolias AG, Sen J, Belli A (2009) Pathogenesis of cerebral vasospasm following aneurysmal subarachnoid hemorrhage: putative mechanisms and novel approaches. *J Neurosci Res* 87:1-11.

Linn FH, Rinkel GJ, Algra A, van Gijn J (1996) Incidence of subarachnoid hemorrhage: role of region, year, and rate of computed tomography: a meta-analysis. *Stroke* 27:625-629.

Macdonald RL, Curry DJ, Aihara Y, Zhang ZD, Jahromi BS, Yassari R (2004) Magnesium and experimental vasospasm. *J Neurosurg* 100:106-110

Marinov MB, Harbaugh KS, Hoopes PJ, Pikus HJ, Harbaugh RE (1996) Neuroprotective effects of preischemia intraarterial magnesium sulfate in reversible focal cerebral ischemia. *J Neurosurg* 85:117-124.

McKee JA, Brewer RP, Macy GE, Phillips-Bute B, Campbell KA, Borel CO, Reynolds JD, Warner DS (2005) Analysis of the brain bioavailability of peripherally administered magnesium sulfate: A study in humans with acute brain injury undergoing prolonged induced hypermagnesemia. *Crit Care Med* 33:661-666

Miles AN, Majda BT, Meloni BP, Knuckey NW (2001) Postischemic intravenous administration of magnesium sulfate inhibits hippocampal CA1 neuronal death after transient global ischemia in rats. *Neurosurgery* 49:1443-1450.

Miura K (1988) [Changes in Mg++ concentration of CSF after subarachnoid hemorrhage and Mg++--effects on the contractions of bovine cerebral artery]. *No Shinkei Geka* 16:1251-1259.

Molyneux A, Kerr R, Stratton I, Sandercock P, Clarke M, Shrimpton J, Holman R (2002) International Subarachnoid Aneurysm Trial (ISAT) of neurosurgical clipping versus endovascular coiling in 2143 patients with ruptured intracranial aneurysms: a randomised trial. *Lancet* 360:1267-1274.

Moniz E (1927) L'encéphalographie artérielle, son importance dans la localisation des tumeurs cérébrales. *Rev Neurol (Paris)* 48:72-90.

Moniz E (1933) Anévrysme intra-cranien de la carotide interne droite rendu visible par l'artériographie cérébrale. *Rev Oto-Neuro-Ophthal* 11:198-203.

Muir KW (1998) New experimental and clinical data on the efficacy of pharmacological magnesium infusions in cerebral infarcts. *Magnes Res* 11:43-56.

Muir KW, Lees KR, Ford I, Davis S (2004) Magnesium for acute stroke (Intravenous Magnesium Efficacy in Stroke trial): randomised controlled trial. *Lancet* 363:439-445.

Muroi C, Terzic A, Fortunati M, Yonekawa Y, Keller E (2008) Magnesium sulfate in the management of patients with aneurysmal subarachnoid hemorrhage: a randomized, placebo-controlled, dose-adapted trial. *Surg Neurol* 69:33-39.

Nieuwkamp DJ, Setz LE, Algra A, Linn FH, de Rooij NK, Rinkel GJ (2009) Changes in case fatality of aneurysmal subarachnoid haemorrhage over time, according to age, sex, and region: a meta-analysis. *Lancet Neurol* 8:635-642.

Pearson PJ, Evora PR, Seccombe JF, Schaff HV (1998) Hypomagnesemia inhibits nitric oxide release from coronary endothelium: protective role of magnesium infusion after cardiac operations. *Ann Thorac Surg* 65:967-972.

Pluta RM, Afshar JK, Boock RJ, Oldfield EH (1998) Temporal changes in perivascular concentrations of oxyhemoglobin, deoxyhemoglobin, and methemoglobin after subarachnoid hemorrhage. *J Neurosurg* 88:557-561

Prevedello DM, Cordeiro JG, de Morais AL, Saucedo NS, Jr., Chen IB, Araujo JC (2006) Magnesium sulfate: role as possible attenuating factor in vasospasm morbidity. *Surg Neurol* 65 Suppl 1:S1.

Pyne GJ, Cadoux-Hudson TA, Clark JF (2001) Magnesium protection against in vitro cerebral vasospasm after subarachnoid haemorrhage. *Br J Neurosurg* 15:409-415.

Rabinstein AA, Friedman JA, Weigand SD, McClelland RL, Fulgham JR, Manno EM, Atkinson JL, Wijdicks EF (2004) Predictors of cerebral infarction in aneurysmal subarachnoid hemorrhage. *Stroke* 35:1862-1866.

Ram Z, Sadeh M, Shacked I, Sahar A, Hadani M (1991) Magnesium sulfate reverses experimental delayed cerebral vasospasm after subarachnoid hemorrhage in rats. *Stroke* 22:922-927.

Roos YB, de Haan RJ, Beenen LF, Groen RJ, Albrecht KW, Vermeulen M (2000) Complications and outcome in patients with aneurysmal subarachnoid haemorrhage: a prospective hospital based cohort study in the Netherlands. *J Neurol Neurosurg Psychiatry* 68:337-341.

Saris NE, Mervaala E, Karppanen H, Khawaja JA, Lewenstam A (2000) Magnesium. An update on physiological, clinical and analytical aspects. *Clin Chim Acta* 294:1-26.

Saver JL, Kidwell C, Eckstein M, Starkman S (2004) Prehospital neuroprotective therapy for acute stroke: results of the Field Administration of Stroke Therapy-Magnesium (FAST-MAG) pilot trial. *Stroke* 35:e106-e108.

Schmid-Elsaesser R, Kunz M, Zausinger S, Prueckner S, Briegel J, Steiger HJ (2006) Intravenous magnesium versus nimodipine in the treatment of patients with aneurysmal subarachnoid hemorrhage: a randomized study. *Neurosurgery* 58:1054-1065.

Seelig JM, Wei EP, Kontos HA, Choi SC, Becker DP (1983) Effect of changes in magnesium ion concentration on cat cerebral arterioles. *Am J Physiol* 245:H22-H26.

Shechter M (2000) The role of magnesium as antithrombotic therapy. *Wien Med Wochenschr* 150:343-347

Stippler M, Crago E, Levy EI, Kerr ME, Yonas H, Horowitz MB, Kassam A (2006) Magnesium infusion for vasospasm prophylaxis after subarachnoid hemorrhage. *J Neurosurg* 105:723-729.

Torregrosa G, Perales AJ, Salom JB, Miranda FJ, Barbera MD, Alborch E (1994) Different effects of Mg2+ on endothelin-1- and 5-hydroxytryptamine-elicited responses in goat cerebrovascular bed. *J Cardiovasc Pharmacol* 23:1004-1010.

van den Bergh WM, Algra A, Rinkel GJ (2004a) Electrocardiographic abnormalities and serum magnesium in patients with subarachnoid hemorrhage. *Stroke* 35:644-648.

van den Bergh WM, Algra A, Rinkel GJ (2009) Magnesium and aspirin treatment in patients with subarachnoid haemorrhage: comparison of effects after endovascular and neurosurgical aneurysm occlusion. *J Neurol* 256:213-6.

van den Bergh WM, Algra A, van der Sprenkel JW, Tulleken CA, Rinkel GJ (2003) Hypomagnesemia after aneurysmal subarachnoid hemorrhage. *Neurosurgery* 52:276-282.

van den Bergh WM, Algra A, van Kooten F, Dirven CM, van Gijn J, Vermeulen M, Rinkel GJ (2005) Magnesium sulfate in aneurysmal subarachnoid hemorrhage: a randomized controlled trial. *Stroke* 36:1011-1015.

van den Bergh WM, Dijkhuizen RM, Rinkel GJ (2004b) Potentials of magnesium treatment in subarachnoid haemorrhage. *Magnes Res* 17:301-313.

van den Bergh WM, Van de Water JM, Hoff RG, Algra A, Rinkel GJ (2008b) Calcium Homeostasis During Magnesium Treatment in Aneurysmal Subarachnoid Hemorrhage. *Neurocrit Care.*

van den Bergh WM, Zuur JK, Kamerling NA, van Asseldonk JT, Rinkel GJ, Tulleken CA, Nicolay K (2002) Role of magnesium in the reduction of ischemic depolarization and lesion volume after experimental subarachnoid hemorrhage. *J Neurosurg* 97:416-422.

van der Bilt I, Hasan D, Vandertop WP, Wilde AA, Algra A, Visser FC, Rinkel GJ (2009) Impact of cardiac complications on outcome after aneurysmal subarachnoid hemorrhage: a meta-analysis. *Neurology* 72:635-642.

van der Hel WS, van den Bergh WM, Nicolay K, Tulleken KA, Dijkhuizen RM (1998) Suppression of cortical spreading depressions after magnesium treatment in the rat. *Neuroreport* 9:2179-2182

van Gijn J, Kerr RS, Rinkel GJ (2007) Subarachnoid haemorrhage. *Lancet* 369:306-318.

van Norden AG, van den Bergh WM, Rinkel GJ (2005) Dose evaluation for long-term magnesium treatment in aneurysmal subarachnoid haemorrhage. *J Clin Pharm Ther* 30:439-442.

Veyna RS, Seyfried D, Burke DG, Zimmerman C, Mlynarek M, Nichols V, Marrocco A, Thomas AJ, Mitsias PD, Malik GM (2002) Magnesium sulfate therapy after aneurysmal subarachnoid hemorrhage. *J Neurosurg* 96:510-514.

Warren BB, Muizelaar JP, Choi SC (1993) Magnesium's role in cerebral vasospasm and outcome in patients with aneurysmal subarachnoid hemorrhage. In: *Cerebral Vasospasm* (Findlay JM, ed), pp 401-404.

Weir B, Macdonald RL, Stoodley M (1999) Etiology of cerebral vasospasm. *Acta Neurochir Suppl (Wien)* 72:27-46.

Westermaier T, Stetter C, Vince GH, Pham M, Tejon JP, Eriskat J, Kunze E, Matthies C, Ernestus RI, Solymosi L, Roosen K (2010) Prophylactic intravenous magnesium sulfate for treatment of aneurysmal subarachnoid hemorrhage: a randomized, placebo-controlled, clinical study. *Crit Care Med* 38:1284-1290.

Wong GK, Chan MT, Boet R, Poon WS, Gin T (2006) Intravenous magnesium sulfate after aneurysmal subarachnoid hemorrhage: a prospective randomized pilot study. *J Neurosurg Anesthesiol* 18:142-148.

Wong GK, Kwok R, Tang K, Yeung D, Ahuja A, King AD, Poon WS (2010a) Effects of magnesium sulfate infusion on cerebral perfusion in patients after aneurysmal SAH. *Acta Neurochir Suppl* 106:133-135.

Wong GK, Poon WS, Chan MT, Boet R, Gin T, Ng SC, Zee BC (2010b) Intravenous magnesium sulphate for aneurysmal subarachnoid hemorrhage (IMASH): a randomized, double-blinded, placebo-controlled, multicenter phase III trial. *Stroke* 41:921-926.

Wong GK, Poon WS, Chan MT, Boet R, Gin T, Ng SC, Zee BC (2010c) Plasma magnesium concentrations and clinical outcomes in aneurysmal subarachnoid hemorrhage patients: post hoc analysis of intravenous magnesium sulphate for aneurysmal subarachnoid hemorrhage trial. *Stroke* 41:1841-1844.

Wong GK, Yeung DK, Ahuja AT, King AD, Lam CW, Chan MT, Gin T, Poon WS (2009) Intracellular free magnesium of brain and cerebral phosphorus-containing metabolites after subarachnoid hemorrhage and hypermagnesemic treatment: a (31)P-magnetic resonance spectroscopy study. *J Neurosurg.*

Yang Y, Li Q, Ahmad F, Shuaib A (2000) Survival and histological evaluation of therapeutic window of post-ischemia treatment with magnesium sulfate in embolic stroke model of rat. *Neurosci Lett* 285:119-122.

Magnesium in clinical stroke

Jeffrey L. Saver ✉ *and Sidney Starkman*

UCLA Stroke Center and Department of Neurology, University of California, Los Angeles, CA 90095, USA.
✉ jsaver@ucla.edu

Abstract

Stroke is the second leading cause of death and a leading cause of disability worldwide. Unfortunately, current therapies for acute ischemic stroke are of extremely limited effectiveness. The ideal neuroprotective agent for stroke would be inexpensive, readily available, easy to administer and have no significant adverse side effects. Intravenous magnesium sulfate offers promise as just such an agent. In clinical trials to date, administration of magnesium sulfate has shown favorable trends toward neuroprotection in resuscitated cardiac arrest patients, in cardiac bypass surgery and carotid endarterectomy. In acute stroke, eight pilot clinical trials of magnesium sulfate have shown good safety, and the subset of pilot trials with randomized controls have shown favorable effects on clinical outcome point estimates. The first phase 3 trial of magnesium sulfate for focal stroke was the Intravenous Magnesium Efficacy in Stroke (IMAGES) Trial. Hampered by late administration of study agent, IMAGES overall produced a neutral result, but exploratory analyses identified early (under 3 hour), lacunar stroke, hemorrhagic stroke, and severely hypertensive patients as having a potential differential beneficial response to magnesium that deserved further investigation. The Field Administration of Stroke Therapy – Magnesium (FAST-MAG) trial has been specifically designed to test magnesium in the hyperacute time window by initiating therapy in the prehospital setting.

Introduction

Stroke is the second leading cause of death and a leading cause of disability worldwide (Lopez *et al*, 2006). More than 5.3 million individuals die from a stroke each year, and many more survive with permanent incapacities. One in six individuals worldwide will suffer a stroke in their lifetime (Kaste *et al*, 2010). In Western nations, ischemic cerebral infarctions account for about 80% of strokes, intracerebral hemorhages 15%, and subarachnoid hemorrhages 4%.

Unfortunately, current therapies for acute ischemic stroke are of extremely limited effectiveness. To date, the only United States Food and Drug Administration (FDA) - approved pharmacologic treatment for acute ischemic stroke remains intravenous tissue plasminogen activator (tPA), a thrombolytic agent which must be administered within 3 hours of symptom onset, and only after neuroimaging has ruled out intracerebral hemorrhage (Adams *et al*, 2007). tPA carries significant bleeding risks, is costly, and is not being used in most acute stroke patients. Current estimates are that only 3-8% of acute ischemic stroke patients in the US receive tPA (California Acute Stroke Pilot Registry (CASPR) Investigators, 2005; Reeves *et al*, 2005). The only other pharmacologic agent of proven utility in acute ischemic stroke is aspirin, which confers only minimal benefit, helping only one of every 77 patients treated (Sandercock *et al*, 2008). Mechanical embolectomy devices have been developed and approved for the technical indication of removing acute thrombi from the cerebral vasculature, but have not yet been demonstrated in a randomized clinical trial to improve patient outcome and are employed in only a tiny fraction of stroke patients nationally (Smith *et al*, 2008; The Penumbra Pivotal Stroke Trial Investigators, 2009). New, effective, widely applicable treatments for acute ischemic stroke are desperately needed.

Magnesium sulfate: a highly promising neuroprotective therapy for stroke

When focal occlusions disrupt blood flow to the brain, a cascade of molecular events producing cell injury ensues (Schaller and Graf, 2004; Obrenovitch, 1995). Cell death proceeds rapidly in the infarct core, where blood flow is most drastically curtailed, but more slowly in the ischemic penumbra, where blood flow is variably reduced and molecular elaboration of neuronal injury may proceed over 3-12 hours or more. Central molecular events in the ischemic cascade include accumulation of intracellular calcium, release of excitatory amino acid neurotransmitters, generation of oxygen-free radicals, nitric oxide formation, and the release of cytokines by infiltrating polymorphonuclear leukocytes. These and additional events afford numerous targets for pharmacologic blockade. A multitude of neuroprotective drugs interfering with various pathways of ischemic injury reduce infarct volume substantially in focal stroke animal models when administered 10-120 minutes after ischemia onset, including excitatory amino acid antagonists, oxygen free radical scavengers, and voltage sensitive calcium channel blockers (Green and Shuaib, 2006).

The ideal neuroprotective agent for stroke would be inexpensive, readily available, easy to administer and have no significant adverse side effects. An agent demonstrated to be safe and potentially beneficial in both ischemic and hemorrhagic stroke would have the added benefit of potentially earlier administration prior to obtaining a head CT or brain MRI scan. Intravenous magnesium sulfate offers promise as just such an agent.

Laboratory studies have identified multiple neuronal and vascular effects of magnesium that likely contribute to the potent neuroprotective effects observed in stroke models (Muir, 2000). In a wide variety of in vitro systems and animal models, magnesium has been shown to produce cerebral arteriolar vasodilation and increased cerebral blood flow, inhibit presynaptic release of excitatory neurotransmitters, noncompetitively block the N-methyl-D-aspartate (NMDA) receptor, presynaptically potentiate adenosine, block voltage-gated calcium channels, suppress cortical spreading depression and anoxic depolarizations, relax vascular smooth muscle resulting in vasodilation of large and small vascular beds and increased cerebral blood flow, antagonize endothelin-1 and other vasoconstrictors, and replete an underlying and/or ischemia-induced Mg deficient state. Magnesium ions cross the intact blood-brain barrier efficaciously so that intravenous magnesium sulfate significantly raises cerebrospinal fluid and brain extracellular fluid magnesium to supraphysiologic levels (Thurnau *et al*, 1987; Wester *et al*, 1984). The brain penetration of magnesium may increase even further in ischemic regions where the blood-brain barrier is disrupted (Sjostrom and Wester, 1994). Magnesium sulfate is neuroprotective in preclinical models of cerebral and spinal cord ischemia, excitotoxic injury, and head trauma. Magnesium (Mg) is economical, widely available, simple to administer and has a long established safety and tolerability profile in myocardial infarction and eclampsia, as well as in initial human focal stroke studies. Unlike most synthetic neuroprotective compounds, parenteral magnesium has no major adverse effects in doses that achieve serum levels in the range of preclinical neuroprotective concentrations.

Magnesium is neuroprotective in rodent models of reversible and permanent focal cerebral ischemia. In contrast to commercially-supported neuroprotective compounds, magnesium has not been the subject of a systematic preclinical development program. However, academic investigations have demonstrated benefits in diverse models and laboratories, satisfying a key criterion of stroke drug development guidelines often not met by commercially-supported agents (Stroke Therapy Academic Industry Roundtable (STAIR), 1999). At least nine preclinical studies (eight reported) have examined the effect of systemic magnesium sulfate upon final infarct size in animal focal ischemic stroke models (Muir, 2000; 2001). Eight of the nine demonstrated substantial decreases in infarct size in treated animals, with reductions ranging from 26-61% in unconfounded studies. A recent study demonstrated synergistic effects of magnesium when combined with antioxidant and hypothermic therapies in a rat MCAO stroke model, suggesting that magnesium is a promising first agent upon which to build a combination neuroprotection regimen (Scholler *et al*, 2004).

Clinical trials of magnesium sulfate in diverse settings of acute cerebral ischemia

Uniquely among neuroprotective agents being developed for focal stroke, magnesium sulfate has shown signals of potential efficacy in numerous controlled clinical trials in closely allied settings of acute human cerebral ischemia, including 1) delayed cerebral infarction after subarachnoid hemorrhage, 2) newborn hypoxic-ischemic injury, 3) global cerebral ischemia after cardiac arrest, and 4) ischemic brain injury during cardiac and cerebrovascular surgical procedures. For detailed review of the first setting, the reader is referred to Chapter 14 in this volume. We here briefly survey the clinical trial experience with the latter two conditions.

Global cerebral ischemia after cardiac arrest

Paramedic, field-administration of magnesium sulfate showed favorable trends toward neuroprotection in resuscitated cardiac arrest patients in the Brain-Cardiopulmonary Resuscitation (B-CPR) (Longstreth *et al*, 2002). The B-CPR Trial tested magnesium sulfate and diazepam in a 2 x 2 factorial, placebo-controlled design. Paramedic personnel injected study medications to out-of-hospital cardiac arrest patients immediately following return of spontaneous circulation. Three hundred patients were randomized to intravenous magnesium sulfate 2 grams or matching placebo, and then to diazepam 10 mg or matching placebo. The pre-specified primary outcome measure was awakening, defined as having comprehensible speech or following commands. The study was powered to detect only a substantial treatment effect - absolute difference in the primary endpoint of 20%. The magnesium sulfate group showed a trend toward efficacy, with 46.7% awakening among those who received only magnesium versus 37.3% among those who received only placebo (risk difference 9.3%, CI -6.4 to 25.1%). In contrast, the diazepam group showed no evidence of treatment effect. No adverse effects of prehospital administration of magnesium sulfate therapy were noted

Brain ischemic during surgical procedures

The operative setting uniquely allows the administration of neuroprotective agents to occur prior to the onset of ischemia, when benefit will be greatest. Individual randomized controlled trials have suggested benefits of magnesium sulfate for neuroprotection in cardiac bypass surgery and carotid endarterectomy.

In on pump coronary artery bypass graft surgery, neuropsychologic dysfunction occurs in up to 50-80% of patients at the time of discharge, related in part to intra-operative brain ischemia. The Cleveland Clinic trial randomized 350 patients undergoing elective cardiac bypass surgery to magnesium sulfate or placebo during the operation and for the first 24 hours postoperatively. Patients received a 2-gram loading dose and subsequent titration of a continuous infusion to maintain serum magnesium levels at twice normal. Magnesium exerted a benefit on early cognitive function. On the study's primary endpoint of neurologic decline or neurologic death at 96 hours post-operatively, magnesium patients outperformed placebo (p=0.01) (Bhudia *et al*, 2006) By 3 months post-operatively, there were no performance differences between groups, possibly reflecting a test ceiling effect as placebo patients improved.

In carotid endarterectomy, cerebral ischemia due to intraoperative hypoperfusion and microembolic events produces clinical deficits evident on detailed neurocognitive testing. Standardized neuropsychometric evaluation has demonstrated cognitive decline in up to 25% of patients undergoing carotid surgery. The Columbia University trial randomly assigned 108 patients undergoing carotid surgery to placebo infusion or one of three magnesium sulfate dose tiers (Mack *et al*, 2009). The highest magnesium dose tier was a 4 gram loading dose followed by 16 grams over the next 24 hours. On a neuropsychologic test battery the day after surgery, patients treated with intravenous magnesium infusion demonstrated less postoperative neurocognitive impairment than those treated with placebo (OR 0.27, 95% CI 0.10–0.74, p = 0.01).

Pilot clinical trials of magnesium sulfate in focal stroke

There have been eight pilot clinical trials of magnesium sulfate in acute stroke, exploring dose optimization, feasibility, safety, and signals of efficacy. Among these, 6 were randomized and 2 uncontrolled. All showed good safety with each randomized controlled trial (RCT) showing favorable effects on clinical outcome point estimates (Wester *et al*, 1984; Muir and Lees, 1995; Muir and Lees, 1998; Galeas *et al*, 1998; Bradford *et al*, 1998; Lampl *et al*, 2001; Saver *et al*, 2002; Muir *et al*, 2004). A meta-analysis of the four phase 2 RCTs with combinable data (total of 162 patients) found a favorable clinical outcome trend, with late disability or death seen in 44.3%

of magnesium sulfate patients compared with 52.7% of placebo patients (OR. 0.67, 95% CI, 0.35-1.26) (Muir, 2001).

The pilot trial that optimized a dose regimen for subsequent phase 3, pivotal trials was the dose ranging study reported by Muir and Lees (1998). They sought a regimen that efficiently and safely achieved a doubling of the serum magnesium concentration. This target was selected as serum concentrations of 3.48 meq/L and above had been neuroprotective in preclinical models of focal cerebral ischemia, and doubling of serum concentrations was known to be efficacious in the prophylaxis and treatment of seizures in preeclamptic and eclamptic women (the normal range for serum magnesium is 1.4 – 1.7 meq/L). They randomized 25 patients to placebo or one of three magnesium sulfate dose schedules: loading infusions of 8, 12, or 16 mmol, all followed by a maintenance infusion of 65 mmol over 24 hours. All dose tiers were found safe, with no major effects on heart rate, blood pressure, blood glucose, or other physiologic variables. Serum magnesium concentrations rose to target levels most rapidly in the highest loading infusion group and were maintained in all groups for at least 24 hours. The highest loading dose infusion regimen was therefore identified as safe and most efficient, and taken forward to later phase clinical trials.

A distinctive pilot trial was undertaken to demonstrate the feasibility and safety of having paramedics initiate magnesium sulfate in the field, prior to hospital arrival. Magnesium sulfate's properties make it a particularly attractive agent to study in the prehospital setting (Table 1). In the Field Administration of Stroke Therapy – Magnesium (FAST-MAG) Pilot Trial, the primary prespecified feasibility trial endpoint was reduction in time interval from paramedic arrival on scene to start of study agent infusion, compared with a historical control group of ambulance-arriving patients enrolled in standard post-hospital arrival fashion in acute neuroprotective trials (Saver *et al*, 2004). Twenty patients were enrolled, all receiving active therapy of a 4 gram loading dose initiated by paramedics in the field, followed by a 16 gram maintenance infusion administered upon hospital arrival. Substantially more rapid initiation of neuroprotective therapy was found with field administration versus historic controls, with the mean interval from paramedic arrival on scene to initiation of study drug 23 minutes in field-initiation patients vs 141 minutes in hospital-initiated patients, $p < .0001$. Experimental neuroprotective therapy was started 2 hours earlier as a result of the strategy of prehospital initiation of therapy.

The pharmacologic efficacy of field administration of study in the FAST-MAG Pilot Trial was assessed by measuring the serum magnesium level 10 minutes after completion of the bolus loading dose. In the 19 patients completing the loading dose, post bolus serum

Table 1. Properties of Magnesium Sulfate Advantageous for Prehospital Study

Magnesium Sulfate Properties	Import for Prehospital Trial
Stable at room temperature	• Can be stored in rescue vehicles
No major antithrombotic effects	• Can be used in ischemic and hemorrhagic stroke • May be started in ambulance prior to CT or MR scan
Loading intravenous dose quickly achieves target blood levels	• Paramedics can efficiently initiate through standard field intravenous line
Well-established safety record in clinical practice	• Extensive monitoring not required
Neuroprotective in multiple stroke models	• Promising agent for efficacy study

magnesium levels were mean 3.6 mEq/L, range 2.4-5.7, demonstrating successful achievement of target supraphysiologic, neuroprotective levels of magnesium sulfate in all patients completing the loading dose. These results of paramedic loading dose administration were comparable to those of standard in hospital loading dose administration in the dose-optimization clinical trial of Muir and Lees (1998).

Safety and exploratory efficacy endpoints in the FAST-MAG Pilot trial were encouraging. No drug related serious major adverse event was observed. Although conclusions derived from an open-label, small pilot trial must be extremely guarded, clinical efficacy suggested potential beneficial treatment effects. Dramatic early recovery, defined as complete recovery or improvement by 10 or more points on the National Institute of Health Stroke Scale (NIHSS) by 24 hours, occurred in 27% of cerebral infarct patients. This response compares quite favorably with rates of dramatic early recovery noted in the NINDS-tPA Trial 1 placebo group (12%) and approximates the treatment effect of tPA in yielding dramatic early recovery in the NINDS-tPA Trial 1 (27%) (Haley *et al*, 1997).

IMAGES phase 3 trial

The first phase 3 trial of magnesium sulfate for focal stroke was the Intravenous Magnesium Efficacy in Stroke (IMAGES) Trial (Muir *et al*, 2004). Funded by the British Medical Research Council, IMAGES was an international trial that enrolled 2589 patients within 12 hours of onset to receive 4 gram magnesium sulfate bolus followed by 16.25 gram magnesium sulfate maintenance infusion over 24 hours or matched placebo.

The performance of IMAGES demonstrated a worldwide consensus that magnesium sulfate in focal human stroke shows robust promise and merits phase 3 trial testing. However, the design of IMAGES had a critical drawback common among trials of its era: a late enrollment window. IMAGES permitted enrollment of patients up to 12 hours after symptom onset, well after ischemic injury has already reached completion in many patients. Additionally, IMAGES required that a patient's deficit be persistent for at least one hour before enrollment could occur, precluding agent initiation within the first 60 minutes of onset in the trial.

The IMAGES trial overall had a neutral result, but trial data suggest that the nonpositive outcome may have been due to late administration of study agent. The primary efficacy endpoint in IMAGES was death and disability at 3 months, identified by the joint binary outcome of outcome of a Barthel score < 95 and a modified Rankin score > 1. On this endpoint, the point estimate favoring magnesium did not reach statistical significance (OR 0.95, 95% CI 0.80-1.13). However, the vast majority of patients in IMAGES were enrolled late after stroke onset. Median time to treatment was 7 hours. The single hour with a plurality of enrolled patients was hour 12. Only 71 patients (3.1% of the entire IMAGES cohort) were enrolled within 3 hours of onset, only 16 patients (0.6%) were enrolled within 2 hours, and no patients were enrolled within 1 hour.

IMAGES generally confirmed the safety of magnesium sulfate administration in acute stroke. No statistically significant differences were noted in time to first serious adverse event or to mortality. Nominal differences in mortality did not reach statistical significance (OR 1.22, 95% CI 0.98-1.53) and no individual causes of death were in excess in the magnesium group. Mild cardiovascular effects of magnesium were observed, as expected. Magnesium slightly reduced the blood pressure during the period of infusion, on average by 4 points systolic and 3 points diastolic. This reduction disappeared by 24 hous after the end of the infusion. Heart rate was minimally reduced at 12 hours into the infusion, but not at other time points. No increase in clinically reported hypotension, cardiac failure, cardiac conduction block, or flushing was reported n the magnesium group.

Exploratory analyses in IMAGES identified four patient subgroups with potential differential beneficial response to magnesium that deserve further investigation: 1) lacunar stroke, 2) hemorrhagic stroke, 3) severely hypertensive patients, and 4) early, under 3 hour, treated patients. Among 765 patients with lacunar syndromes, unfavorable outcomes were less common in the treatment group, OR 0.70 (0.53-0.92) (Aslanyan *et al*, 2007). This observation is intriguing in light of in vitro models indicating that magnesium has biological protective activities in white matter ischemia (Lecrux *et al*, 2008). Among 1193 patients with initial blood pressures higher than the trial median, unfavorable outcomes also were less common in treated patients, OR 0.78 (0.61-0.99) (Muir *et al*, 2004). The optimal treatment of elevated blood pressure in acute stroke remains uncertain; it is possible that the slight antihypertensive action of magnesium sulfate was beneficial in these patients, in addition to neuroprotective actions. While ischemic stroke patients were the primary target of IMAGES, 7% of enrolled patients had primary supratentorial intracerebral hemorrhages. Among these 168 patients, the OR for an unfavorable outcome was nominally lower among magnesium-treated patients: 0.84 (0.41-1.74) (Muir *et al*, 2004). Primary hemorrhage patients are another group among whom mild antihypertensive effects, as well as neuroprotective effects, could be beneficial.

Few patients were enrolled in IMAGES in the first three hours after stroke onset, the time period when acute stroke treatments are most effective; however, among these patients, results were quite encouraging. There are not enough under 1 or under 2 hour patients to permit analysis of these subgroups, but 79 patients (3.3% of the study cohort) were enrolled within 3 hours. On the IMAGES primary endpoint, the global odds ratio comparing magnesium vs placebo for a favorable death or disability outcome was 0.66 (95%CI 0.25-1.70)(Muir *et al*, 2004). Considering the modified Rankin component of the IMAGES primary endpoint, a non-disabled outcome (mRS 0-1) was achieved in 45.9% of magnesium patients vs 33.3% of placebo patients, a 12.6% absolute difference. Mortality observations in the IMAGES under 3 hour cohort were also favorable, with death observed in 26% of placebo vs. 19% of magnesium patients (OR 0.65, 95% CI 0.23 - 1.92). With the small numbers of patients, these results do not reach statistical significance, but do represent a suggestive signal of potential efficacy of magnesium within very early time windows.

The key variable of time and the prehospital strategy for magnesium sulfate

In the past several decades, more than 100 neuroprotective agents have been tested in randomized controlled clinical trials in acute ischemic stroke (Kidwell *et al*, 2001; Hong *et al*, 2011). Several agents have shown promising findings in safety and preliminary efficacy phase 2 trials. However, no agent has been shown unequivocally to be beneficial in definitive phase 3 trials and none has been approved by the FDA as indicated for ischemic stroke. These results have led many investigators to ask the question, "Why do neuroprotective drugs work in animals but not humans?" (DeGraba and Pettigrew, 2000). Leading basic and clinial neuroscientists have identified 4 key design defects of past human clinical trials of neuroprotective clinical trials: 1) failure to administer study agents at neuroprotective doses in humans because of limiting side effects, 2) failure to select patients for trials who will respond to the known mechanisms of action of study drug, 3) failure to employ sample sizes large enough to detect modest benefits of study agent, and 4) failure to treat patients early enough after stroke onset (DeGraba and Pettigrew, 2000; Stroke Therapy Academic Industry Roundtable II (StairII) 2001; Gorelick, 2000; De Keyser *et al*, 1999; Fisher, 2003; Ovbiagele *et al*, 2003; Wahlgren and Ahmed, 2004; Muir and Teal, 2005).

The NIH Field Administration of Stroke Therapy – Magnesium (FAST-MAG) trial was designed to remedy each of these past difficulties. The trial employs magnesium sulfate at doses known to be both well tolerated and to yield serum levels neuroprotective in animal models. The trial tests an agent likely to be beneficial for both gray and white matter ischemic injury, based on vasodilating effects in both superficial and deep circulations and cytoprotective effects in both gray and white matter. The trial is adequately powered to detect even a modest treatment effect, and will be larger than 95% of all previous phase 3 neuroprotective trials. Most importantly, the FAST-MAG trial is designed to address the crucial factor of delayed time to treatment which has hindered all past human clinical trials of neuroprotective drugs.

Rodent and nonhuman primate experimental studies suggest the duration of the therapeutic window within which neuroprotective intervention can ameliorate bioenergetic failure in the ischemic penumbra is very brief, generally less than 2-3 hours. Most animal studies of neuroprotective agents initiate therapy within 1-60 minutes after ischemia onset. For magensium sulfate specifically, a strong time constraint upon potential benefit was found in a rodent middle cerebral artery occlsuion model. Treating with magnesium sulfate at 2 hours after occlusion reduced infarct size by 61%, while treatment at 6 hours reduced infarct size by 48% and treatment at 8 hours reduced infarct size by 19% (Yang *et al*, 2000).

However, although it is in the first 2 hours of onset that neuroprotective agents in general and magnesium sulfate in particular are most beneficial in focal animal stroke models, no prior human clinical neuroprotective agent trial has enrolled any substantial cohort of patients in this time window (Kidwell *et al*, 2001; Ferguson *et al*, 2004). Early neuroprotective trials permitted initiation of therapy at lengthy intervals after symptom onset, up to 48 hours, well after the critical period for stabilizing the penumbral region had closed. More recent trials have utilized shorter entry windows, but continue to treat few patients within the first 1 or 2 hours. Validating methods to safely initiate experimental neuroprotective therapies more quickly is critical if the dramatic benefits of neuroprotective agents evident in the laboratory are to be achieved in human stroke victims. This perspective is supported by the pooled analysis of the first 6 major intravenous tPA trials (Brott *et al*, 2002). Due to the powerful effect of time to treatment upon benefit of tPA, the sample sizes required to demonstrate treatment benefit escalate rapidly with increasing time window. A trial enrolling patients in the 0-90 minute epoch would require a sample size of only 90 to demonstrate benefit; a 91-180 minute trial would require a sample size of 528; a 181-270 minute trial, 816; and a 271-360 minute trial a sample size of 4007.

Enrolling patients in the field in acute neuroprotective trials is a highly promising approach to the challenge of testing neuroprotective agents in hyperacute time epochs. The FAST-MAG trial is the first phase 3 focal stroke trial in the field, but recent trials in both cardiac and other brain disorders demonstrate the feasibility and advantages of the prehospital treatment approach. In the analogous setting of acute myocardial ischemia, randomized clinical trials have shown that paramedic prehospital diagnosis and initiation of defibrillation and thrombolytic therapy reduces time to treatment start and improves clinical outcome (Bozik *et al*, 2001). In status epilepticus, the Prehospital Treatment of Status Epilepticus (PHTSE) trial showed that paramedic initiation of anticonvulsants in the field is safe, reliable, and yields better clinical outcomes than standard in hospital therapy (Alldredge *et al*, 2001). In global brain ischemia due to cardiac arrest, the Melbourne hypothermia trial demonstrated a benefit of paramedic-initiated, whole body cooling in resuscitated out of hospital cardiac arrest patients (Bernard *et al*, 2002)

Prehospital trials of treatments for focal stroke face several design challenges, including accurate identification of stroke patients, rating of pretreatment stroke severity, elicitation of informed consent in the field prior to hospital arrival, and randomization to appropriate treatment arm. The Field Administration of Stroke Therapy – Magnesium (FAST-MAG) investigators developed several novel methods to address these obstacles, first in a pilot, 20 patient feasibility trial (Saver *et al*, 2004) and then in an ongoing, pivotal, 1700 patient phase 3 trial.

- Stroke identification – LAPSS: Paramedics identify stroke patients using the Los Angeles Prehospital Stroke Screen (LAPSS), an 8 item diagnostic inventory that takes 1-2 minutes to perform, is well validated, and is a standard part of ambulance personnel training worldwide.
- Stroke severity rating – LAMS: The Los Angeles Motor Scale is a 0-5 point rating of motor deficit severity that is derived directly from the face, arm, and grip weakness exam section of the LAPSS. When performing the LAPSS, paramedics also automatically perform the LAMS. Though simple and rapid, the LAMS is a useful assessment of stroke deficit severity, correlating well with concurrently measured 13 item NIH Stroke Scale (NIHSS) scores, and predicting final three month disability, activity of daily living, and neurologic deficit outcomes nearly as well as the full NIHSS (Llanes *et al*, 2004).
- Informed consent elicitation – cellular telemedicine: Most recent prehospital treatment trials have been conducted for

conditions that render patients incompetent to provide consent, such as cardiac arrest, under regulations permitting waiver of explicit consent in emergency circumstances. In acute stroke, however, many patients retain decision-making capacity and require fully informed consent. Having paramedics elicit consent has the drawbacks of having nonstroke experts answering subject queries and of diverting paramedic attention from prehospital duties. In the cellular telemedicine enrollment system developed for FAST-MAG, rescue vehicles carry written informed consent forms and cellular phones that permit instant connection to on-call enrolling physician–investigators (Sanossian *et al*, 2009). The physician–investigator discusses the trial by phone with the patient or their legally authorized representative while paramedics perform prehospital care duties unimpeded.

- Pre-encounter randomization: Keep It Simple and Straightforward (KISS) is an important principle in prehospital research. In the potentially chaotic prehospital setting, complex randomization schemes and multiple drug source bins have a high risk of leading to administration of unintended treatment regimens. To promote reliable and rapid administration of study agent, the randomized phase 3 FAST-MAG trial employs a pre-encounter randomization system. Each ambulance is stocked with only one blinded study kit at a time. When the study kit is used in a patient, the ambulance is restocked within 24 hours with the next kit in that ambulance's permuted block treatment schedule. When given approval to start study procedures by the enrolling physician-investigator, paramedics can quickly and unambiguously proceed with administering the sole, "pre-randomized" kit available in the vehicle.

Using these techniques, the FAST-MAG Phase 3 Trial during its initial years of performance has already enrolled more patients in the hyperacute, under 2 hour period than all prior acute stroke treatment trials combined. By late January of 2011, 1190 patients had been enrolled, with a median time interval from last known well to start of study infusion of 46 minutes (Saver *et al*, 2011). Fully 869 patients (73%) were enrolled within the first hour after onset, and another 286 (24%) in the second hour. In this initial cohort, patient demographics are typical for the stroke population, with average age 69 and 58% of the population male. Stroke mimicking conditions have been enrolled at a low rate, 3%, below the 5% allotted in trial sample size projections. The enrolling event was acute cerebral ischemia in 73% of patients and intracerebral hemorrhage in 24%. These preliminary observations findings indicate that the FAST-MAG trial is accomplishing several innovations in stroke clinical trials, including being: 1) the first prehospital randomized stroke trial, 2) the first treatment trial to enroll a substantial cohort of patients in first 60 minutes after onset (the "golden hour"), and 3) the first trial testing neuroprotective therapy delivery in advance of recanalization therapy, potentially permitting more brain tissue to still be salvageable when reperfusion is achieved.

Commercial sponsors have been reluctant to conduct paramedic administered trials of neuroprotective agents because of perceived regulatory hurdles and because of the lack of established phase 3 trial methodology in the prehospital setting. Successful completion of the FAST-MAG trial may blaze a trail for future neuroprotective field trials, both governmental and commercial, and could lead to a resurgence of research activity in neuroprotection for stroke.

Acute stroke investigators have suggested the desirability of paramedic treatment of acute stroke in the field (Alberts, 1997; The European Ad Hoc Consensus Group, 1998; Rajajee and Saver, 2005). A vision of future stroke care widely shared in the stroke research community is: 1) paramedic administration of a group of complementary neuroprotective agents in the field to protect the brain during transfer and extend the time window for recanalization therapy, 2) definitive thrombolysis or other revascularization procedure on hospital arrival, and 3) in-hospital administration of a second group of neuroprotective agents specifically active against reperfusion injury (Table 2). The FAST-MAG Trial constitutes the first major test of the prehospital element of this stroke treatment strategy. The need for a prehospital neuroprotective agent has become even more urgent with the dissemination of designated Stroke Center

Table 2. Vision for Future Comprehensive Acute Ischemic Stroke Care

Stage	Typical Setting	Diagnostic Steps	Treatment Strategy	Treatment Components
Hyperacute (0-2 hours)	Prehospital and ED	Clinical screens	Stabilize penumbra	• Neuroprotective cocktail, e.g. magnesium
Early Acute (1-4.5 hours)	Primary Stroke Center ED + ICU	Rapid CT	Reperfuse rapidly	• IV thrombolysis
Later Acute (2-10 hours)	Comprehensive Stroke Center	Multimodal MRI or CT	Reperfuse definitively	• Endovascular recanalization • Reperfusion injury cocktail
Early Subacute	Stroke Unit	Complete work-up	Deter reocclusion, recurrence	• Antithrombotics • Secondary prevention
Subacute	Rehabilitation Unit	Functional MRI	Enhance neurorepair	• Nerve growth factors • Stem cells • Transcranial magnetic stimulation • Neural prosthetics (brain-machine interface)

systems throughout the United States (Schwamm *et al*, 2005). At the end of 2010, 18 states and additional counties, encompassing 52% of the American populace, had adopted regulations requiring routing of ambulances directly to designated Stroke Centers (Song and Saver, 2011). Identification of a proven prehospital treatment agent would help mitigate the impact of the resulting slight increase in average prehospital transport time for stroke patients.

Paramedics reach, within 2 hours of onset, 20-50% of the 600,000 ischemic stroke patients in the United States each year. Positive results in the FAST-MAG clinical trial would mean that 120,000 – 300,000 Americans suffering an acute stroke each year could potentially benefit from treatment with magnesium sulfate therapy. This would represent a tremendous advance in reducing the nationwide, and worldwide, burden of stroke.

References

Adams HP, Jr., del Zoppo G, Alberts MJ, et al (2007) Guidelines for the early management of adults with ischemic stroke: a guideline from the American Heart Association/American Stroke Association Stroke Council, Clinical Cardiology Council, Cardiovascular Radiology and Intervention Council, and the Atherosclerotic Peripheral Vascular Disease and Quality of Care Outcomes in Research Interdisciplinary Working Groups: the American Academy of Neurology affirms the value of this guideline as an educational tool for neurologists. *Stroke* 38:1655-711.

Alberts MJ (1997) Hyperacute stroke therapy with tissue plasminogen activator. *Am J Cardiol* 80(4C):29D-34D.

Alldredge BK, Gelb AM, Isaacs SM, Corry MD, Allen F, Ulrich S, Gottwald MD, O'Neil N, Neuhaus JM, Segal

MR, Lowenstein DH (2001) A Comparison of Lorazepam, Diazepam, and Placebo for the Treatment of Out-of-Hospital Status Epilepticus. *N Engl J Med* 345:631-7.

Aslanyan S, Weir CJ, Muir KW, Lees KR (2007) Magnesium for treatment of acute lacunar stroke syndromes: further analysis of the IMAGES trial. *Stroke* 38:1269-73.

Bernard SA, Gray TW, Buist MD, Jones BM, Silvester W, Gutteridge G, Smith K (2002) Treatment of comatose survivors of out-of-hospital cardiac arrest with induced hypothermia. *N Engl J Med* 346:557-63.

Bhudia SK, Cosgrove DM, Naugle RI, Rajeswaran J, Lam BK, Walton E, Petrich J, Palumbo RC, Gillinov AM, Apperson-Hansen C, Blackstone EH (2006) Magnesium as a neuroprotectant in cardiac surgery: a randomized clinical trial. *J Thorac Cardiovasc Surg* 131:853-61.

Bozik M, Bogousslavsky J, Fayad P, et al (2001) POST-010: Efficacy and safety of MaxiPost in patients with acute stroke. *Neurology* 56(suppl 3):A76.

Bradford APJ, Muir KW, Lees KR, IMAGES Study Group (1998) IMAGES pilot study of intravenous magnesium in acute stroke. *Cerebrovasc Dis* 8:86A.

Brott TG, Kaste M, Albers GW (2002) Analysis of the NINDS, ECASS I and ECASS II, and Atlantis data sets. In: *27th International Stroke Conference*, San Antonio, TX.

California Acute Stroke Pilot Registry (CASPR) Investigators (2005) Prioritizing interventions to improve rates of thrombolysis for ischemic stroke. *Neurology* 64:654-9.

De Keyser J, Sulter G, Luiten PG (1999) Clinical trials with neuroprotective drugs in acute ischaemic stroke: are we doing the right thing? *Trends Neurosci* 22:535-40.

DeGraba TJ, Pettigrew LC (2000) Why do neuroprotective drugs work in animals but not humans? *Neurol Clin* 18:475-93.

Ferguson KN, Kidwell CS, Starkman S, Saver JL (2004) Hyperacute treatment initiation in neuroprotective agent stroke trials. *J Stroke Cerebrovas Dis* 13:109-12.

Fisher M, Ratan R (2003) New perspectives on developing acute stroke therapy. *Ann Neurol* 53:10-20.

Galeas T, Ziogas G, Valotasiou B (1998) The role of magnesium (Mg)--a natural calcium (Ca) antagonist in the Ca channels of the platelets--in the treatment of acute ischaemic stroke. In: *Consensus Conference on Stroke*, Edinburgh, UK: Royal College of Physicians of Edinburgh, p. 15.

Gorelick PB (2000) Neuroprotection in acute ischaemic stroke: a tale of for whom the bell tolls? *Lancet* 355:1925-6.

Green AR, Shuaib A (2006) Therapeutic strategies for the treatment of stroke. *Drug Discovery Today* 11:681-93.

Haley EC, Jr., Lewandowski C, Tilley BC (1997) Myths regarding the NINDS rt-PA Stroke Trial: setting the record straight. *Ann Emerg Med* 30:676-82.

Hong KS, Lee SJ, Hao Q, Liebeskind DS, Saver JL (2011) Acute Stroke Trials in the 1st decade of the 21th Century. *Stroke* 42:e314.

Kaste M, Norrving B (2010) From the World Stroke Day to the World Stroke Campaign: one in six: act now! *Int J Stroke* 5:342-3.

Kidwell CS, Liebeskind DS, Starkman S, Saver JL (2001) Trends in acute ischemic stroke trials through the 20th century. *Stroke* 32:1349-59.

Lampl Y, Gilad R, Geva D, Eshel Y, Sadeh M (2001) Intravenous administration of magnesium sulfate in acute stroke: a randomized double-blind study. Clin *Neuropharmacol* 24:11-5.

Lecrux C, McCabe C, Weir CJ, Gallagher L, Mullin J, Touzani O, Muir KW, Lees KR, Macrae IM (2008) Effects of Magnesium Treatment in a Model of Internal Capsule Lesion in Spontaneously Hypertensive Rats. *Stroke* 39:448-54.

Llanes JN, Kidwell CS, Starkman S, Leary MC, Eckstein M, Saver JL (2004) The Los Angeles Motor Scale (LAMS): a new measure to characterize stroke severity in the field. *Prehosp Emerg Care* 8:46-50.

Longstreth WT, Jr., Fahrenbruch CE, Olsufka M, Walsh TR, Copass MK, Cobb LA (2002) Randomized clinical trial of magnesium, diazepam, or both after out-of-hospital cardiac arrest. *Neurology* 59:506-14.

Lopez AD, Mathers CD, Ezzati M, Jamison DT, Murray CJ (2006) Global and regional burden of disease and risk factors, 2001: systematic analysis of population health data. *Lancet* 367:1747-57.

Mack WJ, Kellner CP, Sahlein DH, Ducruet AF, Kim GH, Mocco J, Zurica J, Komotar RJ, Haque R, Sciacca R, Quest DO, Solomon RA, Connolly ES, Heyer EJ (2009) Intraoperative magnesium infusion during carotid endarterectomy: a double-blind placebo-controlled trial. *J Neurosurg* 110:961-7.

Muir KW (2000) Therapeutic potential of magnesium in the treatment of acute stroke. *J Stroke Cerebrovasc Dis* 9:257-67.

Muir KW (2001) Magnesium for neuroprotection in ischaemic stroke: rationale for use and evidence of effectiveness. *CNS Drugs* 15:921-30.

Muir KW (2001) Systematic review of clinical trials of magnesium for acute stroke. *Stroke* 31:379A.

Muir KW, Lees KR (1995) A randomised, double-blind, placebo-controlled pilot trial of intravenous magnesium sulfate in acute stroke. *Stroke* 26:1183-8.

Muir KW, Lees KR (1998) Dose optimization of intravenous magnesium sulfate after acute stroke. *Stroke* 29:918-23.

Muir KW, Lees KR, Ford I, Davis S (2004) Magnesium for acute stroke (Intravenous Magnesium Efficacy in Stroke trial): randomised controlled trial. *Lancet* 363:439-45.

Muir KW, Teal PA (2005) Why have neuro-protectants failed?: lessons learned from stroke trials. *J Neurol* 252:1011-20.

Obrenovitch TP (1995) The ischaemic penumbra twenty years on. *Cerebrovasc Brain Metab Reviews* 7:297-323.

Ovbiagele B, Kidwell CS, Starkman S, Saver JL (2003) Neuroprotective agents for the treatment of acute ischemic stroke. *Curr Neurol Neurosci Rep* 3:9-20.

Rajajee V, Saver J (2005) Prehospital care of the acute stroke patient. *Tech Vasc Interv Radiol* 8:74-80.

Reeves MJ, Arora S, Broderick JP, et al (2005) Acute stroke care in the US: results from 4 pilot prototypes of the Paul Coverdell National Acute Stroke Registry. *Stroke* 36:1232-40.

Sandercock PA, Counsell C, Gubitz GJ, Tseng MC (2008) Antiplatelet therapy for acute ischaemic stroke. *Cochrane Database Syst Rev* CD000029.

Sanossian N, Starkman S, Liebeskind DS, Ali LK, Restrepo L, Hamilton S, Conwit R, Saver JL, FAST-MAG Trial Investigators (2009) Simultaneous ring voice-over-Internet phone system enables rapid physician elicitation of explicit informed consent in prehospital stroke treatment trials. *Cerebrovasc Dis* 28:539-44.

Saver J, Eckstein M, Stratton S, et al (2011) Field Administration of Stroke Therapy – Magnesium (FAST-MAG) Phase 3 Trial. In: *International Stroke Conference*, Los Angeles, CA.

Saver JL, Kidwell C, Eckstein M, Starkman S (2004) Prehospital neuroprotective therapy for acute stroke: results of the Field Administration of Stroke Therapy-Magnesium (FAST-MAG) pilot trial. *Stroke* 35:e106-8.

Saver JL, Kidwell CS, Leary MC, et al (2002) Results of the Field Administration of Stroke Treatment - Magnesium (FAST-MAG) pilot trial: a study of prehospital neuroprotective therapy. *Stroke* 33:363-4.

Schaller B, Graf R (2004) Cerebral ischemia and reperfusion: the pathophysiologic concept as a basis for clinical therapy. *J Cereb Blood Flow Metab* 24:351-71.

Scholler K, Zausinger S, Baethmann A, Schmid-Elsaesser R (2004) Neuroprotection in ischemic stroke--combination drug therapy and mild hypothermia in a rat model of permanent focal cerebral ischemia. *Brain Research* 1023:272-8.

Schwamm LH, Pancioli A, Acker JE, 3rd, et al (2005) Recommendations for the establishment of stroke systems of care: recommendations from the American Stroke Association's Task Force on the Development of Stroke Systems. *Stroke* 36:690-703.

Sjostrom LG, Wester P (1994) Systematically induced hypermagnesemia increases the bioavailability of magnesium in rat brain. *Soc Neurosci Abstr* 20:181.

Smith WS, Sung G, Saver J, et al (2008) Mechanical Thrombectomy for Acute Ischemic Stroke: Final Results of the Multi MERCI Trial. *Stroke* 39:1205-12.

Song S, Saver J (2011) Growth of Regional Stroke Systems of Care in the United States in the First Decade of the 21st Century. *Stroke* 42:e340.

Stroke Therapy Academic Industry Roundtable (STAIR) (1999) Recommendations for standards regarding preclinical neuroprotective and restorative drug development. *Stroke* 30:2752-8.

Stroke Therapy Academic Industry Roundtable II (STAIR-II) (2001) Recommendations for clinical trial evaluation of acute stroke therapies. *Stroke* 32:1598-606.

The European Ad Hoc Consensus Group (1998) Neuroprotection as initial therapy in acute stroke. *Cerebrovasc Dis* 8:59-72.

The Penumbra Pivotal Stroke Trial Investigators (2009) The penumbra pivotal stroke trial: safety and effectiveness of a new generation of mechanical devices for clot removal in intracranial large vessel occlusive disease. *Stroke* 40:2761-8.

Thurnau GR, Kemp DB, Jarvis A (1987) Cerebrospinal fluid levels of magnesium in patients with preeclampsia after treatment with intravenous magnesium sulfate. *Am J Obstet Gynecol* 1987:1435-8.

Wahlgren N, Ahmed N (2004) Neuroprotection in cerebral ischaemia: facts and fancies--the need for new approaches. *Cerebrovasc Dis* 17 (Suppl 1):153-66 .

Wester PO, Asplund K, Eriksson W, Hagg E, Lithner F, Strand T (1984) Infusion of magnesium in patients with acute brain infarction. *Acta Neurol Scand* 70:143.

Yang Y, Li Q, Ahmad F, Shuaib A (2000) Survival and histological evaluation of therapeutic window of post-ischemia treatment with magnesium sulfate in embolic stroke model of rat. *Neurosci Lett* 285:119-22.

Magnesium and cancer: more questions than answers

Marzia Leidi,[1] *Federica Wolf*[2] *and Jeanette A.M. Maier*[1,✉]

[1] Università di Milano, Dipartimento di Scienze Cliniche Luigi Sacco, 20157 Milano, Italy.
[2] Università Cattolica del Sacro Cuore, Istituto di Patologia generale e Centro di Ricerche Oncologiche Giovanni XXIII, Facoltà di Medicina "A. Gemelli", 00168 Roma, Italy.
✉ jeanette.maier@unimi.it

Abstract

The relationship between Mg and cancer is still a hank to disentangle. The knowledge derived from preclinical studies reveals a complex scenario in which low magnesium has both anti- and pro-tumor effects, such as inhibition of tumor growth at its primary site and facilitation of tumor implantation at its metastatic sites. In different cell types, neoplastic transformation dramatically disrupts the controlled and coordinated fluctuations of intracellular magnesium, an event which offers selective advantages to the cells. It is difficult to translate the lesson learnt from experimental models to humans. Based on epidemiological studies, Mg deficiency seems to be linked to increased risk of some types of cancers. The demonstration of an impairment of magnesium homeostasis in oncologic patients further complicates the field. We need more translational and clinical data to draw firm conclusions about the contribution of magnesium to tumors.

Introduction

Although cancer mortality has declined in the last two decades, particularly in western countries (Jemal *et al*, 2010), cancer exacts a very high toll as a leading cause of death all over the world. Great strides have been made to disclose the molecular bases of neoplasia, but how to prevent or cure cancer still remains a largely unanswered question.

There is a general agreement about the environmental origin of cancer. It has been estimated that more than two-thirds of human cancers can be prevented by changes of lifestyle. Statistical and epidemiological data point to diet as responsible for about 35% of human cancer mortality (Doll and Peto, 1981). While many dietary constituents transform normal cells into malignant ones *in vitro* and stimulate the development, growth and spread of tumors *in vivo*, evidence from population and laboratory studies indicate that many microconstituents inhibit, retard or reverse tumorigenesis (Manson, 2003). There is a general agreement about the inverse correlation between regular consumption of fruit, cereals and vegetables and the risk of cancer. Edible plant matter contains many beneficial microconstituents, vitamins and minerals. In particular, magnesium (Mg), which is predominantly obtained by eating unprocessed grains and green leafy vegetables, is an essential micronutrient implicated in a large array of regulatory, metabolic and structural activities (Wolf and Trapani, 2008). Evidence suggests that the occidental diet is relatively deficient in Mg because of preference for calorie-rich, micronutrient-poor foods, low Mg content in water and soil, and processing of many food items (Ford and Mokdad, 2003). Inadequate dietary intake of Mg is not the only cause of Mg deficiency. Mg homeostasis is very tightly tuned in the intestine and in the renal tubules through a complex network of transporters, some of which have recently been defined at the molecular level (Quamme, 2010). Consequently, Mg deficiency accompanies chronic gastrointestinal and renal diseases, and also complicates diabetes mellitus, therapies with some classes of diuretics or anticancer drugs. In addition, it is common in alcoholics and in the elderly (Ford and Mokdad, 2003).

Considerable debate remains about the role of Mg in human tumors, partly due to the lack of reliable and selective analytical procedures to measure Mg. However, there has been a recent resurgence of interest in the relation between

Mg and tumors both in experimental and in clinical oncology, leading to the question whether Mg is Dr Jekyll or Mr Hyde in tumor biology and clinics.

Low magnesium and cancer: insights from human studies

Although not conclusive, a clinical study indicated a potential benefit of Mg deficiency in patients with malignant tumors (Parsons *et al*, 1974). These results have been sustained by the fact that Mg is required in all the steps involved in cell growth, from receptor-mediated intracellular signaling and transphosphorylation reactions to gene transcription, protein synthesis, DNA duplication and cell division (Wolf and Trapani, 2008). Another study showed that the serum level of Mg is frequently decreased in patients with solid tumors independently from therapies and that this decrease correlates to the stage of malignancy (Sartori *et al*, 1992). This finding seems to be due to the avidity of the tumors for Mg, which behave as Mg traps. Also therapies influence Mg homeostasis. It has been shown that serum Mg decreases at the end of the first week of radiotherapy (Cohen and Kitzes, 1985) as well as after treatment with different chemotherapeutics which induce Mg waste. Indeed, cisplatin is nephrotoxic (Yao *et al*, 2007), and cetuximab, a monoclonal antibody against the Epidermal Growth Factor (EGF) receptor, reversibly and specifically inhibits Mg reabsorption in the renal distal convoluted tubule (Muallem and Moe, 2007). An obvious question is whether radiation- or drug-induced hypomagnesemia amplifies the effect of DNA damaging cancer treatments by acting as a chemo- and radiosensitizer. Recently, decreased serum Mg has been suggested to contribute to the therapeutic effects of cetuximab in patients with colon carcinoma (Vincenzi *et al*, 2008). However, it is still controversial whether to supplement or not severely hypomagnesemic oncologic patients with Mg (Wolf *et al*, 2009).

Several epidemiological studies have provided evidence that a correlation exists between dietary Mg and various types of cancer. A high content of Mg in drinking water seems to protect from liver and oesophageal cancer (Tukiendorf and Rybak, 2004; Yang *et al*, 2002). In addition, Mg content in drinking water was inversely correlated with death by breast, prostate, and ovarian cancers, whereas no correlation existed for other tumors (Yang *et al*, 2000; Yang *et al*, 2000; Chiu *et al*, 2004; Yang *et al*, 2002). In particular, a high serum calcium Ca:Mg ratio has been suggested as a novel risk factor which increases the development of postmenopausal breast cancer (Sahmoun and Singh, 2010), the most commonly diagnosed cancer among women in North America and Europe with a mortality which ranks second only to lung cancer (Jemal *et al*, 2010). Indeed, in western populations, and even more in postmenopausal women who are taking Ca supplements to prevent osteoporosis, a high Ca:Mg intake is rather common and determines a negative Mg balance, since the two minerals compete for the same transporters in almost all tissues. Ca and Mg have equally important roles in regulating cell growth (McKeehan and Ham, 1978) and Mg is considered the natural Ca antagonist. It is therefore feasible that alteration in Ca:Mg ratio might lead to dysregulated cell functions. The ratio of Ca:Mg is also to be considered in relation to colon cancer, one of the three big killers, together with breast and lung cancer, in western society. Ca has been indicated as a chemopreventive agent for colon cancer (Lamprecht and Lipkin, 2003).

It should also be pointed that Mg might have a role in colon cancer prevention. Indeed, large epidemiological studies in Sweden, in the Netherlands, in the USA and in Taiwan have demonstrated an association between low intake of Mg and the risk of colon cancer (Larsson *et al*, 2005; Folsom *et al*, 2006; van den Brandt *et al*, 2007; Chiu *et al*, 2010) and a large population-based prospective study in Japan showed a significant inverse correlation between dietary intake of Mg and colon cancer in men but not in women (Ma *et al*, 2010). Intriguingly, the association between low intake of Mg and colon cancer seems to be due, at least in part, to the increased formation of N-nitroso compounds, most of which are potent carcinogens (Chiu *et al*, 2010). That Mg has a role in colon neoplasia is supported by the association of adenomatous and hyperplastic polyps with a genetic polymorphism of Transient Receptor Potential Melastatin (TRPM)-7 (Dai *et al*, 2007), a ubiquitous ion channel with a central role in Mg uptake and homeostasis (Schmitz *et al*, 2003). Indeed, the subjects carrying the Thr1482-Ile variant allele are at high risk of Mg deficiency and, in turn, of colorectal neoplasia (Dai *et al*, 2007). While total Mg consumption has been linked to a significant lower risk of colorectal adenoma and hyperplastic polyps (Dai *et al*, 2007), unequivocal evidence that Mg reduces the risk of cancer will only be obtained by demonstrating that Mg supplementation prevents colorectal cancer.

The role of Mg in lung cancer is rather controversial. A first case-control study correlated low dietary Mg with poor DNA repair capacity and increased lung cancer risk both in men and women (Mahabir *et al*, 2008). This link was more evident in the elderly, current smokers, drinkers and in those with a late-stage disease. Apart from its role in maintaining genomic stability, the authors proposed several additional mechanisms by which Mg might have protected against lung cancer, i.e. by regulating cell multiplication and protecting against oxidative stress, invariably associated with Mg deficiency (Guerrero-Romero and Rodriguez-Moràn, 2006). Unexpectedly, these results were not supported by a recent prospective analysis which showed that dietary Mg intake slightly increased lung cancer risk (Mahabir *et al*, 2010). These contrasting data could result from recall bias. In addition, residual confounding may account for weak associations because smoking is a very strong risk factor for lung cancer, and diet might not be perfectly measured. More studies of dietary Mg and lung cancer risk are required to carefully consider measurement error issues and confounding from smoking.

A last topic to consider is the implication of inflammation in the initiation and development of cancer in Mg deficient individuals. The inflammation-cancer connection is a well-established paradigm (Colotta *et al*, 2009) and low Mg status has been clearly linked to increased inflammatory stress in humans (Nielsen, 2010). While in some context, such as lymphomas, inflammation exerts an anti-neoplastic role, cancer-related inflammation is involved in the early and late steps of the most common solid tumors. Indeed, inflammatory mediators induce genetic instability and contribute to the proliferation of tumor cells, promote invasion, metastasis and angiogenesis as well as an impaired response to therapies (Colotta *et al*, 2009).

In summary, Mg deficiency seems to be linked to an increased risk of some types of cancers in humans, but population studies are rather complicated to interpret. Too many issues need to be considered - genotype, risk factors, interactions among different nutrients and, in particular, the Mg:Ca ratio, the degree of the inflammatory response, etc – to unravel the role of low Mg in the complex, multistep process of human cancerogenesis.

Low magnesium and cancer: highlights from animal models.

Two main questions have been addressed in animal models: i) whether a relationship exists between Mg and sensitivity to various carcinogens; and ii) whether primary tumor growth and metastasis are affected by Mg deficiency. Several studies indicate that Mg exerts a protective effect in the early phases of chemical cancerogenesis. Mg prevents lead and nickel-induced lung tumors in mice (Poirier *et al*, 1984), inhibits nickel-induced carcinogenesis in the rat kidney (Kasprzak *et al*, 1994) and protects against 3-methyl-cholantrene induced fibro-sarcomas in rats (Patiroğlu *et al*, 1997). In analogy with data in humans, Mg acts as a protective agent in colorectal cancer by inhibiting c-myc expression and ornithine decarboxylase activity in the mucosal epithelium of the intestine (Mori *et al*, 1997). Whether Mg acts directly or by controlling inflammation is an issue which has not received adequate consideration until now. However, it should be pointed out that the inflammatory response in Mg deficient rodents is very accentuated (Mazur *et al*, 2007) and, as mentioned above, inflammation markedly contributes to cancer.

Back to the second question, i.e. whether Mg deficiency impacts on tumor growth *in vivo*, a study showed that dietary Mg deprivation inhibited tumor growth in rats by limiting glutathione (GSH) synthesis (Mills *et al*, 1986) for which Mg is an obligatory cofactor. More recently, in mice subcutaneously injected with Lewis lung carcinoma, mammary adeno-carcinoma and colon carcinoma cells, a low Mg containing diet was shown to inhibit primary tumor growth, an effect which was promptly reversed by re-introducing Mg in the diet (Nasulewicz *et al*, 2004). Surprisingly, Mg deficient mice developed far more lung metastases than controls. Some cellular and molecular aspects were investigated to explain how a low Mg diet inhibited the development of primary tumors while enhancing metastatization. Regarding primary tumors, it is noteworthy that Mg deficiency directly inhibited tumor cell growth by downregulating cyclin B and D3, crucial for the progression through the cell cycle, and by upregulating p21, p27 and Jumonji, all involved in braking cell proliferation (Nasulewicz *et al*, 2004; Maier *et al*, 2007). Mg deficiency also affects tumor development indirectly, because it promotes DNA oxidative damage (Maier *et al*, 2007) and impairs angiogenesis, one of the hallmarks of cancer (Hanahan and Weinberg, 2000). Indeed, Mg-deficient mice develop tumors that are significantly less vascularized than the controls (Maier *et al*, 2007). The angiostatic effect of low Mg can be ascribed to two different mechanisms. First, low Mg inhibits endothelial growth and migration, pivotal steps in the formation of new vessels (Bernardini *et al*, 2005). Second, it has recently been shown that Mg deficiency suppresses hypoxia inducible factor (HIF)-1α activity in paraganglion cells (Torii *et al*, 2009). HIF1α is fundamental to initiate the cell response to hypoxia and, therefore, the release of angiogenic factors. If this finding will also be confirmed in *in vivo* models, it might be involved in impairing angiogenesis upon Mg deficiency. *In vitro*, the suppression of HIF-1α activity is due to the upregulation of IPAS, which acts as a dominant negative inhibitor by preventing HIF-1α DNA binding. Intriguingly, IPAS upregulation is caused by the activation of NFkB, the transcription factor orchestrating the inflammatory response and also implicated in tumorigenesis (Karin *et al*, 2006). Inflammation, which is very intense in Mg deficient mice (Mazur *et al*, 2007), might impact both on the growth of primary tumors and on metastases. Indeed, inflammatory mediators induce genetic instability (Colotta *et al*, 2009) and might synergize with low Mg in causing mutations thus allowing the generation of highly aggressive cells. Tumor Necrosis Factor (TNF)α, target of NFkB and prototypical pro-inflammatory cytokine, is increased in the serum of Mg deficient rodents (Mazur *et al*, 2007). In spite of its name, TNFα has several marked pro-tumoral functions, because it facilitates the epithelial to mesenchymal transition, it enhances tumor invasion and recruits leukocytes within the tumor, thus amplifying the inflammatory process (Drutskaya *et al*, 2010). Moreover, TNFα contributes to immune suppression (Drutskaya *et al*, 2010). Together with TNFα, interleukins (IL)1 and 6, both induced under Mg deprivation, augment the capacity of cancer cells to metastatize (Royuela *et al*, 2008). TNFα and IL1s also upregulate endothelial adhesion molecules in lung capillaries, thus facilitating the tethering of metastatic cells to the vessel wall and their subsequent transmigration and colonization in the adjacent tissues. In addition, Mg is an absolute requirement for the function of the metastasis-suppressor gene product NM23-H1 (Ma *et al*, 2008). NM23-H1 knock-out mice showed accelerated metastasis (Boissan *et al*, 2005). It is therefore possible that low Mg availability impairs NM23-H1 anti-metastatic activity in mice.

Briefly, in rodents Mg deficiency seems to participate both in early (initiation) and in late (progression) phases of tumorigenesis. The following scenario is feasible. Low Mg promotes oxidative stress and inflammation which generate genetic instability and, therefore, increases the risk of mutations. Since Mg is an essential cofactor in almost all enzymatic systems involved in DNA synthesis and repair, under low Mg availability mutations may become permanent thus generating the so-called "initiated" cell. The persistence of oxidative stress and inflammation together might generate further mutations, which render the cell immortal and self sufficient in terms of proliferation. Some cells might also acquire an invasive, metastatic phenotype and colonize distant organs (Figure 1).

Magnesium and cancer: lessons from cultured cells

Even though studies on cultured cells can only focus on some isolated aspects of the complex events implicated in the development of tumors, they have produced an extraordinary body of knowledge. The field of Mg research in cancer makes no exception.

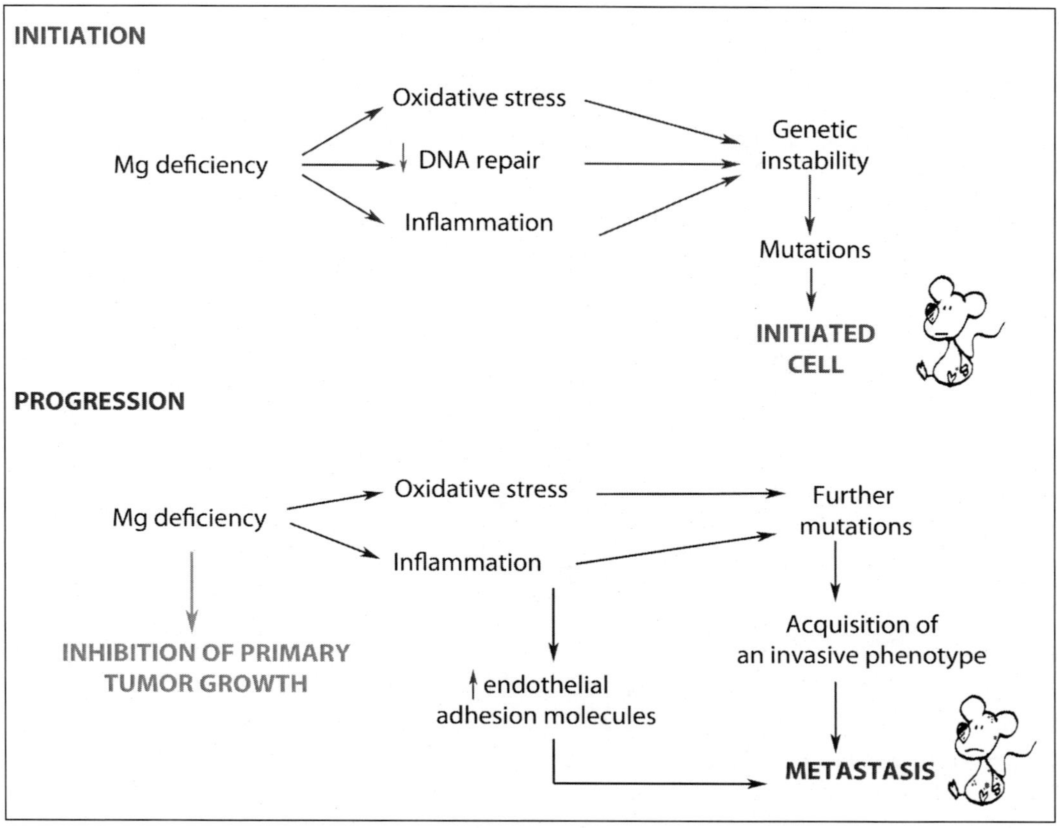

Figure 1. A low Mg content in the diet might influence both early and late steps of tumorigenesis in mice. **Upper panel:** By inducing oxidative stress and inflammation and by inhibiting DNA repair enzyme, low Mg enhances the risk of DNA damage and, therefore, might synergize with carcinogens giving rise to an initiated cell, which is potentially capable of originating a tumor. **Lower panel:** Once the tumor has developed, low Mg facilitates metastasis by further damaging DNA and by inducing inflammatory events, in the face of an inhibition of primary tumor growth.

The impact of extracellular Mg on tumor cells

Based on the results obtained in humans and in animal models, the effects of low extracellular Mg on tumor cells has been investigated. While normal diploid cells are very sensitive to low extracellular Mg and are rapidly growth retarded, neoplastic cells are rather refractory to Mg deprivation (Wolf *et al*, 2009). Indeed, tumor cells require longer times and much lower concentrations of extracellular Mg than normal cells to slow their proliferation rate (Wolf, 2004; Maier *et al*, 2007). Another peculiarity of tumor cells is their avidity for Mg, which accumulates within the cells even when extracellular Mg concentrations are low. The molecular mechanisms involved have not been completely disclosed, but it is known that Na-dependent Mg extrusion is impaired in tumor cells and contributes to elevate intracellular Mg (Wolf *et al*, 2007). In addition, TRPM7 is overexpressed in breast tumors and in neoplastic cultured cells (Guilbert et al, 2009) and this feature may well account for the avidity of cancer cells for extracellular Mg. Also nuclear Mg content is higher in neoplastic than in normal cells (Lukacs *et al*, 1996). Considering that Mg acts a second messenger and activates a vast array of enzymes, it noteworthy that not only intracellular Mg increases but also it is differently distributed in transformed vs normal cells.

The role of intracellular Mg in tumor cells

A very simple question is then raised: does intracellular Mg impact on different aspects of the neoplastic phenotype? Before addressing this issue, it is useful to rapidly review the latest hypotheses proposed to explain the contribution of Mg to normal cell proliferation. Since Mg participates in all the major metabolic processes as well as to redox reactions, it is no surprise that

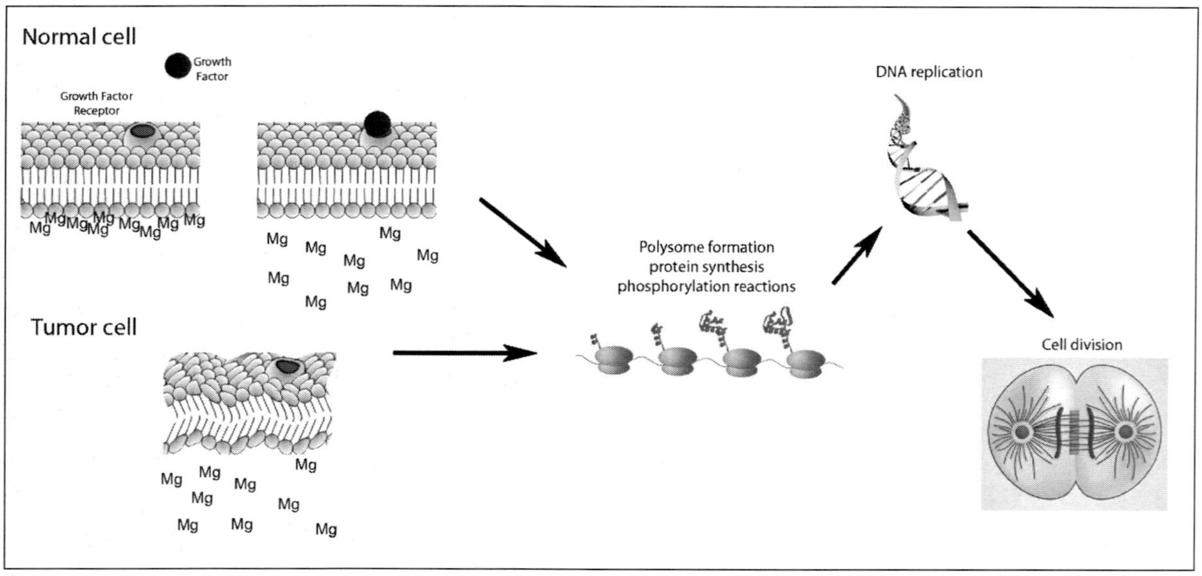

Figure 2. Intracellular Mg controls cell proliferation. In normal cells, the binding of a growth factor to its receptor determines membrane perturbations which decrease Mg binding affinity for negatively charged membrane sites, thus increasing intracellular Mg levels. Increased intracellular Mg promotes polysome formation, protein synthesis, DNA synthesis and ultimately cell division (according to Rubin, 2007). In neoplastic cells, the membranes are altered and differently organized. These modifications decrease the binding affinity for Mg which therefore increases promoting protein and DNA synthesis.

it has a direct role in controlling cell survival and growth. Cell survival is strictly related to attachment to the extracellular matrix. Adhesion and consequent spreading are mediated by diverse molecules, most notably by integrins which require divalent cations such as Ca and Mg to function (Rouslathi and Pierschbacher, 1987). Once the cells adhere and spread, they are alive, metabolically active and ready to respond to growth factors. According to a recently proposed model (Rubin, 2007), intracellular Mg levels vary in quiescent vs growth factor-activated, proliferating cells. In quiescent cells, cytosolic Mg stabilizes the plasma membrane and subcellular organelles by complexing with negatively charged phospholipids (Suh and Halle, 2007), while nuclear Mg stabilizes the double helix and retains the chromatin structure (Figure 2). Binding of growth factors to their cognate receptors perturbs the membranes and, consequently, decreases Mg binding affinity for the membrane, thus resulting in increased focal concentrations of intracellular Mg (Rubin, 2007). Also Mg influx from the extracellular milieu contributes to increase total intracellular Mg in response to growth factors. In particular, EGF regulates Mg transepithelial transport by increasing TRPM6 activity and surface expression (Thebault *et al*, 2009). Intracellular Mg then behaves as a second messenger and regulates a wide variety of reactions ultimately leading to cell division.

Neoplastic transformation dramatically disrupts these controlled and coordinated fluctuations of intracellular Mg (Figure 2). Membrane perturbations that are typically associated with the neoplastic phenotype determine the release of intracellularly bound Mg. Accordingly, a seminal study showed a significant increase of intracellular Mg in human brain tumors by 31P-NMR (Taylor *et al*, 1991).

Having high intracellular Mg might represent a selective advantage for the transformed cells. Mg forms complexes with ATP, ADP and GTP, being necessary for the activity of enzymes implicated in the transfer of phosphate groups such as glucokinase, phosphofructokinase, phosphoglycerate-kinase and pyruvate kinase (Gunther, 2008), enzymes of glycolysis which is known to be the preferential pathway utilized by neoplastic cells to produce energy also in the presence of oxygen. This issue has recently been reappraised. The expression of TRPM7 and, therefore, the capability of the cells to take up Mg has been associated with the transition from a quiescent to a proliferative metabolic state in which it is aerobic glycolysis that generates the energy necessary for cell growth (Sahni *et al*, 2010).

Mg also complexes with DNA polymerase, ribonucleases, adenylcyclase, phosphodiesterases, guanylate-cyclase, ATPases and GTPases, being therefore implicated in the metabolism of nucleic acids and proteins and in signal transduction. In addition, Mg activates telomerase (Lue, 1999), a ribonucleoprotein that is responsible for maintaining the terminal repeats of telomeres and conferring limitless replicative potential. It is because of the reactivation of telomerase activity that transformed cells become immortal (Hanahan and Weinberg, 2000).

Intriguingly, the nuclear Ser/Thr phosphatase PPM1D (also known as WIP1), which is over-expressed in human primary breast, gastric, pancreatic, ovarian and neuroblastoma tumors, requires Mg for its activity. PPM1D is involved in the regulation of several essential signaling pathways that are implicated in cancer pathogenesis (Le Guezennec and Bulavin, 2010). The oncogenic properties of PPM1D were originally thought to stem from its ability to dephosphorylate and, consequently, inactivate the p53 tumor suppressor gene. However, recent studies have shown that PPM1D targets also other key stress response kinases, which function in DNA damage response and repair. In addition, PPM1D complements several oncogenes, such as *Ras*, *Myc*, and *HER-2/neu,* for cellular transformation both *in vitro* and *in vivo.* Therefore, a rise in intracellular Mg might result in a permanent activation of PPM1D and potently contribute to several steps of tumor development.

A last issue needs consideration. Tumors should be regarded as complex tissues in which normal cell types within the stroma serve as active collaborators in cancer progression. Many of the growth signals driving the proliferation and invasion of carcinoma cells originate from the stromal cell components of the tumor mass. Indeed, low Mg modulates the functions of normal cells present in the tumor micro-environment. In particular, endothelial cells cultured in low Mg release higher amounts of metalloproteases and growth factors (Ferrè *et al*, 2010). Similar results were obtained in cultured human fibroblasts (unpublished results). In addition, low Mg promotes endothelial and fibroblast senescence (Killilea and Maier, 2008) and senescent cells can modify the tissue environment in a way that synergizes with oncogenic mutations to promote the progression of cancers (Campisi, 2003). On the other hand, low Mg impairs the acquisition of an angiogenic phenotype *in vitro*. Yet, the question about the role of Mg deficiency in cancer remains: good or bad?

A synthetic view

How to reconcile this wealth of information? Although some results are controversial, it is possible to conclude that most of the data available point to low Mg as a contributing factor to tumorigenesis. Mg deficiency increases oxidative stress, which causes DNA damage, and impairs DNA repair mechanisms. It therefore may lead to mutations that produce oncogenes with dominant gain of function and tumor suppressor genes with recessive loss of function (Hanahan and Weinberg, 2000). Upon transformation, the cells lose the capability to regulate Mg homeostasis. Mg accumulates in the cell also when Mg availability is low, its distribution is altered and is not subjected to coordinated fluctuations in response to various stimuli. Low extracellular Mg also affects normal stromal cells that can release growth factors and proteases, thus potentiating tumor growth and development. In addition, *in vivo* low Mg activates an inflammatory response, which has many tumor-promoting effects.

Big questions

The connection between Mg and cancer is rather strong, but several questions remain. First, it might be asked whether Mg deficiency is sufficient for the development of cancer. Indeed, low Mg increases the levels of reactive oxygen species, which mutate DNA and, therefore, generate genetic instability. Another candidate as a potential carcinogen in Mg deficiency is inflammation. However, it is more likely that a low Mg state only contributes to tumorigenesis by synergizing with many different factors.

A second aspect which is often underevaluated is the effect on the tumor of an aberrant Ca:Mg ratio that is inevitably created in Mg deficiency. Even though Ca and Mg have become the gold standard when discussing nutritional supplements, the balance between the two cations needs to be carefully evaluated both *in vitro* and *in vivo*.

A third question arises about whether outcomes in the cancer mouse model can predict a real human disease mechanism. Mg deficiency retards primary tumor growth but enhances metastases in mice. It would be relevant to consider the balance between cancer-promoting and inhibiting responses by low Mg in humans also.

The last bigger question is whether knowledge about the connection between low Mg and cancer can be translated into useful approaches to prevent and treat cancer. Most of the data available suggest that Mg could be a chemo-preventive agent. Therefore, correcting Mg intake might represent an effective and low cost preventive measure to reduce cancer risk. The picture is different in oncologic patients, because hypomagnesemia might be beneficial since it sensitizes neoplastic cells to radiation or chemotherapeutics. Therefore the "hamletic" doubt remains: to treat or not to treat hypo-magnesemic oncologic patients?

Conclusion

Future research should focus on elucidating how Mg is involved in preventing cancer by modulating crucial events in signal transduction pathways and the cell cycle. Hints might derive from nutrigenomics, i.e. the use of high-throughput genomic methods in nutritional studies, which can provide information about the cross-talk between Mg and genes. The next step should lead to translation of this basic research into nutritional preventive protocols for human tumors, an approach that will involve many scientific disciplines. The challenge is great, but the reward might be enormous.

Acknowledgements
This work is supported by MIUR-PRIN 2007 grant number 2007ZT39FN.

References

Bernardini D, Nasulewicz A, Mazur A, Maier JA (2005) Magnesium and microvascular endothelial cells: a role in inflammation and angiogenesis. *Frontiers Biosci* 10: 1177-1182.

Boissan M, Wendum D, Arnaud-Dabernat S, Munier A, Debray M, Lascu I, Daniel JY, Lacombe ML (2005) Increased lung metastasis in transgenic NM23-Null/SV40 mice with hepatocellular carcinoma. *J Natl Cancer Inst* 97: 836-845.

Campisi J (2003) Cancer and aging: rival demons? *Nat Rev Cancer* 3:339-349.

Chiu HF, Chang CC, Yang CY (2004) Calcium and Magnesium in drinking water and the risk of death from ovarian cancer. *Magnes Res* 17:28–34.

Chiu HF, Tsai SS, Wu TN, Yang CY (2010) Colon cancer and the content of nitrate and magnesium in drinking water. *Magnes Res* 23:81-89.

Cohen L, Kitzes R (1985) Early radiation induced proctosigmoiditis responds to magnesium therapy. *Magnesium* 4:16-19.

Colotta F, Allavena P, Sica A, Garlanda C, Mantovani A (2009). Cancer-related inflammation, the seventh hallmark of cancer: link to genetic instability. *Carcinogenesis* 30: 1073-1081.

Dai Q, Shrubsole J, Ness RM, Schlundt D, Cai Q, Smalley WE, Li M, Shyr Y, Zheng W (2007) The relation of magnesium and calcium intakes and a genetic polymorphism in the magnesium transporter to colorectal neoplasia risk. *Am J Clin Nutr* 86:743-751.

Doll R, Peto R (1981) The causes of cancer: quantitative estimates of avoidable risks of cancer in the US today. *J Natl Cancer Inst* 66:1191-1308.

Drutskaya MS, Efimov GA, Kruglov AA, Kuprash DV, Nedospasov SA (2010) Tumor necrosis factor, lymphotoxin and cancer. *IUBMB Life* 62:283-9.

Ferrè S, Baldoli E, Leidi M, Maier JA (2010) Magnesium deficiency promotes a pro-atherogenic phenotype in cultured human endothelial cells via activation of NFkB. *Biochim Biophys Acta* 1802:952-8.

Folsom AR, Hong CP (2006) Magnesium intake and reduced risk of colon cancer in a prospective study of women. *Am J Epidemiol* 163: 232-235.

Ford ES, Mokdad AH (2003) Dietary magnesium intake in a national sample of US adults. *J Nutr* 133:2879-2882.

Guerrero-Romero F, Rodríguez-Morán M (2006) Hypomagnesemia, oxidative stress, inflammation, and metabolic syndrome. *Diabetes Metab Res Rev* 22:471–476.

Guilbert A, Gautier M, Dhennin-Duthille I, Haren N, Sevestre H, Ouadid-Ahidouch H (2009) Evidence that TRPM7 is required for breast cancer cell proliferation. *Am J Physiol Cell Physiol* 297:C493-502.

Günther T (2008) Comment on the number of magnesium activated enzymes. *Magnes Res* 21:185-187.

Hanahan D, Weinberg RA (2000) The hallmarks of cancer. *Cell* 100:57-70.

Jemal A, Siegel R, Xu J, Ward E (2010) Cancer Statistics, 2010. *CA Cancer J Clin* 60:277-300.

Karin M, Cao Y, Greten FR, Li ZW (2002) NF-kB in cancer: from innocent bystander to major culprit. *Nat Rev Cancer* 2:301-310.

Kasprzak KS, Diwan BA, Rice JM (1994) Iron accelerates while magnesium inhibits nickel-induced carcinogenesis in the rat kidney. *Toxicology* 90:129-140.

Killilea DW, Maier JA (2008) A connection between magnesium deficiency and aging: new insights from cellular studies. *Magnes Res* 21:77-82.

Lamprecht SA, Lipkin M (2003) Chemoprevention of colon cancer by calcium, vitamin D and folate: molecular mechanisms. *Nat Rev Cancer 3*:601-613.

Larsson SC, Bergkvist L, Wolk A (2005) Magnesium intake in relation to risk of colon cancer in women. *JAMA* 293:86–89.

Le Guezennec X, Bulavin DV (2010) WIP1 phosphatase at the crossroads of cancer and aging. *Trends Biochem Sci* 35:109-114.

Lue NF (1999) Sequence-specific and conformation-dependent binding of yeast telomerase RNA to single-stranded telomeric DNA. *Nucleic Acids Res* 1999 27:2560-7.

Lukács GL, Zs-Nagy I, Steiber J, Györi F, Balázs G (1996) Relative intranuclear magnesium and phosphorus contents in normal and tumor cells of the human thyroid gland as revealed by energy-dispersive X-ray microanalysis. *Scanning Microsc* 10:1191-200.

Ma E, Sasazuki S, Inoue M, Iwasaki M, Sawada N, Takachi R, Tsugane S (2010) High dietary intake of magnesium may decrease risk of colorectal cancer in Japanese men. *J Nutr* 140:779-85.

Ma W, Chen J, Xue X, Wang Z, Liu H, Wang T, Bai Y, Tang SC, Zhou Q (2008) Alteration in gene expression profile and biological behavior in human lung cancer cell line NL9980 by MN23-H1 gene silencing. *Biochem Biophys Res Commun* 371:425-430.

Mahabir S, Forman MR, Dong YQ, Park Y, Hollenbeck A, Schatzkin A (2010) Mineral intake and lung cancer risk in the NIH-American Association of Retired Persons Diet and Health study. *Cancer Epidemiol Biomarkers Prev* 19:1976-83.

Mahabir S, Wei Q, Barrera SL, Dong YQ, Etzel CJ, Spitz MR, Forman MR (2008) Dietary magnesium and DNA repair capacity as risk factors for lung cancer. *Carcinogenesis* 29:949-956.

Maier JA, Nasulewicz-Goldeman A, Simonacci M, Boninsegna A, Mazur A, Wolf FI (2007) Insights into the mechanisms involved in magnesium-dependent inhibition of primary tumor growth. *Nutr Cancer* 59:192-198.

Manson MM (2003) Cancer prevention – the potential for diet to modulate molecular signaling. *Trend Mol Med* 9:11-18.

Mazur A, Maier JA, Rock E, Gueux E, Nowacki W, Rayssiguier Y (2007) Magnesium and the inflammatory response: potential physiopathological implications. *Arch Biochem Biophys* 458:48-56.

Mc Keehan, Ham RG (1978) Ca and Mg ions and the regulation of multiplication in normal and transformed cells. *Nature* 275:756-758.

McKeehan WL, Ham RG (1978) Ca and Mg ions and the regulation of multiplication in normal and transformed cells. *Nature* 275:756-758.

Mills BJ, Lindeman RD, Lang CA (1986) Magnesium deficiency inhibits biosynthesis of blood glutathione and tumor growth in the rat. *Proc Soc Exp Biol Med* 181:326-32.

Mori H, Tanaka T, Sugie S, Yoshimi N, Kawamori T, Hirose Y, Ohnishi M (1997) Chemopreventium by naturally occuring and sinthetic agents in oral, liver and large bowel carcinogenesis. *J Cell Biochem Suppl* 27:35–41.

Muallem S, Moe OW (2007) When EGF is offside, magnesium is wasted. *J Clin Invest* 117:2086–9.

Nasulewicz A, Wietrzyk J, Wolf FI, Dzimira S, Madej J, Maier JA, Rayssiguier Y, Mazur A, Opolski A (2004) Magnesium Deficiency Inhibits Primary Tumor Growth But Favors Metastasis In Mice. *Biochim Biophys Acta-Mol Basis Dis*1739:26-32.

Nielsen FH (2010) Magnesium, inflammation, and obesity in chronic disease. *Nutr Rev* 68:333-340.

Parson FM,Edwards GF, Anderson CK, Ahmad S, Clark PB, Hetherington C, Young GA (1974) Regression of malignant tumors in potassium and magnesium depletion induced by diet and haemodialysis. *Lancet* 16:243–244.

Patiroğlu T, Sahin G, Kontaş O, Uzüm K, Saraymen R (1997) Protective effect of magnesium supplementation on experimental 3-methyl cholanthrene-induced fibrosarcoma and changes in tissue magnesium distribution during carcinogenesis in rats. *Biol Trace Elem Res* 56:179-185.

Poirier LA, Theiss JC, Arnold LJ, Shimkin MB (1984) Inhibition by magnesium and calcium acetates of lead subacetate- and nickel acetate-induced lung tumors in strain A mice. *Cancer Res* 44:1520-1522.

Quamme GA (2010) Molecular identification of ancient and modern mammalian magnesium transporters. *Am J Physiol Cell Physiol* 298:C407-C429.

Royuela M, Rodríguez-Berriguete G, Fraile B, Paniagua R (2008) TNF-alpha/IL-1/NF-kappaB transduction pathway in human cancer prostate. *Histol Histopathol* 23:1279-90.

Rubin H (2007) The logic of the Membrane, Magnesium, Mitosis (MMM) model for the regulation of animal cell proliferation. *Arch Biochem Biophys* 458: 16–23.

Ruoslahti E, Pierschbacher MD (1987) New perspectives in cell adhesion: RGD and integrins. *Science* 238:491-97.

Sahmoun AE, Singh BB (2010) Does a higher ratio of serum calcium to magnesium increase the risk for postmenopausal breast cancer? *Med Hypotheses* 75:315-18.

Sahni J, Tamura R, Sweer IR, Scharenberg AM (2010) TRPM7 regulates quiescent/proliferative metabolic transitions in lymphocytes. *Cell Cycle* 9:3565-74.

Sartori S, Nielsen I, Tassinari D, Mazzotta D,Vecchiatti G, Sero A, Abbasciano V (1992) Serum and erythrocyte magnesium concentrations in solid tumors: relationship with stage and malignancy. *Magnes Res* 5:189–92.

Schmitz C, Perraud AL, Johnson CO, Inabe K, Smith MK, Penner R, Kurosaki T, Fleig A, Scharenberg AM (2003) Regulation of vertebrate cellular Mg homeostasis by TRPM7. *Cell* 114:191-200.

Suh BC, Halle B (2007) Electrostatic interaction of internal Mg with membrane PIP2 seen with KCNQ K+ channel. *J General Physiol* 130:241-56.

Taylor JS, Vigneron DB, Murphy-Boesch J, Nelson SJ, Kessler HB, Coia L, Curran W, Brown TR (1991) Free magnesium levels in normal human brain and brain tumors: 31P chemical-shift imaging measurements at 1.5 T. *Proc Natl Acad Sci USA* 88:6810-6814.

Thebault S, Alexander RT, Tiel Groenestege WM, Hoenderop JG, Bindels RJ (2009) EGF increases TRPM6 activity and surface expression. *J Am Soc Nephrol* 20: 78-85.

Torii S, Kobayashi K, Takahashi M, Katahira K, Goryo K, Matsushita N, Yasumoto K, Fujii-Kuriyama Y, Sogawa K (2009) Magnesium deficiency causes loss of response to intermittent hypoxia in paraganglion cells. *J Biol Chem* 284:19077-89.

Tukiendorf A, Rybak Z (2004) New data on ecological analysis of possible relationship between magnesium in drinking water and liver cancer. *Magnes Res* 17:46–52.

van den Brandt PA, Smits KM, Goldbohm RA, Weijenberg MP (2007) Magnesium intake and colon cancer risk in the Netherlands Cohort Study. *Br J Cancer* 96:510-13.

Vincenzi B, Santini D, Galluzzo S, Russo A, Fulfaro F, SillettaM, Battistoni F, Rocci L, Zobel BB, Adamo V, Dicuonzo G, Tonini G. (2008) Early magnesium reduction in advanced colorectal cancer patients treated with cetuximab plus irinotecan as predictive factor of efficacy and outcome. *Clin Cancer Res* 14:4219–24.

Wolf FI, Cittadini AR, Maier JA (2009) Magnesium and tumors: ally or foe? *Cancer Treatment Rev* 35:378-82.

Wolf FI, Maier JA, Nasulewicz A, Feillet-Coudray C, Mazur A, Simonacci M, Cittadini A (2007) Magnesium and neoplasia: from carcinogenesis to tumor growth and progression or treatment. *Arch Biochem Biophys* 458:24-32.

Wolf FI, Trapani V (2008) Cell (patho)physiology of magnesium. *Clin Sci* 114:27-35.

Wolf FI. TRPM7: Channeling the Future of Cellular Magnesium Homeostasis? (2004) *Sci STKE* 233:pe23.

Yang CY, Chiu HF, Cheng MF, Hsu TY, Cheng MF, Wu TN (2000) Calcium and Magnesium in drinking water and the risk of death from breast cancer. *J Toxicol Environ Health A* 60:231–41.

Yang CY, Chiu HF, Tsai SS, Cheng MF, Lin MC, Sung FC (2000) Calcium and Magnesium in drinking water and the risk of death from prostate cancer. *J Toxicol Environ Health A* 60:17–26.

Yang CY, Chiu HF, Tsai SS, Wu TN, Chang CC (2002) Calcium and Magnesium in drinking water and the risk of death from esophageal cancer. *Magnes Res* 15:215–22.

Yao X, Panichpisal K, Kurtzman N, Nugent K (2007) Cisplatin nephrotoxicity: a review. *Am J Med Sci* 334:115–24.

Magnesium in Parkinson's disease: an update in clinical and basic aspects

Kiyomitsu Oyanagi ✉ *and Tomoyo Hashimoto*

Department of Brain Disease Research, Shinshu University School of Medicine, Matsumoto, Nagano 390-8621, Japan.
✉ k123ysm@shinshu-u.ac.jp

Abstract

Magnesium (Mg) is essential for cell functions such as transport of calcium and potassium ions, and modulates signal transduction, energy metabolism, and cell proliferation. Several studies elucidated a reduced concentration of Mg in patients with Parkinson's disease (PD), and experimentally, severe loss of dopaminergic neurons exclusively in the substantia nigra in 1-year-old rats that had been subjected to continuously low Mg intake (one-fifth of the normal level) over generations. A study conducted by the authors revealed a significant and striking effect of Mg to prevent neurite and neuron pathology, and also to ameliorate neurite pathology in a rat Parkinson disease (PD) model involving culture of ventral mesencephalic-striatal cells with 1-methyl-4-phenylpyridinium (MPP^+). Mg is expected to prevent and ameriolate Parkinson's disease in cases where it would be able to cross into the brain in a suitable way.

Introduction

Parkinson's disease (PD) is a neurodegenerative disease occurring in middle-aged and aged humans characterized by clinical symptoms including tremor and rigidity (Parkinson, 1817). It has been reported that almost 90% of the patients are sporadic and 10% are familial. Sporadic PD shows neuropathological features involving the appearance of Lewy bodies (Lewy, 1912; Tretiakoff, 1919) and loss of neurons in the substantia nigra (Figures 1 and 2) and substantia innominata. After establishment of the disease as an entity, it was revealed that dopaminergic neurons in the vetral tegmental area, noradrenergic neurons in the locus coeruleus and motor vagal nucleus, serotonergic neurons in the dorsal raphe nucleus, and neurons in the sympathetic ganglia and visceral autonomic nervous system are involved in the disease with neuronal loss and presence of Lewy bodies (Jellinger, 1999). In the present manuscript, the authors review the role of magnesium (Mg) in the pathogenesis and pathomechanisms in clinical and basic aspects of PD.

Mg in Parkinson's disease and related diseases

Uitti et al (1989) analyzed four brain regions (frontal cortex, caudate nucleus, substantia nigra and cerebellum) for concentrations of 24 metals (Ag, Al, As, B, Be, Ca, Cd, Co, Cr, Cu, Fe, K, Pb, Mg, Mn, Mo, Na, Ni, P, Se, Ti, V, W, Zn) by atomic absorption and atomic emission spectroscopy in brains of 9 patients with PD, 15 patients with other chronic neurological diseases and 12 subjects of controls. The results were that brains of PD and parkinsonism secondary to neurofibrillary tangle disease showed lower concentrations of Mg in the caudate nucleus and copper in the substantia nigra than control brains. Barbiloni et al (1999) performed in vivo phosphorus magnetic resonance spectroscopy on the occipital lobes of 13 patients with PD, 15 patients with multiple system atrophy and 16 age-matched healthy subjects. They reported that patients with PD showed significantly increased contents of inorganic phosphate (Pi), decreased cytosolic free $[Mg^{2+}]$, and unchanged phosphocreatine and pH. Bocca et al (2006) examined concentrations of Ca, Cu, Fe, Mg, Si and Zn by inductively coupled plasma atomic emission spectrometry (ICP-AES) in blood, urine and cerebrospinal fluid (CSF) of 91 PD patients and 18 controls. They concluded that Mg concentration in CSF of PD patients decreased with the duration and severity of the disease.

It has been proposed that Mg deficiency is involved in the pathogenesis of parkinsonism-dementia complex (PDC) and amyotrophic lateral sclerosis (ALS) in the Chamorro population on

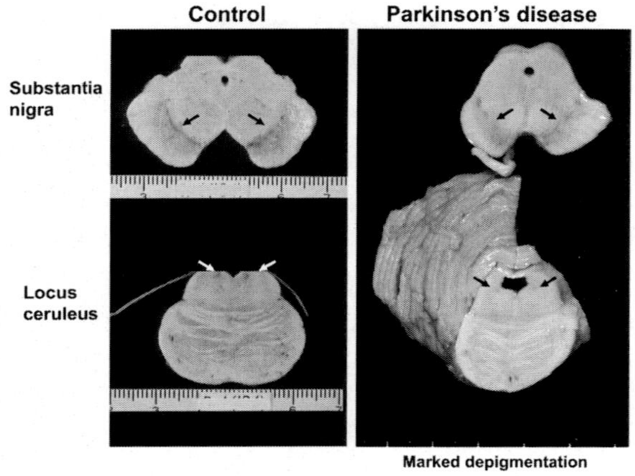

Figure 1. Midbrain and upper pons. The substantia nigra and locus coeruleus in the patient with Parkinson's disease show marked depigmentation as compared with those of controls.

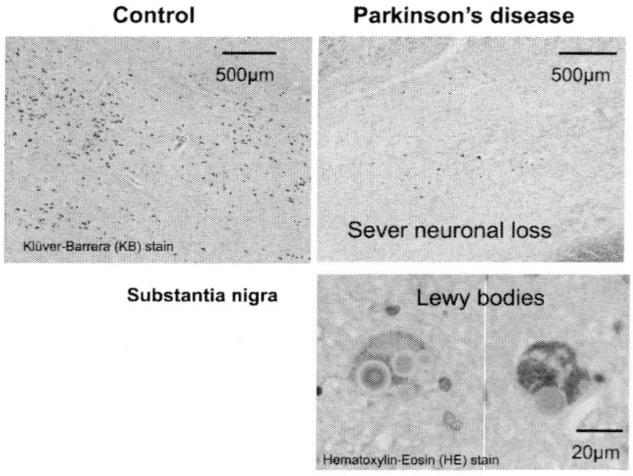

Figure 2. The substantia nigra of a patient with Parkinson's disease shows severe loss of neurons as compared with a control subject. Some remaining neurons represent Lewy bodies.

Guam, which is a member of the Mariana islands in the western Pacific Ocean, as well as in the Kii peninsula of Japan and in West New Guinea (Yase 1978, Garruto *et al,* 1984). PDC is a disease entity that was established by Hirano *et al,* (1961a, 1961b) that affects the neurons in the substantia nigra, brainstem, and temporal and frontal cortex. The disease is characterized by the presence of neurofibrillary tangles in the remaining neurons, and disease-specific granular hazy inclusions in the astrocytes (Oyanagi *et al,* 1997; Oyanagi, 2005), tau-positive fine granules in the cerebral white matter (Yamazaki *et al,* 2005), and widespread TDP-43-immunopositive inclusions (Hasegawa *et al,* 2007). Patients exhibit parkinsonism and dementia, and usually die within about 5 years from infectious diseases (Hirano *et al,* 1961a; 1961b; Chen and Chase, 1985). ALS is a motor neuron disease affecting the Betz cells in the cerebral cortex, and facial and hypoglossal nuclei in the brainstem and anterior horn cells in the spinal cord, and usually patients die of respiratory failure within 5 years after the onset.

Possible pathomechanisms in Parkinson's disease

Mitochondrial damage and oxidative stress

Increased expression of 4-hydroxy-2-nonenal (HNE) (Yoritaka *et al*, 1996), decreased activity of mitochondrial complex I and a decreased amount of alpha-ketoglutarate dehydrogenase complex (KGDHC) in the pigmented neurons of the substantia nigra (Hattori *et al*, 1991; Mizuno *et al*, 1994) have been reported in affected patients. In the substantia nigra, decreased activity of catalase and peroxidase (Ambani *et al*, 1975) and increased amounts of protein carbonyls, 8-hydroxy-2'-deoxyguanosine (8-OHdG)/8-hydroxy-guanine (8-OHG), 4-hydroxynonenal-lysine and malondialdehyde-lysine (MDAL) (Alam *et al*, 1997a,b; Zhang *et al*, 1999; Dalfo *et al*, 2005) have been reported.

1-Methyl-4-phenyl-1,2,3,6-tetrahydropyridine (MPTP) was the first human parkinsonian agent to be characterized. It is converted to 1-methyl-4-phenylpyridinium (MPP^+) by monoamine oxidase B in astrocytes. MPP^+ damages mitochondrial complex I of dopaminergic neurons after transfer by the dopamine transporter, and increased calcium permeability of the mitochondrial membrane induces free radicals (Smeyne *et al*, 2005). MPP^+ has been used to induce selective degeneration of dopaminergic neurons in an experimental model of PD (Nakamura *et al*, 2000). In addition, rotenone, 6-hydroxydopamine (6-OHDA), paraquat and annonacin have been used as noxious agents to create in vivo models of PD (Fornai *et al*, 2003; Champy *et al*, 2004; Bove *et al*, 2005) (Figure 3). Dopamine and dopamine quinones themselves are considered to be causes of oxidative stress. PINK1 (PTEN-induced putative kinase 1) maintains mitochondrial function, and the gene is causative in some familial PD (Valente *et al*, 2004).

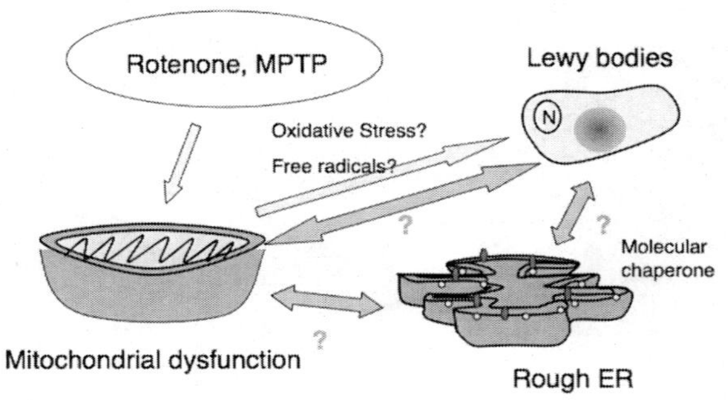

Figure 3. Possible relationship between mitochondria, rough ER and Lewy body formation.

Unfolded protein retention and endplasmic reticulum stress

Alpha-synuclein was found as a main component of the Lewy bodies and the gene was found to be a causative gene of a rare autosomal dominant PD (Polymeropoulos *et al,* 1997). It has been reported that multiplication of the gene was to be the cause of the disease (Singleton *et al,* 2003). It has been suggested that aggregates of alpha-synuclein cause potentiation of oxidative stress, possibly with interaction with iron. Synuclein was considered to be degraded in the proteasome. Knock-out of the 26S proteasome in the dopaminergic neurons induced "pale bodies" which is reported to be a prodrome of the Lewy bodies (Bedford *et al,* 2008).

Parkin and UCHL-1 are considered essential for ubiquitination of the unfolded proteins, and the gene mutations were found in some familial PD. It is considered that an oxidative stress may lead a combination of Parkin and DJ-1, and the combination suffocates unfolded protein degradation (Kitada *et al*, 1998; Bonifati *et al,* 2003). Mg has also been reported to inhibit spontaneous and iron-induced aggregation of alpha-synuclein (Golts *et al,* 2002) (Figure 4).

Low Mg and Parkinson's disease model

In the course of investigations into the pathogenesis of the PDC, the present authors performed an experiment in which rats were exposed to restricted intake of Ca and/or Mg over two generations. This resulted in severe loss of dopaminergic neurons exclusively in the substantia nigra in 1-year-old rats that had been subjected to continuously low Mg intake

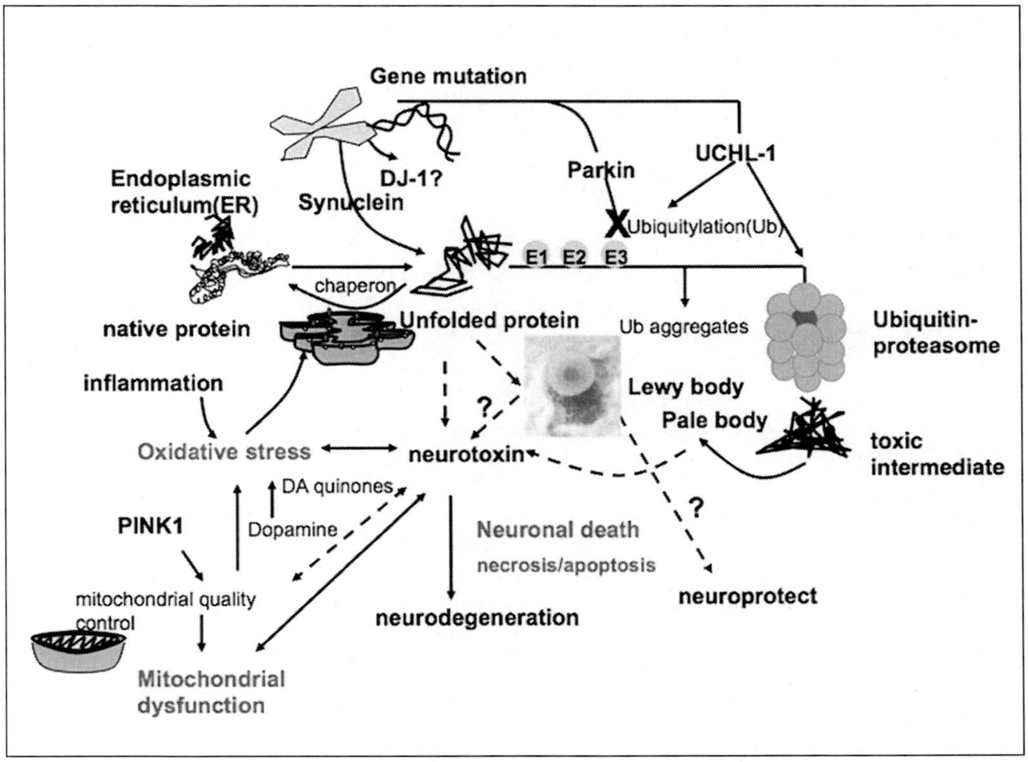

Figure 4. Scheme of possible pathomechanisms of dopaminergic neuron death in Parkinson's disease.

(one-fifth of the normal level) over generations (Oyanagi *et al*, 2006). This finding suggested a deep concern of low Mg intake over several generations to the pathogenesis of degeneration of the substantia nigra in humans.

Therapeutic possibility by Mg for Parkinson's disease

As a blocker of the glutamatergic NMDA receptor

Mg controls cytochrome *c* release in mitochondria (Eskes *et al*, 1998), and decreases the activity of N-methyl-D-aspartate (NMDA) receptors in excitotoxicity (Mayer *et al*, 1984). Mg treatment has also been shown to decrease cerebral infarct volume in rats in vivo (Lyden *et al*, 2000). The mechanism responsible for the neuroprotective effect of Mg has been considered to be reduced presynaptic release of the neurotransmitter glutamate (Lin *et al*, 2002), and blockade of the glutamatergic NMDA receptor (Nowak *et al*, 1984)(Figure 5). A relationship between decreased Mg concentration in serum and migraine has been reported in humans, and it has been suggested that migraine might be caused by hypersensitivity of the NMDA receptor to glutamic acid and certain other neuro-excitatory amino acids due to Mg depletion (Cojocaru *et al*, 2006). A decrease of cytosolic free Mg in the occipital lobe of PD patients has also been demonstrated by phosphorus magnetic response spectroscopy (Barbiroli *et al*, 1999).

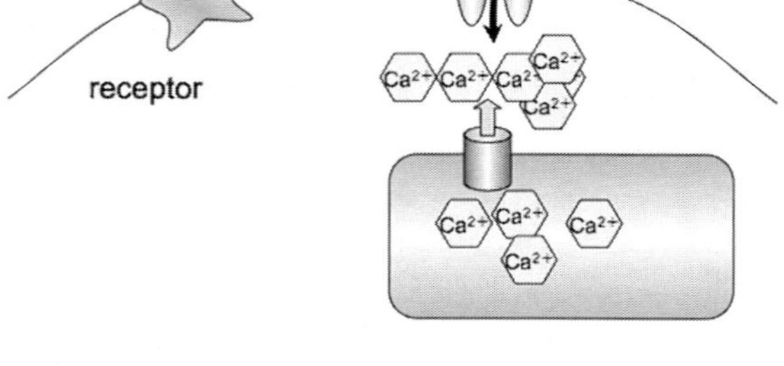

Figure 5. Metallic elements and neuron conduction.

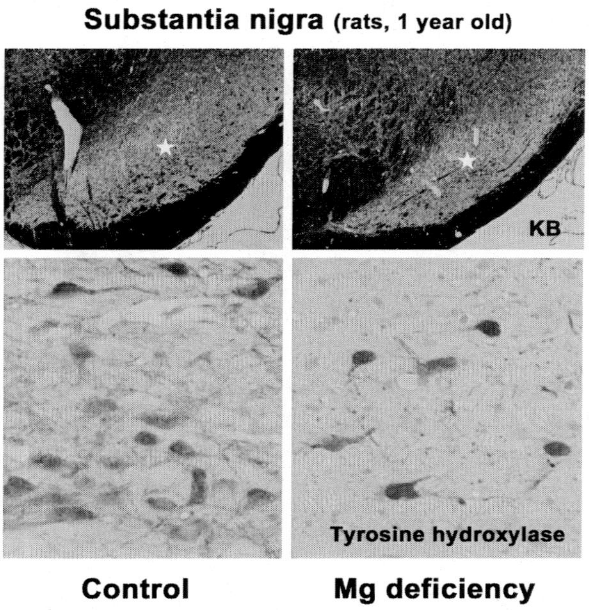

Figure 6. Severe atrophy and selective loss of dopaminergic neurons in the substantia nigra in rats with low Mg over generations (Oyanagi K, *et al*, 2006).

As an inhibiter of oxidative stress

The present authors conducted a study to clarify the effects of Mg administration in a rat PD model involving culture of ventral mesencephalic-striatal cells with 1-methyl-4-phenylpyridinium (MPP^+), based on recent evidence for significant loss of dopaminergic neurons exclusively in the substantia nigra of 1-year-old rats after exposure to low Mg intake over generations (Oyanagi *et al*, 2006) (Figure 6). The results indicated that Mg might protect dopaminergic neurons in the substantia nigra from degeneration. The concentration of Mg in the culture medium varied from 0.8 mM, corresponding to the control condition, to 4.0 mM. Effects were estimated by counting the number of surviving dopaminergic neurons immunopositive for tyrosine hydroxylase and measuring the length of dopaminergic neurites. An increase in the concentration of Mg to 1.2 mM significantly inhibited the toxicity of MPP^+, and a concentration of 4.0 mM completely prevented any decrease in the number of dopaminergic neurons. The length of dopaminergic neurites was significantly preserved in the presence of Mg at 1.2 and 4.0 mM. An increase in the concentration of Mg to 1.2 and 4.0 mM led to a significant amelioration in the length of dopaminergic neurites after MPP^+ toxicity (Figure 7).

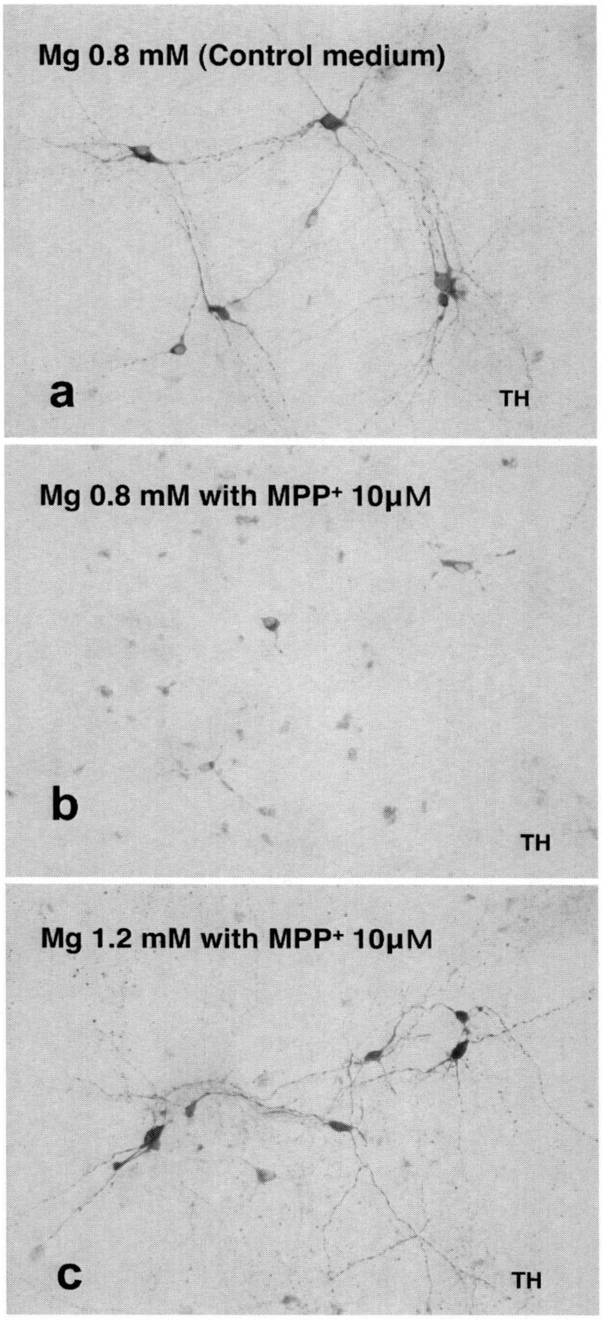

Figure 7. Prevention of MPP^+ toxicity by Mg in a Parkinson model (Hashimoto *et al*, 2008). **a:** normal condition of cultured nigral dopaminergic neurons. **b:** severe loss of dopaminergic neurons and the neuritis after MPP^+ administration. **c:** An increase in the concentration of Mg to 1.2 mM significantly inhibited the toxicity of MPP^+.

This was the first report to document a significant and striking effect of Mg for prevention of neurite and neuron pathology, and also amelioration of neurite pathology in a PD model. In addition, an increase in the Mg concentration to 1.2, 2.0, and 4.0 mM did not induce any degenerative features in the cultured dopaminergic cells, suggesting that a Mg concentration of up to 4.0 mM in the extracellular space might not induce any neuron degeneration in humans. Mg oxide per os has often been used as a laxative for patients with PD, but is reportedly not absorbed in the bowels, thus not affecting the serum concentration of Mg (Sakimura *et al*, 1998). Recent studies by the authors using mice also established that no significant alteration was found in the CSF of B6 mice injected intraperitoneally with Mg, even though the serum Mg concentration was significantly increased (Sun *et al, 2009*). Further research is necessary to find Mg compounds that can easily be absorbed in the bowels and pass through the blood-brain barrier, like Mg-L-threonate (Slutsky *et al*, 2010) and besides, via transporters that can carry Mg through the bowel mucosa, blood-brain barrier and plasma membrane of neurons.

Acknowledgements

The authors are indebted to Dr. M. Yasui, Yasui Clinic, Wakayama, Japan, Dr. K. Nishi, Nishi Clinic, Tokyo, Japan, Dr. J. Nagasao, Ms. E. Kawakami, Dr. L. Sun and Dr. Y. Piao, Department of Neuropathology, Tokyo Metropolitan Institute for Neuroscience, Tokyo, Japan, Dr. S. Takahama, Graduate School of Frontier Biosciences, Osaka University, Osaka, Japan, Ms. Y. Kosugi, Department of Environmental Health and Toxicology, Division of Environmental Health, Tokyo Metropolitan Institute of Public Health, Tokyo, Japan for their valuable advice and technical assistance. This work was supported in part by grants from the Japanese Ministry of Education, Science, Sports and Culture (Basic Research (C) #20500330 to TH), a Yujin Memorial Grant (to KO) and The Salt Science Research Foundation, No. 1028 (to KO).

References

Alam ZI, Daniel SE, Lees AJ, Marsden CD, Jenner P, Halliwell B (1997a) A generalized increase in protein carbonyls in the brain in Parkinson's but incidental Lewy body disease. *J Neurochem* 69:1326-9.

Alam ZI, Jenner A, Daniel SE, Lees AJ, Cairns N, Marsden CD, Jenner P, Halliwell B (1997b) Oxidative DNA damage in Parkinsonian brain; An apparent selective increase in 8-Hydroxyguanine levels in substantia nigra. *J Neurochem* 69:1196-203.

Ambani LM, Van Woert MH, Murphy S (1975) Brain peroxidase and catalase in Parkinson disease. *Arch Neurol* 32:114-8.

Barbiroli B, Martinelli P, Patuelli A, Lodi R, Iotti S, Cortelli P, Montagna P (1999) Phosphorus magnetic resonance spectroscopy in multiple system atrophy and Parkinson's disease. *Mov Disord* 14:430-5.

Bedford L, Hay D, Devoy A, Paine S, Powe DG, Seth R, Gray T, Topham I, Fone K, Rezvani N, Mee M, Soane T, Layfield R, Sheppard PW, Ebendal T, Usoskin D, Lowe J, Mayer RJ. (2008) Depletion of 26SS proteasomes in mouse brain neurons caused neurodegeneration and Lewy-like inclusions resembling human pale bodies. *J Neurosci* 28:8189-98.

Bocca B, Alimonti A, Senofonte O, Pino A, Violante N, Petrucci F, Sancesario G, Forte G (2006) Metal changes in CSF and peripheral compartments of parkinsonian patients. *J Neurol Sci* 248:23-30.

Bonifati V, Rizzu P, van Baren MJ, Schaap O, Breedveld GJ, Krieger E, Dekker MC, Squitieri F, Ibanez P, Joosse M, van Dongen JW, Vanacore N, van Swieten JC, Brice A, Meco G, van Duijn CM, Oostra BA, Heutink P (2003) Mutations in the DJ-1 gene associated with autosomal recessive early-onset parkinsonism. *Science* 299:256-9.

Bove J, Prou D, Perier C, Przedborski S (2005) Toxin-induced models of Parkinson's disease. *Neurotherapeutics* 2:484-94.

Champy P, Hoglinger GU, Feger J, Gleye C, Hocquemiller R, Laurents A, Guerineau V, Laprevote O, Medija F, Lombes A, Michel P P, Lannuzel A, Hirsch EC, Ruberg M (2004) Annonacin, a lipophilic inhibitior of mitochondrial complex I, induces nigral and striatal neurodegeneration in rats. *J Neurochem* 88:63-9.

Chen K-M, Chase TN (1985) Parkinsonism-dementia. In: *Handbook of Clinical Neurology* (Vinken PJ, Bruyn GW, Klawans HL, eds), Vol. 49, Revised series 5, Chap 8, Amsterdam: Elsevier, 167-83.

Cojocaru M, Cojocaru IM, Muuroi C, Botezat M, Lazar L, Duruta A (2006) Serum magnesium concentrations in migraine with aura. *Advances in Magnesium Research: New Data,* 31-5.

Dalfo E, Protero-Otin M, Ayala V, Martinez A, Pamplona R, Ferrer I (2005) Evidence of oxidative stress in the neocortex in incidental Lewy body disease. *J Neuropathol Exp Neurol* 64:816-30.

Eskes R, Antonsson B, Osen-Sand A, Montessuit S, Richter C, Sadoul R, Mazzei G, Nichols A, Martinou JC (1998) Bax-induced cytochrome C release from mitochondria is independent of the permeability transition pore but highly dependent on Mg^{2+} ions. *J Cell Biol* 143:217-24.

Fornai F, Lenzi P, Gesi M, Ferrucci M, Lazzeri G, Busceti CL, Ruffoli R, Soldani P, Ruggieri S, Alessandri MG, Paparelli A (2003) Fine structure and biochemical mechanisms underlying nigrostriatal inclusions and cell death after proteasome inhibition. *J Neurosci* 23:8955-66.

Garruto RM, Yanagihara R, Gajdusek DC. Arion DM (1984) Concentration on heavy metals and essential minerals in garden soil and drinking water in the Western Pacific. In: *Amyotrophic Lateral Sclerosis in Asia and Oceania* (Chen KM, Yase Y, eds), Taipei: National Taiwan University, 265–330.

Golts N, Snyder H, Frasier M, theisler C, Choi P, Wolozin B (2002) Magnesium inhibits spontaneous and iron-induced aggregation of alpha-synuclein. *J Biol Chem* 277:16116-23.

Hasegawa M, Arai T, Akiyama H, Nonaka T, Hiroshi Mori, Hashimoto T, Yamazaki M, Oyanagi K (2007) TDP-43 is deposited in the Guam parkinsonism-dementia complex brains. *Brain* 130:1386-94.

Hattori N, Tanaka M, Ozawa T, Mizuno Y (1991) Immunohistochemical Studies on complexes I, II, III, and VI of mitochondoria in Parkinson's disease. *Ann Neurol* 30:563-71.

Hirano A, Kurland LT, Krooth RS, Lessell S (1961a) Parkinsonism-dementia complex, an endemic disease on the island of Guam. I. Clinical features. *Brain* 84:642-61.

Hirano A, Malamud N, Kurland LT (1961b) Parkinsonism-dementia complex, an endemic disease on the Island of Guam. II. Pathological features. *Brain* 84:662-79.

Jellinger KA (1999) The role of iron in neurodegeneration : prospects for pharmacotherapy of Parkinson's disease. *Drugs Aging* 14:115-40.

Kitada T, Asakawa S, Hattori N, Matsumine H, Yamamura Y, Minoshima S, Yokochi M, Mizuno Y, Shimizu N (1998) Mutations in the parkin *gene cause autosomal recessive juvenile parkinsonism.* Nature *392, 605-8.*

Lewy FH (1912) Paralysis agitans. In: *Pathologische Anatomi* (Lewandowsky M, ed). Handbuch der Neurologie, vol. 3. Berlin, Springer, 920-33.

Lin JY, Chung SY, Lin MC, Cheng FC (2002) Effects of magnesium sulfate on energy metabolites and glutamate in the cortex during focal cerebral ischemia and reperfusion in the gerbil monitored by a dural-probe microdialysis technique. *Life Sci* 71:803-11.

Lyden P, Wahlgren NG (2000) Mechanisms of action of neuroprotectants in stroke. *J Stroke Cerebrovasc Dis* 9:9-14.

Mayer ML, Westbrook GL, Guthrie PB (1984) Voltage-dependent block by Mg^{2+} of NMDA responses in spinal cord neurones. *Nature* 309:261-3.

Mizuno Y, Matuda S, Yoshino H, Mori H, Hattori N, Ikebe S (1994) An immunohistochemical study on alpha-ketoglutarate dehydrogenase complex in Parkinson's disease. *Ann Neurol* 35:204-10.

Nakamura K, Bindokas VP, Marks JD, Wright DA, Frim DM, Miller RJ, Kang UJ (2000) The selective toxicity of 1-methyl-4-phenylpyridinium to dopaminergic neurons: the role of mitochondrial complex I and reactive oxygen species revisited. *Mol Pharmacol* 58: 271-8.

Nowak L, Bregestovski P, Ascher P, Herber A, Prochiantz A (1984) Magnesium gates glutamate-activated channels in mouse central neurons. *Nature* 307:462-5.

Oyanagi K (2005) The nature of the parkinsonism-dementia complex and amyotrophic lateral sclerosis of Guam and magnesium deficiency. *Parkinson Rel Dis* 11:S17-S23.

Oyanagi, K, Kawakami E, Kikuchi-Horie K, Ohara K, Ogata K, Takahama S, Wada M, Kihira T, Yasui M (2006) Magnesium deficiency over generations in rats with special references to the pathogenesis of the parkinsonism-dementia complex and amyotrophic lateral sclerosis of Guam. *Neuropathology* 26:115-28.

Oyanagi K, Makifuchi T, Ohtoh T, Chen K-M, Gajdusek DC, Chase TN(1997) Distinct pathological features of the Gallyas- and tau-positive glia in the parkinsonism-dementia complex and amyotrophic lateral sclerosis of Guam. *J Neuropathol Exp Neurol* 56:308-16.

Parkinson J (1817) *An Essay on the Shaking Palsy*. Neely and Jones, ed. Whittingham and Rowland for Sherwood, London.

Polymeropoulos MH, Lavedan C, Leroy E, Ide SE, Dehejia A, Dutra A, Pike B, Root H, Rubinstein J, Boyer R, StenroosES, Chandrasekharappa S, Asanassiadou A, Papapetropoulos T, Johnston WG, Lazzarini AM, Duvoisin RC, Di Iorio G, Golbe LI, Nussbaum RL (1997) Mutation in the alpha-synuclein gene identified in families with Parkinson's disease. *Science* 276:2045-7.

Sakimura K, Machino H, Miyoshi K, Nakata K, Ueda K, Ide M, Minegishi A, Harada Y (1998) Clinical evaluation of YO-106 (magnesium oxide tablets) in the treatment of Habitual constipation-A cross over study with Magnesium oxide powders (JP)- *Jpn Pharmacol Ther* 26:1027-53.

Saris NE, Mervaala E, Karppanen H, Khawaja JA, Lewenstam A (2000) Magnesium. An update on physiological, clinical and analytical aspects. *Clin Chim Acta* 294:1-26.

Singleton AB, Farrer M, Johnson J, Singleton A, Hague S, Kachergus J, Hulihan M, Peuralinna T, Dutra A, Nussbaum R, Lincoln S, Crawley A, Hanson M, Maraganore D, Adler C, Cookson MR, Muenter M, Baptista M, Miller D, Blancato J, Hardy J, Gwinn-Hardy K (2003) Alpha-synclein locus triplication causes Parkinson's disease. *Science* 302:841

Slutsky I, Abumaria N, Wu LJ, Huang C, Zhang L, Li B, Zhao X, Govindarajan A, Zhao MG, Zhuo M, Tonegawa S, Liu G (2010) Enhancement of learning and memory by elevating brain magnesium. *Neuron* 65:165-77.

Smeyne RJ, Jackson-Lewis V (2005) The MPTP model of Parkinson's disease. *Brain Res. Mol Brain Res* 134:57-66.

Sun L, Kosugi Y, Kawakami E, Piao Y-S, Hashimoto T, Oyanagi K (2009) Magnesium concentration in the cerebrospinal fluid of mice and its response to changes in serum magnesium concentration. *Magnes Res* 22:266-72.

Tretiakoff C (1919) Contribution a l'etude del l'Anatomie pathologique du Locus Niger de Soemmering avec quelques deduction relatives a la pathogenie des troubles du tonus musculaire et de la maladie de Parkinson. *Theses de Paris*.

Uitti Rj, Rajput AH, Rozdilsky B, Bickis M, Wollin T, Yuen WK (1989) Regional metal concentrations in Parkinson's disease, other chronic neurological diseases, and control brains. *Can J Neurol Sci* 16:310-4.

Valente EM, Abou-Sleiman PM, Caputo V, Muqit MMK, Harvey K, Gispert S, Ali Z, Del Turco D, Bentivoglio AR, Healy DG, Albanese A, Nussbaum R, González-Maldonado R, Deller T, Salvi S, Cortelli P, Gilks WP, Latchman DS, Harvey RJ, Dallapiccola B, Auburger G, Wood NW (2004) Hereditary Early-Onset Parkinson's Disease Caused by Mutations in *PINK1. Science* 304:1158-60.

Yamazaki M, Hasegawa M, Mori O, Murayama S, Tsuchiya K, Ikeda K, Chen K-M, Katayama Y, Oyanagi K (2005) Tau-positive fine granules in the cerebral white matter: a novel finding among tauopathies exclusive to parkinsonism-dementia complex of Guam. *J Neuropathol Exp Neurol* 64:1-8.

Yase Y (1978) ALS in the Kii peninsula: one possible etiological hypothesis. In: *Amyotrophic lateral sclerosis* (Tsubaki T, Toyokura Y, eds), Tokyo: University of Tokyo Press, 307-18.

Yoritaka A, Hattori N, Uchida K, Tanaka M, Stadtman ER, Mizuno K (1996) Immunohistochemical detection of 4-hydroxynonenal protein adducts in Parkinson's disease. *Proc Natl Acad Sci USA* 93: 2696-701.

Zhang J, Perry G, Smith MA, Robertson D, Olson SJ, Graham DG, Montine TJ (1999) Parkinson's disease is associated with oxidative damage to cytoplasmic DNA and RNA in substantia nigra neurons. *Am J Pathol* 154:1423-9.

Section 3

Involvement of Magnesium in Psychiatric Diseases

Magnesium in Alzheimer's disease

Dehua Chui,[1,*,✉] *Zheng Chen,*[2,*] *Jia Yu,*[2,*] *Honglin Zhang,*[2] *Weishan Wang,*[2] *Yuetao Song,*[2] *Huan Yang* [1] *and Liang Zhou* [1]

[1] Neuroscience Research Institute & Department of Neurobiology, Key Laboratory for Neuroscience, Ministry of Education & Ministry of Public Health, Health Science Center, Peking University, Beijing 100191, China.
[2] Department of Psychiatry & Institute for Geriatric Clinic and Rehabilitation, Beijing Geriatric Hospital, Beijing 100095, China.
* Dehua Chui, Z. Chen and J. Yu contributed equally to this work.
✉ dchui@bjmu.edu.cn

Abstract

Alzheimer's disease (AD) is the most common form of dementia. It is characterized by a progressive cognitive impairment clinically, and excessive deposits of aggregated amyloid-β (Aβ) peptides pathologically. Environmental factors, including nutrition and metal elements, are implicated in the pathophysiology of AD. Magnesium (Mg) affects many biochemical mechanisms vital for neuronal properties and synaptic plasticity, including the response of N-methyl D-aspartate (NMDA) receptors to excitatory amino acids, stability and viscosity of the cell membrane and antagonism of calcium. Mg levels were found decreased in various tissues of AD patients and negatively correlated with clinical deterioration. Moreover, Mg was demonstrated to modulate the trafficking and processing of amyloid-β precursor protein (APP), which plays a central role in the pathogenesis of AD. Here, we review in vitro and in vivo data that indicated a role for magnesium in many biological and clinical aspects of AD.

Alzheimer's disease

Alzheimer's disease (AD) is the most prevalent neurodegenerative disease in elderly people, affecting approximate 6~8% of all individuals over the age of 65 years. AD is characterized by progressive cognitive impairment and distinct neuropathological lesions in the brain, including intracellular neurofibrillary tangles, extracellular parenchymal and cerebrovascular senile plaques (Braak and Braak, 1991). Senile plaques are mainly constituted of a 39–42 amino acid peptide, amyloid-β protein (Aβ) (Glenner and Wong, 1984; Masters *et al,* 1985), which is generally accepted as being neurotoxic and playing a central role in the pathogenesis of neuronal dysfunction and synaptic failure in Alzheimer's disease (Selkoe, 1991; Hardy and Selkoe, 2002). Aβ is derived from full-length amyloid-β precursor protein (APP) (Kang *et al,* 1987), which is a type I trans-membrane protein composed of a large extra-cellular domain, a short transmembrane domain, and a cytoplasmic tail, by sequential proteolytic cleavages of β-secretase and γ-secretase. The β-cleavage of APP, catalyzed by the well characterized transmembrane aspartyl protease β-site APP-cleaving enzyme (BACE) (Hussain *et al,* 1999; Sinha *et al,* 1999; Yan *et al,* 1999; Haniu *et al,* 2000), cleaves APP at the NH2-terminus of Aβ sequence (Seubert *et al,* 1993) to generates a soluble version of APP (sAPP) and a 99-residue COOH-terminal fragment (CTFβ or C99) which remains membrane bound.

C99 is further cleaved to release Aβ of varying lengths, predominantly Aβ40 andAβ42 (Selkoe, 2001; Hussain *et al,* 1999; Price *et al,* 1998; Sinha *et al,* 1999; Christensen *et al,* 2004), by an atypical aspartyl protease, γ-secretase complex which contains at least four different proteins: Aph-1, nicastrin, presenilin, and Pen-2 (De Strooper, 2003; Edbauer *et al,* 2003). Proteolysis by γ-secretase is heterogeneous: most of the full-length Aβ species produced is a 40-residue peptide (Aβ40), whereas a small proportion is a 42-residue COOH-terminal variant (Aβ42) (Esler and Wolfe, 2001). However, prior processing of APP by α-secretase precludes the formation of the neurotoxic Aβ. It cuts APP within the Aβ region (between residues Lys16 and Leu17 of Aβ), generating a sAPPα and a membrane-anchored 83-residue C-terminal fragment (CTFα or C83) which is also a substrate of γ-secretase (Esch *et al,* 1990; Sisodia, 1992). α-Secretase is thought to be a metalloprotease, such as TNF-α converting enzyme (TACE) or a disintegrin and metalloprotease 10 (ADAM10) (Lammich *et al,* 1999). Secreted APP exerts proliferative actions in a variety of cell types as well as neurotrophic and neuroprotective effects (Mucke *et al,* 1996).

Synaptic failure in AD is caused by accumulation and oligomerization of Aβ42 in limbic and association cortices (Selkoe, 2002). Mutations in the APP gene or presenilins (PS) 1 or 2 genes, which cause an autosomal dominant early onset familial AD (<5% of AD patients), increase the relative production of Aβ42. In the majority of patients with so-called sporadic late-onset AD, an age-dependent accumulation of Aβ, caused by disturbed dynamic balance between anabolic and catabolic activities has been implicated (Selkoe, 2001). Also, environmental factors, such as metallic elements may play a protective or disruptive role in the pathogenesis of AD (for review, see Adlard and Bush, 2006; Shcherbatykh and Carpenter, 2007). Different metals may be involved in multiple aspects of the disease process, such as the regulation of APP gene expression and mRNA translation, the proteolytic processing of APP, the aggregation and degradation of Aβ, and the formation of neuro-fibrillary tangles. Heavy metals (e.g. lead, mercury and cadmium) are neurotoxic and associated with intellectual impairment (Bleecker *et al,* 2005). Recent studies have implicated lead exposure in the subsequent elevation of APP and Aβ in animals (Basha *et al,* 2005a) as well as in the aggregation of synthetic $A\beta_{1-40}$ in vitro (Basha *et al,* 2005b). In the case of aluminum, another "toxic" metal, its relevance to AD is ascribed to the involvement in the formation of paired helical filaments (PHF), the aggregation and toxicity of Aβ, and the generation of oxidative species (for review, see Gupta *et al,* 2005). Transition metals (e.g. copper, zinc, and iron, which are essential in cell biology) can induce Aβ aggregation (Huang *et al,* 2004; Mantyh *et al,* 1993) and are found concentrated in and around the amyloid plaques in the AD brain (Lovell *et al,* 1998). Disturbed homeostasis of these biometals in the AD brain (decreased copper levels, and increased concentrations of iron, zinc, and manganese (Cornett *et al,* 1998; Deibel *et al,* 1996) have been reported. An imbalance of zinc and copper has been shown to significantly alter APP processing and Aβ generation in relevant animal models (Bayer *et al,* 2003; Borchardt *et al,* 1999; Phinney *et al,* 2003; Sparks and Schreurs, 2003; Lee *et al,* 2002; Friedlich *et al,* 2004).

Neurological function of magnesium

The magnesium ion, Mg^{2+}, is the second most abundant intracellular cation, serving to stabilize nucleic acid and protein structure (Subirana *et al,* 2003; Brion *et al,* 1997), and regulating over 300 enzymes as a cofactor (Romni *et al,* 1992 and 2000; Zhao *et al,* 2002), including ATP-related enzymatic reactions (Hirata *et al,* 2002; Ko *et al,* 1999). Physiological concentration of Mg is essential for synaptic conduction, and required for normal functioning of the nervous system. It has various effects at different concentrations on intellectual and neuronal functions via many bio-chemical mechanisms, including NMDA-receptor response to excitatory amino acids and calcium influx (Nowak *et al,* 1984; Mayer *et al,* 1984; Vandenberg *et al,* 1987; Matsuda *et al,* 1987), inhibition of calcium channels (Iseri *et al,* 1984) and glutamate release (Lin *et al,* 2002), cell membrane fluidity and stability (Ebel *et al* 1980), and toxic effects of calcium (Alvarez-Leefmans *et al* 1987). These mechanisms have important roles in chronic neuronal degeneration and subsequent development of dementia.

The role of Mg in degenerative diseases has been the focus of increased attention in recent years. Continuous low Mg intake for two generations induces exclusive loss of dopaminergic neurons in rats (Oyanagi, 2005), and may support the Mg hypothesis in the pathogenesis of parkinsonism-dementia complex (PDC) of Guam. Mg supplementation prevents the loss of dopaminergic neurons and ameliorates neurite pathology in PD model, indicating a role of Mg in protection of dopaminergic neurons in the substantia nigra from degeneration (Oyanagi *et al,* 2006; Hashimoto *et al,* 2008). Also, Mg at concentrations >0.75 mM inhibits the aggregation of α-synuclein induced either spontaneously or by incubation with iron (Golts *et al,* 2002). Microinjection of magnesium into cells caused microtubule disassembly (Prescott *et al,* 1988). Mg^{2+} and Ca^{2+} effectively induced formation of approximately 340 kD aggregates of paired helical filament tau (PHF-tau) obtained from corticobasal degeneration (CBD) and AD but not normal tau proteins isolated from fetal and adult brains as determined by sodium dodecyl sulfate (SDS)-polyacrylamide gel electrophoresis and immunoblotting (Yang *et al,* 1999). This finding suggests regional elevation of these ions may trigger pathological deposition of PHF-tau in certain neurodegenerative disorders.

Magnesium in AD

Recent evidence suggests that Mg was implicated in the pathogenesis of AD. Mg levels were found decreased in the serum and brain tissues of AD patients in clinical, experimental and autopsy studies (Durlach, 1990; Glick, 1990; Lemke, 1995; Andrasi *et al,* 2000; Andrási *et al,* 2005; Vural *et al,* 2010). Moreover, serum Mg levels in AD patients negatively correlated with Global Deterioration Scale (GDS) and Clinical Dementia Rating (CDR) (Cilliler *et al,* 2007). A causal relationship between low Mg in hippocampal neurons and impairment of learning was also demonstrated in aged rats (Landfield *et al,* 1984). Magnesium deficiency can lead to specific impairments in emotional memory (Bardgett *et al,* 2005; Bardgett *et al,* 2007), while magnesium therapy facilitates cognitive function recovery following brain injury; however, there are task and dose-dependent aspects to this recovery (Enomoto *et al,* 2005; Hoane, 2005; Hoane, 2007). Increasing brain magnesium leads to the enhancement of both short-term synaptic facilitation and long-term potentiation and improves learning and memory functions in rats (Slutsky *et al,* 2010). Interestingly, treatment of dementia patients with nutritional Mg support efficiently improved memory and other symptoms (Glick *et al,* 1990b). However, therapeutic administration of Mg is still controversial regarding the treatment of AD, and high dose of Mg may have potential detrimental side effects (Clark and Brown, 1992; Fung *et al,* 1995; Hallak, 1998; Ladner and Lee, 1999).

Neuronal degeneration occurs in PS1 mutant mice without extracellular Aβ deposits, suggesting it is caused by the accumulation of intracellular Aβ42 (Chui *et al,* 1999); deposits of intracellular Aβ42 are correlated with apoptotic cell death in AD brains (Chui *et al,* 2001). The Aβ is derived from APP through sequential cleavages by β-and γ-secretases, whose enzymatic activities are tightly controlled by subcellular localization. Thus, delineation of how the intracellular trafficking of these secretases and APP are regulated is important for understanding AD pathogenesis. Although APP trafficking has been found to be regulated by multiple factors including PS1, a major component of the γ-secretase complex, and phospholipase D1, a phospholipid-modifying enzyme; APP can reciprocally regulate PS1 trafficking; APP deficiency results in faster transport of PS1 from the trans-Golgi network to the cell surface and increased steady state levels of PS1 at the cell surface, which can be reversed by restoring APP levels (Liu *et al,* 2009). However, it is not known whether altered magnesium level may also affect APP trafficking or/and processing. Recently, it has been demonstrated that magnesium modulated APP processing in a time- and dose-dependent manner: extracellular magnesium ($[Mg^{2+}]_o$) at high doses increased CTFα level and sAPPα release; in contrast, $[Mg^{2+}]_o$ at low doses enhanced CTFβ accumulation and Aβ secretion (Yu *et al,* 2010). The mechanism of how varying magnesium concentrations led to shifts between α- and β-secretase cleavage of APP might be partially explained by the evidence that $[Mg^{2+}]_o$ at high doses promoted retention of APP on plasma membrane, whereas $[Mg^{2+}]_o$ at low doses reduced cell surface APP level (Yu *et al,* 2010). All APP family members are predominantly cleaved in the late secretory pathway, including the plasma membrane and endosomes (Yamazaki *et al,* 1996). Further, different secretase activities show distinct subcellular localization, namely α-secretase at the plasma membrane (Lammich *et al,* 1999; Skovronsky *et al,* 2000) and β/γ-secretases within endocytic compartments (Vassar *et al,* 1999; Huse *et al,* 2000 ; Cupers *et al,* 2001 ; Kaether *et al,* 2002; Ray *et al,* 1999). Because targeting of APP to distinct subcellular compartments determines processing into amyloidogenic or non-amyloidogenic products, much attention has been focused on factors that regulate APP trafficking. Interestingly, several adaptor proteins are known to influence APP transport and processing. For example, F-spondin, a secreted factor that binds to the extracellular domain of APP (Ho and Sudhof, 2004), has been shown to increase levels of cell surface APP, promote α-cleavage of APP, and decrease β-cleavage of APP (Hoe *et al,* 2005). Similarly, the extracellular matrix protein Reelin caused increased surface APP and a preference for α-cleavage over β-cleavage (Hoe *et al,* 2006).

These findings suggest that trafficking and proteolysis of APP are regulated together. Thus a function of $[Mg^{2+}]_o$ in APP transport from/to the cell surface might be a possible explanation for its modulation of APP processing. In the light of Mg^{2+} as an antagonist of the NMDA receptor, our finding is corroborated by the previous report that chronic NMDA receptor activation decreased α-secretase-mediated APP processing and increased Aβ production in cultured cortical neurons (Lesne *et al,* 2005). Furthermore, several lines of evidence suggest that APP metabolism and Aβ levels are closely correlated with neural activity in animals (Fazeli *et al,* 1994; Cirrito *et al,* 2005; Cirrito *et al,* 2008) and humans (Buckner *et al,* 2005). It has been demonstrated that decreasing neuronal activity by high $[Mg^{2+}]_o$ (10 mM $MgCl_2$) resulted in significant reduction of Aβ secretion, which may involve a change in APP processing (Kamenetz *et al,* 2003). However, the precise functional mechanism of how magnesium regulates APP transport and whether magnesium interacts with α- and β-secretase or regulates enzyme activity or their subcellular localization remains undetermined but will be part of our future analysis.

The dose dependent response of sAPPα to increasing $[Mg^{2+}]_o$ implies high concentrations of Mg may exert protective effects against AD. Various studies have strongly established that secreted sAPPα possesses potent neurotrophic and neuroprotective activities against excitotoxic and oxidative insults (Mattson *et al,* 1993; Schubert *et al,* 1993), p53-mediated apoptosis (Xu *et al,* 1999), and the proapoptotic action of mutant PS1 by activating the transcription factor NF-κB (Guo *et al,* 1998). Moreover, sAPPα stimulates neurite outgrowth (Small *et al,* 1994), regulates synaptogenesis (Morimoto *et al,* 1998), exerts trophic effects on cerebral neurons in culture (Araki *et al,* 1991), stabilizes neuronal calcium homeostasis and protects hippocampal and cortical neurons against the toxic effects of glutamate and Aβ peptides (Furukawa *et al,* 1996). It also has been shown that intra-cerebroventricular administration of secreted forms of sAPPα to amnestic mice has potent memory-enhancing effects and blocks learning deficits induced by scopolamine (Meziane *et al,* 1998).

Secreted Aβ increased upon low $[Mg^{2+}]_o$ (0.0 and 0.4 mM) compared with physiological concentration of Mg (ie. 0.8 mM), whereas high $[Mg^{2+}]_o$ (1.2, 1.6, 4.0 mM) could not significantly lower total extracellular Aβ level (Yu *et al,* 2010). The data are consistent with several reports showing a dissociation between sAPPα release and Aβ generation both in vitro or in vivo (Loefler *et al,* 1993; Querfurth *et al,* 1994; Dyrks *et al,* 1994; LeBlanc *et al,* 1998; Rossner *et al,* 2000), suggesting that there might be a more complex regulatory mechanism of these two processing events of APP. For instance, constitutive activation of PKC in guinea pig brain increased sAPPα secretion without any effect on secreted Aβ (Rossner *et al,* 2000), suggesting that the a- and β-secretase pathways may be differentially controlled. Because Yu *et al*. examined the effects of Mg only on the pathologically high production of Aβ, the modulation of the physiological Aβ production by Mg needs to be established in future studies. The steady-state level of Aβ peptide is determined by the rate of production from APP via β- and γ-secretases and degradation by the activity of several degradative enzymes, including neprilysin (Hama *et al,* 2001; Iwata *et al,* 2001; Leissring *et al,* 2003; Marr *et al,* 2004; review see Wang *et al,* 2006), insulin degrading enzyme (IDE) (Kurochkin *et al,* 1994; Farris *et al,* 2003), endothelin-converting enzyme (Eckman *et al,* 2003) and MMPs (Roher *et al,* 1994; Backstrom *et al,* 1996; Leissring *et al,* 2003). Yu *et al*. found that Mg deprivation resulted in 50% decrease of neprilysin activity without alteration in the protein level of neprilysin and IDE (Yu *et al,* unpublished data). Thus, the exacerbated accumulation of Aβ induced by $[Mg^{2+}]_o$ at 0.0 mM resulted from both the enhanced production and aberrant catabolism.

Conclusion

Magnesium participates in the biochemical mechanisms of neuronal properties and synaptic functions, which are involved in the pathophysiology of neurodegenerative diseases. Magnesium was demonstrated to modulate APP trafficking and processing, and its level was found decreased in AD patients. Both clinical and experimental data implicated a role of Mg in the pathogenesis of AD. Given the prevalence of magnesium inadequacy in the general population (Ford *et al,* 2003), magnesium supplementation could constitute a potential novel pharmacological target for the treatment of AD via its action on APP processing.

Acknowledgment
This work was supported by the National Natural Science Foundation of China (NSFC; Grants No. 30570533, No. 30670414 and No. 30973145) and the National High Technology Research and Development Program of China (973 Program No. 2006CB500705 and 863 Program No. 0060102A4031).

References

Adlard PA, Bush AI (2006) Metals and Alzheimer's disease. *J Alzheimers Dis* 10; 145-63.

Altura BM, Zhang A, Altura BT (1993) Magnesium, hypertensive vascular diseases, atherogenesis, subcellular compartmentation of Ca2+ and Mg2+ and vascular contractility. *Miner Electrolyte Metab* 19:323-36.

Altura BM, Zhang A, Cheng TP, Altura BT (2001) Extracellular magnesium regulates nuclear and perinuclear free ionized calcium in cerebral vascular smooth muscle cells: possible relation to alcohol and central nervous system injury. *Alcohol* 23:83-90.

Alvarez-Leefmans FJ, Giraldez F, Gamino SM (1987) Intracellular free magnesium in excitable cells: its measurement and its biologic significance. *Can J Physiol Pharmacol* 65:915-25.

Andrasi E, Igaz S, Molnar Z, Mako S (2000) Disturbances of magnesium concentrations in various brain areas in Alzheimer's disease. *Magnes Res* 13:189-96.

Andrási E, Páli N, Molnár Z, Kösel S (2005) Brain aluminum, magnesium and phosphorus contents of control and Alzheimer-diseased patients. *J Alzheimers* Dis 7(4):273-84.

Araki W, Kitaguchi N, Tokushima Y, Ishii K, Aratake H, Shimohama S, Nakamura S, Kimura J (1991) Trophic effect of beta-amyloid precursor protein on cerebral cortical neurons in culture. *Biochem Biophys Res Commun* 181:265-71.

Backstrom JR, Lim GP, Cullen MJ, Tokes ZA (1996) Matrix metalloproteinase-9 (MMP-9) is synthesized in neurons of the human hippocampus and is capable of degrading the amyloid-beta peptide (1-40). *J Neurosci* 16:7910-19.

Bardgett ME, Schultheis PJ, McGill DL, Richmond RE, Wagge JR (2005) Magnesium deficiency impairs fear conditioning in mice. *Brain Res* 1038:100-6.

Bardgett ME, Schultheis PJ, Muzny A, Riddle MD, Wagge JR (2007) Magnesium deficiency reduces fear-induced conditional lick suppression in mice. *Magnes Res* 20:58-65.

Basha MR, Murali M, Siddiqi HK, Ghosal K, Siddiqi OK, Lashuel HA, Ge YW, Lahiri DK, Zawia NH (2005b) Lead (Pb) exposure and its effect on APP proteolysis and Abeta aggregation. *FASEB J* 19, 2083-84.

Basha MR, Wei W, Bakheet SA, Benitez N, Siddiqi HK, Ge YW, Lahiri DK, Zawia NH (2005a) The fetal basis of amyloidogenesis: exposure to lead and latent over-expression of amyloid precursor protein and beta-amyloid in the aging brain. *J Neurosci* 25: 823-29.

Bayer TA, Schafer S, Simons A, Kemmling A, Kamer T, Tepest R, Eckert A, Schussel K, Eikenberg O, Sturchler-Pierrat C, Abramowski D, Staufenbiel M, Multhaup G (2003) Dietary Cu stabilizes brain superoxide dismutase 1 activity and reduces amyloid Abeta production in APP23 transgenic mice. *Proc Natl Acad Sci* USA 100, 14187-92.

Bleecker ML, Ford DP, Lindgren KN, Hoese VM, Walsh KS, Vaughan CG (2005) Differential effects of lead exposure on components of verbal memory. *Occup Environ Med* 62:181-7.

Borchardt T, Camakaris J, Cappai R, Masters CL, Beyreuther K, Multhaup G (1999) Copper inhibits beta-amyloid production and stimulates the non-amyloidogenic pathway of amyloid-precursor-protein secretion. *Biochem J* 344: 461-7.

Braak H, Braak E (1991) Neuropathological stageing of Alzheimer-related changes. *Acta Neuropathol* 82:239-59.

Brion P, Westhof E (1997) Hierarchy and dynamics of RNA folding. *Annu Rev Biophys Biomol Struct* 26:113-37.

Buckner RL, Snyder AZ, Shannon BJ, LaRossa G, Sachs R, Fotenos AF, Sheline YI, Klunk WE, Mathis CA, Morris JC, Mintun MA (2005) Molecular, structural, and functional characterization of Alzheimer's disease: evidence for a relationship between default activity, amyloid, and memory. *J Neurosci* 25:7709-17.

Cai D, Leem JY, Greenfield JP, Wang P, Kim BS, Wang R, Lopes KO, Kim SH, Zheng H, Greengard P, Sisodia SS, Thinakaran G, Xu H (2003) Presenilin-1 regulates intracellular trafficking and cell surface delivery of beta-amyloid precursor protein. *J Biol Chem* 278:3446-54.

Christensen MA, Zhou W, Qing H, Lehman A, Philipsen S, Song W (2004) Transcriptional regulation of BACE1, the beta-amyloid precursor protein beta-secretase, by Sp1. *Mol Cell Biol* 24:865-74.

Chui DH, Dobo E, Makifuchi T, Akiyama H, Kawakatsu S, Petit A, Checler F, Araki W, Takahashi K, Tabira T (2001) Apoptotic neurons in Alzheimer's disease frequently show intracellular Abeta42 labeling. *J Alzheimers Dis* 3: 231-39.

Chui DH, Tanahashi H, Ozawa K, Ikeda S, Checler F, Ueda O, Suzuki H, Araki W, Inoue H, Shirotani K, Takahashi K, Gallyas F, Tabira T (1999) Transgenic mice with Alzheimer presenilin 1 mutations show accelerated neurodegeneration without amyloid plaque formation. *Nat Med* 5: 560-64.

Cilliler AE, Ozturk S, Ozbakir S (2007) Serum magnesium level and clinical deterioration in Alzheimer's disease. *Gerontology* 53(6):419-22.

Cirrito JR, Kang JE, Lee J, Stewart FR, Verges DK, Silverio LM, Bu G, Mennerick S, Holtzman DM (2008) Endocytosis is required for synaptic activity-dependent release of amyloid-beta in vivo. *Neuron* 58:42-51.

Cirrito JR, Yamada KA, Finn MB, Sloviter RS, Bales KR, May PC, Schoepp DD, Paul SM, Mennerick S, Holtzman DM (2005) Synaptic activity regulates interstitial fluid amyloid-beta levels in vivo. *Neuron* 48:913-22.

Clark BA, Brown RS (1992) Unsuspected morbid hypermagnesemia in elderly patients. *Am J Nephrol* 12:336-43.

Cornett CR, Markesbery WR, Ehmann WD (1998) Imbalances of trace elements related to oxidative damage in Alzheimer's disease brain. *NeuroToxicology* 19:339-45.

Cupers P, Bentahir M, Craessaerts K, Orlans I, Vanderstichele H, Saftig P, De SB, Annaert W (2001) The discrepancy between presenilin subcellular localization and gamma-secretase processing of amyloid precursor protein. *J Cell Biol* 154:731-40.

De SB (2003) Aph-1, Pen-2, and Nicastrin with Presenilin generate an active gamma-Secretase complex. *Neuron* 38:9-12.

Deibel MA, Ehmann WD, Markesbery WR (1996) Copper, iron, and zinc imbalances in severely degenerated brain regions in Alzheimer's disease: possible relation to oxidative stress. *J Neurol Sci* 143: 137-42.

Durlach J (1990) Magnesium depletion and pathogenesis of Alzheimer's disease. *Magnes Res* 3:217-18.

Dyrks T, Monning U, Beyreuther K, Turner J (1994) Amyloid precursor protein secretion and beta A4 amyloid generation are not mutually exclusive. *FEBS Lett* 349:210-14.

Ebel H, Gunther T (1980) Magnesium metabolism: a review. *J Clin Chem Clin Biochem* 18:257-70.

Eckman EA, Watson M, Marlow L, Sambamurti K, Eckman CB (2003) Alzheimer's disease beta-amyloid peptide is increased in mice deficient in endothelin-converting enzyme. *J Biol Chem* 278:2081-84.

Edbauer D, Winkler E, Regula JT, Pesold B, Steiner H, Haass C (2003) Reconstitution of gamma-secretase activity. *Nat Cell Biol* 5:486-88.

Enomoto T, Osugi T, Satoh H, McIntosh TK, Nabeshima T (2005) Pre-Injury magnesium treatment prevents traumatic brain injury-induced hippocampal ERK activation, neuronal loss, and cognitive dysfunction in the radial-arm maze test. *J Neurotrauma* 22:783-92.

Hoane MR (2005) Treatment with magnesium improves reference memory but not working memory while reducing GFAP expression following traumatic brain injury. *Restor Neurol Neurosci* 23:67-77.

Esch FS, Keim PS, Beattie EC, Blacher RW, Culwell AR, Oltersdorf T, McClure D, Ward PJ (1990) Cleavage of amyloid beta peptide during constitutive processing of its precursor. *Science* 248:1122-24.

Esler WP, Wolfe MS (2001) A portrait of Alzheimer secretases--new features and familiar faces. *Science* 293:1449-54.

Farris W, Mansourian S, Chang Y, Lindsley L, Eckman EA, Frosch MP, Eckman CB, Tanzi RE, Selkoe DJ, Guenette S (2003) Insulin-degrading enzyme regulates the levels of insulin, amyloid beta-protein, and the beta-amyloid precursor protein intracellular domain in vivo. *Proc Natl Acad Sci USA* 100:4162-67.

Fazeli MS, Breen K, Errington ML, Bliss TV (1994) Increase in extracellular NCAM and amyloid precursor protein following induction of long-term potentiation in the dentate gyrus of anaesthetized rats. *Neurosci Lett* 169:77-80.

Friedlich AL, Lee JY, van Groen T, Cherny RA, Volitakis I, Cole TB, Palmiter RD, Koh JY, Bush AI (2004) Neuronal zinc exchange with the blood vessel wall promotes cerebral amyloid angiopathy in an animal model of Alzheimer's disease. *J Neurosci* 24: 3453-59.

Fung MC, Weintraub M, Bowen DL (1995) Hypermagnesemia. Elderly over-the-counter drug users at risk. *Arch Fam Med* 4:718-23.

Furukawa K, Barger SW, Blalock EM, Mattson MP (1996) Activation of K+ channels and suppression of neuronal activity by secreted beta-amyloid-precursor protein. *Nature* 379:74-78.

Glenner GG, Wong CW (1984) Alzheimer's disease: initial report of the purification and characterization of a novel cerebrovascular amyloid protein. *Biochem Biophys Res Commun* 120:885-90.

Glick JL (1990) Dementias: the role of magnesium deficiency and an hypothesis concerning the pathogenesis of Alzheimer's disease. *Med Hypotheses* 31:211-25.

Glick JL. Use of magnesium in the management of dementias. *Med Sci Res* 1990b;18:831–3.

Golts N, Snyder H, Frasier M, Theisler C, Choi P, Wolozin B (2002) Magnesium Inhibits Spontaneous and Iron-induced Aggregation of a-Synuclein. *J Biol Chem* 277(18):16116–16123.

Guo Q, Robinson N, Mattson MP (1998) Secreted beta-amyloid precursor protein counteracts the proapoptotic action of mutant presenilin-1 by activation of NF-kappaβ and stabilization of calcium homeostasis. *J Biol Chem* 273:12341-51.

Gupta VB, Anitha S, Hegde ML, Zecca L, Garruto RM, Ravid R, Shankar SK, Stein R, Shanmugavelu P, Jagannatha Rao KS (2005) Aluminium in Alzheimer's disease: are we still at a crossroad? *Cell Mol Life Sci* 62: 143-58.

Hallak M (1998) Effect of parenteral magnesium sulfate administration on excitatory amino acid receptors in the rat brain. *Magnes Res* 11:117-31.

Hama E, Shirotani K, Masumoto H, Sekine-Aizawa Y, Aizawa H, Saido TC (2001) Clearance of extracellular and cell-associated amyloid beta peptide through viral expression of neprilysin in primary neurons. *J Biochem* 130:721-6.

Han P, Dou F, Li F, Zhang X, Zhang YW, Zheng H, Lipton SA, Xu H, Liao FF (2005) Suppression of cyclin-dependent kinase 5 activation by amyloid precursor protein: a novel excitoprotective mechanism involving modulation of tau phosphorylation. *J Neurosci* 25:11542-52.

Haniu M, Denis P, Young Y, Mendiaz EA, Fuller J, Hui JO, Bennett BD, Kahn S, Ross S, Burgess T, Katta V, Rogers G, Vassar R, Citron M (2000) Characterization of Alzheimer's beta -secretase protein BACE. A pepsin family member with unusual properties. *J Biol Chem* 275:21099-106.

Hardy J, Selkoe DJ (2002) The amyloid hypothesis of Alzheimer's disease: progress and problems on the road to therapeutics. *Science* 297:353-6.

Hashimoto T, Nishi K, Nagasao J, Tsuji S, Oyanagi K (2008) Magnesium exerts both preventive and ameliorating effects in an in vitro rat Parkinson disease model involving 1-methyl-4-phenylpyridinium (MPP+) toxicity in dopaminergic neurons. *Brain Res* 1197:143-51.

Hirata A, Hirata F (2002) DNA chain unwinding and annealing reactions of lipocortin (annexin) I heterotetramer: regulation by Ca(2+) and Mg(2+). *Biochem Biophys Res Commun* 291:205-9.

Ho A, Sudhof TC (2004) Binding of F-spondin to amyloid-beta precursor protein: a candidate amyloid-beta precursor protein ligand that modulates amyloid-beta precursor protein cleavage. *Proc Natl Acad Sci USA* 101:2548-53.

Hoane MR (2007) Assessment of cognitive function following magnesium therapy in the traumatically injured brain. *Magnes Res* 20:229-36.

Hoe HS, Magill LA, Guenette S, Fu Z, Vicini S, Rebeck GW (2006) FE65 interaction with the ApoE receptor ApoEr2. *J Biol Chem* 281:24521-30.

Hoe HS, Tran TS, Matsuoka Y, Howell BW, Rebeck GW (2006) DAB1 and Reelin effects on amyloid precursor protein and ApoE receptor 2 trafficking and processing. *J Biol Chem* 281:35176-85.

Hoe HS, Wessner D, Beffert U, Becker AG, Matsuoka Y, Rebeck GW (2005) F-spondin interaction with the apolipoprotein E receptor ApoEr2 affects processing of amyloid precursor protein. *Mol Cell Biol* 25:9259-68.

Huang X, Moir RD, Tanzi RE, Bush AI, Rogers JT (2004) Redox-active metals, oxidative stress, and Alzheimer's disease pathology. *Ann NY Acad Sci* 1012: 153-63.

Huse JT, Pijak DS, Leslie GJ, Lee VM, Doms RW (2000) Maturation and endosomal targeting of beta-site amyloid precursor protein-cleaving enzyme. The Alzheimer's disease beta-secretase. *J Biol Chem* 275:33729-37.

Hussain I, Powell D, Howlett DR, Tew DG, Meek TD, Chapman C, Gloger IS, Murphy KE, Southan CD, Ryan DM, Smith TS, Simmons DL, Walsh FS, Dingwall C, Christie G (1999) Identification of a novel aspartic protease (Asp 2) as β-secretase. *Mol Cell Neurosci* 14:419-27.

Iseri LT, French JH (1984) Magnesium: nature's physiologic calcium blocker. *Am Heart J* 108:188-193.

Iwata N, Tsubuki S, Takaki Y, Shirotani K, Lu B, Gerard NP, Gerard C, Hama E, Lee HJ, Saido TC (2001) Metabolic regulation of brain Abeta by neprilysin. *Science* 292:1550-2.

Kaether C, Lammich S, Edbauer D, Ertl M, Rietdorf J, Capell A, Steiner H, Haass C (2002) Presenilin-1 affects trafficking and processing of betaAPP and is targeted in a complex with nicastrin to the plasma membrane. *J Cell Biol* 158:551-61.

Kamenetz F, Tomita T, Hsieh H, Seabrook G, Borchelt D, Iwatsubo T, Sisodia S, Malinow R (2003) APP processing and synaptic function. *Neuron* 37:925-37.

Kang J, Lemaire HG, Unterbeck A, Salbaum JM, Masters CL, Grzeschik KH, Multhaup G, Beyreuther K, Muller-Hill B (1987) The precursor of Alzheimer's disease amyloid A4 protein resembles a cell-surface receptor. *Nature* 325:733-6.

Kim SH, Leem JY, Lah JJ, Slunt HH, Levey AI, Thinakaran G, Sisodia SS (2001) Multiple effects of aspartate mutant presenilin 1 on the processing and trafficking of amyloid precursor protein. *J Biol Chem* 276:43343-50.

Ko YH, Hong S, Pedersen PL (1999) Chemical mechanism of ATP synthase. Magnesium plays a pivotal role in formation of the transition state where ATP is synthesized from ADP and inorganic phosphate. *J Biol Chem* 274:28853-6.

Koo EH, Squazzo SL (1994) Evidence that production and release of amyloid beta-protein involves the endocytic pathway. *J Biol Chem* 269:17386-89.

Kurochkin IV, Goto S (1994) Alzheimer's beta-amyloid peptide specifically interacts with and is degraded by insulin degrading enzyme. *FEBS Lett* 345:33-7.

Ladner CJ, Lee JM (1999) Reduced high-affinity agonist binding at the M(1) muscarinic receptor in Alzheimer's disease brain: differential sensitivity to agonists and divalent cations. *Exp Neurol* 158:451-8.

Lammich S, Kojro E, Postina R, Gilbert S, Pfeiffer R, Jasionowski M, Haass C, Fahrenholz F (1999) Constitutive and regulated alpha-secretase cleavage of Alzheimer's amyloid precursor protein by a disintegrin metalloprotease. *Proc Natl Acad Sci USA* 96:3922-7.

Lammich S, Kojro E, Postina R, Gilbert S, Pfeiffer R, Jasionowski M, Haass C, Fahrenholz F (1999) Constitutive and regulated alpha-secretase cleavage of Alzheimer's amyloid precursor protein by a disintegrin metalloprotease. *Proc Natl Acad Sci* USA 96: 3922-7.

Landfield PW, Morgan GA (1984) Chronically elevating plasma Mg2+ improves hippocampal frequency potentiation and reversal learning in aged and young rats. *Brain Res* 322:167-71.

LeBlanc AC, Koutroumanis M, Goodyer CG (1998) Protein kinase C activation increases release of secreted amyloid precursor protein without decreasing Abeta production in human primary neuron cultures. *J Neurosci* 18:2907-13.

Lee JY, Cole TB, Palmiter RD, Suh SW, Koh JY (2002) Contribution by synaptic zinc to the gender-disparate plaque formation in human Swedish mutant APP transgenic mice. *Proc Natl Acad Sci USA* 99: 7705-10.

Leissring MA, Farris W, Chang AY, Walsh DM, Wu X, Sun X, Frosch MP, Selkoe DJ (2003) Enhanced proteolysis of beta-amyloid in APP transgenic mice prevents plaque formation, secondary pathology, and premature death. *Neuron* 40:1087-93.

Lemke MR (1995) Plasma magnesium decrease and altered calcium/magnesium ratio in severe dementia of the Alzheimer type. *Biol Psychiatry* 37:341-3.

Lesne S, Ali C, Gabriel C, Croci N, MacKenzie ET, Glabe CG, Plotkine M, Marchand-Verrecchia C, Vivien D, Buisson A (2005) NMDA receptor activation inhibits alpha-secretase and promotes neuronal amyloid-beta production. *J Neurosci* 25:9367-77.

Lin JY, Chung SY, Lin MC, Cheng FC (2002) Effects of magnesium sulfate on energy metabolites and glutamate in the cortex during focal cerebral ischemia and reperfusion in the gerbil monitored by a dual-probe microdialysis technique. *Life Sci* 71:803-11.

Liu Y, Zhang YW, Wang X, Zhang H, You X, Liao FF, Xu H (2009) Intracellular trafficking of presenilin 1 is regulated by beta-amyloid precursor protein and phospholipase D1. *J Biol Chem* 284:12145-52.

Loffler J, Huber G (1993) Modulation of beta-amyloid precursor protein secretion in differentiated and nondifferentiated cells. Biochem Biophys Res Commun 195:97-103.

Lovell MA, Robertson JD, Teesdale WJ, Campbell JL, Markesbery WR (1998) Copper, iron and zinc in Alzheimer's disease senile plaques. *J Neurol Sci* 158, 47-52.

Mantyh PW, Ghilardi JR, Rogers S, DeMaster E, Allen CJ, Stimson ER, Maggio JE (1993) Aluminum, iron, and zinc ions promote aggregation of physiological concentrations of β-amyloid peptide. *J Neurochem* 61: 1171-4.

Marr RA, Guan H, Rockenstein E, Kindy M, Gage FH, Verma I, Masliah E, Hersh LB (2004) Neprilysin regulates amyloid Beta peptide levels. *J Mol Neurosci* 22:5-11.

Martin H, Abadie C, Heyd B, Mantion G, Richert L, Berthelot A (2006) N-acetylcysteine partially reverses oxidative stress and apoptosis exacerbated by Mg-deficiency culturing conditions in primary cultures of rat and human hepatocytes. *J Am Coll Nutr* 25:363-9.

Martin H, Richert L, Berthelot A (2003) Magnesium deficiency induces apoptosis in primary cultures of rat hepatocytes. *J Nutr* 133:2505-11.

Masters CL, Simms G, Weinman NA, Multhaup G, McDonald BL, Beyreuther K (1985) Amyloid plaque core protein in Alzheimer disease and Down syndrome. *Proc Natl Acad Sci USA* 82:4245-9.

Matsuda H, Saigusa A, Irisawa H (1987) Ohmic conductance through the inwardly rectifying K channel and blocking by internal Mg2+. *Nature* 325:156-9.

Mattson MP, Cheng B, Culwell AR, Esch FS, Lieberburg I, Rydel RE (1993) Evidence for excitoprotective and intraneuronal calcium-regulating roles for secreted forms of the beta-amyloid precursor protein. *Neuron* 10:243-54.

Mayer ML, Westbrook GL, Guthrie PB (1984) Voltage-dependent block by Mg2+ of NMDA responses in spinal cord neurones. *Nature* 309:261-3.

Meziane H, Dodart JC, Mathis C, Little S, Clemens J, Paul SM, Ungerer A (1998) Memory-enhancing effects of secreted forms of the beta-amyloid precursor protein in normal and amnestic mice. *Proc Natl Acad Sci USA* 95:12683-8.

Morimoto T, Ohsawa I, Takamura C, Ishiguro M, Kohsaka S (1998) Involvement of amyloid precursor protein in functional synapse formation in cultured hippocampal neurons. *J Neurosci Res* 51:185-95.

Mucke L, Abraham CR, Masliah E (1996) Neurotrophic and neuroprotective effects of hAPP in transgenic mice. *Ann N Y Acad Sci* 777:82-8.

Nowak L, Bregestovski P, Ascher P, Herbet A, Prochiantz A (1984) Magnesium gates glutamate-activated channels in mouse central neurones. *Nature* 307:462-5.

Oyanagi K (2005) The nature of the parkinsonism-dementia complex and amyotrophic lateral sclerosis of Guam and magnesium deficiency. *Parkinsonism and Related Disorders* 11:S17–S23.

Oyanagi K, Kawakami E, Kikuchi-Horie K, Ohara K, Ogata K, Takahama S, Wada M, Kihira T, Yasui M (2006) Magnesium deficiency over generations in rats with special references to the pathogenesis of the Parkinsonism-dementia complex and amyotrophic lateral sclerosis of Guam. *Neuropathology* 26(2):115-28.

Phinney AL, Drisaldi B, Schmidt SD, Lugowski S, Coronado V, Liang Y, Horne P, Yang J, Sekoulidis J, Coomaraswamy J, Chishti MA, Cox DW, Mathews PM, Nixon RA, Carlson GA, St George-Hyslop P, Westaway D (2003) In vivo reduction of amyloid-beta by a mutant copper transporter. *Proc Natl Acad Sci USA* 100: 14193-8.

Prescott AR, Comerford JG, Magrath R, Lamb NJC, Warn RM (1988) Effects of elevated intracellular magnesium on cytoskeletal integrity. *J Cell Science* 89:321-9.

Price DL, Sisodia SS, Borchelt DR (1998) Genetic neurodegenerative diseases: the human illness and transgenic models. *Science* 282:1079-83.

Qi-Takahara Y, Morishima-Kawashima M, Tanimura Y, Dolios G, Hirotani N, Horikoshi Y, Kametani F, Maeda M, Saido TC, Wang R, Ihara Y (2005) Longer forms of amyloid beta protein: implications for the mechanism of intramembrane cleavage by gamma-secretase. *J Neurosci* 25:436-45.

Querfurth HW, Selkoe DJ (1994) Calcium ionophore increases amyloid beta peptide production by cultured cells. *Biochemistry* 33:4550-61.

Ray WJ, Yao M, Mumm J, Schroeter EH, Saftig P, Wolfe M, Selkoe DJ, Kopan R, Goate AM (1999) Cell surface presenilin-1 participates in the gamma-secretase-like proteolysis of Notch. *J Biol Chem* 274:36801-7.

Richert L, Binda D, Hamilton G, Viollon-Abadie C, Alexandre E, Bigot-Lasserre D, Bars R, Coassolo P, LeCluyse E (2002) Evaluation of the effect of culture configuration on morphology, survival time, antioxidant status and metabolic capacities of cultured rat hepatocytes. *Toxicol In Vitro* 16:89-99.

Roher AE, Kasunic TC, Woods AS, Cotter RJ, Ball MJ, Fridman R (1994) Proteolysis of A beta peptide from Alzheimer disease brain by gelatinase A. *Biochem Biophys Res Commun* 205:1755-61.

Romani A, Marfella C, Scarpa A (1993) Regulation of magnesium uptake and release in the heart and in isolated ventricular myocytes. *Circ Res* 72:1139-48.

Romani A, Scarpa A (1992) Regulation of cell magnesium. *Arch Biochem Biophys* 298:1-12.
Romani AM, Scarpa A (2000) Regulation of cellular magnesium. *Front Biosci* 5:D720-D734.

Rossner S, Beck M, Stahl T, Mendla K, Schliebs R, Bigl V (2000) Constitutive overactivation of protein kinase C in guinea pig brain increases alpha-secretory APP processing without decreasing beta-amyloid generation. *Eur J Neurosci* 12:3191-200.

Schubert D, Behl C (1993) The expression of amyloid beta protein precursor protects nerve cells from beta-amyloid and glutamate toxicity and alters their interaction with the extracellular matrix. *Brain Res* 629:275-82.

Selkoe DJ (1991) The molecular pathology of Alzheimer's disease. *Neuron* 6:487-98.

Selkoe DJ (1999) Translating cell biology into therapeutic advances in Alzheimer's disease. *Nature* 399:A23-A31.

Selkoe DJ (2001) Alzheimer's disease: genes, proteins, and therapy. *Physiol Rev* 81:741-66.

Selkoe DJ (2001) Clearing the brain's amyloid cobwebs. *Neuron* 32:177-80.

Selkoe DJ (2002) Alzheimer's disease is a synaptic failure. *Science* 298:789-91.

Seubert P, Oltersdorf T, Lee MG, Barbour R, Blomquist C, Davis DL, Bryant K, Fritz LC, Galasko D, Thal LJ, . (1993) Secretion of beta-amyloid precursor protein cleaved at the amino terminus of the beta-amyloid peptide. *Nature* 361:260-63.

Shcherbatykh I, Carpenter DO (2007) The role of metals in the etiology of Alzheimer's disease. J *Alzheimers Dis* 11:191-205.

Shirotani K, Tsubuki S, Iwata N, Takaki Y, Harigaya W, Maruyama K, Kiryu-Seo S, Kiyama H, Iwata H, Tomita T, Iwatsubo T, Saido TC (2001) Neprilysin degrades both amyloid beta peptides 1-40 and 1-42 most rapidly and efficiently among thiorphan- and phosphoramidon-sensitive endopeptidases. *J Biol Chem* 276:21895-901.

Sinha S, *et al.* (1999) Purification and cloning of amyloid precursor protein beta-secretase from human brain. *Nature* 402:537-40.

Sisodia SS (1992) Beta-amyloid precursor protein cleavage by a membrane-bound protease. *Proc Natl Acad Sci USA* 89:6075-9.

Skovronsky DM, Moore DB, Milla ME, Doms RW, Lee VM (2000) Protein kinase C-dependent alpha-secretase competes with beta-secretase for cleavage of amyloid-beta precursor protein in the trans-golgi network. *J Biol Chem* 275:2568-75.

Slutsky I, Abumaria N, Wu LJ, Huang C, Zhang L, Li B, Zhao X, Govindarajan A, Zhao MG, Zhuo M, Tonegawa S, Liu G (2010) Enhancement of learning and memory by elevating brain magnesium. *Neuron* 65(2):165-77.

Small DH, Nurcombe V, Reed G, Clarris H, Moir R, Beyreuther K, Masters CL (1994) A heparin-binding domain in the amyloid protein precursor of Alzheimer's disease is involved in the regulation of neurite outgrowth. *J Neurosci* 14:2117-27.

Soundararajan R, Wishart AD, Rupasinghe HP, rcellana-Panlilio M, Nelson CM, Mayne M, Robertson GS (2008) Quercetin 3-glucoside protects neuroblastoma (SH-SY5Y) cells in vitro against oxidative damage by inducing sterol regulatory element-binding protein-2-mediated cholesterol biosynthesis. *J Biol Chem* 283:2231-45.

Sparks DL, Schreurs BG (2003) Trace amounts of copper in water induce beta-amyloid plaques and learning deficits in a rabbit model of Alzheimer's disease. *Proc Natl Acad Sci USA* 100: 11065-9.

Subirana JA, Soler-Lopez M (2003) Cations as hydrogen bond donors: a view of electrostatic interactions in DNA. *Annu Rev Biophys Biomol Struct* 32:27-45.

Turner AJ, Fisk L, Nalivaeva NN (2004) Targeting amyloid-degrading enzymes as therapeutic strategies in neurodegeneration. *Ann N Y Acad Sci* 1035:1-20.

Vandenberg CA (1987) Inward rectification of a potassium channel in cardiac ventricular cells depends on internal magnesium ions. *Proc Natl Acad Sci USA* 84:2560-4.

Vassar R, Bennett BD, Babu-Khan S, Kahn S, Mendiaz EA, Denis P, Teplow DB, Ross S, Amarante P, Loeloff R, Luo Y, Fisher S, Fuller J, Edenson S, Lile J, Jarosinski MA, Biere AL, Curran E, Burgess T, Louis JC, Collins F, Treanor J, Rogers G, Citron M (1999) Beta-secretase cleavage of Alzheimer's amyloid precursor protein by the transmembrane aspartic protease BACE. *Science* 286: 735-41.

Vassar R, *et al.* (1999) Beta-secretase cleavage of Alzheimer's amyloid precursor protein by the transmembrane aspartic protease BACE. *Science* 286:735-41.

Vural H, Demirin H, Kara Y, Eren I, Delibas N (2010) Alterations of plasma magnesium, copper, zinc, iron and selenium concentrations and some related erythrocyte antioxidant enzyme activities in patients with Alzheimer's disease. *J Trace Elements Med Biol* 24:169–73.

Wang DS, Dickson DW, Malter JS (2006) beta-Amyloid Degradation and Alzheimer's Disease. *J Biomed Biotechnol* 2006:58406.

White AR, Cappai R (2003) Neurotoxicity from glutathione depletion is dependent on extracellular trace copper. *J Neurosci Res* 71:889-97.

White AR, Du T, Laughton KM, Volitakis I, Sharples RA, Xilinas ME, Hoke DE, Holsinger RM, Evin G, Cherny RA, Hill AF, Barnham KJ, Li QX, Bush AI, Masters CL (2006) Degradation of the Alzheimer disease amyloid beta-peptide by metal-dependent up-regulation of metalloprotease activity. *J Biol Chem* 281:17670-80.

Wiltfang J, Esselmann H, Cupers P, Neumann M, Kretzschmar H, Beyermann M, Schleuder D, Jahn H, Ruther E, Kornhuber J, Annaert W, De SB, Saftig P (2001) Elevation of beta-amyloid peptide 2-42 in sporadic and familial Alzheimer's disease and its generation in PS1 knockout cells. *J Biol Chem* 276:42645-57.

Wiltfang J, Smirnov A, Schnierstein B, Kelemen G, Matthies U, Klafki HW, Staufenbiel M, Huther G, Ruther E, Kornhuber J (1997) Improved electrophoretic separation and immunoblotting of beta-amyloid (A beta) peptides 1-40, 1-42, and 1-43. *Electrophoresis* 18:527-32.

Wolf FI, Torsello A, Fasanella S, Cittadini A (2003) Cell physiology of magnesium. *Mol Aspects Med* 24:11-26.

Xu X, Yang D, Wyss-Coray T, Yan J, Gan L, Sun Y, Mucke L (1999) Wild-type but not Alzheimer-mutant amyloid precursor protein confers resistance against p53-mediated apoptosis. *Proc Natl Acad Sci USA* 96:7547-52.

Yamazaki T, Koo EH, Selkoe DJ (1996) Trafficking of cell-surface amyloid beta-protein precursor. II. Endocytosis, recycling and lysosomal targeting detected by immunolocalization. *J Cell Sci* 109 (Pt 5):999-1008.

Yan R, Bienkowski MJ, Shuck ME, Miao H, Tory MC, Pauley AM, Brashier JR, Stratman NC, Mathews WR, Buhl AE, Carter DB, Tomasselli AG, Parodi LA, Heinrikson RL, Gurney ME (1999) Membrane-anchored aspartyl protease with Alzheimer's disease beta-secretase activity. *Nature* 402:533-37.

Yang LS, Ksiezak-Reding H (1999) Ca2+ and Mg2+ selectively induce aggregates of PHF-tau but not normal human tau. *J Neurosci Res* 55:36-43.

Yu J, Sun M, Chen Z, Lu J, Liu Y, Zhou L, Xu X, Fan D, Chui D (2010) Magnesium modulates amyloid-beta protein precursor trafficking and processing. *J Alzheimers Dis* 20(4):1091-106.

Zhao G, Mao G, Tan J, Dong Y, Cui MZ, Kim SH, Xu X (2004) Identification of a new presenilin-dependent zeta-cleavage site within the transmembrane domain of amyloid precursor protein. *J Biol Chem* 279:50647-50.

Zhao J, Wang WN, Tan YC, Zheng Y, Wang ZX (2002) Effect of Mg(2+) on the kinetics of guanine nucleotide binding and hydrolysis by Cdc42. *Biochem Biophys Res Commun* 297:653-658.

Magnesium and stress

Magdalena D. Cuciureanu [1,✉] *and Robert Vink* [2]

[1] Department of Pharmacology, "Gr. T. Popa" University of Medicine and Pharmacy, Iasi, 700115, Romania.
[2] Centre for Neuroscience Research, School of Medical Sciences, The University of Adelaide, South Australia 5005, Australia.
✉ magdacuciur@gmail.com

Abstract

Magnesium status is highly associated with stress levels, with both stress and hypomagnesemia potentiating each other's negative effects. Indeed, hypomagnesemia has been associated with stressful conditions such as photosensitive headache, fibromyalgia, chronic fatigue syndrome, audiogenic stress, cold stress, and physical stress, amongst others. The role of magnesium in these conditions is unclear, although a number of potential mechanisms for magnesium's action have been identified including via the glutamatergic, serotonergic, and adrenergic neurotransmitter systems, as well as via several neuro-hormones. The current review examines the link between magnesium deficiency and stress, focusing on the association between magnesium and various stress pathologies, magnesium's potential interaction with stress pathways, and magnesium's effects on the brain.

Introduction

At the beginning of the twentieth century, Walter Cannon pioneered research concerning the importance of the sympathetic nervous system in adaptation of the body. While Claude Bernard was the first who defined the term of "milieu interieur" as being "the constancy of the internal environment" (see Cameron, 2007), it was Walter Cannon who coined the terms "homeostasis" and "fight-or-flight response" (see Quick, 1994). Subsequently, Hans Selye (see Neylan, 1998) in 1936 adapted a concept from physics describing the resistance of a body to applied pressure in order to define the concept of stress. General adaptation syndrome, as he called it, is the non-specific response of the body to any demand for change. It consists of three stages of adaptation: an initial brief alarm reaction, a prolonged period of resistance, and finally, the stage of exhaustion and death. Although there is no generally accepted definition, stress can be understood to be a complex adaptive biochemical, physiological, psycho-logical and gene expression change of the organism (stress response) triggered by a stimulus (stressor) that was interpreted by the brain as being dangerous (McEwen, 2008b; Kvetnansky, 2009; Kantorovich, 2008). The neuroendocrine response to stress initiates hyperventilation, elevated blood pressure, increased heart rate, sudomotor response (sweating), increased blood flow to skeletal muscles and perturbations of gut function ('fight or flight' defense reaction) in order to enable body survival. More, the amygdala activates neurons in the hippocampus and neocortex, where threatening stimuli are associated with fear, in order to adapt future behavior to avoid danger (Rupniak 2005).

To further refine the stress concept, Sterling and Eyer (1988) proposed the term allostasis to describe the process of achieving stability through change. As compared to homeostatic values (blood oxygen, blood pH, and body temperature), which have to be kept within a narrow range, the allostatic mediators (hormones of the hypothalamic-pituitary-adrenal axis, catechol-amines, and cytokines) may vary during daily and seasonal routines (McEwen, 2008b; Ablin and Buskila; Billard, 2006).

Nowadays, the profound implications of stress in human pathology are unanimously recognized and represent a dynamic field of research. There is a continued interest in identifying new possibilities to alleviate stress and improve quality of life in a fast-changing, modern world.

The idea that magnesium (Mg^{2+}) supplement-ation modifies the effect of chronic stress dates back to 1981 (Classen, 1981). This hypothesis is certainly feasible given the cation's ubiquitous distribution and role throughout the body. Indeed, Mg^{2+} is the fourth most abundant cation in the body and the second most abundant intracellular cation. It is involved in a wide variety of cellular processes including aerobic and anaerobic metabolism, all bioenergetic reactions, regulation of metabolic pathways, signal transduction, ion channels activity, cell proliferation, differentiation, apoptosis, angiogenesis, and membrane stabilization (Nishizawa *et al*, 2007; Szewczyk *et al*, 2008; Turner and Vink 2007; Wolf *et al*, 2007). At a biochemical level, more than 325 enzymes are Mg^{2+} dependent, many of which are nervous system enzymes, thus reflecting the important role potentially played by Mg^{2+} in CNS physiological and pathological function (Eby and Eby, 2006).

Magnesium interaction with stress pathways

Acute stress has been shown to be associated with increased plasma Mg^{2+} levels and increased urinary Mg^{2+} excretion (Murck, 2002; Whyte *et al*, 1987). The shift of Mg^{2+} from the intracellular to extracellular space initially plays a protective role in order to diminish the adverse effects of stress, but extended periods of stress result in progressive Mg^{2+} deficit and deleterious consequences for health (Seelig, 1994). Moreover, stress and hypomagnesemia potentate each other's negative effects in a veritable pathogenic vicious circle. Low Mg^{2+}/Ca^{2+} ratios augment the release of catecholamines in response to stress (Caddell *et al*, 1986; Seelig, 1994). Fatty acids resulting from adrenergic-induced lipolysis form undissociated Mg^{2+} soaps which further exacerbates Mg^{2+} depletion (Seelig, 1994). Mg^{2+} deficiency also favors the release of vasoconstrictive and platelet aggregating factors (derived from fatty acids metabolism and endothelium), increases the thromboxane B2 to prostaglandin I2 (TxB_2/PgI_2) ratio and enhances intravascular blood coagulation (Ceremuzynski *et al*, 1978; Franz 2004; Dong *et al*, 2008; Soma *et al*, 1988; Sontia and Touyz, 2007). Most interestingly, Mg^{2+} deficiency itself doesn't induce specific pathology but reduces the tolerance to secondary stress (Tejero-Taldo *et al*, 2006).

The active transport systems between plasma and cerebrospinal fluid enable elevated and relatively constant Mg^{2+} concentrations in the CSF (typically 1.1 mmol/l in CSF compared to 0.8 mmol/l in plasma) (Oppelt *et al*, 1963; Murck 2002). There are reports that parenteral administration of magnesium sulfate augments cerebrospinal fluid Mg^{2+} concentration by 20%–25% in approximately 4 hours (Ko *et al*, 2001; Muir, 2002), although recent reports suggest that Mg^{2+} may not readily cross the intact blood brain barrier (see Chapter 3).

With respect to mechanisms of action, Mg^{2+} affects a number of neurotransmitter systems. It inhibits the release of excitatory neurotransmitters and also acts as a voltage-gated antagonist at the glutamate, N-methyl-D-aspartate (NMDA) receptor. Mg^{2+} also antagonizes calcium entry via voltage-gated channels of all types. In addition to exhibiting agonist properties at γ-aminobutyric acid A receptors, it is an angiotensin II receptor antagonist. Mg^{2+} inhibits calcium/protein kinase C related neurotransmission, increases reuptake of glutamate via stimulation of Na^+/K^+ATPase and is involved in mitochondrial ATP-dependent potassium channel activity (Bednarczyk *et al*, 2005; Eby and Eby, 2006; Muir 2002; Murck , 2002). Furthermore, Mg^{2+} inhibits the phosphorylation activity of glycogen synthase kinase-3 (GSK-3), increases brain-derived neurotrophic factor (BDNF) expression and enhances the cAMP response element-binding (CREB)/BDNF pathway via the serotonergic system, all mechanisms related to the antidepressant-like activity of this ion (Szewczyk *et al*, 2008).

There is also an increasing body of evidence indicating that psychological stress promotes ***oxidative stress***, mainly by auto-oxidation of catecholamines. Several studies have shown that psychological stress exacerbates lipid peroxidation, increases production of markers of oxidative damage of DNA (8-oxo-7,8-dihydroguanine), and decreases plasma antioxidant activity (Seelig, 1994; Sivonova *et al*, 2004). Many of these processes are antagonized by Mg^{2+} (Cernak *et al*, 2000; Muir, 2002; Nishizawa *et al*, 2007).

A stressor (either physical or psychological event) initially activates the hypothalamic-pituitary-adrenal (HPA) axis and the autonomic nervous system. Activating these systems leads to release of catecholamines from sympathetic nerves and the adrenal medulla, and of

corticotropin-releasing factor (CRF) and vasopressin (AVP) from parvicellular neurons. Seconds later, adrenocorticotropic hormone (ACTH) is secreted from the anterior pituitary gland and stimulates release of glucocorticoids from the adrenal cortex (Rupniak, 2005; Carrasco and Van de Kar, 2003). CRF is a neurotransmitter involved in the coordination of the endocrine, autonomic, behavioral and immune responses to stress, and whose administration elicits stress-like effects (De Souza *et al*, 1991; Carrasco and Van de Kar 2003; Cratty and Birkle, 1999). Magnesium interacts either directly or indirectly with the activity of a number of these neurotransmitters and neurohormones. For example, Cratty and Birkle (1999) showed that glutamate-stimulated CRF release is antagonized by the addition of $MgCl_2$ to the incubation medium. Mg^{2+} stabilizes CRF receptor binding and is directly correlated to the number of CRF binding sites (Perrin *et al*, 1986). On the other hand, Mg^{2+} stimulates the Na^+/K^+ATPase, which decreases CRF-receptor sensitivity (De Souza 1995).

Mg^{2+} also decreases the release of ***ACTH*** and modulates adrenocortical sensitivity to this hormone. As i.c.v. administration of angiotensin II (ATII) increases the secretion of ACTH and AVP via CRF, it is presumed that Mg^{2+} induces a suppression of the HPA-axis activity at least partially through antagonism of ATII effects (Murck, 2002). Intracerebroventricular administration of artificial CSF with low Mg^{2+} concentration induces an increase in cortisol secretion in cats (Garcy and Marotta, 1978). In stressful circumstances, $MgSO_4$ administration reduces the release of ***AVP*** (Jee *et al*, 2009), a neuropeptide that plays an important role in generation of emotions, social behavior (aggression), learning and memory (Neumann *et al*, 2010; Ebner *et al*, 2000).

Low blood Mg^{2+} levels have been associated with raised brain ***norepinephrine*** (NE) content in mice selectively bred for hypomagnesemia (Amyard *et al*, 1995). Such low Mg^{2+} levels in blood have also been associated with increased catecholamine release in response to noise stress in rats, and with significantly increased urinary excretion (+200%) of NE compared to controls (Caddell *et al*, 1986; Henrotte, 1997). Also, it has been proven that Mg^{2+} exerts a direct suppressive effect on locus coeruleus activity and that poor Mg^{2+} status increases sensitivity to stress (Henrotte *et al*, 1997).

Another pathway influenced by Mg^{2+} is the ***serotoninergic*** system. Mg^{2+} acts like a cofactor of tryptophan hydroxylase, intervenes in serotonin receptor binding *in vitro* and exhibits a direct enhancing effect on 5-HT1A serotonin receptor transmission (Szewczyk *et al*, 2008; Mizoguchi *et al*, 2008; Abaamrane *et al*, 2009). Microdialysis studies showed that stressors can change the extracellular levels of serotonin in different brain areas including the hypothalamus, amygdala, frontal cortex and raphe nuclei (Fujino *et al*, 2002; Funada and Hara, 2001). Serotonin is involved in neuroendocrine regulation of stress through actions on prolactin, oxytocin, AVP, CRF and ACTH activity (Jorgensen, 2007). HPA axis dysregulation and sensitization of 5-HT_2 receptor-mediated signaling induced by CRF have implied chronic stress in the etiology of depression and anxiety (Szewczyk *et al*, 2008; Magalhaes *et al*, 2010).

It is also tempting to speculate that the protective effect of the ***estrogens*** in stress are partially mediated by Mg^{2+} (Carrasco and Van de Kar, 2003). For example, It is known that estrogens mediate the shift of Mg^{2+} from plasma to cells and increase intracellular levels of Mg^{2+} (Galland, 1991; Seelig, 1993; Seelig *et al*, 2004). Likewise, serum levels of Mg^{2+} and total magnesium were inversely correlated with estrogen concentration level (Muneyyirci-Delale *et al*, 1999). In postmenopausal women estrogen replacement therapy suppresses HPA axis responses to an emotional stressor (Dayas *et al*, 2000).

Besides cortisol, ***prolactin***, is regarded as a measurable marker of a coping strategy to "psychological stress" (Sobrinho, 2003). Confirming that Mg^{2+} levels can modulate prolactin secretion during stress, pretreatment with Mg^{2+} aspartate significantly decreased, in a dose-dependent manner, the prolactin plasma concentration of turkey pullets exposed to immobilization stress compared to non-treated birds (Marois *et al*, 1985; Ali *et al*, 1987). In addition, Mg^{2+} acts like a positive allosteric modulator for ***oxytocin*** binding to the receptor and in this way facilitates the neuropeptide's action to alleviate stress (Gimpl *et al*, 2008; Labuschagne *et al*, 2010; Uvnas-Moberg and Petersson, 2005).

Magnesium deficiency, stress and miscellaneous pathologies

Clinical manifestations of hypomagnesemia include neuromuscular irritability and weakness (tremors, fasciculations, tetany and positive Chvostek's and Trousseau's signs, although some of these features may be due to concomitant hypocalcemia), headaches, focal seizures, hyper-emotionality, generalized anxiety, panic attack disorders, insomnia, fatigue, asthenia (Touyz, 2004; Wacker and Parisi, 1968; Eby and Eby, 2006; Rayssiguier*et al*, 1990; Durlach *et al*, 1997). For symptomatic patients, plasma magnesium, erythrocyte magnesium, plasma calcium and daily magnesiuria, calciuria and magnesium retention test should be evaluated (Durlach *et al*, 1997; Cundy T 2008). The alleviation of clinical manifestations by oral supplementation with 5 mg of magnesium/ kg/day confirms the diagnosis (Durlach *et al*, 1997).

Experimental data indicate that Mg^{2+}- deficient rats exhibit slightly increased plasma corticosterone levels, increased irritability and aggressive behavior, and higher mortality compared to controls (Caddell, 1991; Henrotte *et al*, 1997). Recent data also indicate that genetic polymorphism of Na^{+}/Mg^{2+} exchanger activity influences Mg^{2+} efflux from erythrocytes (Feillet-Coudray *et al*, 2004). Extensive work regarding the genetic predisposition for Mg^{2+} deficiency has been carried out by Henrotte et al (1990) who showed that both major histocompatibility complex associated genes (MHC; HLA and H-2), and non-MHC genes are important contributing factors for Mg^{2+} status. In humans, Henrotte (Henrotte and Levy-Leboyer, 1985) also found an interesting link between HLA-B35, type A personality and low Mg^{2+} status. HLA-B35 individuals are more frequently found among stress-sensitive type A behavior subjects and exhibit lower red blood cell Mg^{2+} levels than non-carriers. Moreover, these individuals show impaired cytotoxicity and higher titers to antibodies after anti-influenza vaccination, data that establish a connection between genetic background, Mg^{2+} deficiency, stress and autoimmunity (Bobkowski *et al*, 2005). It is generally accepted that, in response to a psychological stressor, type A persons exhibit increased release of catecholamines and cortisol, which consequently lowers Mg^{2+} levels and increases cardiovascular risk as compared to type B behavior (Henrotte *et al*, 1985; Matthews 1982).

Experimental Mg^{2+} deficiency has also been associated with disrupted ***sleep*** patterns. In rats, Mg^{2+} deficiency is associated with increased amplitude in daily variation in sleep and slow-wave sleep delta power, and has been noted to shorten life span and lower reproductive ability (Chollet *et al*, 2001; Motta *et al*, 1998). In humans, chronic sleep deprivation is associated with progressively decreasing levels of intracellular Mg^{2+}, reduced duration of cardiopulmonary exercise and increased hypersensitivity of the chronotropic response to sympathetic nervous stimulation (Omiya *et al*, 2009). Intriguingly, Mg^{2+} depletion is associated with decreased melatonin and its supplementation alleviates the symptoms (Billyard *et al*, 2006; Depoortere *et al*, 1993; Held *et al*, 2002). In elderly subjects, Mg^{2+} administration (10 mmol and 20 mmol each for 3 days followed by 30 mmol for 14 days) significantly increased slow wave sleep, renin levels during the total night, and aldosterone levels in the second half of the night, but decreased cortisol levels in the first part of the night (Held *et al*, 2002).

Photosensitive headache is another condition that is exacerbated by stress and Mg^{2+} deficiency. Even wearing of tinted spectacles indoors is considered to be a valid indicator of psychological distress. Patients most susceptible to develop this condition include photophobic individuals that experience ophthalmological discomfort during visual stress tests. Sarchielli et al (1992) showed that migraine sufferers with and without aura, and tension-type headaches, exhibit significantly lower levels of serum and salivary Mg^{2+} concentrations. Hypomagnesaemia raises the sensitivity of cerebral arteries to CO_2 which in turn favors cerebral vasospasm and headache (Thomas *et al*, 1994). Despite being controversial, some authors recommend intravenous administration of 1 gram of $MgSO_4$ for the treatment of migraine headache (Durlach *et al*, 2005).

Fibromyalgia is considered a stress–related disorder, with both the onset and the exacerbation of the syndrome associated with intensely stressful periods. Patients with fibromyalgia frequently exhibit chronic, widespread pain caused by the increase in the processing and handling of pain by the CNS (Ablin and Buskila, 2010). It has been shown that there is an inverse correlation between Mg^{2+} levels and clinical parameters in patients with fibromyalgia (Sendur *et al*, 2008). The beneficial role of Mg^{2+} in this pathology is presumably based on its antagonistic effect upon NMDA receptors, receptors that are significantly involved in the process of central sensitization (Galland, 1991). Various studies have also shown that patients with a ***chronic fatigue condition*** closely linked to fibromyalgia exhibit low Mg^{2+} levels that are correlated with total antioxidant capacity of blood and GSH concentrations, but not with lipid peroxidation in vitro (Galland, 1991; Manuel y Keenoy *et al*, 2000). In these patients, weekly intramuscular injections of 1g magnesium sulfate resulted in a significant improvement in energy levels, pain, and emotional reactions as measured by the Nottingham health profile score (Cox *et al*, 1991; Murck 2002). Durlach et al (2002) indicated that fibromyalgia and chronic fatigue syndrome are clinical forms of magnesium depletion associated with dysfunction of the biological clock.

An interesting correlation has been reported between Mg^{2+} deficiency and ***attention-deficit/ hyperactivity disorder*** (ADHD). Elevated subjective stress levels and stress intolerance is often mentioned as part of the clinical presentation of ADHD and often these patients present high post-stress cortisol concentrations (Hirvikoski *et al*, 2009). In a study examining 116 children, 95% of children with this pathology exhibited Mg deficiency (Kozielec and Starobrat-Hermelin, 1997). Although evidence regarding the improvement of ADHD symptoms by Mg^{2+} supplementation is mixed, some studies indicate that a Mg-B6 regimen over at least two months significantly alleviated hyperactivity and hyperemotivity/aggressiveness and improved attention at school (Mousain-Bosc *et al*, 2006; Rucklidge *et al*, 2009). Interestingly, ADHD symptoms reappear in a few weeks after the cessation of the treatment, together with a decrease in erythrocyte-Mg^{2+} values (Mousain-Bosc *et al*, 2006). A Mg-B6 regimen has also been shown to be effective in the treatment of ***Tourette's syndrome***. Tourette's syndrome is associated with increased vulnerability to stress, and Mg^{2+} deficit is considered to be a central precipitating event (Carrasco and Van de Kar, 2003; Grimaldi 2002). Hypomagnesemia is linked with exacerbated neural excitability, increased anxiety, orofacial tardive dyskinesia, and migraine, symptoms that are alleviated by the administration of a combination of 0.5 mEq/kg Mg^{2+} and 2mg/kg vitamin B6 (Garcia-Lopez *et al*, 2009; Stendig-Lindberg *et al*, 1998).

An inverse correlation between ***audiogenic stress*** and erythrocyte Mg^{2+} levels has been observed (Galland 1991), and low Mg^{2+} status has been linked to self-reported noise sensitivity, noise-induced emotional lability and noise-induced feelings of tenseness (Galland, 1991). Notably, exposure to long-term road traffic noise in both children and adults leads to elevated nighttime secretion of noradrenaline and cortisol when compared to controls (Ising and Braun 2000). Mg^{2+} administration is effective in diminishing ototoxicity (Abaamrane *et al*, 2009; Ehrenberger and Felix, 1995; Hoane *et al*, 1997 as well as in alleviating ***transportation stress*** (Tang *et al*, 2008) (Peeters *et al*, 2005). ***Cold stress*** also induces a decrease in Mg^{2+} levels in CSF and raises the incidence of clinical manifestations (Matsui, 2007). Interestingly, a correlation has been described between Mg^{2+} levels (in serum and peritoneal fluid) and stress perception (Jung *et al*, 2010; Garalejic *et al*, 2010) in relatively healthy, adult women unable to conceive but without identified organic causes of ***sterility***.

It is now well known that Mg^{2+} deficiency facilitates ***epileptiform discharges*** in hippocampal slices (Gutierrez *et al*, 1999) and in audiogenic seizures (Bac *et al*, 1998). Hippocampal neurons are more sensitive to low Mg^{2+} than neurons from other brain regions and their responses to Mg^{2+} deficiency differ depending on the developmental period (Furukawa *et al*, 2009). Human studies show that stress augments seizure frequency and severity in epileptic patients (Sawyer and Escayg, 2010).

Data from a second examination of the Copenhagen City Heart Study showed that self-reported high stress intensity and weekly stress were associated with almost a doubled risk of fatal ***stroke*** (Truelsen *et al*, 2003). In ischemic or hypoxic tissue, Mg^{2+} antagonizes calcium's effects and decreases reactive oxygen species production through phopholipases, lipoxygenase and cyclooxygenase pathways. Likewise, in conditions associated with cerebral ischemia, Mg^{2+} deficiency promotes vasoconstriction of cerebral and coronary arteries, as well as anoxic depolarizations and cortical spreading depression. Accordingly, Mg^{2+} supplementation potentially plays a neuro-protective role (Pokan *et al*, 2006; Turner *et al*, 2004). Mechanical stress such as membrane stretch or osmotic cell swelling can activate TRPM7-like channels (Numata *et al*, 2007), which are involved in Mg^{2+} transport. These channels are members of the ubiquitously expressed melastatin-related subfamily of transient receptor potential (TRP) channels, and represent essential mediators of anoxic neuronal death (Aarts and Tymianski, 2005; Penner and Fleig, 2007). Low intracellular levels of Mg^{2+}, a process that exacerbates the effects of stress on the organism, also activate TRPM7 channels.

Conscious ***critically ill patients*** experience unprecedented levels of stress, both physical and psychological. However, even unconscious, comatose or sedated patients can exhibit stress initiated by peripheral stimuli that directly activate limbic structures prior to cortical involvement. These patients exhibit multiple organ dysfunction and veritable endocrine chaos (Papathanassoglou *et al*, 2010). In these patients, hypomagnesemia is often associated with hypokalemia and is considered to aggravate the prognosis. Under these conditions, prolongation of QT interval constitutes a useful biomarker of electrolyte imbalance and the requirement for replacement therapy (Whitted *et al*, 2010). It is noteworthy that hypomagnesemia has been linked with a decrease in insulin sensitivity which can also affect the neurological outcome of critically ill patients (Polderman *et al*, 2003). In critically ill patients, a daily Mg^{2+} supplementation index higher than 1g/day is associated with lower mortality rate. Mg supplementation is also recommended for patients exposed to therapeutic hypothermia who often exhibit hypomagnesemia due to polyuresis (Dabbagh *et al*, 2006; Polderman *et al*, 2003).

In a model of ***intraperitoneal sepsis***, $MgSO_4$ administration (750 micromol/kg) attenuated the increased blood–brain barrier permeability and caused a reduction in brain edema formation (Esen *et al*, 2005). Similar results have been observed in experimental ***traumatic brain injury*** (Turner and Vink, 2007) where intravenous administration of $MgSO_4$ (250 μmol/kg) also significantly decreased the incidence of post-traumatic depression/anxiety as compared to non-treated animals (Fromm *et al*, 2004).

Stress also influences the susceptibility to ***neurodegenerative disorders*** such as multiple sclerosis and Alzheimer's disease (Brown *et al*, 2006a; Brown *et al*, 2006b; Esch *et al*, 2002a). Pro-inflammatory effects associated with stress are exacerbated and exert deleterious actions upon the neurons, including increased IL6 levels that initiate microglial activation. Increased iNos levels are also expressed during critical periods and the elevated stress hormones themselves impair hippocampal neurogenesis and memory (Esch *et al*, 2002a; Esch *et al*, 2002b). Moreover, Mg^{2+} deficiency increases neuronal calcium influx and consequently augments NO production that is associated with cytotoxic effects (Eby and Eby, 2006). Recent data also indicate a possible link between acute and sudden psychological stress and the appearance of malignant primitive ***brain tumors*** appearance (Cabaniols *et al*, 2010). Furthermore, long-term survivors of brain cancer continue to experience elevated levels of stress as the fear of recurrence increases with time (Keir *et al*, 2007). Epidemiological data have described an inverse relationship between Mg^{2+} content in drinking water and incidence of some types of cancers (Maier *et al*, 2007). A protective effect of fresh vegetable and fruit intake has also been noted. Although the role of Mg^{2+} in carcinogenesis is yet to be established, it's involvement in DNA stabilization has been described (Anastassopoulou and Theophanides, 2002; Anghileri, 2009; Wolf *et al*, 2009).

Individuals with ***cardiovascular pathology*** are most susceptible to the concerted effects of stress and Mg^{2+} deficiency. The inotropic and chronotropic response induced by catecholamine release produces an oxygen debt in the myocardium. In a hypoxic tissue, Mg^{2+} shifts from the intracellular to the extracellular space, and calcium enters into cells, leading to increased risk of arrhythmias and cardiac deterioration (Seelig, 1989). Interestingly, $MgSO_4$ is successfully used in the treatment of pheochromocytoma, a condition associated with excessive release of catecholamine. In this situation, Mg^{2+} exhibits simultaneous beta-agonist effects and alpha-adrenergic antagonist actions, improves diastolic dysfunction and reduces episodes of arrhythmia (James, 2009). Encouraging results have also been obtained using Mg^{2+} therapy in two newly described cardiomyopathic syndromes: Irukandji syndrome and stress cardiomyopathy. Irukandji syndrome is caused by envenomisation from a jelly-fish (*Carukia barnesi),* which induces excessive release of endogenous catecholamines. Administration of $MgSO_4$ alleviates pain and the cardiovascular response in Irukandji syndrome but there is still need for evidence-based guidelines in management of this condition (Tiong, 2009; Nickson *et al*, 2009; Barnett *et al*, 2005; Corkeron *et al*, 2004). Stress cardio-myopathy (also referred as Takotsubo cardiomyopathy or transient left ventricular apical ballooning syndrome) is an acute reversible apical ventricular dysfunction provoked by elevated levels of catecholamines. These stress hormones enable the shift of β2-adrenoceptor transducing signal from Gs protein to Gi protein causing negative inotropic effects (Lyon *et al*, 2008). While there is no specific treatment for this condition, some authors reported beneficial results with Mg^{2+} administration (Akashi *et al*, 2008).

Considerable evidence now supports the fact that Mg^{2+} presents beneficial effects in different types of ***surgical stress***, including induction and maintenance of pneumoperitoneum, endotracheal intubation, cardiopulmonary bypass, occlusion-reperfusion surgery and middle ear surgery (James 2009; Jee *et al*, 2009; Puri *et al*, 1998; (Ashton *et al*, 1991; Delhumeau *et al*, 1995; Manrique *et al*, 2010; Dorman *et al*, 2000; Kurian and Paddikkala 2010; Ryu *et al*, 2009). Considering the fact that pain induces the release of stress mediators, the blockade of neuronal NMDA receptors by Mg^{2+} provides additional positive effects. Even if Mg^{2+} is not a potent analgesic per se, several authors have shown that Mg^{2+} potentates the analgesic effect of traditionally used pain relievers, reduces their requirements and decreases the incidence of postoperative shivering (Dabbagh *et al*, 2009; Lysakowski *et al*, 2007). Following carotid endarterectomy or cardiac surgery, Mg^{2+} therapy improves cognitive outcome and prevents postoperative arrhythmias, especially in patients with contraindications for beta-blockers (Mack *et al*, 2009; Dabrowski *et al*, 2008; Davis *et al*,).

In athletes who are subjected to severe ***physical stress***, Mg^{2+} favorably stabilizes the membrane integrity by binding with phosphate groups of phospholipids located in cell and organelle membranes (Golf *et al*, 1998). In these subjects, 17 mmol magnesium supplementation per day lowered serum cortisol levels and augmented venous O_2 partial pressure leading to better performance. Recent studies indicated that magnesium intake should be at least 260 mg/day for male and 220 mg/day for female athletes (Nielsen and Lukaski, 2006). According to Couzy and colleagues, Mg^{2+} overdosage in professional sportsmen may lead to hypo-zincemia (Couzy *et al*, 1990; Kantorovich *et al*, 2008). The overtraining syndrome described in athletes is also a stress-related condition that designates the exhaustion stage of Selye's general adaptation syndrome. This syndrome is characterized by impairment of psychological processing, systemic inflammatory response, and HPA dysfunction (Angeli *et al*, 2004). Magnesium deficiency has been reported in this condition.

Stress and the brain

The brain is very susceptible to stress, largely because corticosterone binds at this level to high affinity mineralocorticoid receptors (Abaamrane *et al*, 2009) and to glucocorticoid receptors (GR), albeit with 10-fold lower affinity. The CA1 and dentate gyrus neurons of the hippocampus express high amounts of both receptor types, whereas CA3 pyramidal neurons primarily express MR (Karst and Joels, 2003). A stress-induced rise in corticosteroid levels modulates short-term memory, generally by promoting storage of information that is emotionally related to the stressful event, but by suppressing information that is not associated with it (Lupien and Maheu, 2007). Glucocorticoids contribute to the consolidation of contextual fear conditioning, but can also lead to memory impairments

(Kolber *et al*, 2008; Leon-Carrion *et al*, 2009). The inability to remember important data worsens the individual's stress and makes the subject even more vulnerable. Animal studies also show that stress-induced increases in NE levels modulates declarative memory according to an inverted-U-shaped function by enhancing the memory for information unrelated to the source of stress (Lupien and Maheu, 2007). A strong link between noradrenergic activation, glucocorticoid effects and basolateral amygdala function has been described (McGaugh and Roozendaal, 2002; Baldi and Bucherelli, 2005).

While acute stress affects memory in a reversible way, chronic stress results in deleterious changes in the hippocampus, especially an atrophy of dendrites of pyramidal neurons in the CA3 region of the hippocampus, and in other brain regions (prefrontal cortex, amygdala, brain stem and pons). By antagonising NMDA receptors, Mg^{2+} prevents acute glucocorticoid effects on neurogenesis (Nacher and McEwen, 2006; Cameron *et al*, 1998; McEwen, 2008a; Slutsky *et al*, 2010). Mg^{2+} removal from the extracellular medium produces hyperexcitability and cellular death in cultured hippocampal neurons through a mechanism based on NMDA receptor activation and Raf-MEK-MSK1 signaling pathway (Hughes *et al*, 2003). Moreover, through the effects upon P-glycoprotein, Mg^{2+} modulates the access of corticosteroids to the brain (Murck, 2002). Consistent with these data, Mg^{2+} deficiency represents an important factor in the aethiopathogenesis of aging defined by decreased adaptability to stress, alteration of hippocampus functioning, failure to turn off the hypothalamo-pituitary-adrenal axis and hyperadrenoglucocorticism (Durlach *et al*, 1993; Steptoe, 2007).

Stress exposure results a long-lasting sensitization of the HPA axis to subsequent novel stressors. Exposure to a single stressor induces CRF–dependent depression of postsynaptic NMDA receptors that allows glutamate synapses in the paraventricular nucleus of the hypothalamus to undergo a short-term potentiation (STP) (Kuzmiski *et al*, 2010). There is a growing body of evidence that Mg^{2+} plays an important role in synaptic plasticity and is involved in long-term potentiation (LTP) and long-term depression (LTD) of synaptic transmission (Billard, 2006). LTP is induced by cortical stimulation in Mg^{2+}-free solutions and it is associated with massive calcium influx through NMDA-type receptors (Nakano *et al*, 2010). Diamond et al (2007) suggested that complex interactions between LTP and LTD processes in the hippocampus contribute to the storage of emotional memories and stress-induced amnesia; whether Mg^{2+} can modulate effects of stress on LTP in the hippocampus, amygdala and prefrontal cortex remains to be established. Magnesium-L-threonate administration in rats increases the density of synaptophysin-/synaptobrevin-positive puncta in DG and CA1 subregions of the hippocampus, which contributes to improvement of cognitive functions (learning abilities, working memory, short- and long-term memory in rats) (Slutsky *et al*, 2010). Mg^{2+} also acts synergistically with the NMDA antagonist memantine on hippocampal LTP, and there are data that indicate that Mg^{2+} leads to an improvement of cognitive function in dementia (Danysz *et al*, 2000; Frankiewicz *et al*, 1996).

Mg^{2+} is also involved in long-term memory formation through NE activated pathways. Saturation by free Mg^{2+} increases the affinity of adenylate cyclase for adrenaline and excessive stress affects the stability of this enzyme and produces loss of activity. Moreover, by activating adenylate cyclase in fat tissues, stress increases the production of chelating metabolites like ATP^{4-} or $citrate^{-}$, which reduce the level of free Mg^{2+} (Bennun, 2010).

Magnesium during the developmental period

A number of studies have now suggested that magnesium and stress may play an important regulatory role in the early developmental period. For example, in rhesus monkeys, stressful pregnancy reduced the hippocampal volume and impaired neurogenesis in the dentate gyrus of the offspring (Bac *et al*, 1995; Coe *et al*, 2003). An acoustic startle protocol applied during the 24-weeks gestation time was associated with increased levels of cortisol and reduced exploration behavior of the 3-years-old descendants. Another study examining the newborn's response to moderate surgical trauma showed that neonates are more susceptible to stress than infants (Okur *et al*, 1995). Although there were not significant differences between infants and neonates regarding the elevations of cortisol and growth hormones after surgical stress, Mg^{2+} concentrations declined more in newborns compared to the other group.

Both experimental and clinical data also suggest that fetal Mg^{2+} depletion (as a consequence of maternal deficiency) and stress during critical developmental periods are involved in the pathogeny of sudden infant death syndrome (Caddell, 2001; Durlach *et al*, 2004). Durlach (2002) also emphasize the importance of chrono-pathological stress due to primary hypofunction of the biological clock and the pineal dysfunction. Among the exogenous stressors that may lead to this syndrome, it is worth mentioning parental smoking, maternal alcoholism, environmental pollutants, bottle feeding, sleeping position, bedding, and wrapping and ambient temperature (Durlach *et al*, 2004).

In fetal guinea pig brain, maternal $MgSO_4$ administration during hypoxic stress exhibits neuroprotective effects by ameliorating nuclear membrane peroxidation and nuclear DNA fragmentation (Maulik *et al*, 2001). Additionally, maternal $MgSO_4$ treatment before anticipated early preterm birth has proven to reduce the risk of cerebral palsy in surviving infants (Marlow, 2009). Given the "anti-stress" properties of Mg^{2+}, this discovery once more emphasizes the importance of maternal Mg^{2+} status on the neural, hormonal and behavioral outcome of the progenitors.

Finally, children hospitalized for respiratory pathology and who received sporadic parental visits exhibited lower serum Mg^{2+} level and increased excretion of this cation compared to children who received constant parental support (Bednarek *et al*, 2004). There are also data that suggest Mg^{2+} deficiency in children brought up in stressful orphanage conditions may lead to a lower intelligence quotient (Manrique *et al*, 2010; Papadopol *et al*, 2001).

Magnesium and self-damaging behavior

In order to cope better with stress, individuals exhibit variable behavioral responses ranging from improving lifestyle to self-damage (e.g., smoking, drinking, overeating) or risk-taking. It is well known that susceptibility to stress among the population is diverse and there is a minority who exhibit an extreme response to stress in respect to intensity, features and extension of time. The myriad of individual differences regarding stress responses are mainly a result of genetic background, developmental processes (both prenatal and postnatal), and lifetime experiences (McEwen, 2007).

Individuals exhibiting self-damaging behavior are more likely to present hypomagnesemia as alcohol itself depletes the organism of Mg^{2+} (Romani, 2008). Depletion of Mg^{2+} induced in rat astrocytes by alcohol produces disturbances in cytoplasmic and mitochondrial bioenergetic pathways leading to Ca^{2+} overload, ischemia and stroke (Altura and Altura 1994). Eating disorders are also commonly linked to hypomagnesemia that may or may not be associated with hypokalemia, hypocalcemia and hypophosphatemia (Laird Birmingham 2010; Touyz, 2004). This is particularly concerning where the normal western diet is already low in magnesium. For example, in most countries, the magnesium RDA for women varies from 240 to 400mg/day and for adult men varies from 310 to 420mg/day. However, Mg^{2+} intake in 70% of the western population is less than 400 mg Mg^{2+} per day, and for approximately 20% of the population this cation intake is less than one-half of the recommended dose (Eby and Eby, 2006). Persons with inadequate nutrition that often accompanies chronic stressful lifestyle need Mg^{2+} supplementation as increased intake of carbohydrates, fats, exaggerated consumption of coffee and sodas reduce the Mg^{2+} levels in the organism (Seelig, 1994; Nishimuta, 2007).

Mg^{2+} administration can provide beneficial effects by decreasing the susceptibility of stress-induced drug relapse. Mg^{2+} decreases activity of central glutamatergic synapses, especially those involved in the reward system that is activated by stress (Gilman, 2007; Nechifor, 2008), and displays a modulatory effect for opioid receptor binding (Turner and Vink, 2007). Furthermore, Mg^{2+} administration indirectly influences hippocampal neurogenesis through its effect upon corticosteroid hormones, and in this way may decrease the drug-seeking behavior in drug-addicted persons (Noonan *et al*, 2010).

Magnesium and substance P

Several authors have recently suggested that many of the consequences Mg^{2+} deficiency in stress may be explained by the release of substance P. Substance P is a neuropeptide that preferably activates tachykinin NK1 receptors. It is considered to be involved both in early (4–7 days) and late (3 weeks) phases of the systemic response to Mg^{2+} deficiency. In the early days after the onset of a Mg^{2+}-restricted diet, low concentrations of this cation diminishes the Mg^{2+}-gated blockade of NMDA receptor channels, which leads to the release of substance P and calcitonin gene-related peptide from the sensory C fibres. The increased circulating levels of these neuropeptides initiate an important "neurogenic inflammation" characterized by raised levels of inflammatory cells, inflammatory cytokines and augmented production of reactive oxygen and nitrogen species (Kramer *et al*, 2009; Tejero-Taldo *et al*, 2006). Brain microinjection of substance P activates stress-processing pathways and induces defensive respiratory, cardiovascular, gastrointestinal and psychological changes, as well as stimulating corticosterone secretion by the adrenal glands (Rupniak 2005). Furthermore, in a model of chronic psychosocial stress in shrews, the NK1 receptor antagonist SLV-323 alleviated dentate cytogenesis and diminished the decrease of hippocampal volume induced by stress (Czeh *et al*, 2005). Thus, substance P is now widely considered to be involved in the clinical expression of stress.

Conclusion

Mg^{2+} still represents an emerging research field despite being entered into medicine in the XVIIth century as a constituent of Epsom salts (Durlach 2007). Although much has been discovered, many aspects of magnesium still remain unclear and await discovery. Undoubtedly, the future will uncover new Mg^{2+} compounds of medicinal value, will further characterize Mg^{2+} as a common factor in more stress-related pathologies, and will result in the discovery of more Mg^{2+} transporters, while better methods for the determination of intracellular levels of the cation will pave the way for an improvement in simple diagnosis of Mg^{2+} deficiency.

Acknowledgements
Magdalena Cuciureanu was a recipient of a 2010 Australian Go8 European Fellowship.

References

Aarts MM, Tymianski M (2005) TRPM7 and ischemic CNS injury. *Neuroscientist* 11:116-23.

Abaamrane L, Raffin F, Gal M, Avan P, Sendowski I (2009) Long-term administration of magnesium after acoustic trauma caused by gunshot noise in guinea pigs. *Heart Res* 247:137-45.

Ablin JN, Buskila D (2010) Emerging therapies for fibromyalgia: an update. *Expert Opin Emerging Drugs* 15:521-33.

Akashi YJ, Goldstein DS, Barbaro G, Ueyama T (2008) Takotsubo cardiomyopathy: a new form of acute, reversible heart failure. *Circulation* 118:2754-62.

Ali BH, Silsby JL, el Halawani ME (1987) The effect of magnesium aspartate, xylazine and morphine on the immobilization-induced increase in the levels of prolactin in turkey plasma. *J Vet Pharmacol Ther* 10:119-26.

Altura BM, Altura BT (1994) Role of magnesium and calcium in alcohol-induced hypertension and strokes as probed by in vivo television microscopy, digital image microscopy, optical spectroscopy, 31P-NMR, spectroscopy and a unique magnesium ion-selective electrode. *Alcohol Clin Exp Res* 18:1057-68.

Amyard N, Leyris A, Monier C, Frances H, Boulu RG, Henrotte JG (1995) Brain catecholamines, serotonin and their metabolites in mice selected for low (MGL) and high (MGH) blood magnesium levels. *Magnes Res* 8:5-9.

Anastassopoulou J, Theophanides T (2002) Magnesium-DNA interactions and the possible relation of magnesium to carcinogenesis. Irradiation and free radicals. *Crit Rev Oncol Hematol* 42:79-91.

Angeli A, Minetto M, Dovio A, Paccotti P (2004) The overtraining syndrome in athletes: a stress-related disorder. *J Endocrinol Invest* 27:603-12.

Anghileri LJ (2009) Magnesium, calcium and cancer. *Magnes Res* 22:247-55.

Ashton WB, James MF, Janicki P, Uys PC (1991) Attenuation of the pressor response to tracheal intubation by magnesium sulphate with and without alfentanil in hypertensive proteinuric patients undergoing caesarean section. *Brit J Anaes* 67:741-7.

Bac P, Pages N, Herrenknecht C, Teste JF (1995) Inhibition of mouse-killing behaviour in magnesium-deficient rats: effect of pharmacological doses of magnesium pidolate, magnesium aspartate, magnesium lactate, magnesium gluconate and magnesium chloride. *Magnes Res* 8:37-45.

Bac P, Maurois P, Dupont C, Pages N, Stables JP, Gressens P, Evrard P, Vamecq J (1998) Magnesium deficiency-dependent audiogenic seizures (MDDASs) in adult mice: a nutritional model for discriminatory screening of anticonvulsant drugs and original assessment of neuroprotection properties. *J Neurosci* 18:4363-73.

Baldi E, Bucherelli C (2005) The inverted "u-shaped" dose-effect relationships in learning and memory: modulation of arousal and consolidation. *Nonlinearity Biol Toxicol Med* 3:9-21

Barnett FI, Durrheim DN, Speare R, Muller R (2005) Management of Irukandji syndrome in northern Australia. *Rural Remote Health* 5:369.

Bednarczyk P, Dolowy K, Szewczyk A (2005) Matrix Mg2+ regulates mitochondrial ATP-dependent potassium channel from heart. *FEBS Lett* 579:1625-32.

Bednarek A, Pasternak K, Sztanke M, Boguszewska A (2004) Influence of admission procedure and hospitalization form on the value of magnesium concentration in serum, blood cells and urine in children hospitalizated due to pneumonia or obstructive bronchiolitis. *Magnes Res* 17:94-101.

Bennun A (2010) Characterization of the norepinephrine-activation of adenylate cyclase suggests a role in memory affirmation pathways Overexposure to epinephrine inactivates adenylate cyclase, a causal pathway for stress-pathologies. *Bio Systems* 100:87-93.

Billard JM (2006) Ageing, hippocampal synaptic activity and magnesium. *Magnes Res* 19:199-215.

Billyard AJ, Eggett DL, Franz KB (2006) Dietary magnesium deficiency decreases plasma melatonin in rats. *Magnes Res* 19:157-61.

Bobkowski W, Nowak A, Durlach J (2005) The importance of magnesium status in the pathophysiology of mitral valve prolapse. *Magnes Res* 18:35-52.

Brown RF, Tennant CC, Sharrock M, Hodgkinson S, Dunn SM, Pollard JD (2006a) Relationship between stress and relapse in multiple sclerosis: Part I. Important features. *Mult Scler* 12:453-64.

Brown RF, Tennant CC, Sharrock M, Hodgkinson S, Dunn SM, Pollard JD (2006b) Relationship between stress and relapse in multiple sclerosis: Part II. Direct and indirect relationships. *Mult Scler* 12:465-75.

Cabaniols C, Giorgi R, Chinot O, Ferahta N, Spinelli V, Alla P, Barrie M, Lehucher-Michel MP (2010) Links between private habits, psychological stress and brain cancer: a case-control pilot study in France. *J Neurooncol* [Epub ahead of print].

Caddell J, Kupiecki R, Proxmire DL, Satoh P, Hutchinson B (1986) Plasma catecholamines in acute magnesium deficiency in weanling rats. *J Nutr* 116:1896-901

Caddell JL (2001) A triple-risk model for the sudden infant death syndrome (SIDS) and the apparent life-threatening episode (ALTE): the stressed magnesium deficient weanling rat. *Magnes Res* 14:227-38.

Cameron OG (2007) Pharmacological Treatments of Stress, In: *Encyclopedia of Stress* (Fink G, ed.) 2nd Edn, Oxford: Academic Press, p113-8.

Carrasco GA, Van de Kar LD (2003) Neuroendocrine pharmacology of stress. *Eur J Pharmacol* 463:235-72.

Ceremuzynski L, Herbaczynska-Cedro K, Broniszewska-Ardelt B, Nauman J, Nauman A, Wozniewicz B, Lawecki J (1978) Evidence for the detrimental effect of adrenaline infused to healthy dogs in doses imitating spontaneous secretion after coronary occlusion. *Cardiovasc Res* 12:179-89.

Cernak I, Savic V, Kotur J, Prokic V, Kuljic B, Grbovic D, Veljovic M (2000) Alterations in magnesium and oxidative status during chronic emotional stress. *Magnes Res* 13:29-36.

Chollet D, Franken P, Raffin Y, Henrotte JG, Widmer J, Malafosse A, Tafti M (2001) Magnesium involvement in sleep: genetic and nutritional models. *Behav Genet* 31:413-25.

Classen HG (1981) [Effect of the current magnesium status on the development of stress ulcers and myocardial necroses]. *Fortschr Med* 99:1303-6.

Coe CL, Kramer M, Czeh B, Gould E, Reeves AJ, Kirschbaum C, Fuchs E (2003) Prenatal stress diminishes neurogenesis in the dentate gyrus of juvenile rhesus monkeys. *Biol Psychiatry* 54:1025-34.

Corkeron M, Pereira P, Makrocanis C (2004) Early experience with magnesium administration in Irukandji syndrome. *Anaesth Intensive Care* 32:666-9.

Couzy F, Lafargue P, Guezennec CY (1990) Zinc metabolism in the athlete: influence of training, nutrition and other factors. *Int J Sports Med* 11:263-6

Cox IM, Campbell MJ, Dowson D (1991) Red blood cell magnesium and chronic fatigue syndrome. *Lancet* 337:757-60.

Cratty MS, Birkle DL (1999) N-methyl-D-aspartate (NMDA)-mediated corticotropin-releasing factor (CRF) release in cultured rat amygdala neurons. *Peptides* 20:93-100.

Cundy T GA, Reid I.R., (2008) Calcium, phosphate and magnesium. In: *Clinical biochemistry: Metabolic and Clinical Aspects* (De William J and Marshall SKB, eds.) 2nd edn, Edinburgh: Churchill Livingstone Elsevier.

Czeh B, Pudovkina O, van der Hart MG, Simon M, Heilbronner U, Michaelis T, Watanabe T, Frahm J, Fuchs E (2005) Examining SLV-323, a novel NK1 receptor antagonist, in a chronic psychosocial stress model for depression. *Psychopharmacol (Berl)* 180:548-57.

Dabbagh A, Elyasi H, Razavi SS, Fathi M, Rajaei S (2009) Intravenous magnesium sulfate for post-operative pain in patients undergoing lower limb orthopedic surgery. *Acta Anaesthesiol Scand* 53:1088-91.

Dabbagh OC, Aldawood AS, Arabi YM, Lone NA, Brits R, Pillay M (2006) Magnesium supplementation and the potential association with mortality rates among critically ill non-cardiac patients. *Saudi Med J* 27:821-5.

Dabrowski W, Rzecki Z, Sztanke M, Visconti J, Wacinski P, Pasternak K (2008) The efficiency of magnesium supplementation in patients undergoing cardiopulmonary bypass: changes in serum magnesium concentrations and atrial fibrillation episodes. *Magnes Res* 21:205-17.

Danysz W, Parsons CG, Mobius HJ, Stoffler A, Quack G (2000) Neuroprotective and symptomatological action of memantine relevant for Alzheimer's disease--a unified glutamatergic hypothesis on the mechanism of action. *Neurotox Res* 2:85-97.

Davis EM, Packard KA, Hilleman DE (2010) Pharmacologic prophylaxis of postoperative atrial fibrillation in patients undergoing cardiac surgery: beyond beta-blockers. *Pharmacotherapy* 30:749, 274e-318e.

Dayas CV, Xu Y, Buller KM, Day TA (2000) Effects of chronic oestrogen replacement on stress-induced activation of hypothalamic-pituitary-adrenal axis control pathways. *J Neuroendocrinol* 12:784-94.

De Souza EB, Grigoriadis DE, Webster EL (1991) Role of brain, pituitary and spleen corticotropin-releasing factor receptors in the stress response. *Methods Achiev Exp Pathol* 14:23-44.

De Souza EB (1995) Corticotropin-releasing factor receptors: physiology, pharmacology, biochemistry and role in central nervous system and immune disorders. *Psychoneuroendocrinol* 20:789-819.

Delhumeau A, Granry JC, Cottineau C, Bukowski JG, Corbeau JJ, Moreau X (1995) [Comparison of vascular effects of magnesium sulfate and nicardipine during extracorporeal circulation]. *Annales Francaises d'anesthesie et de Reanimation* 14:149-53.

Depoortere H, Francon D, Llopis J (1993) Effects of a magnesium-deficient diet on sleep organization in rats. *Neuropsychobiol* 27:237-45.

Diamond DM, Campbell AM, Park CR, Halonen J, Zoladz PR (2007) The temporal dynamics model of emotional memory processing: a synthesis on the neurobiological basis of stress-induced amnesia, flashbulb and traumatic memories, and the Yerkes-Dodson law. *Neural Plast* 2007:60803.

Dong JF, Cruz MA, Aboulfatova K, Martin C, Choi H, Bergeron AL, Martini SR, Kroll MH, Kent TA (2008) Magnesium maintains endothelial integrity, up-regulates proteolysis of ultra-large von Willebrand factor, and reduces platelet aggregation under flow conditions. *Thromb Haemost* 99:586-93.

Dorman BH, Sade RM, Burnette JS, Wiles HB, Pinosky ML, Reeves ST, Bond BR, Spinale FG (2000) Magnesium supplementation in the prevention of arrhythmias in pediatric patients undergoing surgery for congenital heart defects. *Amer Heart J* 139:522-8.

Durlach J, Durlach V, Bac P, Rayssiguier Y, Bara M, Guiet-Bara A (1993) Magnesium and ageing. II. Clinical data: aetiological mechanisms and pathophysiological consequences of magnesium deficit in the elderly. *Magnes Res* 6:379-94.

Durlach J, Bac P, Durlach V, Bara M, Guiet-Bara A (1997) Neurotic, neuromuscular and autonomic nervous form of magnesium imbalance. *Magnes Res* 10:169-95.

Durlach J, Pages N, Bac P, Bara M, Guiet-Bara A, Agrapart C (2002) Chronopathological forms of magnesium depletion with hypofunction or with hyperfunction of the biological clock. *Magnes Res* 15:263-8.

Durlach J, Pages N, Bac P, Bara M, Guiet-Bara A (2004) New data on the importance of gestational Mg deficiency. *Magnes Res* 17:116-25.

Durlach J, Pages N, Bac P, Bara M, Guiet-Bara A (2005) Headache due to photosensitive magnesium depletion. *Magnes Res* 18:109-22

Durlach J (2007) Overview of magnesium research: history and current trends. In: *New Perspectives in Magnesium Research: Nutrition and Health* (Nishizawa Y, Mori H, Durlach J, eds.) London: Springer-Verlag, p3-10.

Eby GA, Eby KL (2006) Rapid recovery from major depression using magnesium treatment. *Med Hypotheses* 67:362-70.

Ehrenberger K, Felix D (1995) Receptor pharmacological models for inner ear therapies with emphasis on glutamate receptors: a survey. *Acta Otolaryngol* 115:236-40.

Esch T, Stefano GB, Fricchione GL, Benson H (2002a) Stress-related diseases -- a potential role for nitric oxide. *Med Sci Monit* 8:RA103-18.

Esch T, Stefano GB, Fricchione GL, Benson H (2002b) The role of stress in neurodegenerative diseases and mental disorders. *Neuro Endocrinol Lett* 23:199-208.

Esen F, Erdem T, Aktan D, Orhan M, Kaya M, Eraksoy H, Cakar N, Telci L (2005) Effect of magnesium sulfate administration on blood-brain barrier in a rat model of intraperitoneal sepsis: a randomized controlled experimental study. *Crit Care* 9:R18-23.

Feillet-Coudray C, Coudray C, Wolf FI, Henrotte JG, Rayssiguier Y, Mazur A (2004) Magnesium metabolism in mice selected for high and low erythrocyte magnesium levels. *Metabolism* 53:660-5.

Frankiewicz T, Potier B, Bashir ZI, Collingridge GL, Parsons CG (1996) Effects of memantine and MK-801 on NMDA-induced currents in cultured neurones and on synaptic transmission and LTP in area CA1 of rat hippocampal slices. *Br J Pharmacol* 117:689-97.

Franz KB (2004) A functional biological marker is needed for diagnosing magnesium deficiency. *J Amer Coll Nutr* 23:738S-41S.

Fromm L, Heath DL, Vink R, Nimmo AJ (2004) Magnesium attenuates post-traumatic depression/anxiety following diffuse traumatic brain injury in rats. *J Amer Coll Nutr* 23:529S-33S.

Fujino K, Yoshitake T, Inoue O, Ibii N, Kehr J, Ishida J, Nohta H, Yamaguchi M (2002) Increased serotonin release in mice frontal cortex and hippocampus induced by acute physiological stressors. *Neurosci Lett* 320:91-5.

Funada M, Hara C (2001) Differential effects of psychological stress on activation of the 5-hydroxytryptamine- and dopamine-containing neurons in the brain of freely moving rats. *Brain Res* 901:247-51.

Furukawa Y, Kasai N, Torimitsu K (2009) Effect of Mg2+ on neural activity of rat cortical and hippocampal neurons in vitro. *Magnes Res* 22:174S-81S

Galland L (1991) Magnesium, stress and neuropsychiatric disorders. *Magnesium Trace Elements* 10:287-301.

Garalejic E, Bojovic-Jovic D, Damjanovic A, Arsic B, Pantic I, Turjacanin-Pantelic D, Perovic M (2010) Hamilton anxiety scale (HAMA) in infertile women with endometriosis and its correlation with magnesium levels in peritoneal fluid. *Psychiatria Danubina* 22:64-7.

Garcia-Lopez R, Perea-Milla E, Garcia CR, Rivas-Ruiz F, Romero-Gonzalez J, Moreno JL, Faus V, Aguas Gdel C, Diaz JC (2009) New therapeutic approach to Tourette Syndrome in children based on a randomized placebo-controlled double-blind phase IV study of the effectiveness and safety of magnesium and vitamin B6. *Trials* 10:16.

Garcy AM, Marotta SF (1978) Effects of cerebroventricular perfusion with monovalent and divalent cations on plasma cortisol of conscious cats. *Neuroendocrinol* 26:32-40.

Gilman S (2007) *Neurobiology of Disease*, 1st edn, Elsevier Academic Press, New York.

Gimpl G, Reitz J, Brauer S, Trossen C (2008) Oxytocin receptors: ligand binding, signalling and cholesterol dependence. *Prog Brain Res* 170:193-204.

Golf SW, Bender S, Gruttner J (1998) On the significance of magnesium in extreme physical stress. *Cardiovas Drugs Therapy* 12 Suppl 2:197-202.

Grimaldi BL (2002) The central role of magnesium deficiency in Tourette's syndrome: causal relationships between magnesium deficiency, altered biochemical pathways and symptoms relating to Tourette's syndrome and several reported comorbid conditions. *Med Hypotheses* 58:47-60.

Gutierrez R, Armand V, Schuchmann S, Heinemann U (1999) Epileptiform activity induced by low Mg2+ in cultured rat hippocampal slices. *Brain Research* 815:294-303.

Held K, Antonijevic IA, Kunzel H, Uhr M, Wetter TC, Golly IC, Steiger A, Murck H (2002) Oral Mg(2+) supplementation reverses age-related neuroendocrine and sleep EEG changes in humans. *Pharmacopsychiatry* 35:135-43.

Henrotte JG, Levy-Leboyer C (1985) [Is type A behavior modulated by genetic factors regulating magnesium and zinc metabolism? Working hypotheses and preliminary results]. *Magnesium* 4:295-302.

Henrotte JG, Plouin PF, Levy-Leboyer C, Moser G, Sidoroff-Girault N, Franck G, Santarromana M, Pineau M (1985) Blood and urinary magnesium, zinc, calcium, free fatty acids, and catecholamines in type A and type B subjects. *J Amer Coll Nutr* 4:165-72.

Henrotte JG, Pla M, Dausset J (1990) HLA- and H-2-associated variations of intra- and extracellular magnesium content. *Proc Natl Acad Sci USA*:1894-8.

Henrotte JG, Franck G, Santarromana M, Frances H, Mouton D, Motta R (1997) Mice selected for low and high blood magnesium levels: a new model for stress studies. *Physiol Behav* 61:653-8.

Hirvikoski T, Lindholm T, Nordenstrom A, Nordstrom AL, Lajic S (2009) High self-perceived stress and many stressors, but normal diurnal cortisol rhythm, in adults with ADHD (attention-deficit/hyperactivity disorder). *Horm Behav* 55:418-24.

Hughes JP, Staton PC, Wilkinson MG, Strijbos PJ, Skaper SD, Arthur JS, Reith AD (2003) Mitogen and stress response kinase-1 (MSK1) mediates excitotoxic induced death of hippocampal neurones. *J Neurochem* 86:25-32.

Ising H, Braun C (2000) Acute and chronic endocrine effects of noise: Review of the research conducted at the Institute for Water, Soil and Air Hygiene. *Noise Health* 2:7-24.

James MF (2009) Magnesium: an emerging drug in anaesthesia. *Brit J Anaesth* 103:465-7.

Jee D, Lee D, Yun S, Lee C (2009) Magnesium sulphate attenuates arterial pressure increase during laparoscopic cholecystectomy. *Brit J Anaesth* 103:484-9.

Jorgensen HS (2007) Studies on the neuroendocrine role of serotonin. *Dan Med Bull* 54:266-88.

Jung KI, Ock SM, Chung JH, Song CH (2010) Associations of serum Ca and Mg levels with mental health in adult women without psychiatric disorders. *Biol Trace Element Research* 133:153-61.

Kantorovich V, Eisenhofer G, Pacak K (2008) Pheochromocytoma: an endocrine stress mimicking disorder. *Annals NY Acad Sci* 1148:462-8.

Karst H, Joels M (2003) Effect of chronic stress on synaptic currents in rat hippocampal dentate gyrus neurons. *J Neurophysiol* 89:625-33.

Keir ST, Swartz JJ, Friedman HS (2007) Stress and long-term survivors of brain cancer. *Support Care Cancer* 15:1423-8

Kimura (2007) Overview of magnesium nutrition. In: *New Perspectives in Magnesium Research:Nutrition and Health* (Nishizawa Y, Mori H, Durlach J, eds.) 1st edn, London: Springer-Verlag, p69-93.

Ko SH, Lim HR, Kim DC, Han YJ, Choe H, Song HS (2001) Magnesium sulfate does not reduce postoperative analgesic requirements. *Anesthesiol* 95:640-6.

Kolber BJ, Roberts MS, Howell MP, Wozniak DF, Sands MS, Muglia LJ (2008) Central amygdala glucocorticoid receptor action promotes fear-associated CRH activation and conditioning. *Proc Natl Acad Sci USA* 105:12004-9.

Kozielec T, Starobrat-Hermelin B (1997) Assessment of magnesium levels in children with attention deficit hyperactivity disorder (ADHD). *Magnes Res* 10:143-8.

Kramer JH, Spurney C, Iantorno M, Tziros C, Mak IT, Tejero-Taldo MI, Chmielinska JJ, Komarov AM, Weglicki WB (2009) Neurogenic inflammation and cardiac dysfunction due to hypomagnesemia. *Am J Med Sci* 338:22-7.

Kurian GA, Paddikkala J (2010) N-acetylcysteine and magnesium improve biochemical abnormalities associated with myocardial ischaemic reperfusion in South Indian patients undergoing coronary artery bypass grafting: a comparative analysis. *Singapore Med J* 51:381-8.

Kuzmiski JB, Marty V, Baimoukhametova DV, Bains JS (2010) Stress-induced priming of glutamate synapses unmasks associative short-term plasticity. *Nat Neurosci* 13:1257-64.

Labuschagne I, Phan KL, Wood A, Angstadt M, Chua P, Heinrichs M, Stout JC, Nathan PJ (2010) Oxytocin attenuates amygdala reactivity to fear in generalized social anxiety disorder. *Neuropsychopharmacol* 35:2403-13.

Laird Birmingham CJ (2010) Complications of nutritional therapy. In: *Medical Management of Eating Disorders*): Cambridge: University Press, 59-72.

Leon-Carrion J, Atutxa AM, Mangas MA, Soto-Moreno A, Pumar A, Leon-Justel A, Martin-Rodriguez JF, Venegas E, Dominguez-Morales MR, Leal-Cerro A (2009) A clinical profile of memory impairment in humans due to endogenous glucocorticoid excess. *Clin Endocrinol (Oxf)* 70:192-200.

Lupien SJ, Maheu FS (eds) (2007) *Memory and Stress*. Academic Press: Oxford.

Lyon AR, Rees PS, Prasad S, Poole-Wilson PA, Harding SE (2008) Stress (Takotsubo) cardiomyopathy--a novel pathophysiological hypothesis to explain catecholamine-induced acute myocardial stunning. *Nat Clin Pract Cardiovasc Med* 5:22-9.

Lysakowski C, Dumont L, Czarnetzki C, Tramer MR (2007) Magnesium as an adjuvant to postoperative analgesia: a systematic review of randomized trials. *Anesthes Analges* 104:1532-9.

Mack WJ, Kellner CP, Sahlein DH, Ducruet AF, Kim GH, Mocco J, Zurica J, Komotar RJ, Haque R, Sciacca R, Quest DO, Solomon RA, Connolly ES, Heyer EJ (2009) Intraoperative magnesium infusion during carotid endarterectomy: a double-blind placebo-controlled trial. *J Neurosurg* 110:961-7

Magalhaes AC, Holmes KD, Dale LB, Comps-Agrar L, Lee D, Yadav PN, Drysdale L, Poulter MO, Roth BL, Pin JP, Anisman H, Ferguson SS (2010) CRF receptor 1 regulates anxiety behavior via sensitization of 5-HT2 receptor signaling. *Nat Neurosci* 13:622-9.

Maier JA, Nasulewicz-Goldeman A, Simonacci M, Boninsegna A, Mazur A, Wolf FI (2007) Insights into the mechanisms involved in magnesium-dependent inhibition of primary tumor growth. *Nutr Cancer* 59:192-8.

Manrique AM, Arroyo M, Lin Y, El Khoudary SR, Colvin E, Lichtenstein S, Chrysostomou C, Orr R, Jooste E, Davis P, Wearden P, Morell V, Munoz R (2010) Magnesium supplementation during cardiopulmonary bypass to prevent junctional ectopic tachycardia after pediatric cardiac surgery: a randomized controlled study. *J Thorac Cardiovasc Surg* 139:162-9 e2.

Manuel y Keenoy B, Moorkens G, Vertommen J, Noe M, Neve J, De Leeuw I (2000) Magnesium status and parameters of the oxidant-antioxidant balance in patients with chronic fatigue: effects of supplementation with magnesium. *J Amer Coll Nutr* 19:374-82.

Marlow N (2009) Review: antenatal magnesium sulphate prevents cerebral palsy in preterm infants. *Evid Based Med* 14:141.

Marois G, Henrotte JG, Elie C, Franck G (1985) [Changes in plasma prolactin and magnesium in male rats treated with thioproperazine and/or bromocriptine]. *Ann Endocrinol (Paris)* 46:399-405.

Matsui T (2007) Significance of Magnesium in Animals (Yoshiki Nishizawa, Mori H, Durlach J, eds.) London: Springer-Verlag.

Matthews KA (1982) Psychological perspectives on the type A behavior pattern. *Psychol Bull* 91:293-323.

Maulik D, Qayyum I, Powell SR, Karantza M, Mishra OP, Delivoria-Papadopoulos M (2001) Post-hypoxic magnesium decreases nuclear oxidative damage in the fetal guinea pig brain. *Brain research* 890:130-6.

McEwen BS (2007) Stress, Definitions and Concepts of. In: *Encyclopedia of Stress* (Fink, ed.) 2nd ed., vol. 3: Oxford: Academic Press, 653.

McEwen BS (2008a) Central effects of stress hormones in health and disease: Understanding the protective and damaging effects of stress and stress mediators. *Eur J Pharmacol* 583:174-85.

McEwen W (2008b) Allostasis and Allostatic Load. In: *Encyclopedia of Stress* (Fink G, ed.) 2nd ed., vol. I: Oxford: Academic Press, 135-41.

McGaugh JL, Roozendaal B (2002) Role of adrenal stress hormones in forming lasting memories in the brain. *Curr Opin Neurobiol* 12:205-10.

Mizoguchi K, Shoji H, Ikeda R, Tanaka Y, Tabira T (2008) Persistent depressive state after chronic stress in rats is accompanied by HPA axis dysregulation and reduced prefrontal dopaminergic neurotransmission. *Pharmacol Biochem Behav* 91:170-5.

Motta R, Louis JP, Frank G, Henrotte JG (1998) Unexpected association between reproductive longevity and blood magnesium levels in a new model of selected mouse strains. *Growth Dev Aging* 62:37-45.

Mousain-Bosc M, Roche M, Polge A, Pradal-Prat D, Rapin J, Bali JP (2006) Improvement of neurobehavioral disorders in children supplemented with magnesium-vitamin B6. I. Attention deficit hyperactivity disorders. *Magnes Res* 19:46-52.

Muir KW (2002) Magnesium in stroke treatment. *Postgrad Med J* 78:641-5.

Muneyyirci-Delale O, Nacharaju VL, Dalloul M, Altura BM, Altura BT (1999) Serum ionized magnesium and calcium in women after menopause: inverse relation of estrogen with ionized magnesium. *Fertil Steril* 71:869-72

Murck H (2002) Magnesium and affective disorders. *Nutr Neurosci* 5:375-89

Nakano T, Doi T, Yoshimoto J, Doya K (2010) A kinetic model of dopamine- and calcium-dependent striatal synaptic plasticity. *PLoS Comput Biol* 6:e1000670.

Nechifor M (2008) Magnesium in drug dependences. *Magnes Res* 21:5-15.

Neumann ID, Veenema AH, Beiderbeck DI (2010) Aggression and anxiety: social context and neurobiological links. *Front Behav Neurosci* 4:12.

Neylan (1998) Hans Selye and the Field of Stress Research. *J Neuropsychiatry Clin Neurosci* 10:230-1.

Nickson CP, Waugh EB, Jacups SP, Currie BJ (2009) Irukandji syndrome case series from Australia's Tropical Northern Territory. *Ann Emerg Med* 54:395-403.

Nielsen FH, Lukaski HC (2006) Update on the relationship between magnesium and exercise. *Magnes Res* 19:180-9.

Nishimuta M KN, Morikuni E, Matsuzaki N, Yoshioka YH, Yamada H, Kitajima H, Takeyama H (2007) Magnesium Requirement and Affecting Factors (Nishizawa Y, Mori H, Durlach J, eds.) London: Springer-Verlag, p94-103.

Nishizawa Y, Morii H, Durlach J (2007) New Perspectives in Magnesium Research, Nutrition and Health (Nishizawa Y, Mori H, Durlach J, eds.) London: Springer-Verlag.

Noonan MA, Bulin SE, Fuller DC, Eisch AJ (2010) Reduction of adult hippocampal neurogenesis confers vulnerability in an animal model of cocaine addiction. *J Neurosci* 30:304-15.

Numata T, Shimizu T, Okada Y (2007) Direct mechano-stress sensitivity of TRPM7 channel. *Cell Physiol Biochem* 19:1-8.

Okur H, Kucukaydin M, Ustdal KM (1995) The endocrine and metabolic response to surgical stress in the neonate. *J Pediatr Surg* 30:626-5.

Omiya K, Akashi YJ, Yoneyama K, Osada N, Tanabe K, Miyake F (2009) Heart-rate response to sympathetic nervous stimulation, exercise, and magnesium concentration in various sleep conditions. *Int J Sport Nutr Exercise Metabol* 19:127-35.

Oppelt WW, MacIntyre I, Rall DP (1963) Magnesium exchange between blood and cerebrospinal fluid. *Am J Physiol* 205:959-62.

Papadopol V, Tuchendria E, Palamaru I (2001) Magnesium and some psychological features in two groups of pupils (magnesium and psychic features). *Magnes Res* 14:27-32

Papathanassoglou ED, Giannakopoulou M, Mpouzika M, Bozas E, Karabinis A (2010) Potential effects of stress in critical illness through the role of stress neuropeptides. *Nurs Crit Care* 15:204-16.

Peeters E, Neyt A, Beckers F, De Smet S, Aubert AE, Geers R (2005) Influence of supplemental magnesium, tryptophan, vitamin C, and vitamin E on stress responses of pigs to vibration. *J Animal Sci* 83:1568-80.

Penner R, Fleig A (2007) The Mg2+ and Mg(2+)-nucleotide-regulated channel-kinase TRPM7. *Handb Exp Pharmacol*:313-28.

Perrin MH, Haas Y, Rivier JE, Vale WW (1986) Corticotropin-releasing factor binding to the anterior pituitary receptor is modulated by divalent cations and guanyl nucleotides. *Endocrinol*118:1171-9.

Pokan R, Hofmann P, von Duvillard SP, Smekal G, Wonisch M, Lettner K, Schmid P, Shechter M, Silver B,

Bachl N (2006) Oral magnesium therapy, exercise heart rate, exercise tolerance, and myocardial function in coronary artery disease patients. *Brit J Sports Med* 40:773-8.

Polderman KH, van Zanten AR, Girbes AR (2003) The importance of magnesium in critically ill patients: a role in mitigating neurological injury and in the prevention of vasospasms. *Intensive Care Med* 29:1202-3.

Puri GD, Marudhachalam KS, Chari P, Suri RK (1998) The effect of magnesium sulphate on hemodynamics and its efficacy in attenuating the response to endotracheal intubation in patients with coronary artery disease. *Anesthes Analges* 87:808-11.

Quick S (1994) Walter Bradford Cannon: Pioneer of stress research. *Int J Stress Management* I:141-3

Rayssiguier Y, Guezennec CY, Durlach J (1990) New experimental and clinical data on the relationship between magnesium and sport. *Magnes Res* 3:93-102.

Romani AM (2008) Magnesium homeostasis and alcohol consumption. *Magnes Res* 21:197-204.

Rucklidge JJ, Johnstone J, Kaplan BJ (2009) Nutrient supplementation approaches in the treatment of ADHD. *Expert Rev Neurother* 9:461-76.

Rupniak NMJ (2005) Substance P (NK1 receptor) antagonists. In: *Handbook of Stress and the Brain - Part 2: Stress: Integrative and Clinical Aspects* (Steckler T, Kalin NH, Reul JMHM, eds) Elsevier, New York, 423-35.

Ryu JH, Sohn IS, Do SH (2009) Controlled hypotension for middle ear surgery: a comparison between remifentanil and magnesium sulphate. *Brit J Anaesthes* 103:490-5.

Sarchielli P, Coata G, Firenze C, Morucci P, Abbritti G, Gallai V (1992) Serum and salivary magnesium levels in migraine and tension-type headache. Results in a group of adult patients. *Cephalalgia* 12:21-7.

Sawyer NT, Escayg A (2010) Stress and epilepsy: multiple models, multiple outcomes. *J Clin Neurophysiol* 27:445-52.

Seelig M (1989) Cardiovascular consequences of magnesium deficiency and loss: pathogenesis, prevalence and manifestations--magnesium and chloride loss in refractory potassium repletion. *Amer J Cardiol* 63:4G-21G.

Seelig MS (1993) Interrelationship of magnesium and estrogen in cardiovascular and bone disorders, eclampsia, migraine and premenstrual syndrome. *J Amer Coll Nutr* 12:442-58.

Seelig MS (1994) Consequences of magnesium deficiency on the enhancement of stress reactions; preventive and therapeutic implications (a review). *J Amer Coll Nutr* 13:429-46.

Seelig MS, Altura BM, Altura BT (2004) Benefits and risks of sex hormone replacement in postmenopausal women. *J Amer Coll Nutr* 23:482S-96S.

Sendur OF, Tastaban E, Turan Y, Ulman C (2008) The relationship between serum trace element levels and clinical parameters in patients with fibromyalgia. *Rheumatol Int* 28:1117-21.

Sivonova M, Zitnanova I, Hlincikova L, Skodacek I, Trebaticka J, Durackova Z (2004) Oxidative stress in university students during examinations. *Stress (Amsterdam, Netherlands)* 7:183-8

Slutsky I, Abumaria N, Wu LJ, Huang C, Zhang L, Li B, Zhao X, Govindarajan A, Zhao MG, Zhuo M, Tonegawa S, Liu G (2010) Enhancement of learning and memory by elevating brain magnesium. *Neuron* 65:165-77.

Sobrinho LG (2003) Prolactin, psychological stress and environment in humans: adaptation and maladaptation. *Pituitary* 6:35-9.

Soma M, Cunnane SC, Horrobin DF, Manku MS, Honda M, Hatano M (1988) Effects of low magnesium diet on the vascular prostaglandin and fatty acid metabolism in rats. *Prostaglandins* 36:431-41.

Sontia B, Touyz RM (2007) Role of magnesium in hypertension. *Arch Biochem Biophys* 458:33-9.

Stendig-Lindberg G, Moran D, Shapiro Y (1998) How significant is magnesium in thermoregulation? *J Basic Clinical Physiol Pharmacol* 9:73-85.

Steptoe A (2007) Stress Effects, Overview. In: *Encyclopedia of Stress* (Fink G, ed.) 2nd edn, vol. 3: Oxford: Academic Press, 599-600.

Szewczyk B, Poleszak E, Sowa-Kucma M, Siwek M, Dudek D, Ryszewska-Pokrasniewicz B, Radziwon-Zaleska M, Opoka W, Czekaj J, Pilc A, Nowak G (2008) Antidepressant activity of zinc and magnesium in view of the current hypotheses of antidepressant action. *Pharmacol Rep* 60:588-9.

Tang R, Yu B, Zhang K, Chen D (2008) Effects of supplementing two levels of magnesium aspartate and transportation stress on pork quality and gene expression of micro-calpain and calpastatin of finishing pigs. *Arch Animal Nutr* 62:415-25.

Tejero-Taldo MI, Kramer JH, Mak Iu T, Komarov AM, Weglicki WB (2006) The nerve-heart connection in the pro-oxidant response to Mg-deficiency. *Heart Failure Rev* 11:35-44.

Thomas J, Tomb E, Thomas E, Faure G (1994) Migraine treatment by oral magnesium intake and correction of the irritation of buccofacial and cervical muscles as a side effect of mandibular imbalance. *Magnes Res* 7:123-7.

Tiong K (2009) Irukandji syndrome, catecholamines, and mid-ventricular stress cardiomyopathy. *Eur J Echocardiogr* 10:334-6.

Touyz RM (2004) Magnesium in clinical medicine. *Front Biosci* 9:1278-93.

Truelsen T, Nielsen N, Boysen G, Gronbaek M (2003) Self-reported stress and risk of stroke: the Copenhagen City Heart Study. *Stroke* 34:856-62.

Turner R, Vink R (2007) Magnesium in the Central Nervous System. In: *New Perspectives in Magnesium Research: Nutrition and Research* (Yoshiki Nishizawa HM, Mori, H, Durlach J, eds.) London: Springer-Verlag, p338-58.

Turner RJ, Dasilva KW, O'Connor C, van den Heuvel C, Vink R (2004) Magnesium gluconate offers no more protection than magnesium sulphate following diffuse traumatic brain injury in rats. *J Am Coll Nutr* 23: 541S-4S.

Uvnas-Moberg K, Petersson M (2005) [Oxytocin, a mediator of anti-stress, well-being, social interaction, growth and healing]. *Z Psychosom Med Psychother* 51:57-80.

Wacker WE, Parisi AF (1968) Magnesium metabolism. *N Engl J Med* 278:712-7.

Whitted AD, Stanifer JW, Dube P, Borkowski BJ, Yusuf J, Komolafe BO, Davis RC, Jr., Soberman JE, Weber KT (2010) A dyshomeostasis of electrolytes and trace elements in acute stressor states: impact on the heart. *Am J Med Sci* 340:48-53.

Whyte KF, Addis GJ, Whitesmith R, Reid JL (1987) Adrenergic control of plasma magnesium in man. *Clin Sci (Lond)* 72:135-8.

Wolf FI, Maier JA, Nasulewicz A, Feillet-Coudray C, Simonacci M, Mazur A, Cittadini A (2007) Magnesium and neoplasia: from carcinogenesis to tumor growth and progression or treatment. *Arch Biochem Biophys* 458:24-32.

Wolf FI, Trapani V, Cittadini A, Maier JA (2009) Hypomagnesaemia in oncologic patients: to treat or not to treat? *Magnes Res* 22:5-9.

Magnesium in neuroses and neuroticism

Victoria Papadopol [1,✉] *and Mihai Nechifor* [2]

[1] Regional Centre of Public Health, Iasi, Romania.
[2] Department of Pharmacology, "Gr. T. Popa" University of Medicine and Pharmacy, Iasi, Romania.
✉ vicpapadopol@yahoo.com

Abstract

Neuroses are a frequently encountered group of psychiatric diseases with a symptomatology including neuronal hyperexcitability, anxiety, panic, phobic reactions, quite frequent tiredness, attention deficit, anorexia or bulimia, and sleep disorders, amongst others. The main pathogenic mechanisms involved in neurosis are increased activity of the glutamatergic cerebral systems (the increased synthesis, presynaptic release and action upon NMDA receptors), an intense catecholamine release, and the decrease of GABAergic cerebral systems activity. In most neurotic patients there is a reduction of plasma and intracellular magnesium concentration. Magnesium administration decreases anxiety, panic and phobia and ameliorates the attention deficit and sleep disorders. We consider that magnesium acts mainly by: a) the reduction of presynaptic glutamate release; b) the reduction of NMDA receptor activity by competing with calcium at NMDA receptor coupled calcium channels; c) the positive allosteric modulator effect at the level of some metabotropic presynaptic glutamate receptors, thereby decreasing presynaptic glutamate release and stimulating GABA release; and d) the decrease of catecholamine release by a direct presynaptic effect under the action of some factors including calcium. The stimulation of catecholamine release under stressful conditions leads to increased magnesium waste that is an essential event in the appearance of the functional cerebral changes characteristic of neurosis symptomatology. Unlike neuroses, neuroticism is not pathologic, but rather a normal state characterized by the dominance of some neuropsychic symptoms. There are data that show that the level of magnesium concentration is lower in subjects with high scores of neuroticism compared with other subjects.

Introduction

Magnesium is a nutrient essential for the health of the whole organism, including the brain. It is the fourth most abundant mineral in the body. Due to its relationships with more than 300 biochemical reactions, it is possible that magnesium is involved in more aspects of human body make-up and metabolism than any other mineral. Because the usual diet has drifted away from green leafy vegetables and unprocessed grains in favor of more refined and often nutrient-poor food options, magnesium inadequacy has become quite common in many areas of the world. One study shows that 68 % of Americans are magnesium deficient (www.usda.gov).

The role of magnesium is complex and its deficiency is implicated in a number of nonspecific neuropsychological changes such as agitation, fear, anxiety, depression, dizziness, poor attention, insomnia, and restlessness. Some of these symptoms characterize the mental illness known as neurosis.

Neuroses

Neuroses - characteristics and classification

Neurosis is a functional disorder of the central nervous system (CNS) generally characterized by excessive anxiety without evidence of neurologic disease, sometimes accompanied by defensive or immature behaviors. It is a general term describing a group of widespread mental illnesses also known as neurotic disorders, and thus, those suffering from them are said to be neurotics. It is also an emotional disorder that affects a part of the personality. Neuroses include a large variety of psychiatric disorders exhibiting a range of symptoms such as phobias, anxiety, tics and others. These disorders are a quite heterogeneous entity, difficult to delimit. The myriad of implicated factors makes the outline of a single psychopathological theory of neurosis difficult and this convinced some modern authors to remove the term. Although the American Diagnostic and Statistic Manual of Mental Disorders (DSM) have eliminated the category of neurosis, many authors still refer to them. Sometimes it is named anxiety neurosis or anxiety and phobic disorders. Anxiety, one of the most common symptoms of neurosis, is a physical symptom frequently including palpitations, nausea, chest pain, sweating, trembling and others.

Some authors consider that the main characteristics of neuroses are existence of some psychic, somatic and behavioral troubles without anatomical and psychological changes, the patient being aware of the pathology of their symptoms but unable to control them (although social adaptation is satisfactory excepting in serious forms) and obvious but variable sensibility to therapy (medicines, psychotherapy, relaxing techniques, hypnosis). Definition and classification of neuroses were frequently restructured according to different explicative theories. Therefore, the neuroses-related terminology is very variable. Essentially, neurotic symptoms are considered as a symbolic expression of an internal drama that the subject is unable to control because its essential elements drop out of their consciousness. Some authors include the social phobias, agoraphobias, hypochondria, panic disorder and even hysteria in neuroses. Generally, neurosis means poor ability to adapt to ones environment, an inability to change one's life pattern, and the inability to develop a richer, more complex, more satisfying personality (Boeree, 2002). Some professionals use the term to describe anxious symptoms and associated behavior, or to describe the range of mental illnesses outside of the psychiatric disorders. Others use the term neurosis to describe the internal process itself that triggers the anxiety characteristics.

The International Classification of Diseases (ICD) 10 (1992) grouped the neurotic disorders together with stress and somatophorm disturbances because of their historical association with the term neurosis, and because of their association with psychological causes. The concept of neurosis was not the major organizing principle. The combination of symptoms is common (most frequent being the associated depression-anxiety) especially in the less serious variants of these disturbances met in the first instance. ICD-10 introduces this type of disorder in the chapter "Neurotic, stress-related and somatoform disorders":

a- phobic anxiety disorders: agoraphobia with panic attacks, agoraphobia without panic attacks, social phobia, specific phobia, other phobic anxiety disorders (specified and unspecified)
b- other anxiety disorders: panic disorder, generalized anxiety disorder, mixed anxiety and depressive disorder, other anxiety disorders (specified and unspecified)
c- obsessive-compulsive disorders
d- reactions to severe stress, and adjustment disorders
e- dissociative disorders
f- somatoform disorders
g- other neurotic disorders.

Excessive anxiety and fear are common symptoms of neurotic disorders. According to Boeree (2002), the signs and symptoms of neurosis refer to a variety of psychological problems involving persistent experience of negative affect including anxiety, sadness and depression, anger, irritability, mental confusion, low sense of self-worth, behavioral symptoms such as phobic avoidance, vigilance, impulsive and compulsive acts, lethargy, etc., cognitive problems such as unpleasant and disturbing thoughts, repetition of thoughts and obsessions, habitual fantasizing, negativity and cynicism. Neurosis or neurotic disorder can vegetatively affect the person's ability to function affecting the activities of daily living. Some factors (education, culture) may serve to override any predisposing physiological conditions, or to exacerbate them. An essential point concerns the triggering stressors in a person's life, which lead to the various emotional, behavioral, and cognitive symptoms of neurosis.

Relationship between magnesium and neuroses

There are studies that show the involvement of magnesium in the pathogeny of most symptoms that can appear in neuroses. The magnesium level in the brain is more stable and decreases more slowly than in other tissues, but small decreases have important influences on neuron functioning. Taking into account the existence of some symptoms both in magnesium deficiency and in neurosis (latent tetany, hyperventilation syndrome, anxiety, hyper emotionality, fatigue and sometimes migraine, dizziness, nervous fits – panic attack particularly, sensation of "lump in the throat"), one can think that a relationship between magnesium deficiency and neurosis exists.

The most frequent and characteristic form of magnesium deficit disorders in the central nervous system is *nervous hyperexcitability* (Durlach, 1998; Durlach *et al*, 1997) and hence nervous forms of magnesium deficiency represent the most commonly seen form in clinical practice whatever the age. Nervous hyperexcitability is, at the same time, one of the most frequent features of neuroses. Magnesium oral administration determines the correction of the symptomatology and the normalization of the electropolygraphic modifications, ECG and other static and dynamic investigations.

Panic is an essential symptom of neuroses. There are a few studies that have determined the plasma concentration of magnesium and other bivalent cations of panic disorder patients. Nahar et al (2010) did not find significant differences in the magnesium plasma concentration in panic disorders patients versus the control group, but the intracellular concentrations were not determined. ATPase was studied in the erythrocytes of the patients with *phobic* neurosis. Sechenov (1975) found an increased activity of Mg^{2+} ATPase in these patients but a decreased activity of $Na^{+}K^{+}$ATP-ase as compared with the control group. The significance of these changes is not clear.

In *anxiety* neurosis, there was not only a decrease in magnesium concentration but also modified quantitative proportions between magnesium and other blood plasma or cytoplasmic components. It was proven that the blood fatty acids/magnesium ratio was increased and the magnesium level was decreased in anxiety neurotic patients (Iakushev *et al*, 1989).

Regarding the *mechanism* by which magnesium reduces panic and anxiety, we consider that the main elements are decreased glutamate action and increased action of the GABAergic systems. Magnesium reduces anxiety by a number of mechanisms (Figure 1). These include reducing

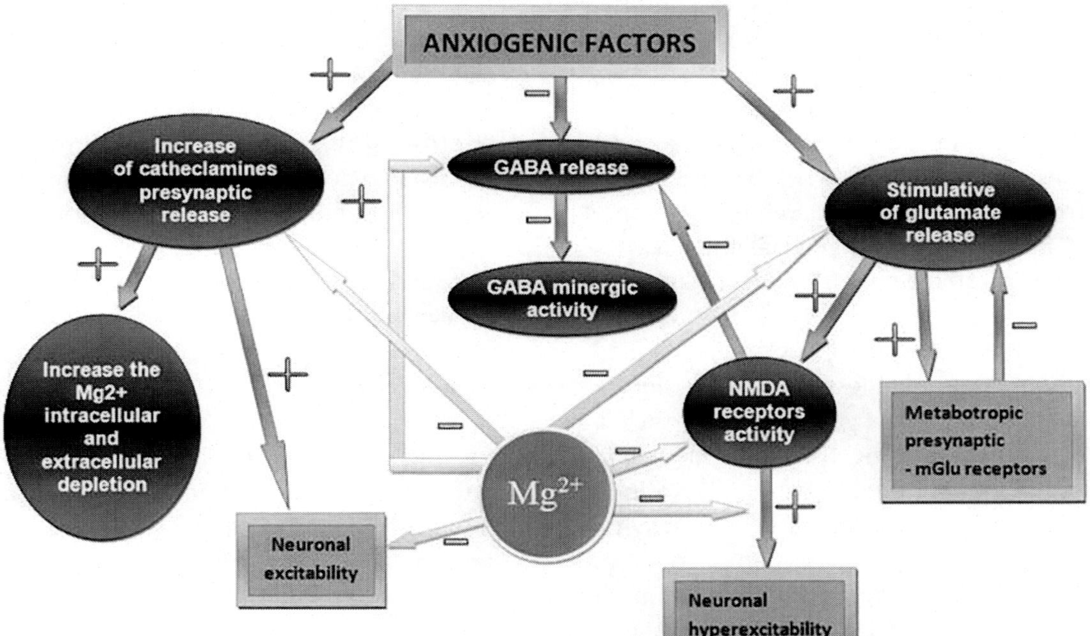

Figure 1. Magnesium mechanisms of action in anxiety and panic. -, inhibition; +, stimulation (increase).

the postsynaptic NMDA receptor activity by acting at the level of the calcium channel coupled with NMDA receptors, reducing the presynaptic cerebral release of epinephrine and norepinephrine, increasing GABA concentration in some brain areas, and acting as a modulator of glutamate release at the presynaptic level.

Glutamate is the most important excitatory neurotransmitter in mammalian brain. It acts at three major receptor types including the NMDA ionotropic receptor coupled with a Ca^{2+} channel, the AMPA (alpha-amino-3 hydroxy-5 methyl-4-isoxazole propionic acid) receptor, and the metabotropic glutamate receptor (mGluR) group (at least 8 subtypes). Glutamate metabotropic receptors are divided into three groups, group I including mGluR1 and mGluR5 subtypes, group II including mGluR2 and mGluR3 subtypes, and group III including mGluR4, mGluR6, mGluR7 and mGluR8 subtypes.

The most important postsynaptic receptor population for glutamate is the NMDA receptors. Dorsomedial hippocampal neurons express both NMDA and AMPA receptors for glutamate (Bailey *et al*, 2003; Goren *et al*, 2003). Magnesium doesn't have a noticeable influence upon AMPA receptors and the existing data implicate the NMDA hypothalamic receptors in producing anxiety and panic disorders. Magnesium does reduce the effect of NMDA receptor stimulation and this is the main mechanism of its anxiolytic effect (Coan and Collingridge, 1985). Chronic stress involved in the pathogeny of some neuroses increases the hypothalamic NMDA receptor expression (Lee *et al*, 2003).

The mGluRs are a family of G-protein coupled receptors that have a widespread expression in CNS (Niswender and Conn, 2010). They have a modulator role in synaptic transmission and in normal excitability in brain, playing a key role in the modulation of glutamatergic activity, glutamate secretion and presynaptic release, GABAergic system activity and in regulation of neuroendocrine activity. The normal and pathological implications of the activation of these receptors are very different. Glutamate action on these brain receptors is important in normal and in pathologic situations such as fear, anxiety, addiction, panic, withdrawal syndrome, and posttraumatic stress disorders. Notably, divalent cations modulate the activity of mGluRs (Francesconi and Duvoisin, 2004). A mounting and important role in not only anxiety but also in other CNS disorders is attributed to malfunction of the mGluRs. Regarding the symptoms in neurosis (anxiety, fear, cognitive impairment, working memory), the mGluR2 and the mGluR7 are the most important types of mGluRs and they are well expressed in hippocampus (Desai, 1992). MGluR7 in particular has a wide distribution in the brain, and in the amygdala and hippocampus, is preferentially localized to presynaptic axon terminals (Masugi *et al*, 1999). This receptor has a low affinity for glutamate, and Niswender and Conn (2010) consider that it reduces glutamatergic activity and only activates in the case of overstimulation by glutamate. Selective stimulation of mGluR7 induced anxiolytic-like effects in mice by enhancement of GABAergic neurotransmission, and by reduction of glutamate synthesis and action (Stachowicz *et al*, 2008). The lack of mGluR7 caused a deficit in fear response and conditioned taste aversion (Masugi *et al*, 1999). Magnesium is important for mGluR7 receptor activity and may explain the enhancement of anxiety in hypomagnesemia (Niswender and Conn, 2010).

The agonists of some mGluRs are promising future drugs in the treatment of some psychiatric disorders. The agonists and positive allosteric modulators of group I mGluRs might treat anxiety disorders (Krystal *et al*, 2010). The mGluR group II agonists block fear learning when they are administrated into the amygdala prior to training (Walker and Davis, 2002). Mares et al (2010) showed in immature rats that some mGluRs are involved in production of anxiolysis. Magnesium is also a positive allosteric modulator for some mGluRs.

The ratio between glutamate-induced excitatory activity and GABAergic inhibition in some brain areas (such as the amygdala, dorsomedial hypothalamus and cortex) plays an essential role in behavior and its imbalances are involved in the pathogenic mechanism of anxiety, panic disorder and phobia. Experimental chronic inhibition of GABA synthesis and enhancement of glutamatergic activity in the dorsomedial hypothalamus induced panic-like responses in rats (Johnson and Shekhar, 2006). Glutamate NMDA receptors are the most important receptor group involved in experimental lactate-induced panic-like response in rats, but other receptors for glutamate are also involved.

Carbamazepine, an antiepileptic drug, is also used for the treatment of many nonepileptic disorders, including anxiety. The anxiolytic effects of carbamazepine seem to be mediated (partly at least) by interactions with GABAergic system because muscimol (a $GABA_A$ receptor agonist) enhanced the carbamazepine anxiolytic effect. The anxiogenic effect of NMDA administration was also reversed by carbamazepine (Rezvanfard *et al*, 2009). In our studies (Nechifor *et al*, 2005; 2007), carbamazepine administration in therapeutic doses in human subjects increased the intracellular magnesium level. We believe that, the anxiolytic effect of carbamazepine is due, at least in part, to the increased intracellular magnesium concentration.

GABA antagonizes the glutamate hyperexcitation in some brain regions such as dorsomedial hypothalamus and protects against anxiety and panic disorders (Millan, 2003). Favoring the idea that the GABAergic system plays an important role in preventing and reducing panic and anxiety, a low GABA concentration in brain has been associated with anxiety behaviors in rats and mice. In rats, chronic administration of 1-allylglicine (a GABA synthesis inhibitor) in the dorsomedial hypothalamus induced panic disorder and enhanced panic-like behavior produced by sodium lactate infusion (Schekhar *et al*, 1996; 2003). The reduction of GABAergic system activity has also been shown in un-medicated panic disorder patients. The subjects without major depression had a 22% reduction of the total occipital cortex GABA concentration compared with the normal control group (Goddard *et al*, 2001). Crestani et al (1999) and Goddard et al (2001) also showed that the impaired brain GABA and benzodiazepine receptor activity is involved in phobic behaviors in mice.

The glutamatergic systems hyperactivity is also involved in other neurosis symptoms, for example the dysregulation of the fear memory, the extinction of the fear memory and post stress neuroses. An NMDA receptor agonist, D-cycloserine (5 mg/kg) blocked fear extinction in rats (Yang *et al*, 2007).

The catecholamines are also involved in fear and panic disorders. The injection of an α1-blocker in the dorsomedial hypothalamus blocks panic-like responses of animals (Johnson and Shekhar, 2006). The systemic administration of yohimbine induced panic-like responses, by blocking presynaptic α2-receptors and increasing epi-nephrine and norepinephrine release (Lowry *et al*, 2003). Yohimbine administration in healthy subjects increased the plasma level of norepinephrine, the adrenergic activity and resulted in increased anxiety and nervousness in the patients. Charney et al (1984) found a significant positive correlation between the plasma level of the norepinephrine metabolite 3-methoxy-4-hydroxyphenylglicol (MHPG) and patient anxiety and panic attacks. Notably, magnesium reduces epinephrine and nor-epinephrine synthesis and release, decreases anxiety and could prevent the panic attacks.

Magnesium deficiency, even when mild, increases susceptibility to various types of neurologic and psychological stressors in healthy human subjects and diverse groups of patients. Repletion of deficiency reverses this increased stress sensitivity and pharmacologic loading of magnesium salts induces resistance to neuropsychological stressors. Mild magnesium deficiency appears to be common among patients with disorders considered functional or neurotic and appears to contribute to a symptom complex that includes asthenia, sleep disorders, irritability, hyperarousal, spasm of striated and smooth muscle and hyperventilation (Galland, 1991-1992). Stress, being a frequent cause of neurosis, influences magnesium concentration in the organism. Adrenergic stress induces a shift of magnesium from the intracellular to the extracellular space and increases urinary magnesium loss. In contrast, magnesium deficiency increases the vulnerability of human body to stress and the damage induced by stress (Galland, 1991-1992). Magnesium deficiency also increases neuronal excitability, not only by increasing the excitatory effect of glutamate mediated by NMDA receptors, but possibly by increasing the calcium current in pre- and postsynaptic membranes and by alteration of the Na^+/K^+ ATPases (Moris, 1992).

Glutamate induces a powerful stimulation of norepinephrine release in amygdala and hippocampal slices (Fink *et al*, 1992). Mg^{2+} ions and MK-801 (dizocilpine, an NMDA receptor antagonist) reduced the NMDA-evoked overflow of norepinephrine. Norepinephrine release related to the stimulation of AMPA receptors by glutamate does not seem to be influenced by Mg^{2+}. Since the activation of mGluR4 and mGluR7 induces a decrease of glutamate release from presynaptic areas (Schrader and Tasker, 1997), it is possible that presynaptic mGluRs can thereby influence norepinephrine release.

Another important problem is the frequency of *sleep disturbances* in patients with neurosis. There are data that sustain the possible involvement of magnesium in sleep regulation. In rats, magnesium deficiency is associated with a decrease in sleep time. Magnesium content in four brain areas were also highly and positively correlated with the length of sleep periods (Chollet *et al*, 2000). Erythrocyte magnesium concentrations are low in adult human subjects with chronic sleep deprivation (1.1 +/- 0.4 mg/dl) versus a control group (1.8 +/- 0.4 mg/dl) (Tanabe et al, 1997). The reduction of sleep time is frequently associated with chronic fatigue. Chronic sleep deprivation is associated with an increase of plasma catecholamine release and with a decrease of intracellular magnesium level. These changes occur relatively quickly. In healthy male students (20-24 years aged), 4 weeks of partial sleep deprivation was sufficient time for the appearance of these changes in the intracellular concentration of magnesium, and in the plasma epinephrine and norepinephrine concentrations. The students with chronic sleep deprivation over the 4-week period (sleep was <80% than in ordinary days), had significantly decreased intracellular magnesium levels (Takase *et al*, 2004a; 2004b).

Experimental magnesium restricted diets in rats also increases the cerebral dopamine and norepinephrine concentration. This rise is associated with a decrease of sleep time and an increase in electroencephalographic wakefulness (Poenaru *et al*, 1984). Magnesium deficiency is accompanied by a decrease of sleep duration and by an increase of brain dopamine level (Chollet *et al*, 2000). These data strongly support the reduction of cerebral catecholamine release by magnesium. The effect of $MgSO_4$ (0.5 mg Mg SO_4/h between 20.30 hours till 7.00 hours) on sleep electroencephalogram (EEG, recorded between 23.00 and 7.00 hours) in healthy adult men showed an increase of the third sleep cycle with unchanged delta power throughout the night (Murch and Steiger, 1998). The activation of GABA receptors is very important for the initiation and maintenance of nor-rapid-eye movement sleep (NREM). Magnesium stimulates the activity cerebral GABAergic systems by behaving as a modulator of GABA receptors, increasing their activity.

Mg^{2+} has a favorable effect with respect to sleep onset and maintenance and also tiredness, which appears as a consequence of sleep deprivation. In their studies of chronic sleep deprivation, Tanabe et al (1998) reported a reduction of intracellular magnesium level. This reduction was associated with a decreased exercise tolerance. Specifically, when subjects were submitted to a bicycle ergometer cardiopulmonary exercise test, the sleep-deprived subjects had a decreased exercise tolerance. The administration of 100 mg magnesium orally per day for 1 month improved the exercise tolerance. There was no difference between the sleep-deprived patients and the normal sleep patients regarding the peak oxygen uptake and anaerobic threshold. The mechanism through which the chronic sleep deprivation can reduce intracellular magnesium concentration is unknown, but we consider that the excess catecholamines that appear in sleep deprivation could accelerate the magnesium disposal. Hornyak et al (1998) showed that magnesium therapy can be useful in periodic leg movements related to insomnia. Magnesium was administered orally 12.4 mmol in the evening during 4-6 weeks. After magnesium administration, periodic limb movements during sleep decreased significantly and the total sleep duration increased.

Attention deficit and hyperactivity disorders (ADHD) are only found in school children and in many patients with neurosis. In these patients the plasma and erythrocyte magnesium level is low. In an animal experimental model of attention deficit, the hippocampal glutamate-stimulated release of norepinephrine was significantly higher. The glutamate stimulatory effect on norepinephrine release was reduced by CNQX (1mμM) (an AMPA receptor antagonist) suggesting that in this case the AMPA receptor stimulation by glutamate plays an important role.

The NMDA receptor antagonist MK-801 (10µM) did not reduce the glutamate-stimulated release of norepinephrine (Howells and Russell, 2008). An involvement of dopamine in attention deficit disorder from the neurotic patient is also possible, because in patients with ADHD there are dysfunctions of the dopaminergic system. In an experimental rat model for ADHD, glutamate-stimulated dopamine release in the substantia nigra is higher. Warton et al (2009) consider that abnormal dopaminergic system function in ADHD could be the result of a change in dopamine central neurons (dopamine synthesis, dopamine transporters or dopamine receptors) or an indirect effect of imbalanced glutamate regulation of dopaminergic neurons. We think that a similar process also occurs in the case of deficit attention of the neurotic patients. Magnesium can directly reduce dopamine release at the presynaptic level and also can reduce the stimulatory effect of glutamate on dopamine release.

The treatment with Mag-B6 was useful in attention deficit syndrome and in hyperactivity treatment (Nogovitsina and Levitina, 2006; 2007). Mag-B6 improved behavior, decreased the level of anxiety and aggression, increased attention and corrected the magnesium homeostasis in children with ADHD.

Both *bulimia and anorexia* are also symptoms found in patients with neurosis. In patients with anorexia nervosa (DSM-IV criteria), a decreased magnesium level was found versus the control group. About 60% of the patients had low serum magnesium (Birmingham et al, 2004).

In neurotic and stressed patients, *sexual dysfunction* (reduced libido and sexual potency) is frequently present. This dysfunction is largely caused by increased prolactin (PRL) synthesis. It was experimentally showed that immobilization and other forms of stress (implicated also in the pathogeny of some cases of neuroses) increased PRL secretion. Pretreatment of the animals with magnesium aspartate in dose of 100 mg, 200 mg and 400 mg significantly decreased the stress-induced PRL secretion in a dose-dependent manner (Ali *et al*, 1987). D-aspartate increased PRL secretion by stimulation of NMDA receptors. In the fish S.Mossambicus, Mg^{2+} also lowered PRL secretion (Bonga *et al*, 1983).

There are a number of mechanisms by which magnesium may reduce the PRL level in neurosis, thereby lowering or preventing the effects of this anterior pituitary hormone. It can directly reduce secretion of PRL at the level of secretary cells, it can decrease PRL secretion by inhibiting stimulation by prolactin releasing hormone at the pituitary level (Kasahara et al, 1993), it can reduce the stimulatory effect of glutamate on pituitary PRL release, and finally, magnesium can reduce the stimulatory effect of calcium ions on PRL secretion. In cultures of adult female rats, pituitary cell glutamate significantly increased the rate of PRL release. This release was augmented 4-fold after elimination of magnesium from the perfusate (Login, 1990). Both NMDA (100 µM) and kainate (100 µM) increased PRL secretion by NMDA receptor stimulation, whereas AMPA receptor agonists did not modify PRL secretion and release. The antagonism between magnesium and the calcium channels coupled to the NMDA receptors is the essential factor in reduction of PRL secretion by this bivalent cation.

Magnesium treatment of neuroses

There are a limited number of studies that show a beneficial effect of magnesium in the treatment of different symptoms of the diseases known as neurotic disorders. Using mice, Poleszak et al (2004) demonstrated that doses of 20 and 30 mg magnesium/ kg (doses which did not affect locomotor activity) produced anxiolytic-like effects measured using the plus-maze test. These doses were acutely or chronically administered and resulted in at least a 58% increase in serum magnesium concentration. Magnesium induced the anxiolytic-like effects without tolerance to these activities, suggesting a potential anxiolytic activity in these disorders in human.

Singewald et al (2004) showed in an animal experiment (mice) that magnesium depletion leads to enhanced depression- and anxiety-related behavior which was further validated by the reversibility of the behavioral changes by known antidepressant and anxiolytic substances. Using a rat model, Fromm et al (2004) demonstrated a reduced incidence of anxiety after traumatic brain injury using magnesium sulfate as an interventional treatment. The study of Bockova et al (1992) demonstrated that the combination of an anxiolytic with a magnesium salt (lactate) resulted in a more rapid reduction of the symptoms of anxious depressive neurosis.

Taborska (1995) showed the curative effect of magnesium salts in patients suffering panic disorders and latent tetany. The symptoms of panic disorder are, with few exceptions, virtually identical with those of latent tetany. The author examined 20 patients treated in a psychiatric outpatient unit for panic disorder, examining latent tetany including serum and red blood cell magnesium. He found a concomitant incidence of latent tetany with decreased level of intracellular magnesium and a remission, in 90 % of cases, of problems common to both nosological entities using therapy with magnesium salts.

A double-blind, randomized, placebo-controlled study evaluated the efficacy and safety of a fixed combination containing two plant extracts and magnesium in treatment of 264 patients presenting generalized anxiety of mild-to-moderate intensity. It demonstrated that the preparation was safe and more effective than placebo (Hanus *et al*, 2004).

The studies of Durlach et al (1997) concluded that the primary or secondary, acute or chronic nervous forms of magnesium deficiency induced by insufficient magnesium intake remain reversible over a long period by simply normalizing the magnesium intake. Untreated chronic forms may however bring irreversible organic disorders.

Physiological oral magnesium supplementation (5mg /kg/day) is simple and can be carried out in the diet or with magnesium salts. This treatment is able to cure all the functional symptoms of magnesium deficiency: signs of neuromuscular hyperexcitability and psychiatric symptoms, which frequently mimic a neurotic pattern. It is necessary to highlight the curative and preventive importance of oral physiological maternal magnesium supplementation, not only during pregnancy, but also in the child throughout life from infancy to older age, to possibly prevent the so-called constitutional factor of neurolability.

It is imperative to emphasize that the nervous consequences of magnesium deficiency remain functional with an atomical integrity for a long time. They are completely reversible since they can be restored to normal with simple oral physiological magnesium supplementation (Durlach *et al*, 1987; 1997).

Neuroticism

Neuroticism is a fundamental personality trait in the study of psychology. Unlike neurosis, it is not pathological in itself but is a tendency that can become pathological in certain conditions. It is also a risk factor for "internalizing" mental disorders such as phobia, depression, panic disorders and other anxiety disorders, traditionally called neuroses (Hettema *et al*, 2006). Neuroticism is an enduring tendency to experience negative emotional states like hyperemotivity, hyperexcitability, anxiety, anger, impulsivity and other psychosomatic manifestations. It is sometime called emotional instability. Individuals who score high on neuroticism are more likely than the average to experience such feelings as anxiety, anger, guilt and, depressed mood (Matthews and Deary, 1998). They are emotionally reactive and respond to events that would not affect most people. Moreover, their reactions tend to be more intense than normal. They are more likely to interpret ordinary situations as threatening, and minor frustrations as hopelessly difficult. Their negative emotional reactions tend to persist for unusually long periods of time, which means they are often in a bad mood. These problems in emotional regulation can diminish a neurotic's ability to think clearly, make decisions, and cope effectively with stress. Neuroticism appears to be related to physiological differences in the brain. Hans Eysenck theoretized that neuroticism is a function of activity in the limbic system, and his research suggests that people who score highly on measures of neuroticism have a more reactive sympathetic nervous system, and are more sensitive to environmental stimulation (Eysenck and Eysenck, 1985). Behavioral genetics researchers have found that a significant portion of the variability on measures of neuroticism can be attributed to genetic factors (Viken *et al*, 1994). As Boeree (2002) shows, neuroticism may be a predisposing physiological condition for neurosis.

Relationship between magnesium and neuroticism

As has already been shown, magnesium deficiency

Table 1. Mean magnesium values (mmol/L) in children from an orphanage (Group I) and a state school (Group II). Adapted from Papadopol *et al*, 2001.

	Group I	Group II	t-test	p
Serum magnesium	0.83 +/- 0.09*	0.78 +/- 0.06	3.76	< 0.001
Erythrocyte magnesium	1.82 +/- 0.18	1.91 +/- 0.18	3.75	< 0.001

*: mean ± standard deviation; p: significance level

Table 2. Comparison of outcomes of personality traits. Adapted from Papadopol *et al*, 2001.

	Steps of personality traits	Group I (number of cases)	Group II (number of cases)	
Psychoticism	Pathological	12	11	χ^2=7.87
	Pathological tendencies	9	19	**p=0.019**
	Normal	63	39	
Neuroticism	Pathological	18	6	χ^2=8.75
	Pathological tendencies	23	12	**p=0.012**
	Normal	43	51	
Extraversion	Pathological	15	14	χ^2=0.53
	Pathological tendencies	25	17	p=0.766
	Normal	44	38	

p: significance level.

manifests at the central nervous system level as hyperemotivity, hyperexcitability, anxiety, and impulsivity, amongst others, and these are also observed in neuroticism. So, a relationship between magnesium deficiency and neuroticism is suggested. Some studies (Tuchendria *et al*, 1998) suggest that magnesium deficiency can be a causal factor of neurotic tendencies in elderly persons. In a group of 80 aged persons, all cases with erythrocyte magnesium deficit presented two or more neurotic tendencies, most frequent being the depressive ones.

There are also a few studies on magnesium deficiency in children and its relationship with personality traits. Specifically, this relationship in children and teenagers was examined in two groups of pupils from different socio-economic backgrounds, namely an orphanage (group I) and a regular state school (group II) (Papadopol *at al*, 2001). Magnesium level and personality features were compared, including psychoticism, neuroticism and extraversion. With regard to the magnesium level (Table 1), one can see a discord between serum magnesium levels and erythrocyte levels. It is known that serum values of magnesium are less stable than erythrocyte values, being quite easily influenced by factors such as stress or physical activity that increases magnesium requirements. Serum magnesium may be normal in spite of a significant magnesium deficiency. The children from the orphanage had a more uniform lifestyle, with a more regular program of eating, sleeping and physical activities. Nutrition is also very important for the tissue magnesium levels. The nutrition of the children from the orphanage is characterized by a satisfactory, uniform level for all the children, while the nutrition of the children who live with their families is very variable but generally better because of socio-economic differences.

Table 3. Relationship between magnesium deficit and neuroticism in children from an orphanage (Group I) and a state school (Group II). Adapted from Papadopol *et al*, 2001.

	Group	r	n	p
Serum magnesium	I	+0.25	84	**0.023**
Erythrocyte magnesium	II	+0.26	67	**0.035**

r: Pearson correlation index; n: number of subjects; p: significance level.

The distribution of the subjects with respect to personality features in the two groups differed significantly in psychoticism and neuroticism tendencies (Table 2). The more numerous pathological tendencies of group I were probably the consequences of the unfavorable emotional climate from the institutionalized milieu. An investigation of the relationship between magnesium levels and personality features pointed out only a significant difference between the two groups, which refers to neuroticism (Table 3). The positive correlation in magnesium deficit-neuroticism suggests that magnesium deficit may be a causal factor in this negative aspect of personality.

In a study by Nizankovska-Blaz et al (1993) on 249 girls and boys aged 5-15 years, serum magnesium level was decreased in 24 children and neurotic reactions or concentration disturbances were observed in 21 of them.

In conclusion, all the available clinical and experimental data prove the involvement and importance of magnesium in neuroses and neuroticism.

References

Ali BH, Silsby JL, el Halawani ME (1987) The effect of magnesium aspartate, xylazine and morphine on the immobilization-induced increase in the levels of prolactin in turkey plasma. *J Vet Pharmacol Ther* 10:119-26.

Bailey TW, Nicol GD, Schild JH, DiMicco JA (2003) Synaptic and membrane properties of neurons in the dorsomedial hypothalamus. *Brain Res* 985:150-62.

Birmingham CL, Puddicombe D, Hlynsky J (2004) Hypomagnesemia during refeeding in anorexia nervosa. *Eat Weight Disord* 9:236-7.

Bockova E, Hronek J, Kolomaznik M, Polackova J, Curdova NO (1992) Popentiation of the effects of anxiolytics with magnesium salts. *Cesk Psychiatr* 88:141-4.

Boeree G (2002) A bio-social theory of neurosis. http: //webspace.ship.edu/cgboer/genpsyneurosis.html.

Bonga W, Löwik CJ, van der Meij JC (1983) Effects of external Mg2+ and Ca2+ on branchial osmotic water permeability and prolactin secretion in the teleost fish Sarotherodon mossambicus. *Gen Comp Endocrinol* 52:222-31.

Charney DS, Heninger GR, Breier A (1984) Noradrenergic function in panic anxiety. Effects of yohimbine in healthy subjects and patients with agoraphobia and panic disorder. *Arch Gen Psychiatry* 41:751-63.

Chollet D, Franken P, Raffin Y, Malafosse A, Widmer J, Tafti M (2000) Blood and brain magnesium in inbred mice and their correlation with sleep quality. *Am J Physiol Regul Integr Comp Physiol* 279:R2173-8.

Coan EJ, Collingridge GL (1985) Magnesium ions block an N-methyl-D-aspartate receptor-mediated component of synaptic transmission in rat hippocampus. *Neurosci Lett* 53:21-6.

Crestani F, Lorez M, Baer K, Essrich C, Benke D, Laurent JP, Belzung C, Fritschy KM, Lucher IH (1999) Decreased GABA receptor clustering results in enhanced anxiety and a bias for treatment. *J Neurosci* 2:833-9.

Desai MA, Smith TS, Conn PJ (1992) Multiple metabotropic glutamate receptors regulate hippocampal function. *Synapse* 12:206-13.

Durlach J, Bac P, Durlach V, Bara M, Guiet-Bara A (1997) Neurotic, neuromuscular and autonomic nervous form of magnesium imbalance. *Magnes Res* 10:169-95

Durlach, J., Poenaru, S., Rouhani, S., Bara, M. & Guiet-Bara, A (1987) The control of central neural hyper-0excitability in magnesium deficiency. In: *Nutrients and Brain Function.* (Essman WB, ed), Basel: Karger, 48-71

Durlach J (1998) Aetiology and pathophysiology of central nervous hyperexcitability due to various type of magnesium deficit: magnesium deficiency and magnesium depletion. *Abstr 6th Europ Magnes Congress*, Budapest (Abstract)

Duvoisin RM, Pfankuch T, Wilson JM, Grabell J, Chhajlani V, Brown DG, Johnson E, Raber J (2010) Acute pharmacological modulation of mGluR8 reduces measures of anxiety. *Behav Brain Res* 212:168-73.

Eysenck HJ, Eysenck MW (1985) *Personality and individual differences: A natural science approach. Perspectives on individual differences*. Plenum Press (Springer)

Fink K, Schultheiss R, Göthert M (1992) Stimulation of noradrenaline release in human cerebral cortex mediated by N-methyl-D-aspartate (NMDA) and non-NMDA receptors. *Br J Pharmacol* 106:67-72.

Francesconi A, Duvoisin RM (2004) Divalent cations modulate the activity of metabotropic glutamate receptors. *J Neurosci Res* 75:472-9.

Fromm L, Heath DL, Vink R, Nimmo AJ (2004) Magnesium attenuates post-traumatic depression/anxiety following diffuse traumatic brain injury in rats. *J Am Coll Nutr* 23:529S-533S.

Galland L (1991-1992) Magnesium, stess and neuropsychiatric disorders. Magnes Trace Elem 10 (2-4): 287-301.

Goddard AW, Mason GF, Almai A, Rothman DL, Behar KL, Petroff OA, Charney DS, Krystal JH (2001) Reductions in occipital cortex GABA levels in panic disorder detected with 1h-magnetic resonance spectroscopy. *Arch Gen Psychiatry* 58:556-61.

Gören MZ, Yananli HR, Berkman K, Onat F, Aker R (2003) The influence of dorsomedial hypothalamic nucleus on contralateral paraventricular nucleus in NMDA-mediated cardiovascular responses. *Brain Res* 968:219-26.

Hanus M, Lafon J, Mathieu M (2004) Double-blind, randomised, placebo-controlled study to evaluate the efficacy and safety of a fixed combination containing two plant extracts (Crataegus oxyacantha and Eschscholtzia californica) and magnesium in mild-to-moderate anxiety disorders. *Curr Med Res Opin* 20:63-71.

Hettema JM, Neale MC, Myers JM, Prescott CA, Kendler KS (2006) A population-based twin study of the relationship between neuroticism and internalizing disorders. *Am J Psychiatry* 163:857-64.

Hornyak M, Voderholzer U, Hohagen F, Berger M, Riemann D (1998) Magnesium therapy for periodic leg movements-related insomnia and restless legs syndrome: an open pilot study. *Sleep* 21:501-5.

Howells FM, Russell VA (2008) Glutamate-stimulated release of norepinephrine in hippocampal slices of animal models of attention-deficit/hyperactivity disorder (spontaneously hypertensive rat) and depression/anxiety-like behaviours (Wistar-Kioto rat) *Brain Res* 1200:107-15.

Iakushev VS, Ruzhov AA, Mironova EV (1989) Changes in the concentration of nonesterified fatty acids and magnesium in emotional stress. *Fiziol Zh SSSR Im I M Sechenova* 75:1146-50.

International Classification of Diseases-10 (1992), World Health Organization, Geneva.

Johnson PL, Shekhar A (2006) Panic-prone state induced in rats with GABA dysfunction in the dorsomedial hypothalamus is mediated by NMDA receptors. *J Neurosci* 26:7093-104.

Kasahara K, Tasaka K, Masumoto N, Nishizaki T, Mizuki J, Tahara M, Miyake A, Tanizawa O (1993) High magnesium concentration inhibits ligand-stimulated calcium influx and hormone secretion in rat pituitary lactotropes with involvement of intracellular free magnesium. *Biochem Biophys Res Commun* 197:92-9.

Krystal JM, Mathew SJ, D'Souza DC, Garakani A, Gunduz-Bruce H, Charney DS (2010) Potential psychiatric applicationms of metabotropic glutamate receptor agonists and antagonists. *CNS Drugs* 24: 669-93.

Lee PR, Brady D, Koenig JI (2003) Corticosterone alters N-methyl-D-aspartate receptor subunit mRNA expression before puberty. *Brain Res Mol Brain Res* 115:55-62.

Login IS (1990) Direct stimulation of pituitary prolactin release by glutamate. *Life Sci* 47:2269-75.

Lowry CA, Plant A, Shanks N, Ingram CD, Lightman SL (2003) Anatomical and functional evidence for a stress-responsive, monoamine-accumulating area in the dorsomedial hypothalamus of the adult rat brain *Horm Behav* 43:254-62.

Mares P, Mikulecká A, Tichá K, Lojková-Janecková D, Kubová H (2010) Metabotropic glutamate receptors as a target for anticonvulsant and anxiolytic action in immature rats. *Epilepsia* 51, Suppl 3:24-6.

Masugi M, Yokoi M, Shigemoto R, Muguruma K, Watanabe Y, Sansig G, van der Putten H, Nakanishi S (1999) Metabotropic glutamate receptor subtype 7 ablation causes deficit in fear response and conditioned taste aversion. *J Neurosci* 19:955-63.

Matthews G, Deary IJ (1998) *Personality Traits*, Cambridge University Press, Cambridge.

Millan MJ (2003) The neurobiology and control of anxious states. *Prog Neurobiol* 71:83-244.

Morris ME (1992) Brain and CSF magnesium concentrations during magnesium deficit in animals and humans: neurological symptoms. *Magnes Res* 5:303-13.

Murck H, Steiger A (1998) Mg2+ reduces ACTH secretion and enhances spindle power without changing delta power during sleep in men -- possible therapeutic implications. *Psychopharmacology (Berl)* 137:247-52.

Nahar Z, Azad MA, Rahman MA, Rahman MA, Bari W, Islam SN, Islam MS, Hasnat A (2010) Comparative analysis of serum manganese, zinc, calcium, copper and magnesium level in panic disorder patients. *Biol Trace Elem Res* 133:284-90.

Nechifor M (2007) Magnesium in Psychoses. In: *New perspectives in Magnesium Research – Nutrition and Health* (Yoshiki Nishizuwa, Hirotoshi Mori, Jean Durlach J eds) London, SpringenVerlag, 369-377.

Nechifor M, Vaideanu C, Mindreci I, Palamaru I, Boistenu P (2005) Research on plasmatic and tissular concentration of some bivalent cations in patients with bipolar disorders. In: *Abstract book of 5th International Symposium on Trace Elements in Human-New Perspectives* (Ermidon Pollet S, Pollet S, eds) Athens Publishing House, p.18.

Niswender CM, Conn PJ (2010) Metabotropic glutamate receptors: physiology, pharmacology, and disease. *Annu Rev Pharmacol Toxicol* 50:295-322.

Nizankowska-Blaz T, Korczowski R, Zys K, Rybak A (1993) Level of magnesium in blood serum in children from the province of Rzesz,ow. *Wiad Lek* 46:120-2.

Nogovitsina OR, Levitina EV (2006) Effect of MAGNE-B6 on the clinical and biochemical manifestations of the syndrome of attention deficit and hyperactivity in children. *Eksp Klin Farmakol* 69:74-7.

Nogovitsina OR, Levitina EV (2007) Neurological aspects of the clinical features, pathophysiology, and corrections of impairments in attention deficit hyperactivity disorder. *Neurosci Behav Physiol* 37:199-202.

Papadopol V, Tuchendria E, Palamaru I (2001) Magnesium and some psychological features in two groups of pupils (magnesium and psychic features). *Magnes Res* 14:27-32.

Poenaru S, Rouhani S, Durlach J, Aymard N, Belkahla F, Rayssiguier Y, Iovino M (1984) Vigilance states and cerebral monoamine metabolism in experimental magnesium deficiency. *Magnesium* 3:145-51.

Poleszak E, Szewczyk B, Kedzierska E, Wlaź P, Pilc A, Nowak G (2004) Antidepressant- and anxiolytic-like activity of magnesium in mice. *Pharmacol Biochem Behav* 78:7-12.

Rezvanfard M, Zarrindast MR, Bina P (2009) Role of ventral hippocampal GABA(A) and NMDA receptors in the anxiolytic effect of carbamazepine in rats using the elevated plus maze test. *Pharmacology* 84:356-66.

Schrader LA, Tasker JG (1997) Presynaptic modulation by metabotropic glutamate receptors of excitatory and inhibitory synaptic inputs to hypothalamic magnocellular neurons. *J Neurophysiol* 77:527-36.

Sechenov SI (1975) Activity of Mg 2+, N+ and K+ stimulated ATP-ase in erythrocytes of patients with phobic neurosis and the effect of lithium carbonate in enzymatic activity. *Vopr Med Khim* 21:283-5.

Shekhar A, Keim SR, Simon JR, McBride WJ (1996) Dorsomedial hypothalamic GABA dysfunction produces physiological arousal following sodium lactate infusions. *Pharmacol Biochem Behav* 55:249-56.

Shekhar A, Sajdyk TJ, Gehlert DR, Rainnie DG (2003) The amygdala, panic disorder, and cardiovascular responses. *Ann N Y Acad Sci* 985:308-25.

Singewald N, Sinner C, Hetzenauer A, Sartori SB, Murck H (2004) Magnesium-deficient diet alters depression- and anxiety-related behavior in mice--influence of desipramine and Hypericum perforatum extract. *Neuropharmacology* 47:1189-97.

Stachowicz K, Brañski P, Kłak K, van der Putten H, Cryan JF, Flor PJ, Andrzej P (2008) Selective activation of metabotropic G-protein-coupled glutamate 7 receptor elicits anxiolytic-like effects in mice by modulating GABAergic neurotransmission. *Behav Pharmacol* 19:597-603.

Takase B, Akima T, Satomura K, Ohsuzu F, Mastui T, Ishihara M, Kurita A (2004a) Effects of chronic sleep deprivation on autonomic activity by examining heart rate variability, plasma catecholamine, and intracellular magnesium levels. *Biomed Pharmacother* 58 Suppl 1:S35-9.

Takase B, Akima T, Uehata A, Ohsuzu F, Kurita A (2004b) Effect of chronic stress and sleep deprivation on both flow-mediated dilation in the brachial artery and the intracellular magnesium level in humans. *Clin Cardiol* 27:223-7.

Tanabe K, Osada N, Suzuki N, Nakayama M, Yokoyama Y, Yamamoto A, Oya M, Murabayashi T, Yamamoto M, Omiya K, Itoh H, Murayama M (1997) Erythrocyte magnesium and prostaglandin dynamics in chronic sleep deprivation. *Clin Cardiol* 20:265-8.

Tanabe K, Yamamoto A, Suzuki N, Osada N, Yokoyama Y, Samejima H, Seki A, Oya M, Murabayashi T, Nakayama M, Yamamoto M, Omiya K, Itoh H, Murayama M (1998) Efficacy of oral magnesium administration on decreased exercise tolerance in a state of chronic sleep deprivation. *Jpn Circ J* 62:341-6.

Taborska V (1995) Incidence of latent tetany in patients with panic disorder. *Cesk Psychiatr* 91:183-90.

Tuchendria E, Palamaru I, Papadopol V, Duda R, Laszlo S, Rusu L (1996) Magnesium deficit: a possible causal factor of csome neurotic tendencies in elderly persons. (Abstract) *Magnes Res* 9:232-3.

Viken RJ, Rose RJ, Kaprio J, Koskenvuo M (1994) A developmental genetic analysis of adult personality: extraversion and neuroticism from 18 to 59 years of age. *J Pers Soc Psychol* 66:722-30.

Walker DL, Davis M (2002) The role of amygdala glutamate receptors in fear learning, fear-potentiated startle, and extinction. *Pharmacol Biochem Behav* 71:379-92.

Warton FL, Howells FM, Russell VA (2009) Increased glutamate-stimulated release of dopamine in substantia nigra of a rat model for attention-deficit/hyperactivity disorder--lack of effect of methylphenidate. *Metab Brain Dis* 24:599-613.

Yang YL, Chao PK, Ro LS, Wo YY, Lu KT (2007) Glutamate NMDA receptors within the amygdala participate in the modulatory effect of glucocorticoids on extinction of conditioned fear in rats. *Neuropsychopharmacology* 32:1042-51.

Magnesium, hyperactivity and autism in children

Marianne Mousain-Bosc,[1,✉] *Christian Siatka* [1] *and Jean-Pierre Bali* [2]

[1] Ecole de l'ADN, Museum d'Histoire Naturelle de Nîmes, 19, Grand'rue, 30000 Nimes, France.
[2] Université Montpellier I, 34000 Montpellier, France.
✉ mariannemousain@yahoo.fr

Abstract

For many years, magnesium has been described as a crucial factor for cellular activity. In this chapter, a brief overview of pharmacology and genetics of magnesium transport will be followed by a review of clinical and biological studies of Mg^{2+}/VitB6 supplementation in attention deficit/hyperactivity disorder (ADHD) and autism (autistic spectrum disorders family, ASD) in children. Although to date, no study carried out on a rational basis has been published, some experimental and/or clinical works support the hypothesis of a positive effect of such therapy in these pathologies. All the individual observations report a decrease in hyperactivity and a stabilization of scholarly behaviour with treatment. These data strongly support the need for a controlled study to confirm or invalidate these assumptions.

Introduction

Magnesium is the second most abundant intracellular cation in the body; its main action is to regulate enzyme activity, to control the activity of various calcium and potassium channels, and to promote membrane stabilization. It is also responsible for the maintenance of the transmembrane gradients of sodium and potassium. Magnesium depletion is known to be associated with many clinical diseases including hypocalcemia, hypokalemia, cardiac arrhythmias, neuromuscular excitability, hypertension, atherosclerosis, and osteoporosis. Some evidence indicates that magnesium could also be involved in neurological diseases such as attention deficit/hyperactivity disorder and autism. However, no direct study has been published to confirm this assumption.

Attention deficit/hyperactivity disorder (ADHD) and autism (autistic spectrum disorders, ASD; pervasive developmental disorders, PDD) are different neurological disorders which have been described for many years, and in which the involvement of a deficient magnesium pathway could be suspected given the presence of active transport for such cations through transient receptor potential melastatin (TRPM) channels in brain.

ADHD is the most common neurobehavioral disorder presenting for treatment in youth. Children with ADHD are "a group at risk" as far as their further emotional and social development and educational possibilities are concerned (Spencer *et al*, 2002). An effective intervention for many hyperactive children, beside methylphenidate and other psycho-stimulant drugs, is the use of vitamin B6 (pyridoxine) and magnesium (Mg^{2+}). For over 30 years, parents have given high doses of pyridoxine and Mg^{2+} to their children and have observed decreased physical aggression and improved social responsiveness. However, up until today, very few studies have reported a possible association between magnesium supplementation, ADHD (attention deficit hyperactivity disorders) symptoms, and Mg^{2+} status of the children. The first such study from Liebscher et al (Liebscher and Liebscher, 2003) suggested that patients with ADHD should be considered as potentially Mg-deficient as opposed to a wrong interpretation of the serum Mg test (tetanic patients have lower Mg values than normals). Other studies from Kozielec et al reported for the first time an intra-erythrocyte magnesium deficiency in ADHD children (Kozielec and Starobrat-Hermelin, 1997; Mousain-Bosc *et al,* 2004). We also published similar data (Mousain-Bosc *et al,* 2004, 2006). However, it is not a true "Mg deficiency" with clinically associated respiratory repletion, as that observed in the familial hypomagnesaemia with secondary hypocalcemia (Shalev *et al,* 1998; Mousain-Bosc *et al,* 2004). More precisely, it may be called "intracellular Mg deficiency", affecting mainly neural transmission, which is very sensitive to such ionic variations.

Another group of neuronal diseases in which magnesium has been implicated is ASD/PDD/ autism. Studies from 18 different research groups have shown that B6 and Mg^{2+} are beneficial to about half of autistic individuals, with no significant adverse effects. Eleven of these studies involved a double-blind placebo design and have documented decreases in behavioral problems, improvements in appropriate behavior, and normalization of brain wave activity and urine biochemistry. There is also evidence that B6 and Mg^{2+} may reduce seizure activity. Parent reports confirm improvement in attention, learning, speech/language, and visual contact. More recently, in a pilot study of a moderate dose multivitamin/mineral supplement for children with autistic spectrum disorder, Adams and Holloway (2004) found significant improvements in sleep and gastrointestinal problems compared to the placebo group. Despite all these data, the intervention of Mg-B6 remains controversial and contradictory studies have been published (Vink, 2001; Helpern, 1993; Mousain-Bosc *et al,* 2006; Shalev *et al,* 1998).

So, new data concerning a possible association between Mg-B6 supplementation, neurobehavioral symptoms, and the Mg^{2+} status of children have been published, opening a new way of research in this domain. This chapter will present a review of essential works published in this domain.

Magnesium transport and pharmacology of magnesium

Magnesium transport

The protein involved in Mg permeable channels belongs to the family of TRPM proteins (Schmidt and Taylor 1988; Chubanov *et al,* 2004). The transient receptor potential (TRP) superfamily consists of a large number of cation channels that are mostly permeable to both monovalent and divalent cations. The 28 mammalian TRP channels can be subdivided into six main subfamilies: the TRPC (canonical), TRPV (vanilloid), TRPM (melastatin), TRPP (polycystin), TRPML (mucolipin) and the TRPA (ankyrin) groups. TRP channels are expressed in almost every tissue and cell type and play an important role in the regulation of various cell functions. Currently, significant scientific effort is being devoted to understanding the physiology of TRP channels and their relationship to human diseases. At this point, only a few channelopathies in which defects in TRP genes are the direct cause of cellular dysfunction have been identified. In addition, mapping of TRP genes to susceptible chromosome regions (e.g., translocations, breakpoint intervals, increased frequency of polymorphisms) has been considered suggestive of the involvement of these channels in hereditary diseases. Moreover, strong indications of the involvement of TRP channels in several diseases come from correlations between levels of channel expression and disease symptoms. Finally, TRP channels are involved in some systemic diseases due to their role as targets for irritants, inflammation products, and xenobiotic toxins. The analysis of transgenic models allows further extrapolations of TRP channel deficiency to human physiology and disease.

Two receptors, TRPM6 and TRPM7, have been identified as Mg^{2+} permeable ion channels and their specificity is due to their link with protein kinase. This is the reason why they are defined as chanzymes. Theses chanzymes are involved in Mg^{2+} reabsorption in kidney and intestine. The intake of Mg^{2+} is driven by a transmembrane potential that facilitates the entry of the cation through the TRPM6 channel at the apical part of epithelial cells. The hypothesis is in favor of a Na-dependent flux through ATP-dependent mechanisms (De Franceschi *et al,* 2000; Nilius *et al,* 2007).

In the kidney, different transport pathways for magnesium exist along the nephron. The majority of filtered magnesium is reabsorbed in the thick ascending limb of Henle`s loop via the paracellular route. Observations using genetic studies in affected individuals disclosed the first molecular components of epithelial magnesium transport: the tight junction protein Paracellin-1 (Claudin-16) which was discovered as a key player in paracellular magnesium and calcium reabsorption in the thick ascending limb of Henle`s loop in the distal convoluted tubule (De Franceschi *et al,* 2000; Nilius *et al,* 2007). Mutations of this protein lead to familial hypomagnesemia with hypercalciuria and nephrocalcinosis, a combined urinary magnesium and calcium wasting which almost invariably leads to progression to end stage renal disease.

The discovery of TRPM receptors involved in Mg^{2+} homeostasis (Borella *et al*, 1993; Montell, 2003) serves to identify by genetic engineering and molecular cloning the genes involved in primary inherited hypomagnesaemia. Several genes encoding proteins are directly involved in renal magnesium handling. The family of protein paracellin 1 (PCLN-1) is directly involved in magnesium and calcium reabsorption in the distal convulated tubule (DCT). So diseases such as hypomagnesaemia with secondary hypocalcaemia (HSH) are observed. Reabsorption of magnesium in the DCT is active and transcellular. The renal magnesium leak in HSH patients is due to the role of TRPM6 for active transcellular magnesium reabsorption in the DCT. So the strong interaction between TRPM6 and TRPM7 involves the apical magnesium channel responsible for its uptake from urine into DCT cells. In HSH patients, renal magnesium wasting not only contributes to the development of hypomagnesemia in the postnatal period, but also prevents an adequate conservation of the absorbed magnesium under supplementation.

Hypocalcemia is due to an inhibition of parathyroid hormone caused by a profound hypomagnesemia. Affected children typically manifest during the first months of life with generalized convulsions or signs of increased neuromuscular excitability like muscle spasms or tetany. Reduced clinical symptoms and the normalization of calcium homeostasis are guaranteed by an immediate intravenous administration of magnesium followed by a long substitution with high oral doses of magnesium.

HSH can be also characterized as an autosomal recessive disease due to the gene mapped on chromosome 9q22. Mutational studies on TRPM 6 receptor have shown the same type of HSH; so TRPM 6 is identified as a Mg^{2+} permeable ion channel that causes a combined defect of intestinal and renal magnesium transport.

TRPM6 protein homologous at 52% to TRPM7 was studied together in order to study their regulation. They were functionally characterized as a constitutively active ion channel permeable to a variety of cations like calcium and magnesium. So, TRPM6 and TRPM7 are closely related members of the TRPM transient receptor potential ion channel family named after its founding member melastatin. The pathophysiologic consequences of a TRPM6 defect for magnesium transport in intestine and distal convoluted tubule are important. In the intestine, an active transcellular transport and a passive paracellular pathway were identified. Theses proteins share the unique feature of an atypical kinase domain at their C-terminus for which they have been termed chanzymes (Basso *et al*, 2000; Schlingmann and Gudermann, 2005). The uptake on apical entry into the epithelial cell is a basolateral extrusion mechanism that couples magnesium export to sodium influx. These transport processes yield a curvilinear kinetic for intestinal magnesium absorption. In addition, it has been described that an increased intake of oral magnesium enhances passive paracellular absorption. So, it can be supposed that HSH patients with defective transcellular magnesium transport are able to achieve relief of symptoms and at least subnormal serum magnesium levels.

The electrophysiological and biochemical analyses identified TRPM7 as an important player in cellular magnesium homeostasis; the critical role of TRPM6 for epithelial magnesium transport emerged from the discovery of loss-of-function mutations in patients with a severe form of hereditary hypomagnesemia, called primary hypomagnesemia with secondary hypocalcemia or HSH. TRPM6 plays an important role as an influx pathway for Mg^{2+} (Schmidt and Taylor, 1988; Chubanov *et al*, 2004).

So, TRP channels have a multifunctional role and are involved in many fundamental cell functions investigated in physiopathology and diseases. The TRP superfamily was related to channelopathies, and involves an activation of membrane cation channel. The TRPM subfamilies are distinct families, whereas both TRPM6 and TRPM7 (serine /threonine kinase) exhibit high/variable permeability to Ca^{2+} and Mg^{2+} and are regulated through intracellular levels of Mg^{2+} and Mg-ATP. The defects in these ions channels is supposed to cause various diseases describes as channelopathies. The genetic defect in TRP channels is identified as the direct cause of hereditary disease. Mutations on the TRPM6 gene are liked to human proteinuric kidney disease. TRPM7, the closest relative of TRPM6, is implicated in some neurodegenerative diseases such as amyotrophic lateral sclerosis and Parkinson's disease.

Involvement of magnesium in membrane stability and gene expression

Membrane stability is influenced by many parameters including ionic conductance, ionic fluxes and magnesium (Ebel and Gunther, 2005; Wolf *et al*, 2009). The effect of Mg^{2+}, due to the activity of the superfamily of TRPs channels, is observed on many membranes. It has been reported that the concentration of extracellular Mg^{2+} can affect blood flow, blood pressure and vascular reactivity in intact mammals (Schmidt and Taylor, 1988, Van der Wiijst et al, 2009). The red cell membrane properties have also been explored: Mg^{2+} regulates stability and extends the gross elasticity of the red cell membrane. Magnesium-depleted cells also undergo structural changes on heating below the temperature at which vesiculation sets in.

There is drastic change in ionic flux through the outer and inner cell membranes both in the impaired membranes of cancer, and in Mg deficiency. Researchers from the School of Public Health at the University of Minnesota have just concluded that diets rich in magnesium reduced the occurrence of colon cancer (Chakraborti *et al,* 2002; Aaron, 2006). In another study (Macdonald *et al,* 2004; Susanna *et al,* 2005) women with the highest magnesium intake evidenced a 40% lower risk of developing cancer than those with the lowest intake of the mineral.

Magnesium linked to the phospholipids and more particularly to phosphatidylserine reduces membrane fluidity, and increases the stability of the membrane of pre-synaptic vesicles. Lecithines (phosphatidylcholines) and phosphatidylserines are brain nutrients, which modulate acetylcholine metabolism, and act stimulating memory. A 2003 study (Demougeot *et al,* 2004) describes the lecithins as promoting the synthesis and the working of neurotransmitters involved in memory processes. The mechanism of beneficial action would be linked to activation by choline of phospholipase systems in the hippocampus.

In obstetric and embryonic research, different magnesium salts were studied, such as $MgCl_2$, Mg-acetate and Mg-citrate; they are known to increase and decrease the membrane stability on the two faces of the amnion. $MgSO_4$, Mg-lactate and Mg-nitrate increased the stability on the maternal side, but decreased it on the fetal side. So, addition of magnesium salts modified the human amniotic membrane stability.

In response to a magnesium deficiency, five genes could be identified by using DNA arrays: osteopontin, the cholecystokinin A receptor, connexin 45, a growth hormone receptor and BAG1. Other fundamental studies characterized in bacteria an 'M-box'. It is a genetic switch that is sensitive to Mg^{2+} cellular levels through the conformation of its newly synthesized RNA. This Mg^{2+} sensing riboswitch controls transcription termination in front of a Mg^{2+} transporter gene. So magnesium acts directly as a genetic regulator in genetic expression of RNA in order to control metal ion homeostasis (De Rose, 2007). As magnesium has been shown to activate gene expression, the mitochondrial genome must be affected. A mild mitochondrial dysfunction, and the treatment, may include administration of the mitochondrial cofactors like magnesium (Martin *et al,* 2007).

Action of magnesium on synaptic facilitation

In 2006, a review article (Billiard, 2006; Demougeot *et al*, 2010, 2004) indicated that magnesium is involved in age-related deficits in transmitter release, neuronal excitability, and some forms of synaptic plasticity such as long-term depression of synaptic transmission. Further studies presented by Slutsky et al (2010) show that magnesium is essential for maintaining normal body and brain functions.

Learning and memory are fundamental brain functions affected by dietary and environmental factors. Increasing brain magnesium using a newly developed magnesium compound (magnesium-L-threonate) leads to the enhancement of learning abilities, working memory, and short and long-term memory in rats. Functionally, magnesium increased the number of functional pre-synaptic release sites, while it reduced their release probability. These findings suggest that an increase in brain magnesium enhances both short-term synaptic facilitation and long-term potentiation and improves learning and memory functions. Magnesium impacts upon the release of neurotransmitters, and other mediators or modulators (Slutsky *et al,* 2010).

Magnesium in blood

The study of the regulation of magnesium has gained particular interest in the last decades thanks to the molecular characterization of specific magnesium transporters and the exploitation of molecular biology techniques to clarify their cellular and physiological function(s). Magnesium could be detected both in the plasma in the cationic form (Mg^{2+}) and in blood cells, namely in erythrocytes. All these assays are today well described and can be realized in many laboratories.

In contrast, experimental tools to trace cellular magnesium and to define its homeostasis in living cells have not witnessed a corresponding progress. It was not until recently that efforts were paid to design more appropriate fluorescent indicators that could translate the advances of live imaging techniques into the field of magnesium research (Trapani *et al,* 2010).

Phosphorus magnetic resonance spectroscopy also offers an opportunity to measure *in vivo* the free cytosolic magnesium [Mg^{2+}] of different tissues. In particular, this technique has been employed in human brain and in skeletal muscle providing new hints on Mg^{2+} homeostasis and on its involvement in cellular bioenergetics. In skeletal muscle it has been shown that the changes in free Mg^{2+} concentration occurring during contraction and in post-exercise recovery are mainly due to the influence of cytosolic pH. The possibility of assessing the free cytosolic [Mg^{2+}] in the human brain offered the chance of studying the involvement of Mg^{2+} in different neurological pathologies, and particularly in those where defective mitochondrial energy production represents the primary causative factor in the pathogenesis. Moreover, it has also been shown that the measurement of brain Mg^{2+} can help in the differential diagnosis of neurodegenerative diseases sharing common clinical features, such as Multiple System Atrophy and Parkinson's disease (Ebel *et al,* 2004; Iotti and Malucelli, 2008).

The magnesium concentrations in plasma and cells could be affected by diet, disease and genetic factors. It is known that carcinogenesis induces magnesium distribution disturbances, which cause magnesium mobilization through blood cells and magnesium depletion in non-neoplastic tissues. Magnesium deficiency seems to be carcinogenic, and in the case of solid tumors, a high level of supplemental magnesium inhibits carcinogenesis. Both carcinogenesis and magnesium deficiency increase the plasma membrane permeability and fluidity. Scientists have in fact found out that there is much less Mg^{2+} binding to membrane phospholipids of cancer cells, than to normal cell membranes (Wolf *et al*, 2008).

A progressive elevation in external Mg^{2+} levels in blood will produce a progressive inhibition of most contractile substances. The contractile response observed upon withdrawal of external Mg^{2+} are dependent upon Ca^{2+} concentrations and polarity of the membrane. This response is not related to an inhibition of Na^{+}, K^{+} ATPase. So, it is known that Mg^{2+}, combined with Na^{+} and K^{+}, play a major role in regulating blood pressure and arteriolar tone (Altura *et al*, 1978).

Moreover, magnesium concentrations in plasma and cells could be affected by genetic disease. The genetic factors involved in the regulation of magnesium homeostasis were studied in low (MgL) and high (MgH) magnesium status strains of mice. In this model, magnesium-deficiency affects both plasma, erythrocyte and urine magnesium concentrations in similar proportions in the two strains (Schlingmann *et al,* 2002; Montell, 2005; Günter, 2007; Ozgo *et al*, 2007)

Clinical symptoms of ADHD syndrome

Clinical cases

ADHD has been described since the beginning of the twentieth century and was called hyperkinesia or "psycho-motor instability". It would represent 3 to 9 % of the population of children and adults (Feillet-Coudray, 2005; Biederman, 2006). The clinical picture is that of a hyperirritable, impulsive, aggressive child with an attention deficit; the diagnosis was basically done at the sixth year, when the child presented at primary school. These symptoms impair the emotional development and can lead to serious social and family disorders. In adults, statistics show a powerful link between ADHD and serious problems of life. These findings support the idea that, when diagnosed in the community, ADHD is a clinically significant and highly disabling disorder in adults and must be treated very early in children. However, parents' and children's histories should be studied. In parents: behavioral disorders, such as hyperactivity, aggressiveness, emotional lability, stress, or maternal spasmophilia. During the pregnancy, several symptoms can be observed: weariness, stress, anxiety and breakdown, arterial hypertension, muscle cramps, contractions, sleeping disorders, diet deficiency, and twin pregnancy.

The first signs of ADHD generally appear during the first year of life: sleeping disorders (short sleeping and waking to a small noise), spasm of the sob, tremor of the hands and the arms, intense emotionality, frequent tears, hyper-excitability, often fidgets or squirms, doesn't keeps one's seat, inclination to put in danger their life, climbs, doesn't see the danger. Rapidly, the adaptation to the nursery school at three or four years becomes difficult, with hyper-excitability, impulsivity and difficulty to be a good listener.

At six years, all the clinical symptoms of ADHD as described in DMS-IV manual (Findling *et al*, 1997) are present:
- hyperactivity: fidgets with hands or feet, or squirms in seat; gets up from seat when remaining seated is expected; runs about or climbs when it is not appropriate; is "on the go" or often acts as if "driven by a motor"; talks excessively; blurts out answers before questions have been finished; has difficulties in awaiting their turn; interrupts or intrudes on others; has inclination to put their life in danger.
- impulsivity: becomes aggressive, doesn't control their movements; get angry and stops this aggressiveness with difficulty.
- attention deficit: symptoms of inattention should be present for at least six months and when children are at the primary school; does not give close attention to details or makes careless mistakes in schoolwork or other activities; has trouble keeping attention on tasks or play activities; does not follow instructions and fails to finish schoolwork, chores or duty in the work place (not due to opposite behavior or lack of understanding instructions but due to slowness to execute the tasks); has trouble organizing activities; avoids dislikes or does not want to do things that take a lot of mental effort for a long period of time; loses things needed for tasks and activities (toys, pencils, books or tools); is often easily inattentive; is often forgetful in daily activities and has memory difficulties.

In addition, other clinical symptoms occur frequently and must been considered as main symptoms. These include:
- sleeping disorders: mild sleeping problems; cannot put to sleep; has nightmares, broken sleep; is frightened by the night, and awakes weary; very frequent abdominal pains occurring with stress.
- unexplained weariness: weariness begins in the morning with slowness to stand up, to get dressed, and abnormal weariness in sports activities.
- feeling of faintness with or without losing consciousness; twitches in the face or in the breathing reflect hyper-excitability; gnaws one's nails; anxiety, stress, mood disorders, easily upset; loss of trust and loss of respect of oneself; often breakdown; is afraid of people and frightened to die. The medical examination reveals a Chvostek's signs in 66% sign of hyper-excitable children.

In the clinical description of ADHD, biological data are usually not evoked. However, for instance, hyper-excitability can be revealed by an intracellular magnesium deficiency since magnesium was shown to be involved in the control of some nervous system processes.

Clinical Case Study 1
In the first months of her life, patient OCE presents signs of hyper-excitability; she twiddles her fingers, jumps to a lower noise and wakes often. A prescribed calcium therapy was not effective and the tremors persist. But, alternate calcium and magnesium therapy improves all the signs.

At five years, before beginning primary school, patient OCE again presents signs of hyper-excitability; she is fidgety and doesn't stay in her seat; sleeping disorders have reappeared where she awakes very often and sleeps very little; she was impulsive and slaps children, although it was not intentional; she doesn't control herself and was subject to terrible fist of anger. The possibility of magnesium deficiency is raised since her mother has suffered from "spasmophilia" for some years. Both OCE and her mother showed a decrease in erythrocyte magnesium levels.

After two months of Mg^{2+}/vitB6 treatment, OCE feels better. She has become cool, good, less capricious, doesn't play the fool, and her sleeping is calm. Erythrocyte magnesium is increased and the therapy was accordingly stopped. Rapidly, some months later, all the ADHD signs reappeared including attention deficit, hyperactivity, sleeping disorders and impulsiveness. Biological control confirms the diagnosis of magnesium metabolism disorder (magnesium imbalance) a "genetic disease". The treatment was taken up again with symptoms resolving. However, each time where OCE wants to stop taking the treatment, ADHD symptoms return! OCE received magnesium therapy during eight years: magnesium 6mg/kg/day and vitamin B6 0.6 mg/kg/day (Figure 1).

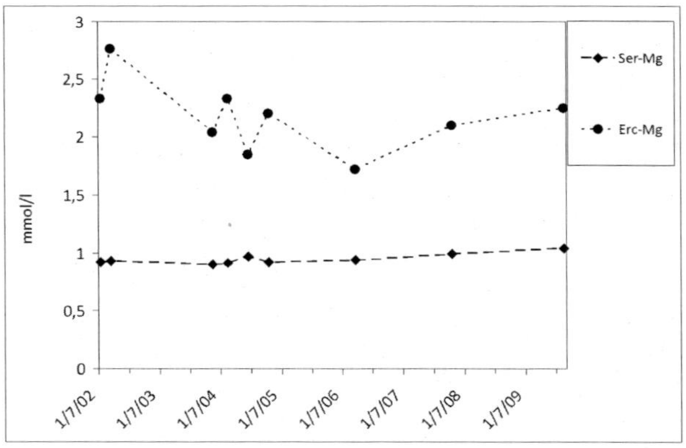

Figure 1. Evolution of biological parameters for magnesium in the case of patient OCE (born February, 1997) during the follow-up (ADHD syndrome). Ser-Mg: total serum magnesium concentrations in mmol/l; Erc-Mg: magnesium concentrations in erythrocytes (obtained after red cell lysis) in mmol/l.

Clinical Case Study 2

Patient NIC was seventeen years old when he came to the consulting office. In the first years of his life, he demonstrated sleeping disorders, a restless sleep, frequent tears, had a delay with communication, was an emotional child, uneasy, over-excitable, and a little aggressive. Upon admission to secondary school, behavioral disorders persisted. He was impulsive, didn't control himself, was aggressive and also had dyslexia.

A diagnosis of ADHD was made and psycho-stimulant treatment was prescribed over three years. He never took the prescribed dosage because his physician (his grand-father) and his pharmacist had warned his parents of the risks of this medication (methylphenidate) listed in the drug category. Rapidly, he presented side effects of this treatment, including sleeping disorders, muscular pains, weariness, "feeling lethargic", behavioral disorders, "became as a zombie", headaches, palpitations, anxiety attacks, breakdowns, and "was frightened to die". His parents were worried by these side effects, and read our publications at the beginning of 2007. The rates of erythrocyte magnesium, calcium, and ionized calcium had dramatically decreased. The parents decided to stop the psycho-stimulant treatment. A magnesium supplementation (300 mg) spectacularly improved patient NIC's behavior: in some weeks, NIC became cool and more relaxed. An excellent participation in scholarly activities and a better concentration in tasks resulted in excellent scholar results in four months. NIC received the "congratulations of the school-board" at the end of the scholar year 2007! NIC could control himself, was not aggressive, had no behavioral disorders, and had self-confidence. In six months, all the biological disturbances were normalized. At the school of "stone cutter for the historic monuments", NIC has excellent assessments: "good student, hardworker"! NIC received a magnesium supplementation for more than three years and each time when he tried to decrease the dose, clinical symptoms reappeared.

The disease, called "*hypomagnesemia with secondary hypocalcemia*", is heritable. NIC's sister was also emotional and hypersensitive while his brother was hyper-excitable, always "on the go " and had both sleeping and behavioral disorders. He had magnesium deficiency and now feels better with magnesium therapy. His mother presented with cramps, muscular pains, pins and needles in the hands, stress and migraines. A biological profile showed an erythrocyte magnesium deficiency; after six months of magnesium therapy, the signs disappeared. The maternal grandfather suffers from Alzheimer disease. His father was emotionally stressed, uneasy and for several years experienced sleeping disorders, heart disease, attention deficit, and above all memory disorders. He is only forty years of age! He had an erythrocyte magnesium deficiency and after six months of the same treatment, the memory improved (Figure 2).

In March 2007, the methylphenidate treatment was stopped and the magnesium therapy was set up. A clear behavioral improvement was observed. However, after the three years of magnesium therapy, all biological data remain

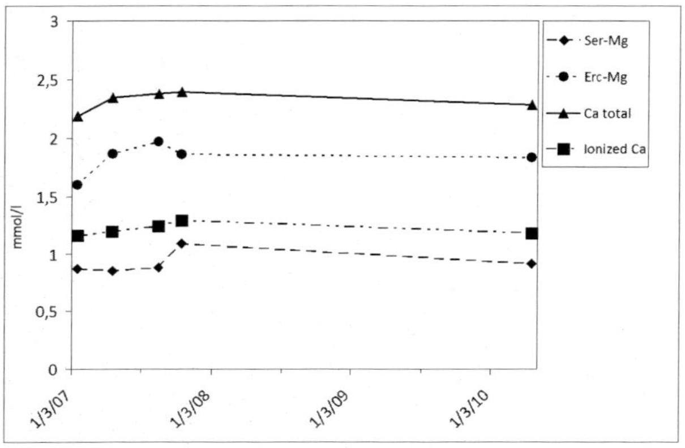

Figure 2. Evolution of biological parameters for magnesium and calcium in the case of patient NIC during the follow-up (ADHD syndrome). Ser-Mg: total serum magnesium concentrations in mmol/l; Erc-Mg: magnesium concentrations in erythrocytes (obtained after red cell lysis) in mmol/l; Total Ca: total serum calcium concentrations in mmol/l; Ionized calcium concentrations in mmol/l in serum.

stable. This result could suggest an alteration of the magnesium transport; it encouraged us to perform additional experiments on magnesium channels in order to check their expression in various tissues.

Experimental Study Number 1

In order to study relationships between hyperactivity symptoms and Erc-Mg levels, we designed an open study on 40 children with ADHD syndrome. For ethical reasons, we chose not to perform a double-blind study against either psychostimulants (methylphenidate) or placebo: parents would not support such a design. In addition, psychostimulants were found to alter magnesium homeostasis (Tolbert *et al*, 1993). Our results (Mousain-Bosc *et al*, 2004) showed a statistically significant improvement of the symptoms after Mg-B6 supplementation, together with a rise in Erc-Mg values.

In this study, a slight but significant intra-erythrocyte Mg^{2+} depletion was evidenced in ADHD patients together with a concomitant decrease in i-Ca concentrations. As we know, Mg^{2+} is essential for normal central activity and Erc-Mg could be representative of intracellular Mg concentrations. A decrease in Erc-Mg without changes in s-Mg concentrations could be interpreted as an alteration of a magnesium transporter (Na^+/Mg^{2+} exchanger) in erythrocytes with concomitant incidences on neuronal Mg concentrations. The impairment to get normal Erc-Mg values under Mg-B6 treatment supports this hypothesis. In addition, Mg pidolate supplementation was found to decrease Na^+/Mg^{2+} exchanger activity with a concomitant rise in Mg^{2+} and K^+ contents of erythrocytes in sickle cell disease (DMS-IV). Erc-Mg was described as a controversial biological parameter for the monitoring of Mg^{2+} deficiency, in contrast to others (Borella *et al*, 1993; Vink *et al*, 2009) who consider Erc-Mg as a suitable index. Moreover, Basso et al (2000) and Helpern et al (1998) present Erc-Mg as not useful for the monitoring of individual changes. We think that in this last study, a 3-week treatment with Mg^{2+} without B6 was too short to induce a durable increase in Erc-Mg (vitamin B6 was described to enhance Mg^{2+} entry through the cell). In any case, in our hands, Erc-Mg measurements were standardized and it appears as a potent indicator of cellular magnesium deficiency.

Ca^{2+} and Mg^{2+} cellular contents classically followed the same pathway: when Mg^{2+} increased, Ca^{2+} also increased. This can explain the significant correlation between Erc-Mg and i-Ca values as well as the fact that in children who have low i-Ca values, Mg therapy increased i-Ca levels. It can be hypothesized that a genetic factor, which modulates Na^+/Mg^{2+} exchanger activity, may be important in the regulation of Mg metabolism (Heath and Vink, 1998).

We also found that increased hyperactivity and decreased scholar attention were associated with decreased Erc-Mg values. This observation was supported by the fact that Mg-B6 supplementation induced a rise in Erc-Mg values and a concomitant improvement of the clinical symptoms. What are the respective roles of pyridoxine and Mg^{2+} in these observations? It was classically accepted that Mg^{2+} is associated with pyridoxine to decrease irritable side-effects of the B6 therapy. We show here evidence of the role of Mg^{2+} itself in this therapy. Previous data support this observation. In ADHD disorders, in which disruptive behavior with hyperactivity was found, psychostimulants are used to improve mental health, probably by increasing synaptic noradrenaline activity. In children who received methylphenidate, a significant increase (6%) in plasma Mg^{2+} concentrations was found depending on the dosage of the drug, showing a relationship between improvement of hyperactivity and Mg^{2+} metabolism (Schmidt *et al*, 1994 (Tolbert *et al*, 1993). More recently, in autistic children with behavioral disorders and hyperactivity (Zilbovicius *et al*, 2000; Schmidt and Taylor, 1988; Chakraborti *et al*, 2002) positive emission tomography (PET) has shown a significant decrease in cerebral blood flow localized at the temporal lobes level in 76% of the children examined. Taken together with the fact that intra-erythrocyte free Mg^{2+} is associated with increased blood pressure (Zilbovicius *et al*, 2000) and that brain from rats fed with low Mg^{2+} diet are more susceptible to permanent brain focal ischemia (Gervais *et al*, 2004), we can hypothesize that intracellular Mg^{2+} deficiency could be responsible, at least in part, of some central activity disorders observed in these children.

The duration of the treatment to get significant improvements seems to be about 8 weeks. Since the cause of this deficiency is yet unknown, and since the symptoms reappeared when the Mg-B6 diet was stopped, the treatment must be maintained for a long time. In addition, while it was difficult to find an evident biological link between central disorders and Erc-Mg values, this biological parameter could be used to select, among the large population of children with hyperactive symptoms, a small population with behavioral abnormalities that is relevant for a Mg-B6 diet. It is evident that another accessible Mg^{2+} store, more significant for central disorders, has to be found.

In conclusion, this study provides additional information about the therapeutic role of a Mg-B6 regimen in children with ADHD. This effect seems to be associated, at least in part, to a cellular Mg^{2+} deficiency, as evidenced by intraeythrocyte Mg^{2+} measurements. Installing a Mg-B6 supplementation for some weeks restored higher intraerythrocyte Mg^{2+} values and significantly reduced the clinical symptoms of these diseases. As chronic magnesium deficiency was shown to be associated to hyperactivity, irritability, sleep disturbances, and low scholar attention, beside other traditional therapeutic treatments, a magnesium supplementation could be required in children with ADHD.

Etiology and risk factors for ADHD

The etiology of ADHD is not yet known. The causes are multifactorial:

- genetics: twin studies indicate that heritability ranges from 60 % to 90 %; various genes are currently being studied (magnesium is involved in gene expression and essential for membrane stability) (Ozgo *et al*, 2007).
- brain abnormalities: it is believed that the dopaminergic system is involved in ADHD. Magnesium has an impact by reducing the release of neurotransmitters and other mediators. Magnesium also stabilizes the membranes (Nemoto *et al*, 2006).
- environmental and peri-natal factors: studies in rats suggest that a magnesium-deficient diet influences not only mineral metabolism but also protein metabolism. Growth retardation results from the low food intake that is induced by magnesium deficiency, which provokes an alteration in energy metabolism. But the protein nutritional status in magnesium-deficient rats is restored by dietary magnesium supplementation in seven days. In women, maternal magnesium intake has an immediate effect on placental vascular flow. Magnesium sulphate reduces the vasoconstriction effect of angiotensin II in human placenta. Reduced placental vascular flow is at least, in part, responsible of placental insufficiency and intrauterine growth retardation. Magnesium deficiency increases the risks of miscarriage symptoms, premature delivery, fetal growth retardation, twin pregnancy, and stress (due illness/depression leading to a loss of magnesium by the kidneys, and increased magnesium requirements); thyroid dysfunction (Takaya *et al*, 2006).
- essential fatty acid imbalance: nutritional factors such as essential fatty-acid (EFA) deficiencies have been associated with ADHD. The principal omega-3 fatty-acid in the brain, DHA, is highly accumulated in nervous tissue membranes and is important for neural function. Studies of diet showed that children with ADHD consumed equal amounts of omega-3 and omega-6 fatty-acid, compared to control children. However, ADHD children had significantly lower levels of DHA and total omega-3 fatty-acids, higher omega-6 fatty-acids, and lower ratios of omega-3/omega-6 fatty-acids, compared to control children. These results suggest that adolescents with ADHD have abnormal EFA profiles, which are not explained by

differences in intake. The role of magnesium will be evoked in the hypothesis of imbalance of essential fatty-acids. Vitamin B6 is also an important cofactor for numerous metabolic reactions including metabolism of serotonin, GABA (gamma-amino-butyric acid) and dopamine (Colter *et al,* 2008, Gonon, 2009).

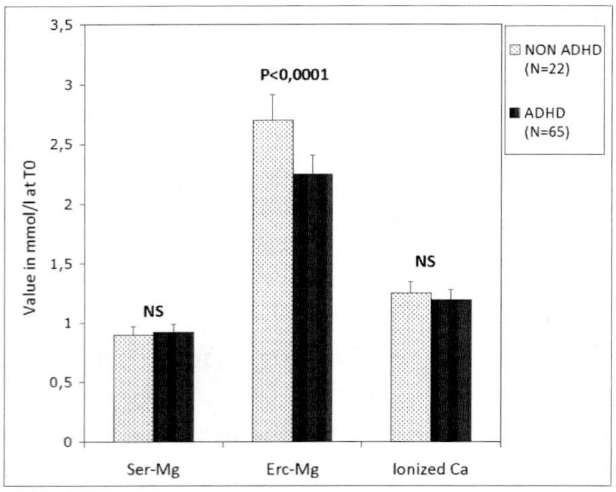

Figure 3. Biological data obtained at the first visit for 65 ADHD and 22 non-ADHD children. Ser-Mg: total serum magnesium concentrations in mmol/l; Erc-Mg: magnesium concentrations in erythrocyte (obtained after red cell lysis) in mmol/l. Only Erc-Mg appeared to be significantly lower than before treatment (statistically significant at $p<0.05$).

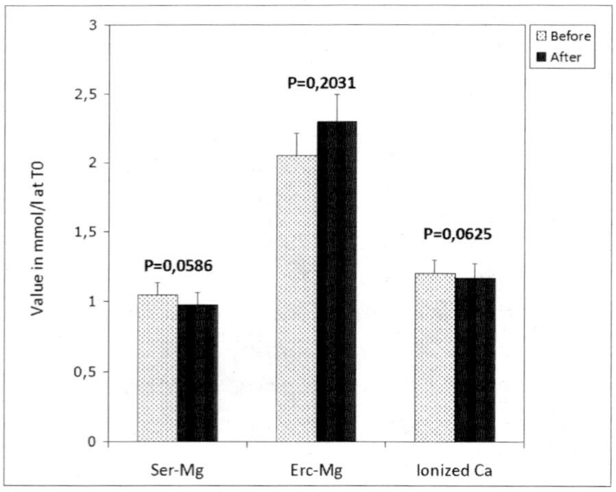

Figure 4. Biological data obtained 3 months after the first visit for the same children. Ser-Mg: total serum magnesium concentrations in mmol/l; Erc-Mg : magnesium concentrations in erythrocyte (obtained after red cell lysis) (in mmol/l). Erc-Mg recovered normal values (statistically significant at $p<0.05$).

Treatment of ADHD

Conventional therapy is often multimodal including behavioral therapies and medications. Approved drugs for ADHD are psychostimulants (amphetamine derivatives), including methylphenidate. Psychostimulant medications approved by the U.S. Food and Drug Administration (FDA) include methylphenidate (Ritalin^R, Concerta^R), and, more recently, atomoxetine (Strattera^R).

In 2008, a study by the National Center of Scientific Research (CNRS) in France (Gonon, 2009) concluded that "*although psychostimulants alleviate the core symptoms of attention deficit hyperactivity disorder (ADHD), recent studies confirm that their impact on the long-term outcomes of ADHD children is null. Psychostimulants enhance extracellular dopamine*". Numerous review articles assert that they correct an underlying dopaminergic deficit of genetic origin. This dopamine-deficit theory of ADHD is often based upon an overly simplistic dopaminergic theory of reward. Psychostimulant medication does not improve long-term academic outcomes of the ADHD children. Therefore, this hypothesis should not be put forward to bias ADHD management towards psychostimulants. The American Journal of Psychiatry in June 2009 published a study "Sudden death and use of Stimulant Medications in Youths". This study was funded, in part, by the FDA and the National Institute for Mental Health (Gould *et al,* 2009). Side effects are described for psychostimulant medications over some years.

As we have seen previously, dietary factors and magnesium deficiency can play a significant role in the etiology of ADHD syndrome. In our study, magnesium deficiency was found in 89% of children with ADHD, whereas only 23% of non-ADHD children present a low erythrocyte Mg^{2+} deficiency (Table1).

Clinical symptoms of autistic spectrum disorders (ASD)

The prevalence of autism increases continuously. It remains an extreme challenge to clinical researchers. It is a neurobiological condition having its origin in a disturbance of the cellular structure of the brain during pregnancy. Generally speaking, there is no "cure" for such children and

Table 1.

Value in mmol/l		Non ADHD (N=22)	ADHD (N=85)
Threshold value		% children < threshold	
Ser-Mg	0.85	0.00	27.69
Erc-Mg	2.46	22.73	81.54
Ionized Ca	1.18	0.00	19.05
At least one criterion under threshold		23.81 (5/21)	88.89 (56/63)

the holy grail of finding a neuropharmacological reversal of symptoms is currently being researched worldwide.

For some years, one must insist on the screening of the early signs of autism during the two first years of the life as described in DMS-IV manual:

- Relationship disorders; too good child with very few smiles.
- Visual contact disorders; missing or poor visual attention; doesn't look at the parents; look is shifty.
- Difficulty in listening; seems not to hear; delayed communication; doesn't repeat words.
- Motor affectation; doesn't take the toys; stereotyped movements of the hands; sits and walks belatedly; hypo-tonicity or hyper-tonicity.
- Sleeping disorders; broken sleep; crying.
- Feeding difficulties; slobbers; cannot swallow; refuses food.

The major feature of autism spectrum disorder is that they only manifest themselves after the age of eighteen months and before the age of three. it is considered like a regression of the development (Burn, 2009). So, we can explain that ASD are disorders of brain function and not of brain structure.

After three years, the clinical picture of ASD becomes typical:

- Impairment of social interactions:
  - visual contact: doesn't look at the parents and the siblings; gives a blank look; look is shifty
  - connection with equals: has no interest with the parents, with the friends at the primary school; seems to be "in their bubble"
  - delight partitions: has no emotional relation with the family, cannot express their pleasure for the event. Social reciprocity: has no answer to a human presence.
- Loss of communication:
  - delayed communication; speaks belatedly; some sounds or some syllables are emitted late; few spontaneous verbal exchanges; lack of creativity in thought.
  - no communication: doesn't repeat words.
  - Stereotypical language: repeats the same word sometimes without significance.
  - social mimicking: cannot reproduce something after a long time earnestly trying.
- Stereotyped restricted behavior:
  - stereotyped interest: he has very poor interest or repeats the same answer for something.
  - customs.
  - handling things: difficulty to take the things, to take toys, and can have abnormal movements.
  - motor affectation: to walk, moves with difficulty; to bring something to somebody, cannot take initiative.
- Abnormal or delayed functioning:
  - language.
  - social interactions.
  - symbolic games: doesn't understand the rules of the game; cannot dream up the game.
  - behavioral disorders like sleeping disorders, aggressiveness, impulsivity; attention deficit cannot listen.

Magnesium metabolism could be involved in autism, autism spectrum disorder or pervasive developmental disorder (Rimland *et al*, 1978): magnesium prevents against encephalopathy and developmental delay (Doyle *et al*, 2008).

Clinical Case Study 3
Patient ARN, three years old, presents all the clinical signs of ASD (Autistic Symptoms Disorder), an autistic disorder that began after two years. The adaptation at the nursery school became difficult. His mother describes behavioral disorders, with incessant restlessness, doesn't listen, puts own life in danger; in the street, let's go the mother's hand; crosses the street without looking around; has important sleeping and communication disorders; he doesn't speak, is always squealing; his glance is shifty. At school, the headmaster's evidence was spectacular: "ARN become isolated, doesn't draw, has no interest with the activities, doesn't listen about the forbidden subjects. He doesn't speak, expresses himself by shouting, his glance is shifty". During the examination, patient ARN was nervous, restless, tetanized, he clench's his fists and shakes h.is hands. In front of all these clinical symptoms, the possibility of a magnesium deficiency is raised; his mother has presented a magnesium deficiency for several years.

With a Mg^{2+}/vitB6 therapy, (6 mg/kg/day of magnesium and 0.6 mg/kg/day of vitamin B6), ARN improved quickly month after month, probably because magnesium supplementation was set up before the age of four years, very early in life. ARN becomes cool, obedient, wants to get dressed alone, put his shoes on, takes interest in the family activities, is looking to manipulate the computer, begins drawing, doesn't cry, says some words and some sentences. At school, he begins to participate in the games, takes a book, shows the pictures and repeats the words. The improvements are spectacular. After six months treatment, he can pronounce "complete sentences" and draws. After eighteen months therapy, the parents stopped therapy, however the behavioral disorders reappeared with incessant restlessness at home and at school in two weeks. Another attempt to stop the treatment was also unsuccessful where he became tired and depressed. The parents now do not want to stop the treatment anymore.

Today, patient ARN is twelve, doesn't present a behavioral disorder and communication and language is almost normal. He begins high school and has taken Mg^{2+}/vitB6 supplementation for eight years (additional biological data: karyotype is 46 XY; fragile X negative).

Clinical Case Study 4
Patient FLO was four years old when the diagnosis of "typical autism" was made. When he was seven years old, the parents were informed about our work on magnesium and autism. He presented communication disorders, could not emit sounds, didn't talk, had abnormal visual reactions, didn't look someone in the eyes, had a blank look and his look was shifty. The behavioral disorders were important with many anxiety attacks, difficulty to calm, impulsiveness and always moving with fits of anger. He had no creativity for the games and didn't know how to play. Erythrocyte magnesium was low. The same observation was made in his parents (Figures 5-7), despite them having a balanced diet including fishes, meats, fruits and vegetables.

After two months treatment, (magnesium 6 mg/kg/day and vitamin B6 0.6 mg/kg/day), patient FLO was more cool, stayed at school with pleasure, began to talk with little sentences, was less in "his bubble", and was looking for his father when he came back from work. He was beginning to play with friends. After three years of treatment, FLO talks appropriately, understands the language, goes to a normal school where reading skills have developed. During the first discussion, the parents advise that they want a third child. They both have evidence of important magnesium depletion. A preventive magnesium supplementation both before the desired pregnancy and during the pregnancy seems to be essential, and indeed allowed good development of the baby without baby blues in the mother. The little sister is now two years old, bright, very much smiling and is always in a good mood! (Additional biological data: search for mutation in the gene neuroligine NLGN3 was negative; search for mutation in the gene neuroligine NLGN 4 X was also negative).

Experimental Study Number 2
In order to study the effect of Mg-B6 for treating social, communication and behavioral responses of children with pervasive developmental disorders (PDD) or autism in connection with the designed an open study on 33 children with PDD magnesium/calcium status of the child, we

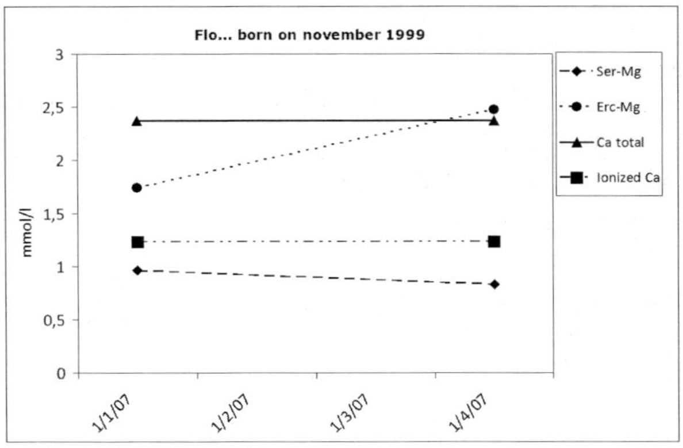

Figures 5. Evolution of biological parameters for magnesium and calcium in the case of patient FLO (born November 1999) during the follow-up (ASD/PED syndrome). Ser-Mg: total serum magnesium concentrations in mmol/l; Erc-Mg: magnesium concentrations in erythrocytes (obtained after red cell lysis) in mmol/l; Total Ca: total serum calcium concentrations in mmol/l; Ionized calcium concentrations in mmol/l in serum.

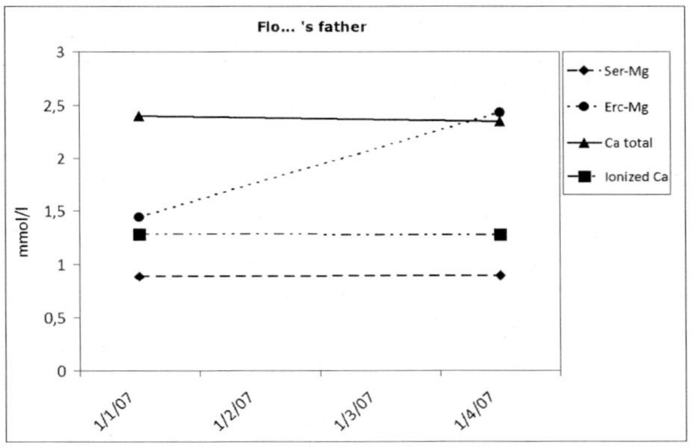

Figure 6. Evolution of biological parameters for magnesium and calcium in the case of patient FLO's father during the follow-up. Ser-Mg: total serum magnesium concentrations in mmol/l; Erc-Mg: magnesium concentrations in erythrocytes (obtained after red cell lysis) in mmol/l; Total Ca: total serum calcium concentrations in mmol/l; Ionized calcium concentrations in mmol/l in serum.

designed an open study on 33 children with PDD syndrome. Our results showed a statistically significant improvement of the symptoms after Mg-B6 supplementation together with a rise in Erc-Mg values (Mousain-Bosc *et al*, 2006).

Intraerythrocyte Mg^{2+} (Erc-Mg), serum Mg^{2+} (s-Mg) and blood ionized Ca^{2+} (i-Ca) were measured

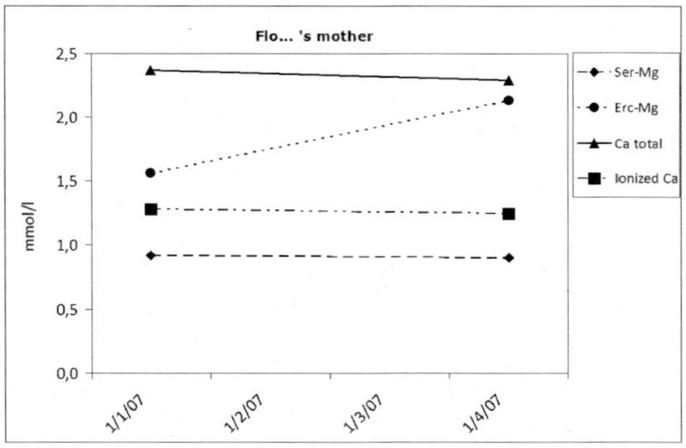

Figure 7. Evolution of biological parameters for magnesium and calcium in the case of patient FLO's mother during the follow-up. Ser-Mg: total serum magnesium concentrations in mmol/l; Erc-Mg: magnesium concentrations in erythrocytes (obtained after red cell lysis) in mmol/l; Total Ca: total serum calcium concentrations in mmol/l; Ionized calcium concentrations in mmol/l in serum.

at different times. Clinical symptoms of PDD were scored (0 to 4). In contrast to s-Mg or i-Ca, PDD children exhibited significantly lower Erc-Mg values than controls (1.26 times; 16/33). The Mg-B6 regimen led to an increase in Erc-Mg values (1.18 times, 11/17) and this supplementation improved PDD symptoms in a large majority of children with no adverse effects: social interactions (23/33, $p<0.0001$), communication (24/33, $p<0.0001$), stereotypical restricted behavior (18/33, $p<0.0001$), and abnormal/ delayed functioning (17/33, $p<0.0001$); 15/33 children improved in the first three groups of symptoms. When the Mg-B6 treatment was stopped, PDD symptoms reappeared in a few weeks. A statistically significant relationship was found in Erc-Mg values from children before treatment and their mothers.

The neurobiological basis of a Mg^{2+}/vit B6 supplementation supposes the existence of an impaired neuronal Mg^{2+} pathway which could be reversed with Mg-B6 therapy. As we have previously discussed, Mg^{2+} acts as an ionic membrane regulator and modulator of ion transfer through membrane channels. In brain, it has been shown that traumatic injury causes a decline in Mg^{2+} concentrations, focally as well as in blood circulation, and contributes to the development of neurologic deficit (Vink *et al*,

2009). Similarly, brain ischemia caused a decline in intracellular free Mg^{2+} concentrations (Basso *et al,* 2000) and magnesium salt administration improves motor outcome in this situation (Ebel and Gunther, 2005). One of its most important modes of action is to inhibit the glutamate N-methyl-D-aspartate (NMDA) channel (Zilbovicius *et al,* 2000). The activity of this channel generates an influx of calcium and, in turn, leads to excitotoxic cell death and apoptosis (Borella *et al,* 1993). In the same way, abnormal dietary deficiency of Mg^{2+} as well as abnormalities in Mg^{2+} metabolism play important roles in different types of heart diseases, and Mg^{2+} influences catecholamine signalling in such diseases (Gervais *et al*, 2004).

Recently, in primary autistic children, positive emission tomography (PET) has been used to demonstrate a significant decrease in cerebral blood flow localized to the temporal lobes in 16/21 of children (Zilbovicius *et al,* 2000; Macdonald *et al*, 2004; Demougeot *et al,* 2004). Taken together with the fact that Mg^{2+} has been shown to increase blood pressure (Macdonald *et al*, 2004) and that brain from rats fed with low Mg^{2+} diet are more susceptible to permanent brain focal ischemia (Demougeot *et al*, 2004), we can hypothesize that intracellular Mg^{2+} depletion could be responsible, at least in part, of some central activity disorders observed in PDD/autistic children.

In our study, an intra-erythrocyte Mg^{2+} depletion was evidenced in almost half of the PDD children. To explain such a phenomenon, two hypotheses can be proposed: (i) a metabolic inhibition of membrane Na^+/K^+ ATPase (observed in autism (Kurup and Kurup, 2003) with concomitant rise in intracellular Ca^{2+} and decrease in intracellular Mg^{2+}; (ii) a genetic defect in magnesium transport through plasma membrane (Na^+-Mg^{2+} exchanger (Ebel et al, 2004; Ebel and Gunther, 2005) or TRPM chanzymes (Montell, 2005). As Erc-Mg can be considered as representative of some intracellular Mg concentrations, a decrease in Erc-Mg without changes in serum Mg concentration could be interpreted as an alteration of Mg^{2+} transport through the plasma membrane. The demonstration that TRPM7 is critical for Mg^{2+} homeostasis evoked the possibility that mutation of TRPM channels may cause disease in humans as a result of reduced intracellular Mg^{2+} levels. Indeed, mutations were found in the case of hypomagnesemia with secondary hypocalcemia disease (Schlingmann *et al,* 2008) and, in this case, symptoms associated with TRPM6 mutations were improved by supplementation with high Mg^{2+} doses, in agreement with increased Mg^{2+} entry through a passive mode of Mg^{2+} influx. This genetic hypothesis was also supported by our own data showing a positive correlation between low Erc-Mg values in PDD children and their mothers. Similarly, Feillet-Coudray et al (2006) have found that, in mice genetically selected for low magnesium levels, Mg efflux from erythrocytes was significantly increased. The genetic regulation of erythrocyte Mg^{2+} content depends on the modification of Mg^{2+} influx (Schlingmann *et al,* 2002). To confirm such a hypothesis, a genetic study of PDD children's family has clearly to be developed.

When PDD children were supplemented with Mg-B6 treatment, Erc-Mg values more or less increased in only 65% of children. The impairment to get normal Erc-Mg values under Mg-B6 treatment supports the hypothesis of a defect in Mg^{2+} transport in erythrocytes. In sickle cell disease, Mg pidolate supplementation was found to decrease Na^+/Mg^{2+} exchanger activity with a partial rise in Mg^{2+} and K^+ contents of erythrocytes (De Franceschi *et al*, 2000). Doses of Mg-B6 and the duration of treatment, which have not been taken into account in our study, could also explain such an observation. Concerning the respective roles of pyridoxine and Mg^{2+} in these observations, it was classically accepted that Mg^{2+} is associated with pyridoxine to decrease irritable side-effects of the B6 therapy and that B6 is the main factor involved in the improvement of clinical symptoms in autistic patients. Following Erc-Mg values during Mg-B6 treatment, we bring here evidence of the role of Mg^{2+} itself in this therapy.

Mg-B6 treatment of PDD children was shown to improve symptoms of the disease. Three of the four main groups of clinical signs described in DSM-IV were significantly reduced and we found for the first time that 8/12 of children who improved under treatment showed higher Erc-Mg values. Persons only slightly deficient in magnesium become irritable, high-strung, sensitive to noise, hyperexcitable, apprehensive and beligerent. If the deficiency is more severe or prolonged, they may develop twitching, tremors, irregular pulse, insomnia, muscle weakness, jerkiness, and leg and foot cramps. These symptoms can also be found in some cases of PDD/autism. Although this study was an open non-controlled study, we found a relationship between clinical signs of PDD/autism and a biological parameter, namely Erc-Mg. However, we were unable to establish any correlation between improvement of symptoms and increase in Erc-Mg. Various possibilities can explain this lack of correlation: (i) Erc-Mg is probably not the best biological parameter to follow the relationship between magnesium homeostasis and neurological dysfunctions of PDD/autism. Contradictory reports have been published on the use of Erc-Mg as index of Mg^{2+} status (Borella *et al*, 1993, Basso *et al*, 2000) and new biological tests that could help to study genetic alterations of magnesium transport (lymphocytes, etc) have to be tested. (ii) Other neurofunctional disorders may be involved in autism, such as a decrease in temporal blood flow. Even if low Erc-Mg levels have been shown to be related to decrease in blood pressure, there is no evidence to associate blood pressure and cerebral blood flow in all cases.

In conclusion, this study brings new information about the therapeutic role of a Mg-B6 regimen in children with PDD syndrome. This effect seems to be associated, at least in part, to a cellular Mg^{2+} depletion as evidenced by intraeythrocyte Mg^{2+} measurements. Children with pervasive developmental disorders (including autism) exhibit low Erc-Mg levels. Parents frequently showed similar low Erc-Mg values suggesting a genetic defect in Mg^{2+} transport. Installing a Mg-B6 supplementation for some weeks restored higher intraerythrocyte Mg^{2+} values and significantly reduced the clinical symptoms of these diseases.

Etiology: role of magnesium during pregnancy

Since developmental disorders appear early during fetal development, magnesium therapy could be justified even during pregnancy. The efficacy of magnesium supplementation is more important if treatment is in the early years of life. Magnesium activates protein synthesis and amino acid synthesis and magnesium deficiency leads to fetal growth retardation by reducing the nutritive utilization of protein as a result of decreased protein absorption and synthesis. Another study found a low cerebral blood flow in the temporal lobe probably due to a low magnesium level in the cells. (Zilbovicius *et al*, 2000)

Effect of magnesium in fragile-X syndrome

Fragile-X syndrome is an X-linked disorder characterized primarily by speech delay and moderate mental retardation and neurobehavioral disorders. The incidence of fragile X syndrome is estimated at 1/4000-1/6000 males and half that for females (Wiesner *et al*, 2004). This disease is linked to the mutation of the FMR1 gene located on the X chromosome, characterized by expansion (CGG amplification) at the FRAXA site (Xq27.3) in the non coding region of the first exon (Weisman-Shomer *et al*, 2002). In 2002, Weisman Shomer revealed two factors indispensable to the stabilization of the CGG tetraplex : magnesium and ATP.

We report a single case of a child referred to our pediatrics unit for a behavioral disorder and for whom Fragile X syndrome had previously been genetically confirmed. Considering the genetic origin of this disease, our work was completed by the clinical and biological evaluation of the patient's family. Both the patient and his affected family members were given a magnesium and vitamin B6 supplementation and evaluated over three years. A couple of family, including children with mental retardation, pervasive development disorder or attention deficit hyperactivity disorder, were followed clinically and biologically for three years. All children carried a mutation produced by expansion at the FRAXA site at Xq 27.3 and showed magnesium and calcium disorders (normal serum Mg^{2+} concentration, but decreased erythrocyte Mg^{2+} and plasma ionized Ca^{2+}). The mother presented a premutation by expansion at the FRAXA site at Xq 27.3 with symptoms of magnesium depletion (emotivity, asthenia, stress). Mg^{2+}/vitB6 supplementation (magnesium 6mg/kg/day and vitamin B6 0.6 mg/kg/day, orally) for three years reduced clinical symptoms in the mother and improved the behavior of the children (aggressiveness, lack of attention at school) concomitant with an increase of intraerythrocyte Mg^{2+}. When the Mg^{2+}/vitB6 treatment was stopped for two months in one of the children, clinical symptoms reappeared.

In 2007, the hypothesis was put forward that Fragile X syndrome (Fra-X) is caused by the transcriptional silencing of the FMR1 gene that encodes the Fra-X mental retardation protein (FMRP) (Dolen *et al*, 2007; Hayashi *et al*, 2007). However, the pathogenesis of this disease is unknown. According to one proposal, many psychiatric and neurological symptoms of Fra-X result from the unchecked activation of mGluR5, a metabotropic glutamate receptor. To test this hypothesis, FMR1 mutant mice presenting a 50% reduction in mGluR5 expression were generated and studied in terms of the range of phenotypes with relevance to the human disorder. Results demonstrated that mGluR5 contributes significantly to the pathogenesis of the disease, a finding that has significant therapeutic implications for Fragile X and related developmental disorders. In line with this observation, Hou et al (2006) demonstrated that mGluR-LTD induces a transient, translation-dependent increase in FMRP that is rapidly degraded by the ubiquitin-proteasome pathway.

The successful management of this disease by magnesium and vitamin B6 supplementation observed in the present study, with an early and late evaluation at 3 years, supports the argument that a deficit in Mg^{2+} influences the appearance of Fra-X and that by replacing this magnesium, the disease symptoms may be managed. Berthelot's group (Martin *et al,* 2007) has previously demonstrated in rats that a deficit in magnesium acts by reducing the level of proteasomes, protein complexes which act at the level of the mGluR5 receptor already implicated in this disease. Conversely, Picado (Picado *et al*, 1994) noted an increase in the levels of Mg^{2+}/NA in patients with behavioral problems and for whom hypertension was diagnosed. It has been demonstrated that for behavioral disorders in which hyperactivity and autism in particular are involved, for which current treatment regimens are difficult to standardize, management of disease symptoms with magnesium and vitamin B6 supplementation is possible (Mousain-Bosc *et al*, 2006). Magnesium depletion represents one possible explanation for the appearance of Fra-X syndrome. Studies show that magnesium-vitamin B6 supplementation given to subjects improved their behavioral disorders. The presence of a genetic mutation together with magnesium deficiency in mothers may constitute an indication for regular evaluation of magnesium status and Mg^{2+}/vitB6 supplementation during pregnancy. We present herein some unpublished data obtained with 3 cases of Fra-X abnormality (poster presentation in Gordon Research Conference, Ventura, CA, March 2008).

Conclusions

This review brings additional information about the therapeutic role of a Mg^{2+}/vitB6 regimen in children with ADHD or ASD/autism syndrome. This effect seems to be associated, at least in part, to a cellular Mg^{2+} depletion as evidenced by intraeythrocyte Mg^{2+} measurements. Children with ADHD or PDD/ASD (pervasive developmental disorders/autistic spectrum disorders), including autism, exhibit low Erc-Mg levels. Parents frequently showed similar low Erc-Mg values suggesting a genetic defect in Mg^{2+} transport. Installing a Mg^{2+}/vitB6 supplement-ation for some weeks restored higher intraerythrocyte Mg^{2+} values and significantly reduced the clinical symptoms of these diseases.

However, in a recent meta-analysis of all studies, Nye et al (2010) arrived at the same conclusion as what they published in 2005: *"Due to the small number of studies, the methodological quality of studies, no recommendation can be advanced regarding the use of B6-Mg as a treatment for autism. There is simply not sufficient evidence to demonstrate treatment efficacy"*. Together with the fact that both the American Psychiatric Association and the American Academy of Pediatrics have stated that megavitamin treatment for learning disabilities and autism is not justified, it helps explain the dearth of clinical studies investigating the use of magnesium and vitamin B6 (Mg-B6) in the treatment of autism and autistic spectrum disorders.

Magnesium is known to be crucial for brain activity and its involvement in the prevention of neurobehavioral diseases seems to be established. As a clinical double-blind study with Mg^{2+}/vitB6 treatment over placebo cannot be accepted for regulatory and ethical reasons, it was suggested to put children under an "alternative treatment" before the conventional drug therapy. We hope that the combined use of new tools to measure intracerebral magnesium levels as proposed by the group of Iotti et al (2008) and a more specific clinical evaluation will help to improve the outcome of children with these pathologies.

Acknowledgements

The authors would like to express their thanks to Professor J.P. Rapin (Dijon) who help them in the conception of the work.

References

Adams JB, Holloway C (2004) Pilot study of a moderate dose multivitamin/mineral supplement for children with autistic spectrum disorder. *J Altern Complement Med* 10:1033-9.

Alexander RT, Hoenderop JG, Bindels RJ (2008) Molecular determinants of magnesium homeostasis: insights from human disease. *J Am Soc Nephrol* 19:1451-8.

Altura BM, Altura BT (1978) Magnesium and vascular tone and reactivity. *Blood Vessels* 15:5-16.

Association AP. (1994). *Diagnostic and Statistical Manual of Mental Disorders DSM-IV-TR Fourth Edition*: American Psychiatric Association.

Basso LE, Ubbink JB, Delport R (2000) Erythrocyte magnesium concentration as an index of magnesium status: a perspective from a magnesium supplementation study. *Clin Chim Acta* 291:1-8.

Biederman J, Faraone SV, Spencer TJ, Mick E, Monuteaux MC, Aleardi M (2006) Functional impairments in adults with self-reports of diagnosed ADHD: A controlled study of 1001 adults in the community. *J Clin Psychiatry* 67:524-40.

Billard JM (2006) Ageing, hippocampal synaptic activity and magnesium. *Magnes Res* 19:199-215.

Borella P, Ambrosini G, Concari M, Bargellini A (1993) Is magnesium content in erythrocytes suitable for evaluating cation retention after oral physiological supplementation in marginally magnesium-deficient subjects? *Magnes Res* 6:149-53.

Burn R (2009) *The Effect of Magnesium Deficiency on Brain Function*: Autism Spectrum Disorder, Neurology, Genetics and Remedial Solutions. The Autism Centre, Carmarthenshire, UK.

Chakraborti S, Chakraborti T, Mandal M, Mandal A, Das S, Ghosh S (2002) Protective role of magnesium in cardiovascular diseases: a review. *Mol Cell Biochem* 238:163-79.

Chubanov V, Waldegger S, Mederos y Schnitzler M, Vitzthum H, Sassen MC, Seyberth HW, Konrad M, Gudermann T (2004) Disruption of TRPM6/TRPM7 complex formation by a mutation in the TRPM6 gene causes hypomagnesemia with secondary hypocalcemia. *Proc Natl Acad Sci USA* 101:2894-9.

Colter AL, Cutler C, Meckling KA (2008) Fatty acid status and behavioural symptoms of attention deficit hyperactivity disorder in adolescents: a case-control study. *Nutr J* 7:8.

De Franceschi L, Bachir D, Galacteros F, Tchernia G, Cynober T, Neuberg D, Beuzard Y, Brugnara C (2000) Oral magnesium pidolate: effects of long-term administration in patients with sickle cell disease. *Br J Haematol* 108:284-9.

De Jesus Moreno Moreno M (2003) Cognitive improvement in mild to moderate Alzheimer's dementia after treatment with the acetylcholine precursor choline alfoscerate: a multicenter, double-blind, randomized, placebo-controlled trial. *Clin Ther* 25:178-93.

Demougeot C, Bobillier-Chaumont S, Mossiat C, Marie C, Berthelot A (2004) Effect of diets with different magnesium content in ischemic stroke rats. *Neurosci Lett* 362:17-20.

DeRose VJ (2007) Sensing cellular magnesium with RNA. *Nat Chem Biol* 3:693-4.

Dolen G, Osterweil E, Rao BS, Smith GB, Auerbach BD, Chattarji S, Bear MF (2007) Correction of fragile X syndrome in mice. *Neuron* 56:955-62.

Doyle LW, Crowther CA, Middleton P, Marret S (2007) Magnesium sulphate for women at risk of preterm birth for neuroprotection of the fetus. *Cochrane Database Syst Rev*:CD004661.

Ebel H, Kreis R, Gunther T (2004) Regulation of Na+/Mg^{2+} antiport in rat erythrocytes. *Biochim Biophys Acta* 1664:150-60.

Ebel H, Gunther T (2005) Na+/Mg^{2+} antiport in erythrocytes of spontaneously hypertensive rats: role of Mg^{2+} in the pathogenesis of hypertension. *Magnes Res* 18:175-85.

Feillet-Coudray C, Coudray C, Wolf FI, Henrotte JG, Rayssiguier Y, Mazur A (2004) Magnesium metabolism in mice selected for high and low erythrocyte magnesium levels. *Metabolism* 53:660-5.

Feillet-Coudray C, Trzeciakiewicz A, Coudray C, Rambeau M, Chanson A, Rayssiguier Y, Opolski A, Wolf FI, Mazur A (2006) Erythrocyte magnesium fluxes in mice with nutritionally and genetically low magnesium status. *Eur J Nutr* 45:171-7.

Fergusson JW RJ, O'Laughlin JW, Banks CV (1964) Simultaneous spectrophotometric determination of calcium and magnesium with chlorophosphonazo III. *Anal Chem* 36:796-99.

Findling RL, Maxwell K, Scotese-Wojtila L, Huang J, Yamashita T, Wiznitzer M (1997) High-dose pyridoxine and magnesium administration in children with autistic disorder: an absence of salutary effects in a double-blind, placebo-controlled study. *J Autism Dev Disord* 27:467-78.

Folsom AR, Hong CP (2006) Magnesium intake and reduced risk of colon cancer in a prospective study of women. *Am J Epidemiol* 163:232-5.

Gervais H, Belin P, Boddaert N, Leboyer M, Coez A, Sfaello I, Barthelemy C, Brunelle F, Samson Y, Zilbovicius M (2004) Abnormal cortical voice processing in autism. *Nat Neurosci* 7:801-2.

Gonon F (2009) The dopaminergic hypothesis of attention-deficit/hyperactivity disorder needs re-examining. *Trends Neurosci* 32:2-8.

Gould MS, Walsh BT, Munfakh JL, Kleinman M, Duan N, Olfson M, Greenhill L, Cooper T (2009) Sudden death and use of stimulant medications in youths. *Am J Psychiatry* 166:992-1001.

Gunther T (2007) Na+/Mg^{2+} antiport in non-erythrocyte vertebrate cells. *Magnes Res* 20:89-99.

Hayashi ML, Rao BS, Seo JS, Choi HS, Dolan BM, Choi SY, Chattarji S, Tonegawa S (2007) Inhibition of p21-activated kinase rescues symptoms of fragile X syndrome in mice. *Proc Natl Acad Sci USA* 104:11489-94.

Heath DL, Vink R (1998) Neuroprotective effects of MgSO4 and MgCl2 in closed head injury: a comparative phosphorus NMR study. *J Neurotrauma* 15:183-9.

Helpern JA, Vande Linde AM, Welch KM, Levine SR, Schultz LR, Ordidge RJ, Halvorson HR, Hugg JW (1993) Acute elevation and recovery of intracellular [Mg^{2+}] following human focal cerebral ischemia. *Neurology* 43:1577-81.

Hou L, Antion MD, Hu D, Spencer CM, Paylor R, Klann E (2006) Dynamic translational and proteasomal regulation of fragile X mental retardation protein controls mGluR-dependent long-term depression. *Neuron* 51:441-54.

Iotti S, Malucelli E (2008) In vivo assessment of Mg^{2+} in human brain and skeletal muscle by 31P-MRS. *Magnes Res* 21:157-62.

Jordt SE, Ehrlich BE (2007) TRP channels in disease. *Subcell Biochem* 45:253-71.

Kidd PM (2002) Autism, an extreme challenge to integrative medicine. Part 2: medical management. *Altern Med Rev* 7:472-99.

Kozielec T, Starobrat-Hermelin B (1997) Assessment of magnesium levels in children with attention deficit hyperactivity disorder (ADHD). *Magnes Res* 10:143-8.

Kuriyama S, Kamiyama M, Watanabe M, Tamahashi S, Muraguchi I, Watanabe T, Hozawa A, Ohkubo T, Nishino Y, Tsubono Y, Tsuji I, Hisamichi S (2002) Pyridoxine treatment in a subgroup of children with pervasive developmental disorders. *Dev Med Child Neurol* 44:284-6.

Lelord G, Callaway E, Muh JP (1982) Clinical and biological effects of high doses of vitamin B6 and magnesium on autistic children. *Acta Vitaminol Enzymol* 4:27-44.

Liebscher D H LDE (2004) About the misdiagnosis of magnesium deficiency. J Am Coll Nutr 23:730S-1S.

Macdonald RL, Curry DJ, Aihara Y, Zhang ZD, Jahromi BS, Yassari R (2004) Magnesium and experimental vasospasm. *J Neurosurg* 100:106-10.

Martin H, Staedtler F, Lamboley C, Adrian M, Schumacher MM, Chibout SD, Laurant P, Richert L, Berthelot A (2007) Effects of long-term dietary intake of magnesium on rat liver transcriptome. *Magnes Res* 20:259-65.

Martineau J, Barthelemy C, Cheliakine C, Lelord G (1988) Brief report: an open middle-term study of combined vitamin B6-magnesium in a subgroup of autistic children selected on their sensitivity to this treatment. *J Autism Dev Disord* 18:435-47.

Montell C (2003) Mg^{2+} homeostasis: the Mg^{2+}nificent TRPM chanzymes. *Curr Biol* 13:R799-801.

Montell C (2005) The TRP superfamily of cation channels. *Sci STKE* 2005:re3.

Mousain-Bosc M, Roche M, Rapin J, Bali JP (2004) Magnesium VitB6 intake reduces central nervous system hyperexcitability in children. *J Am Coll Nutr* 23:545S-8S.

Mousain-Bosc M, Roche M, Polge A, Pradal-Prat D, Rapin J, Bali JP (2006) Improvement of neurobehavioral disorders in children supplemented with magnesium-vitamin B6. II. Pervasive developmental disorder-autism. *Magnes Res* 19:53-62.

Murza KA, Pavelko SL, Malani MD, Nye C (2010) Vitamin B 6-magnesium treatment for autism: the current status of the research. *Magnes Res* 23:115-7.

Nemoto T, Matsuzaki H, Uehara M, Suzuki K (2006) Magnesium-deficient diet-induced reduction in protein utilization in rats is reversed by dietary magnesium supplementation. *Magnes Res* 19:19-27.

Nilius B (2007) TRP channels in disease. *Biochim Biophys Acta* 1772:805-12.

Nilius B, Owsianik G, Voets T (2008) Transient receptor potential channels meet phosphoinositides. *EMBO J* 27:2809-16.

Nye C, Brice A (2005) Combined vitamin B6-magnesium treatment in autism spectrum disorder. *Cochrane Database Syst Rev*:CD003497.

Ozgo M, Bayle D, Zimowska W, Mazur A (2007) Effect of a low magnesium diet on magnesium status and gene expression in the kidneys of mice selected for high and low magnesium erythrocyte levels. *Magnes Res* 20:148-53.

Picado MJ, de la Sierra A, Aguilera MT, Coca A, Urbano-Marquez A (1994) Increased activity of the Mg^{2+}/Na+ exchanger in red blood cells from essential hypertensive patients. *Hypertension* 23:987-91.

Rimland B, Callaway E, Dreyfus P (1978) The effect of high doses of vitamin B6 on autistic children: a double-blind crossover study. *Am J Psychiatry* 135:472-5.

Sanjad SA, Hariri A, Habbal ZM, Lifton RP (2007) A novel PCLN-1 gene mutation in familial hypomagnesemia with hypercalciuria and atypical phenotype. *Pediatr Nephrol* 22:503-8.

Schlingmann KP, Weber S, Peters M, Niemann Nejsum L, Vitzthum H, Klingel K, Kratz M, Haddad E, Ristoff E, Dinour D, Syrrou M, Nielsen S, Sassen M, Waldegger S, Seyberth HW, Konrad M (2002) Hypomagnesemia with secondary hypocalcemia is caused by mutations in TRPM6, a new member of the TRPM gene family. *Nat Genet* 31:166-70.

Schlingmann KP, Gudermann T (2005) A critical role of TRPM channel-kinase for human magnesium transport. *J Physiol* 566:301-8.

Schmidt CJ, Taylor VL (1988) Release of [3H]norepinephrine from rat hippocampal slices by N-methyl-D-aspartate: comparison of the inhibitory effects of Mg^{2+} and MK-801. *Eur J Pharmacol* 156:111-20.

Schmidt ME, Kruesi MJ, Elia J, Borcherding BG, Elin RJ, Hosseini JM, McFarlin KE, Hamburger S (1994) Effect of dextroamphetamine and methylphenidate on calcium and magnesium concentration in hyperactive boys. *Psychiatry Res* 54:199-210.

Schmitz C, Perraud AL, Johnson CO, Inabe K, Smith MK, Penner R, Kurosaki T, Fleig A, Scharenberg AM (2003) Regulation of vertebrate cellular Mg^{2+} homeostasis by TRPM7. *Cell* 114:191-200.

Shalev H, Phillip M, Galil A, Carmi R, Landau D (1998) Clinical presentation and outcome in primary familial hypomagnesaemia. *Arch Dis Child* 78:127-30.

Slutsky I, Abumaria N, Wu LJ, Huang C, Zhang L, Li B, Zhao X, Govindarajan A, Zhao MG, Zhuo M, Tonegawa S, Liu G (2010) Enhancement of learning and memory by elevating brain magnesium. *Neuron* 65:165-77.

Spencer TJ, Biederman, J., Wilens, T.E. & Faraone, S.V (2002) Overview and neurobiology of attention-deficit/hyperactivity disorder. *J Clin Psychiatry* 63:3-9.

Starobrat-Hermelin B, Kozielec T (1997) The effects of magnesium physiological supplementation on hyperactivity in children with attention deficit hyperactivity disorder (ADHD). Positive response to magnesium oral loading test. *Magnes Res* 10:149-56.

Takaya J, Yamato F, Kaneko K (2006) Possible relationship between low birth weight and magnesium status: from the standpoint of "fetal origin" hypothesis. *Magnes Res* 19:63-9.

Tolbert L, Haigler T, Waits MM, Dennis T (1993) Brief report: lack of response in an autistic population to a low dose clinical trial of pyridoxine plus magnesium. *J Autism Dev Disord* 23:193-9.

Trapani V, Farruggia G, Marraccini C, Iotti S, Cittadini A, Wolf FI (2010) Intracellular magnesium detection: imaging a brighter future. *Analyst* 135:1855-66.

Van der Wiijst J, Hodenrop, JGJ, Bindels, RJM (2009) Epithelial Mg^{2+} channel TRPM6: insight into the molecular regulation. *Magnes Res* 22:127-32.

Vink R (2001) Magnesium in traumatic brain injury: past findings and future directions, In: *Advances in Magnesium Research: Nutrition and Health* / Y. Rayssiguier, A. Mazur, J. Durlach (eds.) John Libbey and Company, London, pp. 405-12.

Vink R, Cook NL, van den Heuvel C (2009) Magnesium in acute and chronic brain injury: an update. *Magnes Res* 22:158S-62S.

Voets T, Nilius B, Hoefs S, van der Kemp AW, Droogmans G, Bindels RJ, Hoenderop JG (2004) TRPM6 forms the Mg^{2+} influx channel involved in intestinal and renal Mg^{2+} absorption. *J Biol Chem* 279:19-25.

Walder RY, Landau D, Meyer P, Shalev H, Tsolia M, Borochowitz Z, Boettger MB, Beck GE, Englehardt RK, Carmi R, Sheffield VC (2002) Mutation of TRPM6 causes familial hypomagnesemia with secondary hypocalcemia. *Nat Genet* 31:171-4.

Weisman-Shomer P, Cohen E, Fry M (2002) Distinct domains in the CArG-box binding factor A destabilize tetraplex forms of the fragile X expanded sequence d(CGG)n. *Nucleic Acids Res* 30:3672-81.

Wiesner GL, Cassidy SB, Grimes SJ, Matthews AL, Acheson LS (2004) Clinical consult: developmental delay/fragile X syndrome. *Prim Care* 31:621-5.

Wolf FI, Trapani V, Cittadini A (2008) Magnesium and the control of cell proliferation: looking for a needle in a haystack. *Magnes Res* 21:83-91.

Wolf FI, Trapani V, Cittadini A, Maier JA (2009) Hypomagnesaemia in oncologic patients: to treat or not to treat? *Magnes Res* 22:5-9.

Zilbovicius M, Boddaert N, Belin P, Poline JB, Remy P, Mangin JF, Thivard L, Barthelemy C, Samson Y (2000) Temporal lobe dysfunction in childhood autism: a PET study. Positron emission tomography. *Am J Psychiatry* 157:1988-93.

Magnesium in psychoses (schizophrenia and bipolar disorders)

Mihai Nechifor

Department of Pharmacology, "Gr.T.Popa" University of Medicine and Pharmacy, Iasi, Romania.
✉ mnechif@yahoo.com

Abstract

Schizophrenia and bipolar disorders are two of the most severe CNS conditions. Changes in plasma and intracellular magnesium concentration, as well as other bivalent cations, have been found in both psychoses. Our data, as well as that of other authors, has shown that schizophrenic paranoid patients admitted in the acute state and without previous treatment, have significantly decreased intracellular magnesium levels compared to healthy subjects. Therapy with haloperidol (a typical antipsychotic) or with risperidone (an atypical antipsychotic) both significantly raised the intracellular magnesium concentration without causing significant changes in plasma magnesium concentration. The increase in intracellular magnesium concentration was positively correlated with the improvement in clinical symptomatology. We consider that Mg^{2+} acts foremost by reducing glutamate release and by its action upon NMDA receptors, and results in an augmentation in the activity of the GABAergic systems. Unlike the hypothesis that only implicates zinc deficits in the pathogeny of schizophrenia, we consider that both intracellular magnesium and extracellular zinc deficits are equally involved in schizophrenia pathogeny. In patients with untreated bipolar disorder, our data showed a significant decrease in intracellular magnesium concentration and plasma zinc concentration during the manic episode. Therapy with mood modulators (carbamazepine and valproic acid) increased total intracellular magnesium and plasma zinc concentrations without having a significant effect on total plasma magnesium concentration. Other data showed that lithium also increases intracellular magnesium concentration. The fact that mood modulators with different mechanisms of action have in common the increase of intracellular magnesium concentration is an argument to consider this augmentation as an important element of their mechanism of action.

Introduction

Psychoses are amongst the most severe diseases of the CNS. They are diseases in thought processes and behavior leading to a loss of contact with reality. Various neurological and psychiatric pathologies are associated with changes of plasma and intracellular magnesium and other bivalent cations. Such changes in magnesium concentrations have been observed in brain injury, stroke, headaches, epilepsy, major depression and others (Altura and Altura, 1999; Durlach and Bac, 1997). Schizophrenia and bipolar psychosis present an increasing incidence.

Schizophrenia

Schizophrenia is a chronic and severe brain disorder whose incidence is quite difficult to evaluate. Nonetheless, there are data that show that the prevalence of this disease could arrive at 0.5% of population (Kirkbride *et al*, 2008; Takei *et al*, 1992. It is a psychiatric illness that results in difficulty in telling the difference between real things and ideas and non-real ideas, which causes disturbed thinking and strong and inappropriate emotions. Four basic types of schizophrenia have been described:

1. catatonic schizophrenia;
2. disorganized schizophrenia (hebephrenic schizophrenia);
3. paranoid schizophrenia;
4. undifferentiated schizophrenia.

Identifying the changes in magnesium concentration in schizophrenic patients can be difficult and sometimes contradictory as a result of several factors including diversity of types of disease, unknown time of onset of the disease, and particularities of the disease evolution with periods of reduced intensity in symptoms occurring. In all circumstances, the association of other diseases can also modify intra- and extra-cellular concentrations of magnesium and other bivalent cations.

Some authors have shown increased plasma Mg^{2+} concentrations in schizophrenic patients. Specifically, Jabotinsky-Rubin et al (1993) consider that schizophrenic patients present increased Mg^{2+} plasma concentrations but haloperidol administration reduces Mg^{2+} levels. These authors also show that decreased Mg^{2+} concentration is involved in generation of extrapyramidal side effects of haloperidol, and consider that in schizophrenia, hyper-magnesemia might be correlated with some failure of catecholamine systems in the CNS. Gattaz et al (1983) found a higher Mg^{2+} level in the CSF of the schizophrenic patients. It was stated that schizophrenia appears to increase magnesium concentration in CSF which was associated with decreased neuronal cGMP concentration.

In contrast, other authors didn't find differences in magnesium concentration between healthy subjects and schizophrenic patients. In the studies of Kornhuber et al (1994), postmortem determination of Mg^{2+} concentrations in brain didn't show any differences between the schizophrenic patient group and a control group. Athanassesnas (1983) indicated that there was no difference in plasma Mg^{2+} and Ca^{2+} concentrations in drug free schizophrenic patients.

Finally, other research has shown low Mg^{2+} concentration in the CSF of acute schizophrenic patients but that the levels increase in remitted schizophrenics (Levine *et al*, 1996). Other authors indicated that patients with chronic schizophrenia present magnesium deficiency (Kirov *et al*, 1990; Kanofsky and Sandyk, 1991). Magnesium deficiency was also noted in psychosis induced by cancer chemotherapy (Matzen and Martin, 1985).

Our studies (Nechifor *et al*, 2004) showed that intraerythrocyte total magnesium concentration is significantly lower in patients with paranoid schizophrenia before treatment as compared to normal subjects. The level of intraerythrocyte magnesium was 4.82±0.32 mg/dl in acute paranoid schizophrenia patients as compared to 5.82±0.11 mg/dl in the normal control group ($p<0.05$). In this study, there were no differences between plasma magnesium concentrations of schizophrenic patients and the healthy subjects (18.2±11 mg/L in schizophrenic patients; 18.7 ±2.17 mg/L in the control group).

Kirov and Tsachev (1990) observed a raise in plasma magnesium level in schizophrenic patients in clinic remission, but other studies haven't found any correlation between the decrease in plasma magnesium concentration and the symptoms of schizophrenic patients (Kirov *et al*, 1994).

The analysis of extracellular magnesium and other bivalent cation concentrations in postmortem schizophrenic patients in a variety of cerebral areas (hippocampus, amygdala, caudate nucleus, cortex) showed significant differences between the drug-free schizophrenic group and treated schizophrenic patients. There weren't significant differences regarding magnesium concentration but drug-free schizophrenic patients presented an increased copper level and a reduced zinc level.

We tested the effect of two different anti-psychotic drugs (haloperidol and risperidone) in therapeutic doses on plasma and erythrocyte total magnesium concentrations in acute paranoid adult schizophrenic patients. Our data (Nechifor *et al*, 2004) showed that both typical antipsychotic drugs (haloperidol and risperidone) induced a raise in the intraerythrocyte magnesium concentration and also improved the clinical symptoms in paranoid schizophrenia patients. The data indicated a raise in erythrocyte magnesium concentration after haloperidol treatment from 4.82±0.32mg/dl to 5.46± 0.19mg/dl ($p<0.05$) and after risperidone treatment to 5.28±0.21 mg/dl ($p<0.05$). The antipsychotic drugs tested have very different mechanisms of action. Haloperidol is a strong blocker of D1, D2 and α1 receptors and a weak blocker of 5-HT2A receptors. Risperidone is a strong blocker of D2 receptors and 5-HT2A receptors, but a very weak blocker of D1 receptors.

Renn et al (2010) also found an increased magnesium level in schizophrenic patients treated with antipsychotics, which is in agreement with our data. These data favor the idea that an increase in magnesium concentration is not a peripheral phenomenon, but an essential element for the mechanism of action of the antipsychotic drugs utilized in schizophrenia treatment. However, there is also contrary information whereby treatment with classic neuroleptics decrease plasma concentrations of magnesium and chronic treatment with neuroleptics may even produce hypomagnesemia in some schizophrenics (Alexander et al 1979).

Regarding the involvement of variations in magnesium concentrations in the etiopathogeny of psychosis, we should take into account that intracellular magnesium plays more roles than extracellular magnesium and intracellular total magnesium and free Mg^{2+} are compartmentalized between cells organelles and the cytosol (*Gunther et al*, 2006). In terms of the glutamatergic hypothesis of schizophrenia that involves the imbalance between glutamate and dopamine with an excess of glutamate (Krebs, 1992), an increase in magnesium concentration induced by typical and atypical neuroleptic administration is mainly involved in reduction of NMDA receptor activation by glutamate. In this circumstance, Mg^{2+} reduces the neuronal Ca^{2+} entrance through Ca^{2+} channels coupled with NMDA receptors. We suppose that Mg^{2+} acts in the same way in experimental phencyclidine model of psychosis. We believe that the increase of cell Mg^{2+}level is important for antipsychotic action of haloperidol and risperidone. The effect of magnesium could be produced by decreasing neuronal response to glutamate stimulation of NMDA receptors, decreasing the presynaptic release of glutamate, decreasing formation of peroxide radicals, and increasing GABAergic activity and glycine synthesis; glycine inhibits catecholamine release (Johnson *et al*, 1994).

The increase in magnesium concentration can reduce anxiety, hallucinations and agitation whereas hypomagnesemia could exacerbate anxiety and hallucinations. Ang et al (1993) considered that hypomagnesemia is one of the causes of antipsychotic treatment resistance. The improvement of the clinical state and the increase in intracellular magnesium concentration leads to the idea that magnesium might be involved in the development of the antipsychotic drugs therapeutic effect. The positive effect of increased magnesium concentration could be explained by the decreased activity of NMDA receptors in the same measure in which the excessive activity of some glutamatergic brain systems are involved in some psychotic symptoms.

Some postmortem studies in human subjects have also showed abnormalities of GABAergic systems in schizophrenia patients. There is evidence for a deficit in GABA-containing interneurons in the prefrontal cortex (Beasley *et al*, 2002; Reynolds *et al*, 2001). There are biochemical and morphological arguments for a deficit in GABAergic systems in schizophrenia and this deficit is limited to the parvum-albumin class of GABAergic interneurons (Blum and Mann, 2002). It is possible that by increasing neuronal magnesium concentration with antipsychotic drugs, GABAergic systems are activated and the partial deficit of the GABAergic cortical systems are corrected. Regarding the mechanisms by which magnesium can increase the activity of the GABAergic systems, there are at least two possibilities: by enhancement of vesicular GABA-transporter activity (Gerstein *et al*, 2005) or by modulation of $GABA_A$ receptor activity (Stanley *et al*, 1995). There is evidence that magnesium potentiates the function of native and recombinant $GABA_A$ receptors and Moykkyven et al (2001) suggested a putative Mg^{2+} binding site on the $GABA_A$ receptor complex.

One of the most promising therapeutic prospects is the use of drugs acting at metabotropic glutamate receptors. Krystal et al (2010) described the potential of mGluR2 and mGluR5 agonists and allosteric positive modulators in the treatment of schizophrenia. Magnesium has a positive modulator effect at the level of some mGlu receptors. We believe that the increase of intracellular magnesium concentration after antipsychotic drug treatment allows magnesium to exert this modulator role, especially at mGluR5 and mGluRz and possible at mGluR7 level. By these means, magnesium not only reduces the glutamate action at the level of NMDA receptors but also can increase the GABAergic activity and reduce presynaptic glutamate release.

Autism is one of the main symptoms of schizophrenia but there are also patients with autism (especially children) who are not considered to be schizophrenic. In autistic children that are not schizophrenic, Strambi et al (2006) showed that there are no differences in intracellular Mg in autistic children versus normal children. Unlike autistic children, patients with schizophrenia have significantly lower plasma Mg and intracellular concentration compared with normal subjects. We consider this fact as an argument for a different pathogeny of autism compared with schizophrenia. Regarding the effect of treatment with vitamin-B6-magnesium in children with autism syndrome (non-schizophrenic), there are contradictory data. Nyl and Brice (2002) maintain that in these children (a small number of cases studied), a favorable effect of this treatment might exist. However, Findling (1997) showed no significant differences between the treated and placebo group.

Eating disorders and cognitive dysfunction has also been identified in schizophrenia (Wobrock *et al*, 2009). The serum levels of glutamate and glutamine in schizophrenic people with anorexia and cognitive impairment were significantly higher than those in the control group. Based on these findings, Nakazato et al (2010) hypothesized that change in the glutamate concentrations are involved in the mechanism of cognitive impairment and anorexia of schizophrenic patients. We are in agreement with this point of view and we consider that magnesium, decreasing the action of glutamate upon NMDA receptors, could contribute in the improvement of these symptoms in schizophrenic patients.

Although the etiopathogeny of schizophrenia is not sufficiently known, we consider that \increase in magnesium concentration by antipsychotic therapy is not a secondary phenomena but is part of the mechanism of action of antipsychotics. We consider that these data indicate that the changes of intracellular magnesium concentration are important for neuroleptic drug action in schizophrenic patients, and the fact that antipsychotic drugs with different chemical structures and mechanisms of action induce the increase in intracellular magnesium levels further supports the previous idea. Contrary to Andrews (1992), who supported only the zinc deficiency theory of schizophrenia, we consider that intracellular magnesium and plasma zinc deficiency play an important role in the pathogenic mechanism of schizophrenia. The increase in intracellular magnesium concentration is important, and is not just a side effect of the therapeutic action of typical and atypical antipsychotics.

Bipolar disorders

Bipolar disorder (BD), also called manic-depressive psychosis, is an affective psychosis. It is a recurrent and severe psychiatric disease characterized by episodes of mania followed by depression and by mood instability. Without adequate treatment BD is associated with high rates of mortality. BD is considered a relatively frequent psychiatric disease. Vacheron-Trystan et al (2004) consider that the prevalence of BD over a lifetime is around 1% in the general population. There are several forms of BD. According to DSM IV the first type of BD (the most frequent one) has a dominance of manic symptoms, associated with depression periods. After DSM IV, there are two main subtypes of BD: type I BD with at least one manic episode or several manic and depressive episodes; type II BD is related to patients enduring recurrent depressive episodes.

There are a few data, sometimes contradictory, regarding magnesium and other bivalent cation concentrations in patients with bipolar disorder, although they haven't all been made in the same type of BD or at the same stage of this disease. Decreasing Mg^{2+} level could exacerbate anxiety, weakness and other symptoms in BD patients (Kirov and Tsachev, 1990). Frazer et al (1983) found an increased level of erythrocyte magnesium concentration in patients with bipolar disorder before hospitalization. Contrary to this, George et al (1994) highlight significant changes of magnesium concentration in CSF of BD patients and cannot establish a correlation between the disease outcome and this cation concentration. Some authors have reported a decreased plasma magnesium concentration in BD patients compared to healthy control (Herzberg and Herzberg, 1977) while others found a disturbed ratio between plasma calcium and magnesium concentrations. An increased calcium/magnesium ratio was correlated with manic agitation (Carman *et al*, 1979).

The current medication is mood modulators, the most commonly used drug from this category being lithium, and some anticonvulsive substances that have proven to be effective in BD, such as carbamazepine, sodium valproate, lamotrigine and lamotrigine (Arban *et al*, 2005). More rarely used in the treatment of BD are gabapentine and topiramate. Also, some atypical antipsychotics such as olanzapine, clozapine and risperidone have been administered in BD.

Lithium was and remains one of the most utilized mood modulators in BD therapy, especially in patients with the dominance of manic symptoms, although its therapeutic utility has a tendency to diminish (Gay and Olie, 2005). The data regarding the influence of lithium administration upon serum magnesium concentrations are variable. Most studies show that repeated lithium salt administration increases magnesium concentration. Lithium increases the intracellular magnesium concentration by competing with magnesium for some intracellular binding sites (Leyden *et al*, 2000). Some data demonstrate Li^+/Mg^{2+} competition at therapeutic intracellular Li^+ concentration (after treatment) in human neuroblastoma SH-SY5Y cells (Abukhdeir *et al*, 2003). After experimental loading of neuroblastoma cells with 1-2 mM of extracellular Li^+, the intracellular free magnesium concentration was significantly higher. With respect to Li^+ and Mg^+ competition at some intracellular sites, the existing data have identified the following molecules as sites of competition: G-protein transducin in the guanosine 5'-diphosphate bound conformation (Srinivasan *et al*, 2004); inositol monophosphatase; glycogen synthase kinase 3 (GSK-3); fructose 1,6 biphosphatase; biphosphate nucleotidase (Gould *et al*, 2004); and finally, ATP and ADP phosphate binding sites. It is also possible that other intracellular binding sites for Li^+/Mg^{2+} competition exist. Rybakowski and Szaynerman (1976), hypothesized that magnesium could increase the lithium intracellular influx. This could be another magnesium involvement in the mechanism by which lithium reduces the clinical symptoms from bipolar disorders.

Our data (Nechifor *et al*, 2006; 2007) show that adult patients with bipolar disorder type I presenting acute manic attacks and with no previous treatment exhibit lower intracellular magnesium levels than the control group. Plasma zinc concentration was also significantly lower (0.72±0.02 mg/l versus 89±0.12 mg/l ($p<0.05$). There were no significant differences between patients with bipolar disorder type I and the control group with respect to plasma total magnesium concentration.

Carbamazepine treatment (600mg/day per os 4 weeks) and respectively sodium valproate (900mg/day 4 weeks) significantly increased intracellular magnesium levels from 45.0±1.87 mg/l before treatment to 52.02±0.9 mg/l after sodium valproate, and 53.72±2.18 mg/l after carbamazepine ($p<0.05$). Plasma magnesium concentration wasn't significantly modified but there was a significant rise in plasma zinc concentration (Nechifor *et al,* 2005; 2006). Walden et al (1993) showed that magnesium deficiency decreased the beneficial effect of carbamazepine in the treatment of epilepsies but we think that hypomagnesemia also decreases the effect carbamazepine in the treatment of affective disorders. Magnesium oxide increases the verapamil maintenance therapy in mania (Giannini *et al,* 2000). This fact favors the idea that an increase in magnesium concentration is an important fact, maybe essential for the therapeutic effect of some drugs used in BD treatment. Magnesium valproate reduces the hyperactivity in an animal model of mania. This effect of magnesium valproate could be abolished by bicuculline, suggesting that actions on postsynaptic GABA may also be involved in the antimanic action of magnesium valproate (Cao and Peng, 1993).

We consider that the increase in intracellular magnesium concentration is an important feature of carbamazepine, valproic acid and other mood modulators used in BD treatment. We also consider that transmembrane calcium influx plays an important role in the development of some psychiatric disorders. The calcium channel antagonists (verapamil and others) increase the carbamazepine effect. Magnesium, acting like a natural calcium antagonist on some ionic channels, is a factor that contributes at the pharmacodynamic effect of some mood modulators. In contrast, calcium ions have an antagonistic effect on carbamazepine action. Carbamazepine reduces the neuronal excitability and glutamate release and we consider that this effect is due at least in part by increasing magnesium concentration.

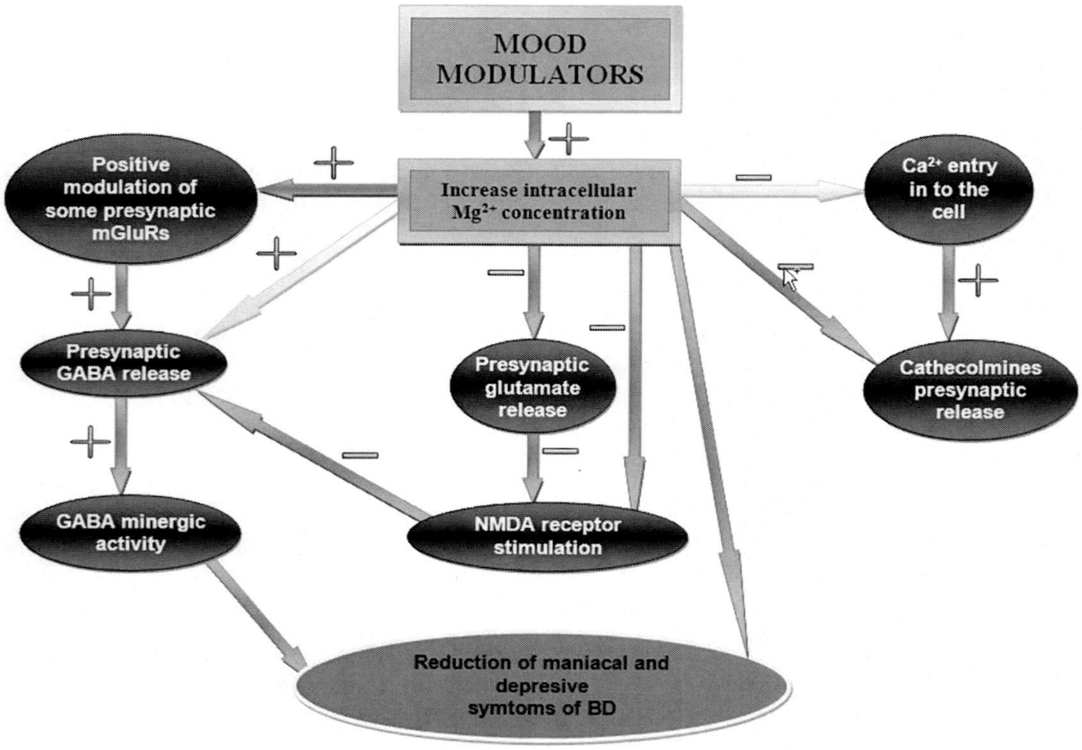

Figure 1. The mechanism of magnesium's involvement in mood modulator action. + = stimulation; - = inhibition

The increase in intracellular magnesium concentration at the neuronal level is important for all the mood modulator drugs utilized in BD therapy and not only for lithium (Nechifor *et al*, 2008). Some of the possible mechanisms describing magnesium's involvement in mood modulator action are presented in Figure 1. Gobbi and Janiri, 2006 showed that magnesium valproate significantly modulates the response induced by NMDA-receptor stimulation. Chuinard et al (1990) showed that magnesium aspartate administration was effective in stabilizing the mood of rapid-cycling BD, which favors the idea that the increase in magnesium concentration is an important factor of lithium and other mood modulators mechanism of action. Heiden et al (1999) administered magnesium sulphate iv as supplementary treatment in severe acute mania.

In conclusion, we suggest that the increase in plasma zinc level and the erythrocyte magnesium level is not a peripheral phenomenon but is involved in the mechanism by which some mood modulators can reduce clinical symptoms of bipolar disorders, not only the manic episodes of BD but also the depressive periods. The changes in intra and extracellular plasma magnesium concentrations and other bivalent cations are an important part of the mechanism of action of some mood modulators and other psychotropic drugs.

References

Abukhdeir AM, Layden BT, Minadeo N, Bryant FB, Stubbs EB Jr, Mota De Freitas D (2003) Effect of chronic Li^+ treatment on free intracellular Mg^{2+} on human neuroblastoma SH-SY5Y cells. *Bipolar Disord* 5(1):6-13.

Alexander DR, Deeb M, Bitar F, Antun F (1986) Sodium-potassium, magnesium and calcium ATP-ase activities in erythrocyte membranes from maniac-depressive patients responding to lithium. *Biol Psychiatry* 21:997-1007.

Altura BM, Altura BT (1999) Association of alcohol in brain injury, headaches and stroke with brain-tissue and serum levels of ionized magnesium. *Alcohol* 19:119-130.

Andrew RC (1992) An update of the zinc deficiency theory of schizophrenia. Identification of the sex determininig system as the site of action of reproductive zinc deficiency. *Med Hypotheses* 38:284291.

Ang AN, Ko SM, Tan CH (1995) Calcium, magnesium and psychotic symptoms in a girl with idiopathic hypoparathyroidism. *Psychoso. Med* 57:299-302.

Athanassenas G, Papadopoulos E, Kourkoubas A, Tsitourides S, Gabriel Hoidas E, Frangos E (1983) Serum calcium and magnesium levels in chronic schizophrenics. *J Clin Psychopharmacol* 3:212-216.

Arban R, Marian G, Brackenborough K, Winyard L, Wilson A, Gerard P, Large C (2005) Evaluation of the effects of lamotrigine, valproate and carbamazepine in a rodent model of mania. *Behav Brain Res* 158(1):123-132.

Beasley CL, Zhang ZJ, Patten I, Reynolds GP (2002) Selective deficits in prefrontal cortical GABAergic neurons in schizophrenia defined by the presence of calcium-binding proteins. *Biol. Psychiatry* 52(7):708-715.

Blum BP, Mann JJ (2002) The GABAergic system in schizophrenia. *Int J Neuropsychopharmacol* 5:159-179.

Cao BJ, Peng NA.(1993) Magnesium valproate attenuates hyperactivity induced by dexamphetamine-chlordiazepoxide mixture in rodents. *Eur J Pharmacol* 237: 177-181.

Carman JS, Post R, Runkle DC, Bunney Jr. WE, Wyatt RJ (1979) Increased serum calcium and phosphorus with the switch into maniac or excited psychotic state. *Br J Psychiatry* 135:55-61.

Chouinard G, Beauclai I, Geiser R, Etienne P (1990) A pilot study of magnesium aspartate hydrochloride (Magnesiocard) as a mood stabilized for a rapid cycling bipolar affective disorder patients. *Prog Neuropsychopharmacol Biol Psychiatry* 14(2):171-180.

Durlach J, Bac P (1997) Mechanisms of action in the nervous system in Magnesium deficiency and dementia, In *Mineral and Neurotoxicity* (Yasui M, Strong MJ, Ota K, Verit MA, eds) CRR Press, Boca Raton, 27-38.

Frazer A, Ramsey TA, Swann A (1983) Plasma and erythrocyte in affective disorders. *J Affect Disorder* 5:103-113.

Findling RL, Maxwell K, Scotese-Wojtila L, Huang J, Yamashita T, Wiznitzer M (1997) High-dose pyridoxine and magnesium administration in children with autistic disorder: an absence of salutary effect sin a double-blind placebo-controlled study. *J Autism Dev Disord* 27:467-478.

Gattaz WF, Kattermann R, Gattaz D, Beckmann H (1983) Magnesium and calcium in the CSF of schizophrenic patients and healthy controls: correlations with cyclic GMP. *Biol Psychiatry* 18:935-939.

Gay C, Olie JP (2005) Management of bipolar disorders. *Rev Prat* 55(5):513-522.

George MS, Rosenstein D, Rubinow DR, Kling MA, Post RM (1994) CSF magnesium in affective disorders lack correlation with clinical course of treatment. *Psychiatry Res* 5:139-146.

Giannini AJ, MacKenzie AM, Melemis SM, Ventresco J, Condon M (2000) Magnesium oxide augmentation of verapamil maintenance therapy in mania. *Psychiatry Res* 93(9):83-87.

Gerstein M, Huleihel M, Mane R, Stilman M, Kashtuzki I. Hallak M, Golan H (2005) Remodelling of hippocampal GABAergic system in adult offspring after maternal hypoxia and magnesium sulphate load: immunohistochemical study. *Exp Neurol* 196:18-29.

Gobbi G. Janiri L (2006) Sodium and magnesium valproate in vivo modulate glutamatergic and GABAergic synapses in the medial prefrontal cortex. *Psychopharmacol* 185(2):255-262.

Gould TD, Quiroz JA, Singh J, Zarate CA, Manji HK (2004) Emerging experimental therapeutics for bipolar disorder: insights from the molecular and cellular actions of current mood stabilizers. *Mol Psychiatry* 9:734-755.

Gunther T (2006) Concentration, compartmentation and metabolic function of intracellular free Mg^{2+}. *Magnes Res* 19:225-236.

Heiden A, Frey R, Presslich O, Blasbichle T, Smetana R, Kasper S (1999) Treatment of severe mania with intravenous magnesium sulphate as a supplementary therapy. *Psychiatry Res* 3:236-246.

Herzberg L, Herzberg B (1977) Mood change and magnesium. A possible interaction between magnesium and lithium. *J New Ment Dis* 163:423-426.

Jabotisky-Rubin K, Durst R, Levitin LA (1993) Effects of haloperidol on human plasma magnesium. *J Psychiatry Res* 27:155-159.

Johnson D, Blandina P, Goldfarb J (1994) Glycine inhibition of glutamate evoked release of norepinephrine in hypothalamus is strycnine-insensitive. *Brain Res* 650:70-74.

Kanofsky JD, Sandyk R (1991) Magnesium deficiency in chronic schizophrenia. *Int J Neurosci* 61:87-90.

Kirkbride JB, Boydell J, Ploubidis GB, Morgan C, Dazzan P, McKenzie K, Murray RM, Jones PB (2008) Testing the association between the incidence of schizophrenia and social capital in an urban area. *Psychol Med* 38:1083-1094.

Kirov GK, Birch NJ, Steadman P, Ramsey RG (1994) Plasma magnesium levels in a population of psychiatric patients: correlation with symptoms. *Neuropsychobiology* 30:73-78.

Kirov GK, Tsachev KN (1990) Magnesium, schizophrenia and maniac-depressive disease, *Neuropsychobiology* 23:79-81.

Kornhuber J, Lange KW, Kruzik P, Rausch WD, Gabriel E, Jellinger K, Riederer P (1994) Iron, copper, zinc, magnesium and calcium in postmortem brain tissue from schizophrenic patients. *Biol Psychiatry* 36:31-34

Krebs MO (1995)Glutamatergic hypothesis of schizophrenia: psychoses induced by phencyclidine and cortical-subcortical imbalance. *Encephale* 21:581-588.

Krystal JH, Mathew SJ, D'souza DC. Garakani A, Gunduz-Bruce H, Charney DS (2010) Potential psychiatric applications of metabotropic glutamate receptor agonists and antagonists. *CNS Drugs* 24:669-693.

Layden B, Diven C, Minadeo N, Bryant FB, Mota de Freitas D (2000) Li^{+}/Mg^{2+} competition at therapeutic intracellular Li^{+} levels in human neuroblastoma SH-SY5Y cells. *Bipolar Dis* 2:2000-2004.

Levine J, Rapoport A, Mashiah M, Dolev E (1996) Serum and cerebrospinal levels of calcium and magnesium in acute versus remitted schizophrenic patients. *Neuropsychobiology* 33:169-172.

Matzen TA, Martin RL (1985) Magnesium deficiency in psychosis induced by cancer chemotherapy. *Biol Psychiatry* 20:788-794.

McLean MJ, McDonald RL (1986) Sodium valproate but not ethosuximide produces use and voltage dependent limitation of high-frequency repetitive firing of action-potentials of mouse central neurons in cell culture. *J Pharmacol Exp Ther* 238:727-738.

Moykkyen T, Uusi-Oukari M, Heikkla J, Lovinger DM, Luddens H, Korpi ER (2001) Magnesium potentiation of the function of native and recombinant GABA A receptors, *Neuroreport* 12:2175-2179.

Murck H (2002) Magnesium and affective disorders, *Nutr Neurosci* 5:375-389.

Nakazato M, Hashimoto K, Schmidt U, Tchanturia K, Campbell IC, Collier DA, Iyo M, Treasure J (2010) Serum glutamine, set-shifting ability and anorexia nervosa. *Ann Gen Psychiatry* 9: 29-43.

Nechifor M (2007) Magnesium in Psychoses, in *New Perspectives in Magnesium Research – Nutrition and Health*, (Nishizawa Y, Mori H, Durlach J, eds) Springer-Verlag, London, 369-377.

Nechifor M, Vaideanu C, Mindreci I, Borza C (2006) Variation of magnesium concentrations in psychoses, In: *Advances in Magnesium Research-New Data* (Porr P J, Nechifor M, Durlach J, eds) John Libbey Eurotext, Paris. 25-30.

Nechifor M, Vaideanu C, Palamaru I, Borza C, Mindreci I (2004) The influence of some antipsychotics on erythrocyte magnesium and plasma magnesium, calcium, copper and zinc in patients with paranoid schizophrenia. *J Am Coll Nutr* 23:5493-5519.

Nechifor M, Vaideanu C, Mandreci I, Palamaru I, Boisteanu P (2005) Research on plasma and erythrocyte concentration of some bivalent cations in patients with bipolar disorders, In (Ermidu-Pollet S., Pollet S. eds.) *Proceedings Book of 3rd International Symposium on Trace Elements in Humans - New Perspectives*, Athens 150-159.

Nechifor M (2008) Interaction between magnesium and psychotropic drugs. *Magnes Res* 21:97-100.

Nye C, Brice A (2005) Combined vitamin B6-magnesium treatment in autism spectrum disorder. *Cochrane Database Syst Rev* 19(4):CD003497.

Renn JH, Yang NP, Choup P (2010) Effects of plasma magnesium and prolactin in quantitative ultrasound measurements of heel bone among schizophrenic patients. *Muscoloskeletal Disord* I:35-52.

Reynolds GP, Zhang ZJ, Beasley CL (2001) Neurochemical correlates of cortical GABAergic deficits in schizophrenia: selective losses of calcium binding protein immunoreactivity. *Brain Res Bull* 55:579-584.

Rybakowski J, Szaynerman Z (1974) Lithium-magnesium relationship in red blood cells during lithium prophylaxis. *Pharmakopsychiatr Neuropsychopharmacol* 9:242-246.

Srinivasan C, Toon J, Amari L, Abukhdeir AM, Hamm H, Geraldes CF, Ho YK, Mota De Freitas D (2004) Competition between lithium and magnesium ions for the G-protein transducin in the guanosine 5'-diphosphate bound conformation. *J Inorg Bioche*m 98:691-701.

Staley KJ, Soldo BL, Proctor WR (1995) Ionic mechanisms of neuronal excitation by inhibitory $GABA_A$ receptors. *Science* 269:977-981.

Stambi M, Longini M, Hayek J, Berni S, Macucci F, Scalacci E, Vezzosi P (2006) Magnesium profile in autism. *Biol Trace Elem Res* 109:97-104.

Takei N, Lewis G, Sham PC, Murray RM (1992) Age-period-cohort analysis of the incidence of schizophrenia. *Br J Psychiatry* 26: 963-973.

Vacheron-Trystram MN, Braitman A, Cheref S, Affray L (2004) Antipsychotics in Bipolar disorders. *Encephale* 30:417-424.

Warden J, Grunze H, Mayer A, Dusing ., Schirrmacher K, Liu Z, Bingmann D. (1993)Calcium antagonistic effects of carbamazepine in epileptics and affective psychoses. *Neuropsychobiology* 27:171-175.

Wobrock T, Ecker UK, Scheerk H, Schneider-Axmann T, Falkdi P, Gruber O (2009) Cognitive impairment of executive function as a core symptom of schizophrenia. *World J Biol Psychiatry* 10:442-451.

Magnesium and major depression

George A. Eby,[1,✉] *Karen L. Eby* [1] *and Harald Murck* [2]

[1] George Eby Research Institute, 14909-C 2109 Paramount Avenue, Austin, Texas 78704, USA.
[2] Clinic of Psychiatry and Psychotherapy, University of Marburg, 35043 Marburg, Germany.
✉ george.eby "at" george-eby-research.com

Abstract

The treatment of major depression is still a major unmet medical need in the majority of patients. Sixty percent of cases of MD are treatment-resistant depression (TRD), showing that classical treatments for MD are poorly effective to non-effective. Magnesium has been largely removed from processed foods, especially refined grains, in the Western world harming the brain and causing mood disorders. Magnesium deficiency causes N-methyl-D-aspartate (NMDA) coupled calcium channels to be biased towards opening which causes neuronal injury and neurological dysfunction, which we believe results in MD. Oral administration of Mg to animals produced antidepressant-like effects that were comparable to those of antidepressant drugs. Cerebral spinal fluid (CSF) Mg has been found low in suicidal TRD. The first report of Mg treatment for agitated depression was published in 1921 showing success in 220 out of 250 cases. One 2008 randomized clinical trial showed that Mg was as effective as the tricyclic antidepressant imipramine in treating MD. Intravenous and oral Mg protocols have been reported to rapidly terminate MD safely and without side effects. Brain Mg deficiency reduces serotonin levels, and antidepressant drugs have been shown to have the action of raising brain Mg. Excessive calcium, glutamate and aspartate intake can greatly worsen MD. We believe that – when taken together – there is more than sufficient evidence to implicate inadequate dietary Mg as contributing to the cause of MD, and we suggest that physicians prescribe Mg for its prevention and treatment.

Incidence of major depression

Neuropsychiatric disorders account for 36% of all non-communicable illnesses. They are the leading cause of all disability (more than twice that of cardiovascular diseases and malignant neoplasms) in the United States and Canada. Depressive disorders cause 40% of all neuropsychiatric disorders (World Health Report, 2004). Without magnesium (Mg) treatment, major depression (MD) is expected to affect up to 25 percent of the American population at some point in their lives. Besides core symptoms of depression, i.e. depressed mood and lack of energy, other symptoms may vary, but nevertheless have strong effects on patient quality of life. These include increased or decreased appetite and weight and sleep disturbances, in particular difficulties falling asleep, maintaining sleep and, in melancholic depression, early morning awakening. Emotional reactivity can be very different with increases in sensitivity to social challenges, easy upset, sadness on the one hand and an unresponsive mood, which leaves patients with "feelings of feelinglessness" on the other hand. Feelings of guilt and sadness can be very pronounced, leading to suicidal ideation and finally suicide itself.

Increasing incidence of depression

Americans are developing MD at higher rates and younger ages than ever before. People born around 1900 rarely had childhood or early adult depression and only about one percent ever developed depression. People born between 1935 and 1944 had a one percent incidence of depression by age 15, a 2 percent rate of depression by age 25 and 9 percent incidence by age 45. People born in 1955, had a one percent incidence of depression by age 15, a 6 percent incidence by age 25, and a lifetime incidence of 25 percent (Meyer and Quenzar, 2005).

The onset of depression has greatly increased in incidence, and it is affecting people much earlier in their lives during the late 20th century and early 21st century than before the 20th century (Meyer and Quenzar, 2005). The reasons for these findings are not quite clear, but inadequate dietary Mg is prevalent in America and is the most likely cause. There is probably a real increase in depression, coupled with a change in diagnostic habits, which has to do with the element of stigma. Lower stigma leads to a higher rate of diagnosis. Modern antidepressant drugs are better tolerated than first generation antidepressive treatments which, in terms of a risk-benefit analysis, makes less severely affected subjects candidates for psychopharmacological intervention. Unfortunately, antidepressant and anti-anxiety medications commonly in use have a tendency to promote suicide, especially in young people (Stone, 2009).

Classical depression treatments

Among those who seek professional help for clinical depression, some patients find relief for their condition using therapies based on modification of monoaminergic systems. Newer generation antidepressants are now used and they include selective serotonin reuptake inhibitors (SSRIs), combined serotonin/noradren-aline reuptake inhibitors, and drugs which interact with monoaminergic receptors such as mirtazapine. First generation antidepressants like monoamine oxidase inhibitors (MAOIs) and tricyclic antidepressants are now rarely used because they are not well tolerated.

Treatment-resistant depression

A large proportion of the burden caused by depression is attributable to treatment-resistant depression (TRD). Only half of patients who are treated with a first line pharmacological therapy of an SSRI respond and only 30% experience remission (Trivedi *et al*, 2006). If a second drug also fails, a commonly used criterion for TRD is fulfilled. Treatment-resistant depression is highly recurrent with as many as 80% of those requiring multiple treatments relapsing within a year of achieving remission. For those with a more protracted illness, the probability of recovery within 10 years is about 40%. Patients with TRD are more likely to suffer from comorbid physical and mental disorders, to experience marked and protracted functional impairment, and to incur higher medical and mental healthcare costs. Thus, in order to reduce the substantial burden caused by depression, TRD is a central focus of medical research (Fekadu *et al*, 2009). Apart from the complete non-responders there are many patients who fulfill criteria of "remission" but still have symptoms severe enough to interfere with their quality of life, i.e. residual symptoms (Nierenberg *et al*, 2010). Besides quality of life implications of residual symptoms, their presence predicts relapse of depressive disorders. This shows that even in the group of remitted subjects an unmet medical need remains.

Markers and risk factors of major depression

Major depression is a disorder which has both psychological and physiological causes and risk factors. Because psychological causes may trigger pathophysiologic mechanisms, there is overlap. In this article we are focusing primarily on physiology of MD with some reference of MD as a stress-related disorder. We also focus on systems which may be related to Mg-dependent regulation.

Biological markers of depression or depression-vulnerability

There are certain biomarkers which have been described in patients with depression and in "high risk" populations; meaning those who never have had MD, but who have a close relative that does (Lauer *et al*, 1995; Modell *et al*, 1998). These biomarkers include an increased stress hormone axis (HPA-axis), a higher density of rapid eye movements in sleep EEGs and less slow-wave sleep (SWS), particularly in the first sleep cycle (Krieg *et al*, 2001). Lower SWS and higher HPA axis activity were also identified as risk factors for a relapse in patients, who were in remission after a depressive episode (Hatzinger *et al*, 2004). Not all studies confirm these points, in particular with regard to HPA axis findings (Ising *et al*, 2005). This suggests biological variability in subjects with a risk for depression.

A more recently indentified potential marker for depression is aldosterone, which is increased in patients with depression (Emanuele *et al*, 2005; Murck *et al*, 2003). This may be of importance, as aldosterone is a primary regulator of Mg. As both aldosterone and cortisol are regulated by ACTH there could be a correlation between the two phenomena (Murck, 2002).

Typical sleep disturbances occur in MD including falling asleep, staying asleep and early morning awakening, or hypersomnia and excessive napping. Sleep EEG patterns have been indentified for MD. Rapid eye movement (REM) sleep changes occur with a shorter latency to the first occurrence of REM, a higher number of eye movements during REM sleep, i.e. a higher REM density, and in some subjects reduced duration of slow wave sleep (Steiger and Kimura, 2010; Thase *et al*, 1997). Subjective reports of sleep disturbances may also be predictive of a depressive episode. A review of eight epidemiological studies concluded that insomnia, lasting for a period of 2 weeks, was predictive for development of depression in the subsequent 1 - 3 years (Riemann and Voderholzer, 2003). Insomnia at baseline and 1 year post-baseline compared with those with no sleep complaints was strongly predictive of a future MD (adjusted odds ratio, OR=39.8; P<0.01) (Ford and Kamerow, 1989). Another study (van den Berg *et al*, 2007) found a similar association for hypersomnia. Sleep disturbances and neuroendocrine data are correlated, in particular hypercortisolism is correlated with the number of awakenings and reduced SWS (Hubain *et al*, 1998).

Several cardiovascular factors, especially low systolic blood pressure, are risk factors for MD (Gilmore *et al*, 1995; Paterniti *et al*, 2000). Subjects with MD show lower heart rate variability (HRV) (Udupa *et al*, 2007). Insomnia is related to a lower HRV (Spiegelhalder *et al*, 2010). Heart rate variability appears to increase with successful treatment. Reduced HRV is a risk factor for depression in patients with coronary heart disease (Pizzi *et al*, 2008).

Inflammatory markers are an additional area of potentially useful predictive markers for depression. Plasma IL-6, TNFα and prostaglandin E2 (PDE2) are of relevance (Murck *et al*, 2004; Zorrilla *et al*, 2001). Elevated inflammatory markers are related to non-response to the most frequently used antidepressants today, i.e. SSRIs (Eller *et al*, 2008; O'Brien *et al*, 2007). Anti-inflammatory agents appear to have anti-depressant effects, as in the case of TNFα-antagonists (Uguz *et al*, 2009), cyclooxygenase inhibition (Muller *et al*, 2006) and omega-3 fatty acids (Murck *et al*, 2004).

Changes in dietary magnesium

Against the wide-spread belief that Western countries have the best fed people on planet Earth, there is evidence that serious deficits in dietary Mg in the Western world are related to an increased risk for MD and biological markers of depression. For a long time it was not accepted that food could have any influence on brain structure or its function including cognitive, mood and intellectual development. It is now absolutely certain that Mg plays vital roles in all major metabolisms in oxidation-reduction and in ionic regulation among its other roles in the brain (Bourre, 2006) and in mood disorders Dietary magnesium intake has steadily declined over the preceding century, due to: (1) the practice of refining grain to make processed foods, (2) making dietary choices low in magnesium-rich foods such as whole grains, rice and wheat bran, nuts, seeds, chocolate, peanuts, peanut butter and green leafy vegetables, (3) strong chemical sequestration of metals during food processing and (4) complete removal of minerals from drinking water processed by distillation, de-salination and reverse osmosis so prevalent in the Middle East, Australia and elsewhere. Only 16% of the original Mg and 24% of the original zinc found in whole wheat remain in refined wheat (Anonymous, 2002). These circumstances reduced average bioavailable Mg consumption from 450 mg in the 19th century and before to 250 mg per day or less in the 20th and early 21st centuries, resulting in significant and unhealthy Mg deficiency in the majority of the population (Seelig and Rosanoff, 2003). Approximately 68% of U.S. adults consume less than the U.S. recommended daily allowance (RDA) of Mg (420 mg / day for men, 320 mg / day for women), with 19% consuming less than half of the RDA (Jacka *et al*, 2009). Deficiency of dietary Mg has been related to depressive disorders (Rasmussen *et al*, 1989; Hashizume and Mori, 1990). The pathological signs of Mg-deficiency and possible reasons for its development have been reviewed earlier (Morris, 1992; Durlach, 1984; Durlach *et al*, 1995; Durlach *et al*, 1997; Durlach, 2002). A recent study confirmed the epidemiological relationship between low dietary Mg intake and the risk of developing depression (Jacka *et al*, 2009).

Conversely, extensive marketing and resultant consumption of excitotoxic glutamates and aspartates have very greatly increased over the same period, even though there is a strong connection between dietary and endogenous excitotoxin excess and neurological dysfunction and mental illness (Blaylock, 1999; Walton *et al*, 1993).

Regulation of brain magnesium

The concentration of Mg within the brain results from a highly regulated process. Its concentration in cerebrospinal fluid (CSF) is higher than that in plasma, pointing to the existence of active transport systems between these compartments (Morris, 1992). Magnesium moves out of CSF into blood by passive diffusion and bulk filtration (Oppelt *et al*, 1963). These dynamics result in relative stability of intra-cerebral Mg concentration even in case of Mg depletion. Up to 40 days of Mg depletion led only to a small global intra-cerebral decrease in Mg concentration in rats, however important regional differences existed (Poenaru *et al*, 1997). The brainstem seemed particularly vulnerable to Mg depletion. Increasing Mg administration had no strong influence on CSF Mg concentrations. Only small changes in CSF Mg after prolonged supplementation were reported in dogs (Kemeny *et al*, 1961; Schain, 1964). However, chronic dietary Mg deficits led to proportional changes in CSF and brain cellular Mg (Chutkow, 1974).

It is of importance to note that metabolism of Mg depends on endocrine parameters. Administration of aldosterone led to an enhancement of urinary excretion of Mg in humans (Horton and Biglieri, 1962). Acute β-adrenergic stimulation with adrenaline or salbutamol reduced plasma Mg in humans (Whyte *et al*, 1987), pointing to an adrenergic mechanism of Mg regulation. The parathyroid is influenced by Mg in its function, and it regulates Mg levels and distribution (Zofkova and Kancheva, 1995). Inadequate central nervous system (CNS) concentration of Mg^{2+} has a critical level below which neurological dysfunction occurs (Yasui *et al*, 1997; Langley, 1991).

Acute emotional stress, which involves an activation of the SNS and the HPA axis, led to an increase in Mg excretion in humans (Grases *et al*, 2006) and experimental animals (Altura *et al*, 1992), the latter resulting from reduced tissue and serum Mg. Swim stress in animals led to an activation of several stress hormone systems and an increase in Mg in plasma, but a decrease in brain Mg (Poleszak *et al*, 2005). This shows that tissue Mg is more relevant than plasma Mg. Stress induced decrease in brain Mg could be counteracted with additional administration of the tricyclic antidepressant imipramine. This finding is complicated by observation that co-administration of both imipramine and Mg has a beneficial behavioral effect, but does not counteract the reduction of brain Mg-concentration resulting from swim stress. Therefore, increased sympathetic nervous system (SNS) activity could lead to increased Mg excretion. This suggests that stressful activities result in lowered Mg content of the CNS and potentially and increased risk of depression.

Similarly, thyroid function is related to Mg regulation. In 135 un-medicated patients with mild to moderate major depressive disorder, a significant correlation between mean serum Mg^{2+} levels and mean circulating T4 thyroid level was observed. There was no significant correlation between any other thyroid indices and either serum Mg^{2+} or Ca^{2+}. The thyroid axis is known to regulate Mg metabolism possibly by regulation of transport of Mg^{2+} from extracellular to intra-cellular fluid compartments. For T4, and to a lesser extent serum Mg^{2+}, the most consistent changes were observed with response to anti-depressant treatment (Joffe *et al*, 1996).

Changes of serum magnesium in major depression

Our following review of serum Mg and depression shows greatly conflicting results, perhaps because 99% of Mg is intracellular with only 1% being found in serum (Mann and Truswell, 2002), and perhaps because some of the work used magnesium oxide, which is not bioavailable (Firoz and Graber, 2001; Lindberg *et al*, 1990; Walker *et al*, 2003; Enya *et al*, 2004).

In patients with low serum Mg, depressive symptoms have been observed (Hashizume and Mori, 1990). Deficits of Mg may result from inadequate intake, malabsorption, or renal loss of Mg that occurs in certain disease states such as alcoholism and diabetes, and with certain drug therapies (antidiuretics, aminoglycosides, fluoroquinolones, cisplatin, digoxin, cyclosporin, amphotericin B) (Morris, 1992). Resulting Mg-deficiencies may lead to depressive symptoms which are secondary to an underlying somatic disease, like diabetes mellitus (Barragan-Rodriguez *et al*, 2007). In depressed patients, an early study reported a decrease in total plasma Mg, but not in ionized Mg, with an increase in total Mg occurring after treatment with electroconvulsive therapy or tryptophan (Frizel *et al*, 1969). Higher serum (Bjorum, 1972) and plasma Mg levels have been reported in patients with recurrent depression independent from their actual state, i.e. as a trait marker (Cade, 1964; Widmer *et al*, 1992). Widmer stressed the importance of gender and clinical subtypes of depressive disorder. They also reported an association between increases in plasma Mg and severity of depression and of plasma cortisol (Widmer *et al*, 1995). Another group reported that depressive symptoms were positively correlated with serum Mg in longstanding depression and remission, but not in acute depression (Linder *et al*, 1989). A further study shows the same relation in patients with unipolar depression (Hasey *et al*, 1993). In other studies, this finding could not be confirmed (Naylor *et al*, 1972; George *et al*, 1994). A further study compared serum Mg and serum Ca/Mg ratio of 145 drug free patients with MD. They compared MD patients to a group of non-mood disordered patients without finding any difference between groups (Young *et al*, 1996). In another study no changes in absolute values of plasma Mg concentration could be observed in patients with a variety of psychiatric disorders. An association between the amount of Mg plasma disturbance (either higher or lower than normal) and severity of clinical disturbance was shown (Kirov *et al*, 1994). Research subjects, who did not meet criteria of any specific psychiatric disorder, were studied to explore their experiences with depression, anxiety and stress in relation to Mg-levels. Subjects were not differentiated on the basis of high vs. low Ca/Mg ratios, but on the basis of Mg tertiles. The group in the middle tertile had the lowest levels of depression and stress in comparison to upper and lower tertiles (Jung *et al*, 2010). A more recent study found a decreased serum Mg concentration in patients with more severe depression (Hamilton depression score > 23), whereas no change was observed for less severely affected subjects (Nechifor, 2009). The studies of Kirov *et al*, 1994 and Jung *et al*, 2010 could point to the fact that closer specification of depressive disorders may be required. Gender differences (with lower concentrations in women) exist in plasma Mg concentrations in patients with depression (Herzberg and Herzeberg, 1977; Herzberg and Bold, 1972; George *et al*, 1994), possibly contributing to the variability seen in the mentioned studies. Furthermore, it appears that medication should be controlled, as anti-depressant compounds have been reported to influence Mg-metabolism, as measured as changes in erythrocyte Mg concentration in the course of antidepressant treatment (Nechifor, 2009). It is unclear if this is a direct effect of the compounds (sertraline and amitriptyline) or an indirect effect of clinical improvement of subjects.

In patients with depression an increase in aldosterone concentration has been observed (Murck *et al*, 2002a). Under physiologic conditions an increase in aldosterone concentration should lead to an increased excretion of Mg . Reports of an increase in serum Mg points to a disturbance in Mg regulation in these patients, which may also involve a higher grade of Mg mobilization from intracellular pools. On the other hand a deceased sensitivity of mineralocorticoid receptors (MR), which are the primary responsible receptor for aldosterone regulation in the kidney, has been reported. This points to a potentially complex Mg dysregulation. It would be of importance to determine the relationship between Mg and aldosterone concentration in order to clarify this issue.

In contrast to peripheral changes in plasma or serum, changes within the CNS point to a brain Mg-deficiency. In subjects with MD, a decrease in CSF Mg concentration has been confirmed (Banki *et al*, 1986; Banki *et al*, 1985). A more recent study found an increase in the Ca/Mg ratio of CSF in patients with depression (Levine *et al*, 1999). Most recently, postmortem studies in patients that had depression showed a reduced Mg concentration in brain tissue (Nowak *et al*, 2010). Human brain Mg measurements by phosphorus nuclear magnetic resonance spectroscopy (NMR) have demonstrated a reduced Mg concentration in depressed patients who were refractory to treatment with an SSRI (Iosifescu *et al*, 2005).

This method provides the best means to determine Mg-concentrations in specific anatomical areas in living brains.

Functional impact of magnesium

An examination of the role of Mg in neurons provides some insight into the cause and possible treatment of MD. Weston in 1921 reported that Meltzer and Auer first showed in 1905 that the primary effect of Mg treatment upon nerve cells was that of paralysis without any preceding excitation, and the effect seemed to be exclusively of an inhibitory character (Weston, 1921-22).

Monoaminergic systems and magnesium

The locus coeruleus (LC) is the principal anatomical structure of the noradrenergic system. Its activity is related to that of the SNS, and it shows overactivity in melancholic depression. Magnesium infusion led to an increase in circulating norepinephrine (NE) in humans in one study (Leppert *et al*, 1994), whereas no changes in catecholamines were reported in another (Zofkova *et al*, 1993). Magnesium-deficiency on the other hand increased plasma catecholamines in response to noise stress in rats (Caddell *et al*, 1986). Mice selectively bred for low blood Mg levels showed a significantly higher brain NE content without a change in dopamine, HVA, and serotonin compared to those with high Mg levels (Amyard *et al*, 1995). This was interpreted as a higher sensitivity to stress in mice with low blood Mg content. A suppressive effect of Mg on LC activity has been demonstrated (Shiekhattar and Aston-Jones, 1992) and interpreted as an NMDA antagonistic mechanism. Magnesium deficiency reduced behavioral activity from dopaminergic activation by amphetamine and apomorphine (Kantak, 1988). The antidepressant-like effects of Mg are dependent on its interaction with serotonergic, noradrenergic and dopaminergic receptors (Cardoso *et al*, 2009).

Glutamatergic system and magnesium

Magnesium depletion is specifically deleterious to neurons by causing NMDA-coupled calcium channels to be biased towards opening (Sapolsky, 1992) At normal neuronal resting membrane potentials, pores of the NMDA glutamate-gated ion channels are blocked by Mg^{2+} ions (Bear *et al*, 2001; Mark *et al*, 2001; Kandel *et al*, 1995; McMenimen, 2006). The ion channel of the NMDA receptor complex is subject to voltage-dependent regulation by Mg ions (Mark *et al*, 2001; Alberts *et al*, 2002; Decollogne *et al*, 1997). Importantly, different types of NMDA receptors exist, on the basis of their constitution subunits. Besides NR1 subunits, which are constitutional for all subtypes, NR2 elements define their diversity. NR2 exists in flavors of NR2A, NR2B, NR2C and NR2D. Of particular interest, NMDA receptors which contain NR2A and NR2B receptors, are more sensitive to voltage sensitive Mg block (Kuner and Schoepfer, 1996). This direct interaction of Mg with the NMDA receptor intracellular mechanism influences its activity. In hippocampal synaptosomes, the Mg block of the NMDA dependent ion channel is removed by activation of protein kinase C (PKC) without changing membrane potential (Pittaluga *et al*, 2000). Intracellular administration of a PKC agonist accordingly potentiated NMDA receptor function in cultured hippocampal neurons (Xiong *et al*, 1998). This could lead to a feed-forward cycle; an NMDA dependent Ca^{2+} current may increase PKC activity leading to further release of the Mg-block of the NMDA dependent ion-current. Mg also has a direct influence on PKC function. The catalytic subunit of PKC requires Mg as a cofactor (Hannun and Bell, 1990), and deactivation of PKC by adenosine triphosphate (ATP) depends on presence of Mg (Wolf *et al*, 1985). Besides influencing NMDAergic neurotransmission, Mg depletion affects hippocampal excitability via non-NMDAergic Ca currents, which can also be suppressed by verapamil, a Ca-channel blocker (Pohl *et al*, 1992; Walden *et al*, 1992). These findings, when put together, illustrate several possible mechanisms for Mg to limit the kindling state via modulation of different elements of the Ca–PKC-second messenger system.

Normally operating NMDA receptors admit into neurons only the amount of Ca^{2+} that is vital to their function, but abnormally functioning NMDA receptors (due to inadequate Mg) increase influx of cellular Ca^{2+} beyond manageable levels leading to the generation of toxic reactive oxygen species and of toxic amounts of nitric oxide (NO) radicals (Blaylock, 1999; Mark, 2001; Carafoli, 2005).

Stress hormone systems (HPA and RAAS) and magnesium

Acute intravenous Mg administration decreased adrenocorticotrophic hormone (ACTH) secretion in healthy subjects (Murck and Steiger, 1998), but did not lead to a change in cortisol secretion (Zofkova *et al*, 1993; Murck and Steiger, 1998). Subchronic oral administration of Mg in healthy elderly subjects led to a decrease in cortisol concentration without a change in ACTH (Held *et al*, 2002). Chronic oral administration of high-dose Mg leads to considerable reductions in cortisol and lowered stress responsiveness. Both effects are in line with a decrease in central corticotropin-releasing hormone release, but differential effects occur at the level of the adrenal cortex. The possibility of an NMDA antagonistic effect of Mg has been discussed in context of hippocampal function. Both systems also influence endocrine regulation and hypothalamic activity.

Inflammatory system and magnesium

Magnesium depletion has been studied for its effects on inflammatory markers. Feeding rats Mg-depleted food led to a nearly 3-fold increase in plasma interleukin 6 (IL-6), a significant increase of fibrinogen and other acute phase proteins and a significant reduction in Zn (Malpuech-Brugere *et al*, 2000). Mg-deficiency also amplifies endotoxin-induced lethality in rats, which was correlated with increased TNFα production (Malpuech-Brugere *et al*, 1999). In rat models Mg deficiency led to an increase in thromboxane TBX2 and prostaglandin E2 (PGE2) (Nigam *et al*, 1986; Soma *et al*, 1988). For a review of the correlation between Mg-deficiency and inflammatory changes, see Nielsen *et al*, 2010. Of considerable importance is that NMDA-ergic mechanisms may activate inflammatory mechanisms (Muller *et al*, 2009).

Magnesium in animal and human research

In the following sections we summarize data concerning effects of Mg in animals and preliminary findings in humans. One important issue to keep in mind is the unresolved question: Does Mg treat a Mg deficit or is Mg to be regarded as a pharmacological agent, i.e. independent of a preexisting deficit? We will not be able to answer this question on the basis of current data. Nevertheless, in the long run it is important to identify specific characteristics of subjects who may benefit from Mg treatment. Most subjects having MD treatable with magnesium also have, or have had, other disorders which are also treatable with magnesium (Eby, 1999-2010).

The functional systems described above have been recognized as potential pharmacological targets for treatment of depression. All current commercial antidepressants are based on the hypothesis of a monoamine-dysfunction. On the other hand, NMDA receptor antagonists, and in particular those for the NR2B subtype, have demonstrated clinical efficacy (Berman *et al*, 2000; Preskorn *et al*, 2008). The HPA axis has long been recognized as a potential target for antidepressants (Flores *et al*, 2006; Holsboer, 2000; Jahn *et al*, 2004). More recently anti-inflammatory mechanism-like COX-2 inhibitors (Muller *et al*, 2006) and TNFα-antagonists (Uguz *et al*, 2009) have been demonstrated. In the following text we report behavioral effects by Mg in animal models as well as human clinical data. The specific mechanism of these effects by Mg has yet to be elucidated.

Animal Models and magnesium

Animal models have provided insight into roles of stress on Mg status, effects of Mg deficiency, and effects of Mg treatment in depression.

Mg is involved in behavioral control in rats. Mg deficiency led to a reduction in offensive behavior and an increase in defensive behavior (Kantak, 1988). Apomorphine- and L-amphetamine mediated behavior was suppressed by Mg deficiency, suggesting that Mg is an important factor for the stimulatory action of catecholamines possibly at the postsynaptic site. In the forced swim test, a screening test for possible antidepressive potency of substances, Mg reduced immobility similar to the norepinephrine reuptake inhibitor imipramine (Decollogne *et al*, 1997). Compared to control mice fed a normal diet, mice receiving a low Mg diet (10% of daily requirement) for several weeks displayed increased immobility time in the forced swim test, indicating enhanced depression-like behavior. In addition, partial magnesium-depletion feed increased anxiety-related behavior in the light/dark and open field test, while locomotor activity and motor coordination was not influenced. Magnesium depletion led to depression and anxiety-related behavior in mice. These changes due to Mg deficiency were prevented by coadministration of desipramine or hypericum extract (Singewald *et al*, 2004). A dependency of intracellular Mg and behavioral regulation appears to exist. Mice selected for low vs. high erythrocyte Mg levels showed pronounced neurobiological differences (Henrotte *et al*, 1997). Low Mg mice showed a more restless behavior, a more aggressive behavior under stressful conditions and higher brain and urine NE levels compared to mice with high erythrocyte Mg. It is not clear if a correlation between intraerythrocyte and intraneuronal Mg concentration exists.

Of importance is that Mg deficiency leads to depression-like changes and that Mg administration has "therapeutic" effects on depression-like behavior. Magnesium administration led to anxiolytic effects in the elevated plus-maze, and antidepressant like effects in the forced swim test (Poleszak *et al*, 2004). In stressed rats Mg and imipramine acted synergistically on immobility time as measured in the forced swim test, i.e. non-efficacious doses of both compounds combined led to a positive behavioral response (Poleszak *et al*, 2006). The mechanism is complex and appears to involve NMDAergic (Poleszak *et al*, 2008), GABAergic (Poleszak 2008) and serotoninergic (Poleszak 2007) modulation.

Human studies and magnesium

There are a number of open label studies on therapeutic effects of Mg administration in treating depression, depression-like and anxiety illnesses. As early as 1921 a report on the therapeutic effect of Mg was published in the first issue of the American Journal of Psychiatry (and immediately forgotten). In 220 out of 250 doses of magnesium sulfate (one or two cc of a 25 or 50 percent solution) given hypodermically to 50 patients having agitated depression, with several having various other agitated states, treatment caused patients to relax and sleep from four to six hours resulting in a 90% success rate for Mg (Weston, 1921-22). The sedative side effects from giving too much Mg were quickly and easily reversed by giving similar amounts of calcium chloride given hypodermically.

Later studies showed a beneficial effect of Mg in treatment of rapid cycling bipolar disorder in ten patients (Chouinard *et al*, 1990) in an open label study for periods up to 32 weeks. Magnesium was found to produce clinical results at least equivalent to those of lithium in 50% of patients. The possibility that Mg could replace or improve efficacy of lithium without side effects as a preventive treatment of manic-depressive illness was suggested.

In tests of magnesium lactate and vitamin B6 (pyridoxine) in treatment of 25 patients with anxiety-depression and epilepsy, the combination exerted positive non-specific influences on patient's mental state, especially with regard to affective disorders. Effects emerged on day 14 of treatment and achieved a statistically significant level by day 28. Treatment was well tolerated and did not cause any side effects (Kalim *et al*, 2004).

Further support comes from improvement of a subject with the rare hereditary disorder of Gitelman's syndrome, which leads to a lack of reabsorption of electrolytes including Mg. Intravenous supplement of magnesium sulfate (20 mEq/day dissolved in 100 ml normal saline given over 2 hours each day for 3 days) immediately terminated both depression and paraesthesia, suggesting that hypomagnesemia played a role in clinical manifestations of depression (Enya *et al*, 2004). Oral magnesium oxide treatment was ineffective and promoted diarrhea. Magnesium oxide should not be given in treatment of mental illnesses since it is not bioavailable generally and it does not pass the blood-brain barrier.

Mood stabilizing properties of Mg have been demonstrated in case reports in patients with mania (Pavlinac *et al*, 1979). In an open study with intravenous magnesium sulfate used as a supplementary therapy to lithium, benzodiazepines, and neuroleptics in mania, marked clinical improvement was observed in the 10 patients included. This was accompanied with a significant reduction in requirement for neuroleptic and benzodiazepine (Heiden *et al*, 1999). In a further open trial in mania the effect of a Mg–verapamil combination was compared with that of verapamil alone, and the combination was superior for manic symptoms (Giannini *et al*, 2000).

Four case histories were presented showing rapid recovery (less than 7 days) from MD using 125–300 mg of magnesium (as glycinate and taurinate) with each meal and at bedtime (Eby and Eby, 2006). Related and accompanying mental illnesses in these case histories, which were also benefited, included traumatic brain injury, headache, suicidal ideation, anxiety, irritability, insomnia, cocaine, alcohol and tobacco abuse, hypersensitivity to calcium, short-term memory loss and IQ loss. Post partum depression appeared prevented in several case histories with Mg, wherein the patients had previously had severe PPD without Mg. The possibility that magnesium deficiency is the main cause of most MD and related mental health problems including IQ loss and addiction was described as enormously important to public health and was recommended for immediate further study (Eby and Eby, 2006). Magnesium was claimed usually effective for treatment of depression in general use by depressives reading "Depression Treatment: A Cure for Depression using Magnesium?" on the Internet (Eby, 1999-2010).

To date only one randomized double-blind, controlled trial exists concerning effects of Mg administration on MD. Magnesium chloride ($MgCl_2$) was evaluated in the treatment of newly diagnosed depression. Twenty-three elderly patients with type 2 diabetes and hypo-magnesemia were enrolled and randomly allocated to receive orally either 50 mL of a $MgCl_2$ 5% solution (equivalent to 450 mg of elemental Mg) or 50 mg imipramine daily during 12 weeks. Widowhood or divorce in the previous six months, alcoholism, degenerative illnesses of the nervous central system, previous or current treatment with antidepressants, chronic diarrhea, use of diuretics, and reduced renal function were exclusion criteria. At end of the treatment period, depression scores were identical between groups. Serum Mg levels were significantly higher in subjects receiving $MgCl_2$ than in subjects receiving imipramine, $p = 0.0005$ (Barragán-Rodríguez *et al*, 2008).

Several studies in indications which involve depressed mood exist. In a double-blind, placebo-controlled trial in chronic fatigue syndrome, a disorder related to atypical depression, weekly intramuscular injections of 2ml magnesium sulfate (50%) or placebo for 6 weeks showed significant superiority of Mg over placebo on energy levels, pain, and emotional reactions as measured by the Nottingham health profile score (Cox *et al*, 1991).

In another placebo controlled study of premenstrual syndrome, which has depressive elements, effects of oral Mg for the duration of two menstrual cycles was observed (Facchinetti *et al*, 1991). The medication consisted of 3 x 360mg Mg in the form of Mg–pyrrolidone carboxylic acid. It was administered from day 15 of the menstrual cycle to onset of menstrual flow. Mg showed a significant superiority to placebo in the total score of the Menstrual Distress Questionnaire score and especially the cluster "negative affect". In the same indication, combination of 200mg Mg and 50mg vitamin B6, but not individual treatments alone, administered daily for the duration of one menstrual cycle in a Latin square design was superior compared to placebo on premenstrual symptoms as nervous tension, mood swings, irritability and anxiety (De Souza *et al*, 2000). Another study using a crossover design found only an improvement in symptoms related to fluid retention in women taking 200mg Mg or placebo in the second menstrual cycle (Walker *et al*, 1998).

Adverse effect of calcium in depression

Decreases in CSF calcium accompanied mood elevation and motor activation in depressed patients. Similarly, decreases in CSF calcium occurred during acute psychotic agitation or mania. Periodic recurrences of such agitated states were accompanied at their onset by transient increases in serum calcium and phosphorus. Several observations suggested that such serum ion shifts triggered the more enduring and opposite shifts in CSF calcium and, in turn, manic behavior. Progressive restriction of dietary calcium was earlier reported to mitigate and finally abolish both rhythmic rises in serum calcium and periodic agitated episodes. A modest oral calcium lactate supplement (approximately one additional U.S. Recommended Daily

Allowance) intensified agitation and worsened depression. In manic patients, symptomatology grew significantly and substantially worse during 2 to 6 weeks of oral vitamin D administration.

On the other hand, in 12 patients, subcutaneous injections of synthetic salmon calcitonin decreased serum calcium and phosphorus, increased cerebrospinal fluid calcium, and augmented depressive symptomatology. Salmon calcitonin, which lowers blood calcium levels, also decreased quantified motor activity, frequency and severity of periodic agitated episodes, serum creatine phosphokinase and prolactin, and nocturnal sleep, while vitamin D or calcium lactate raised them (Carman and Wyatt, 1979).
A dietary supplement of 500mg calcium immediately and severely worsened MD, which was extinguishable within one hour by orally treating with 400mg gel capsules of Mg as magnesium glycinate (Eby and Eby, 2006).

In a study of electrolytes in CSF from depressives, a positive correlation was found between calcium concentration and symptom severity in hospitalized depressed patients. CSF calcium levels tended to decrease as patients improved. In rapidly cycling patients, CSF calcium was higher during depression than during mania (Jimersom *et al*, 1979).

Major depression was found to be accompanied by hyperactivity of subcellular calcium signaling, and any means of reducing pathological neuronal calcium ion flow to reduce pathological nitric oxide NMDA neuronal output would have antidepressant effects (Paul, 2001). Hypercalcemia from excessive vitamin D intake, hyperparathyroidism or other causes has been suggested to lead to clinical depression by lowering brain Mg (Keddie, 1987).

Biomarkers of magnesium and magnesium-related functions

Although there is considerable interest in understanding roles of Mg in brain chemistry and explanation of its role there, we found little consensus as to the value of Mg measurements in blood (serum, plasma or cellular) as a diagnostic tool useful in treating depression. CSF concentrations of Mg in depression were also conflicted, although there appeared agreement that CSF Mg^{2+} values were low only in severe depression associated with suicide attempts supporting the notion that Mg would be useful specifically for TRD, which is often much more severe than treatable depression.

Since 99% of Mg is intracellular, serum Mg testing of the remaining 1% in serum produces misleading results (Mann and Truswell, 2002). Although serum values less than 0.9 mmol/Mg demonstrate Mg deficiency in non-depressives (Liebscher and Liebscher, 2004), it is often normal or elevated in depression. Consequently, serum tests are of negative utility due to their misleading nature, and red blood cell tests are also of questionable, perhaps negative, value. Although various tests for Mg deficiency and calcium excess appear desirable; the response to Mg treatment with calcium reduction is always the deciding criteria.

Brain compartments of Mg are isolated from blood and bone compartments requiring different analytical means. Measuring brain Mg can be safely accomplished in humans using phosphorus NMR spectroscopy (Iosifescu *et al*, 2008; Iotti and Maulcelli, 2008). This test needs to be validated by repeated trials as a reliable means to determine low brain Mg in diagnosis of low brain Mg as cause of MD.

A health warning is therefore warranted regarding potential misinterpretation of "normal" serum Mg. In case of doubt restoration of Mg stores in deficient patients is simple, tolerable, and inexpensive and can be clinically beneficial (Ismail *et al*, 2010).

Recommendations concerning magnesium-supplementation

Dietary fibers affect intestinal absorption of Mg. Inulin, a prebiotic that supports bifidobacteria and lactobacilli, has been confirmed to be important in absorption of Mg in the large intestines (Scholz-Ahrens and Schrezenmeir, 2007; Rondón *et al*, 2008) nearly doubling Mg absorption and reducing tendency to diarrhea, but increasing gas, while taking Mg. Large doses of psyllium seed husks greatly reduced absorption of Mg (Asvarujanon *et al*, 2004) and gum arabic significantly increased both intestinal and renal excretion of Mg (Nasir *et al*, 2008), and both should be avoided. Indole-3-carbinol (I3C) (200 mg/meal) was found in a case study to reduce greatly the necessity for frequent Mg treatment to prevent relapse (Eby and Eby, 2006).

Useful Mg compounds are those that have a sufficiently low first stability constant to be bioavailable and include: magnesium acetate, chloride, citrate, gluconate, glycinate, lactate, malate, oxalate, succinate, sulfate and tartarate (Furia, 1968). The bioavailability of magnesium oxide is extremely limited, ranging from 0 - 4% (Firoz and Graber, 2001; Lindberg *et al*, 1990; Walker *et al*, 2003; Enya *et al*, 2004). Studies in which magnesium oxide is used produce misleading results when compared with results obtained using other compounds of Mg for the same indication.

Future clinical research

We are concerned that there were only a few clinical trials of Mg for human depression found. We suggest that future trials be of larger populations in formal, double-blind, placebo-controlled clinical trials, or comparative trials against a proven antidepressant such as imipramine 50 mg daily. Only when evidence of efficacy has become clearer are physicians likely to adopt Mg for MD.

From reports reviewed herein, we suggest that in future clinical research in depression that the initial treatment utilize IV drip magnesium sulfate in the manner of Enya *et al*, 2004, (20 mEq/day dissolved in 100 ml normal saline given over 2 hours each day for 3 days) to provide an expected rapid (<3 days) initial induction of remission. Treatment is to be followed by an oral bioavailable Mg (125 – 300 mg 4 t/d) maintenance treatment in the manner of Eby and Eby 2006 or Barragán-Rodríguez 2008 using bioavailable Mg compounds with emphasis on magnesium glycinate and taurinate. Magnesium oxide must not be used since it is non-bioavailable (Firoz and Graber, 2001; Lindberg *et al*, 1990; Walker *et al*, 2003; Enya *et al*, 2004). During IV administration, cardiac monitoring should be performed. Protocols for IV administration of magnesium sulfate have been widely used for treatment of eclampsia. The antidote to magnesium overdose is calcium gluconate or calcium chloride. Since 99% of Mg is intracellular, serum Mg testing of the remaining 1% found in serum will produce misleading results (Mann and Truswell, 2002) and it should not be used in future research.

Impediments to success and precautions

We are concerned that there are some impediments to proper absorption of Mg in large therapeutic doses by the oral route with intestinal issues, especially inflammatory bowel disease (Galland, 1988) and diarrhea being primary concerns. Large doses of oral Mg without calcium may exponentially increase Candida albicans intestinal growth (Holmes *et al*, 1991), causing or worsening diarrhea and impairing absorption of Mg, while adding calcium may greatly and immediately worsen depression. Candida albicans overgrowth may be prevented or treated naturally by greatly reducing intake of sugars and treating with large amounts of Bacillus Coagulans probiotic and biotin. We are very concerned that magnesium oxide will be given with failure to respond becoming highly evident, thus damaging the reputation of Mg as an effective treatment for depression. Do not give magnesium oxide because it has been shown to be not bioavailable. Additionally, magnesium aspartate and magnesium glutamate have neurotoxic ligands and they must be avoided to prevent worsening depression.

Conclusions

Lack of definitive, large-scale, double-blind, placebo-controlled clinical trials is the limiting factor for making strong treatment recommendations using Mg. Countering that point of view is the good safety of Mg compared to side-effect prone antidepressant and anti-anxiety medications.

From evidence reviewed here and from the 2010 review by Eby and Eby, the relationship between low Mg intake as a risk factor for MD appear to have extremely important preventative and treatment implications. A dietary supplement of 600 to 800 mg/day Mg (other than magnesium oxide) should be a universal prevention strategy.

Mechanisms, which lead to CNS Mg depletion, should be further studied in an effort to discover new targets and medication for MD. Evidence for a Mg-regulation effect of psychoptropic drugs already exists, however the exact mechanism is unclear. Reasonable candidates go beyond monoaminergic mechanisms and may include manipulation of the renin-angiotensin-aldosterone system and, less studied, specific Mg transport mechanisms. The best direct measurement of brain Mg is by phosphorus NMR spectroscopy, but this will probably be reserved for research purposes.

Although more research is clearly needed, we suggest that it is past time to give Mg in appropriate doses and to reduce intake of calcium, glutamate and aspartate for the prevention and treatment of MD, especially TRD, and anxiety, since we can expect rapid improvements in patient health and major reductions in patient expenses without side effects. We did not pay attention to those early Mg and brain pioneers Meltzer and Auer in 1905 and other magnesium researchers over the last 100 years and we may pay the price today.

Acknowledgements
We thank the George and Patsy Eby Foundation for financial support. We thank Mikaila Bell for assistance. We have no financial interests or conflicts of interest in any aspect of this research.

References

ABC Homeopathy (2010) Magnesia Muriatica. http://www.abchomeopathy.com/r.php/Mag-m/mind (accessed August 15, 2010).

Alberts B, Johnson A, Lewis J, Raff M, Roberts K, Walter P (2002) *Molecular Biology of the Cell* 4th ed. New York, NY, Garland Science, 615-658.

Altura BM, Altura BT, Gebrewold A, Ising H, Gunther T (1992) Noise-induced hypertension and magnesium in rats: relationship to microcirculation and calcium. *J Appl Physiol* 72:194-202.

Amyard N, Leyris A, Monier C, Francès H, Boulu RG, Henrotte JG (1995) Brain catecholamines, serotonin and their metabolites in mice selected for low (MGL) and high (MGH) blood magnesium levels. *Magnes Res* 8:5-9.

Anonymous (2002) Heart gains from whole grains. *Harv Heart Lett* 13:2-4.

Asvarujanon P, Ishizuka S, Hara H (2004) Inhibitory effects of psyllium on rat mineral absorption were abolished by reduction of viscosity with partial hydrolysis. *Biosci Biotechnol Biochem* 68:1737-42.

Banki CM, Arato M, Kilts CD (1986) Aminergic studies and cerebrospinal fluid cations in suicide. *Annals of the New York Academy of Sciences* 487:221-230.

Banki CM, Vojnik M, Papp Z, Balla KZ, Arato M (1985) Cerebrospinal fluid magnesium and calcium related to amine metabolites, diagnosis, and suicide attempts. *Biol Psychiatry* 20:163-171.

Barragán-Rodríguez L, Rodríguez-Morán M, Guerrero-Romero F (2008) Efficacy and safety of oral magnesium supplementation in the treatment of depression in the elderly with type 2 diabetes: a randomized, equivalent trial. *Magnes Res* 21:218-23.

Bear MF, Connors BW, Paradiso MA (2001) Neurotransmitter Systems In: *Neuroscience Exploring the brain,* 2nd edn, Baltimore MD. Lippincott Williams & Wilkins, 131-162.

Berman RM, Cappiello A, Anand A, Oren DA, Heninger GR, Charney DS, Krystal JH. (2000) Antidepressant effects of ketamine in depressed patients. *Biol Psychiatry* 47:351-354.

Bjorum N (1972) Electrolytes in blood in endogenous depression. *Acta Psychiatr Scand* 48:59-68.

Blaylock RL (1999) Food additive excitotoxins and degenerative brain disorders. *Medical Sentinel* 4:212-215.

Bourre JM (2006) Effects of nutrients (in food) on the structure and function of the nervous system: update on dietary requirements for brain Part 1: micronutrients. *J Nutr Health Aging* 10:377-85.

Caddell J, Kupiecki R, Proxmire DL, Satoh P, Hutchinson B (1986) Plasma catecholamines in acute magnesium deficiency in weanling rats. *J Nutr* 116:1896-901.

Cade JF (1964) A significant elevation of plasma magnesium levels in schizophrenia and depressive states. *Med J Aust* 1:195-6.

Carafoli E (2005) Calcium--a universal carrier of biological signals. *FEBS J* 272:1073-89.

Cardoso CC, Lobato KR, Binfaré RW, Ferreira PK, Rosa AO, Santos AR, Rodrigues AL (2009) Evidence for the involvement of the monoaminergic system in the antidepressant-like effect of magnesium. *Prog Neuropsychopharmacol Biol Psychiatry* 33:235-42.

Carman JS, Wyatt RJ (1979) Calcium: bivalent cations in the bivalent psychoses. *Biol Psychiatry* 14:295-336.

Chouinard G, Beauclair L, Geiser R, Etienne P (1990) A pilot study of magnesium aspartate hydrochloride (Magnesiocard) as a mood stabilizer for rapid cycling bipolar affective disorder patients. *Prog Neuropsychopharmacol Biol Psychiatry* 14:171-80.

Chutkow JG (1974) Metabolism of magnesium in central nervous system. Relationship between concentrations of magnesium in cerebrospinal fluid and brain in magnesium deficiency. *Neurology* 24:780-7.

Cox IM, Campbell MJ, Dowson D (1991) Red blood cell magnesium and chronic fatigue syndrome. *Lancet* 337(8744):757-60.

Decollogne S, Tomas A, Lecerf C, Adamowicz E, Seman M (1997) NMDA receptor complex blockade by oral administration of magnesium: comparison with MK-801. *Pharmacol Biochem Behav* 58:261-8.

De Souza MC, Walker AF, Robinson PA, Bolland K (2000) A synergistic effect of a daily supplement for 1 month of 200 mg magnesium plus 50 mg vitamin B6 for the relief of anxiety-related premenstrual symptoms: a randomized, double-blind, crossover study. *J Womens Health Gend Based Med* 9:131-9.

Durlach J and Bac P (1997) Mechanisms of action on the nervous system in magnesium deficiency and dementia. Yasui, M Strong, MJ, Ota, K and Verity MA (eds) In: *Mineral and Metal Neurotoxicology* Boca Raton, New York, CRC Press 201-209.

Durlach J, Durlach V, Bara M, Guiet-Bara A (1995) Diverse applications of magnesium therapy In: Berthon G (ed) *Handbook of Metal-Ligand Interactions in Biologic Fluids* – Bioinorganic Medicine New York, NY, Marcel Dekker, 1116-24.

Durlach J, Durlach V (1984) Speculations on hormonal controls of magnesium homeostasis: a hypothesis. *Magnesium* 3:109-31.

Durlach J, Pagès N, Bac P, Bara M, Guiet-Bara A, Agrapart C (2002) Chronopathological forms of magnesium depletion with hypofunction or with hyperfunction of the biological clock. *Magnes Res* 15:263-8.

Eby GA (1999-2010) Depression Treatment: A Cure for Depression using Magnesium? http://george-eby-research.com/html/depression-anxiety.html (accessed August 15, 2010).

Eby GA, Eby KL (2006) Rapid recovery from major depression using magnesium treatment. *Med Hypotheses* 67:362-70.

Eby GA, Eby KL (2010) Magnesium for treatment-resistant depression: a review and hypothesis. *Med Hypotheses* 74:649-60.

Eller T, Vasar V, Shlik J, Maron E (2008) Pro-inflammatory cytokines and treatment response to escitalopram in major depressive disorder. *Prog Neuropsychopharmacol Biol Psychiatry* 32:445-450.

Emanuele E, Geroldi D, Minoretti P, Coen E, Politi P (2005) Increased plasma aldosterone in patients with clinical depression. *Arch Med Res* 36:544-548.

Enya M, Kanoh Y, Mune T, Ishizawa M, Sarui H, Yamamoto M, Takeda N, Yasuda K, Yasujima M, Tsutaya S, Takeda J (2004) Depressive state and paresthesia dramatically improved by intravenous MgSO4 in Gitelman's syndrome. *Intern Med* 43:410-4.

Facchinetti F, Borella P, Sances G, Fioroni L, Nappi RE, Genazzani AR (1991) Oral magnesium successfully relieves premenstrual mood changes. *Obstet Gynecol* 78:177-81.

Fekadu A, Wooderson SC, Markopoulo K, Donaldson C, Papadopoulos A, Cleare AJ (2009) What happens to patients with treatment-resistant depression? A systematic review of medium to long term outcome studies. *J Affect Disord* 116(1-2):4-11.

Firoz M, Graber M (2001) Bioavailability of US commercial magnesium preparations. *Magnes Res* 14:257-62.

Flores BH, Kenna H, Keller J, Solvason HB, Schatzberg AF (2006) Clinical and biological effects of mifepristone treatment for psychotic depression. *Neuropsychopharmacology* 31:628-636.

Ford DE, Kamerow DB (1989) Epidemiologic study of sleep disturbances and psychiatric disorders. An opportunity for prevention? *JAMA* 262:1479-1484.
Frizel D, Coppen A, Marks V (1969) Plasma magnesium and calcium in depression. *Br J Psychiatry* 115:1375-7.

Furia TE. 1968 Sequestrants in Foods - Chapter 7 In: Furia, TA (ed*), Handbook of Food Additives* Cleveland, OH, The Chemical Rubber Co, 289-312.

Galland L (1988) Magnesium and inflammatory bowel disease. *Magnesium* 7:78-83.

George MS, Rosenstein D, Rubinow DR, Kling MA, Post RM (1994) CSF magnesium in affective disorder: lack of correlation with clinical course of treatment. *Psychiatry Res* 51:139-146.

Giannini AJ, Nakoneczie AM, Melemis SM, Ventresco J, Condon M (2000) Magnesium augmentation of verapamil maintenance therapy in mania. *Psychiatry Res* 93:83-7.

Gilmore C, Green BH, Copeland JR, Dewey ME, Davidson IA, Saunders PA, Sharma V (1995) Blood pressure as a risk factor for depression in elderly people: a prospective study. *Acta psychiatrica Scandinavica* 91:126-129.

Grases G, Pérez-Castelló JA, Sanchis P, Casero A, Perelló J, Isern B, Rigo E, Grases F (2006): Anxiety and stress among science students. Study of calcium and magnesium alterations. *Magnes Res* 19:102-6.

Hannun YA, Bell RM (1990) Rat brain protein kinase C. Kinetic analysis of substrate dependence, allosteric regulation, and autophosphorylation. *J Biol Chem* 265:2962-72.

Hasey GM, D'Alessandro E, Cooke RG, Warsh JJ (1993) The interface between thyroid activity, magnesium, and depression: a pilot study. Biol Psychiatry 33:133-5.
Hashizume N, Mori M (1990) An analysis of hypermagnesemia and hypomagnesemia. *Jpn J Med* 29:368-72.

Hatzinger M, Hemmeter UM, Brand S, Ising M, Holsboer-Trachsler E (2004) Electroencephalographic sleep profiles in treatment course and long-term outcome of major depression: association with DEX/CRH-test response. *J Psychiatr Res* 38:453-465.

Heiden A, Frey R, Presslich O, Blasbichler T, Smetana R, Kasper S (1999) Treatment of severe mania with intravenous magnesium sulphate as a supplementary therapy. *J Psychiatry Res* 89:239-46.

Held K, Antonijevic IA, Künzel H, Uhr M, Wetter TC, Golly IC, Steiger A, Murck H (2002) Oral $Mg^{(2+)}$ supplementation reverses age-related neuroendocrine and sleep EEG changes in humans. *Pharmacopsychiatry* 35:135-43.

Henrotte JG, Franck G, Santarromana M, Francès H, Mouton D, Motta R (1997) Mice selected for low and high blood magnesium levels: a new model for stress studies. *Physiol Behav* 61:653-8.

Herzberg L, Bold AM (1972) Sex difference in mean serum-magnesium levels in depression. *Lancet* 1(7760):1128-9.

Herzberg L, Herzeberg B (1977) Mood change and magnesium. A possible interaction between magnesium and lithium? *J Nerv Ment Dis* 165:423-6.

Holmes AR, Cannon RD, Shepherd MG. (1991) Effect of calcium ion uptake on Candida albicans morphology. *FEMS Microbiol Lett* 61:187-93.

Holsboer F (2000) The corticosteroid receptor hypothesis of depression. *Neuropsychopharmacology* 23:477-501.

Hubain PP, Staner L, Dramaix M, Kerkhofs M, Papadimitriou G, Mendlewicz J, Linkowski P (1998) The dexamethasone suppression test and sleep electroencephalogram in nonbipolar major depressed inpatients: a multivariate analysis. *Biol Psychiatry* 43:220-229.

Iosifescu DV, Bolo NR, Nierenberg AA, Jensen JE, Fava M, Renshaw PF(2008) Brain bioenergetics and response to triiodothyronine augmentation in major depressive disorder. *Biol Psychiatry* 63:1127-34.

Iosifescu DV, Nierenberg AA, Mischoulon D, Perlis RH, Papakostas GI, Ryan JL, Alpert JE, Fava M (2005) An open study of triiodothyronine augmentation of selective serotonin reuptake inhibitors in treatment-resistant major depressive disorder. *J Clin Psychiatry* 66:1038-1042.

Iotti S, Malucelli E (2008) In vivo assessment of Mg^{2+} in human brain and skeletal muscle by 31P-MRS. *Magnes Res* 21:157-62.

Ising M, Lauer CJ, Holsboer F, Modell S (2005) The Munich vulnerability study on affective disorders: premorbid neuroendocrine profile of affected high-risk probands. *J Psychiatr Res* 39:21-28.

Ismail Y, Ismail AA, Ismail AA (2010) The underestimated problem of using serum magnesium measurements to exclude magnesium deficiency in adults; a health warning is needed for "normal" results. *Clin Chem Lab Med* 48:323-7.

Jacka FN, Overland S, Stewart R, Tell GS, Bjelland I, Mykletun A (2009) Association between magnesium intake and depression and anxiety in community-dwelling adults: the Hordaland Health Study. *Aust NZ J Psychiatry* 43:45-52.

Jahn H, Schick M, Kiefer F, Kellner M, Yassouridis A, Wiedemann K (2004) Metyrapone as additive treatment in major depression: a double-blind and placebo-controlled trial. *Arch Gen Psychiatry* 61:1235-1244.

Jimerson DC, Post RM, Carman JS, van Kammen DP, Wood JH, Goodwin FK, Bunney WE Jr. (1979) CSF calcium: clinical correlates in affective illness and schizophrenia. *Biol Psychiatry* 14:37-51.

Joffe RT, Levitt AJ, Young LT (1996) The thyroid, magnesium and calcium in major depression. *Biol Psychiatry* 40:428-9.

Jung KI, Ock SM, Chung JH, Song CH (2010) Associations of serum Ca and Mg levels with mental health in adult women without psychiatric disorders. *Biol Trace Elem Res* 133:153-61.

Kalinin VV, Zheleznova EV, Rogacheva TA, Sokolova LV, Polianskiĭ DA, Zemlianaia AA, Nazmetdinova DM (2004) [A use of Magne-B6 in the treatment of anxiety-depressive states in patients with epilepsy]. *Zh Nevrol Psikhiatr Im S S Korsakova* 104:51-5.

Kandel ER, Schwartz JH, Jessell TM (1995) Synaptic integration In: *Essentials of neural science and behavior*. Stamford, CT, Appleton & Lange 219-241.

Kantak KM (1988) Magnesium deficiency alters aggressive behavior and catecholamine function. *Behav Neurosci* 102:304-311.

Keddie KM (1987) Severe depressive illness in the context of hypervitaminosis D. *Br J Psychiatry* 150:394-6.

Kemeny A, Boldizsar H, Pethes G (1961) The distribution of cations in plasma and cerebrospinal fluid following infusion of solution of salts of sodium, potassium magnesium and calcium. *J New Drugs* 7:218-27.

Kirov GK, Birch NJ, Steadman P, Ramsey RG (1994) Plasma magnesium levels in a population of psychiatric patients: correlations with symptoms. *Neuropsychobiology* 30:73-8.

Krieg JC, Lauer CJ, Schreiber W, Modell S, Holsboer F (2001) Neuroendocrine, polysomnographic and psychometric observations in healthy subjects at high familial risk for affective disorders: the current state of the 'Munich vulnerability study'. *J Affect Disord* 62:33-37.

Kuner T, Schoepfer R (1996) Multiple structural elements determine subunit specificity of Mg^{2+} block in NMDA receptor channels. J Neurosci 16:3549-3558.
Langley WF, Mann D (1991) Skeletal buffer function and symptomatic magnesium deficiency. *Med Hypotheses* 34:62-65.

Lauer CJ, Schreiber W, Holsboer F, Krieg JC (1995) In quest of identifying vulnerability markers for psychiatric disorders by all-night polysomnography. *Arch Gen Psychiatry* 52:145-153.

Leppert J, Myrdal U, Hedner T, Edvinsson L, Tracz Z, Ringqvist I (1994) Effect of magnesium sulfate infusion on circulating levels of noradrenaline and neuropeptide-Y-like immunoreactivity in patients with primary Raynaud's phenomenon. *Angiology* 45:637-45.

Levine J, Stein D, Rapoport A, Kurtzman L (1999) High serum and cerebrospinal fluid Ca/Mg ratio in recently hospitalized acutely depressed patients. *Neuropsychobiology* 39:63-70.

Liebscher DH, Liebscher DE (2004) About the misdiagnosis of magnesium deficiency. *J Am Coll Nutr* 23:730S-731S.

Lindberg JS, Zobitz MM, Poindexter JR, Pak CY (1990) Magnesium bioavailability from magnesium citrate and magnesium oxide. *J Am Coll Nutr* 9:48-55.

Linder J, Brismar K, Beck-Friis J, Saaf J, Wetterberg L (1989) Calcium and magnesium concentrations in affective disorder: difference between plasma and serum in relation to symptoms. *Acta Psychiatr Scand* 80:527-37.

Malpuech-Brugère C, Nowacki W, Daveau M, Gueux E, Linard C, Rock E, Lebreton J, Mazur A, Rayssiguier Y (2000) Inflammatory response following acute magnesium deficiency in the rat. *Biochim Biophys Acta* 1501:91-98.

Malpuech-Brugere C, Nowacki W, Rock E, Gueux E, Mazur A, Rayssiguier Y (1999) Enhanced tumor necrosis factor-alpha production following endotoxin challenge in rats is an early event during magnesium deficiency. *Biochim Biophys Acta* 1453:35-40.

Mann J, Truswell AS. (2002*) Essentials of Human Nutrition*. 2nd ed. New York, NY, Oxford University Press 141.

Mark LP, Prost RW, Ulmer JL, Smith MM, Daniels DL, Strottmann JM, Brown WD Hacein-Bey L (2001) Pictorial review of glutamate excitotoxicity: Fundamental concepts for neuroimaging. *Am J Neuroradiol* 22:1813-1824.

McMenimen KA, Dougherty DA, Lester HA, Petersson EJ. (2006) Probing the Mg^{2+} blockade site of an N-methyl-D-aspartate (NMDA) receptor with unnatural amino acid mutagenesis. *ACS Chem Biol* 1:227-34.

Meyer JS, Quenzer LF (2005) *Psychopharmacology: Drugs the Brain and Behavior.* Sunderland MA, Sinauer Associates Inc163-182 386.

Morris ME. (1992) Brain and CSF magnesium concentrations during magnesium deficit in animals and humans: neurological symptoms. *Magnes Res* 5:303-13.

Muller N, Myint AM, Schwarz MJ (2009) The impact of neuroimmune dysregulation on neuroprotection and neurotoxicity in psychiatric disorders--relation to drug treatment. *Dialogues Clin Neurosci* 11:319-332.

Müller N, Schwarz MJ, Dehning S, Douhe A, Cerovecki A, Goldstein-Müller B, Spellmann I, Hetzel G, Maino K, Kleindienst N, Möller HJ, Arolt V, Riedel M (2006) The cyclooxygenase-2 inhibitor celecoxib has therapeutic effects in major depression: results of a double-blind, randomized, placebo controlled, add-on pilot study to reboxetine. *Mol Psychiatry* 11:680-684.

Murck H (2002) Magnesium and affective disorders. *Nutr Neurosci* 5:375-89.

Murck H, Held K, Ziegenbein M, Kunzel H, Koch K, Steiger A (2003) The renin-angiotensin-aldosterone system in patients with depression compared to controls--a sleep endocrine study. *BMC Psychiatry* 3:15.

Murck H, Song C, Horrobin DF, Uhr M (2004) Ethyl-eicosapentaenoate and dexamethasone resistance in therapy-refractory depression. *Int J Neuropsychopharmacol* 7:341-349.

Murck H, Steiger A (1998) Mg^{2+} reduces ACTH secretion and enhances spindle power without changing delta power during sleep in men -- possible therapeutic implications. *Psychopharmacology (Berl)* 137:247-52.

Murck H. (2002) Magnesium and affective disorders. *Nutr Neurosci* 5:375-89.

Nasir O, Artunc F, Saeed A, Kambal MA, Kalbacher H, Sandulache D, Boini KM, Jahovic N, Lang F (2008) Effects of gum arabic (Acacia senegal) on water and electrolyte balance in healthy mice. *J Ren Nutr* 18:230-8.

Naylor GJ, Fleming LW, Stewart WK, McNamee HB, Le Poidevin D (1972) Plasma magnesium and calcium levels in depressive psychosis. *Br J Psychiatry* 120:683-4.

Nechifor M (2009) Magnesium in major depression. *Magnes Res* 22:163S-166S.

Nielsen FH (2010) Magnesium, inflammation, and obesity in chronic disease. *Nutr Rev* 68:333-340.

Nierenberg AA, Husain MM, Trivedi MH, Fava M, Warden D, Wisniewski SR, Miyahara S, Rush AJ. (2010) Residual symptoms after remission of major depressive disorder with citalopram and risk of relapse: a STAR*D report. *Psychological Medicine* 40:41-50.

Nigam S, Averdunk R, Gunther T (1986) Alteration of prostanoid metabolism in rats with magnesium deficiency. *Prostaglandins Leukot Med* 23:1-10.

Nowak G, Poleszak E, Sowa-Kucma M, Pilc A (2010) Magnesium and Glutamate interaction in depression and antidepressant therapy. *Biological Psychiatry* 67:195S.

O'Brien SM, Scully P, Fitzgerald P, Scott LV, Dinan TG (2007) Plasma cytokine profiles in depressed patients who fail to respond to selective serotonin reuptake inhibitor therapy. *J Psychiatr Res* 41:326-331.

Oppelt WW, MacIntyre I, Rall DP (1963) Magnesium exchange between blood and cerebrospinal fluid. *Am J Physiol.* 205:959-62.

Paterniti S, Verdier-Taillefer MH, Geneste C, Bisserbe JC, Alperovitch A (2000) Low blood pressure and risk of depression in the elderly. A prospective community-based study. *Br J Psychiatry* 176:464-467.

Paul IA (2001) Antidepressant activity and calcium signaling cascades. Hum Psychopharmacol 16:71-80.
Pavlinac D, Langer R, Lenhard L, Deftos L (1979) Magnesium in affective disorders. *Biol Psychiatry* 14:657-61.

Pittaluga A, Bonfanti A, Raiteri M (2000) Somatostatin potentiates NMDA receptor function via activation of InsP(3) receptors and PKC leading to removal of the Mg($^{2+}$) block without depolarization. *Br J Pharmacol.* 130:557-66.

Pizzi C, Manzoli L, Mancini S, Costa GM (2008) Analysis of potential predictors of depression among coronary heart disease risk factors including heart rate variability, markers of inflammation, and endothelial function. *Eur Heart J* 29:1110-1117.

Poenaru S, Manicom R, Rouhani S, Aymard P, Bajenaru O, Rayssiguier Y, Emmanouillidis E, Gueux E, Nkanga N, Durlach J, Dall'ava J. (1997) Stability of brain content of magnesium in experimental hypomagnesemia. *Brain Res* 769:329-32.

Pohl M, Straub H, Speckmann EJ (1992) Low magnesium-induced epileptiform discharges in guinea pig hippocampal slices: depression by the organic calcium antagonist verapamil. *Brain Res* 577:29-35.

Poleszak E (2007) Modulation of antidepressant-like activity of magnesium by serotonergic system. *J Neural Transm* 114:1129-1134.

Poleszak E, Szewczyk B, Kedzierska E, Wlaz P, Pil A, Nowak G (2004) Antidepressant- and anxiolytic-like activity of magnesium in mice. *Pharmacol Biochem Behav* 78:7-12.

Poleszak E, Szewczyk B, Wlaź A, Fidecka S, Wlaź P, Pilc A, Nowak G (2008) D-serine, a selective glycine/N-methyl-D-aspartate receptor agonist, antagonizes the antidepressant-like effects of magnesium and zinc in mice. *Pharmacol Rep* 60:996-1000.

Poleszak E, Wlaź P, Kedzierska E, Nieoczym D, Wyska E, Szymura-Oleksiak J, Fidecka S, Radziwoń-Zaleska M, Nowak G (2006) Immobility stress induces depression-like behavior in the forced swim test in mice: effect of magnesium and imipramine. *Pharmacol Rep* 58:746-52.

Poleszak E, Wlaź P, Kedzierska E, Nieoczym D, Wróbel A, Fidecka S, Pilc A, Nowak G (2007) NMDA/glutamate mechanism of antidepressant-like action of magnesium in forced swim test in mice. *Pharmacol Biochem Behav* 88:158-64.

Poleszak E, Wlaź P, Szewczyk B, Kedzierska E, Wyska E, Librowski T, Szymura-Oleksiak J, Fidecka S, Pilc A, Nowak G (2005) Enhancement of antidepressant-like activity by joint administration of imipramine and magnesium in the forced swim test: Behavioral and pharmacokinetic studies in mice. *Pharmacol Biochem Behav* 81:524-529.

Preskorn SH, Baker B, Kolluri S, Menniti FS, Krams M, Landen JW (2008) An innovative design to establish proof of concept of the antidepressant effects of the NR2B subunit selective N-methyl-D-aspartate antagonist, CP-101,606, in patients with treatment-refractory major depressive disorder. *J Clin Psychopharmacol* 28:631-637.

Rasmussen HH, Mortensen PB, Jensen IW (1989) Depression and magnesium deficiency. *Int J Psychiatry* Med 19:57-63.

Riemann D, Voderholzer U (2003) Primary insomnia: a risk factor to develop depression? *J Affect Disord* 76:255-259.

Rondón LJ, Rayssiguier Y, Mazur A (2008) Dietary inulin in mice stimulates Mg^{2+} absorption and modulates TRPM6 and TRPM7 expression in large intestine and kidney. *Magnes Res.* 21:224-31.

Sapolsky RM (1992) *Stress the aging brain and the mechanisms of neuron death*. Cambridge, MA, A Bradford Book, The MIT Press 192.

Schain RJ (1964) Cerebrospinal Fluid and Serum Cation Levels. *Arch Neurol* 11:330-3.

Scholz-Ahrens KE, Schrezenmeir J (2007) Inulin and oligofructose and mineral metabolism: the evidence from animal trials. J Nutr 137(11 Suppl):2513S-2523S.

Seelig MS, Rosanoff A (2003) *The Magnesium Factor*. New York, NY Avery Publishing Group 5.

Shealy CN (1992) The neurochemistry of depression. *Amer J Pain Management* 2:13-16.

Shiekhattar R, Aston-Jones G (1992) NMDA-receptor-mediated sensory responses of brain noradrenergic neurons are suppressed by in vivo concentrations of extracellular magnesium. *Synapse* 10:103-9.

Singewald N, Sinner C, Hetzenauer A, Sartori SB, Murck H (2004) Magnesium-deficient diet alters depression- and anxiety-related behavior in mice--influence of desipramine and Hypericum perforatum extract. *Neuropharmacology* 47:1189-1197.

Soma M, Cunnane SC, Horrobin DF, Manku MS, Honda M, Hatano M (1988) Effects of low magnesium diet on the vascular prostaglandin and fatty acid metabolism in rats. *Prostaglandins* 36:431-441.

Spiegelhalder K, Fuchs L, Ladwig J, Kyle SD, Nissen C, Voderholzer U, Feige B, Riemann D (2010) Heart rate and heart rate variability in subjectively reported insomnia. *J Sleep Res* 20:137-45.

Steiger A, Kimura M (2010) Wake and sleep EEG provide biomarkers in depression. *J Psychiatr Res* 44:242-252.

Stone M, Laughren T, Jones ML, Levenson M, Holland PC, Hughes A, Hammad TA, Temple R, Rochester G (2009) Risk of suicidality in clinical trials of antidepressants in adults: analysis of proprietary data submitted to US Food and Drug Administration. *BMJ* 339:b2880.

Thase ME, Kupfer DJ, Fasiczka AJ, Buysse DJ, Simons AD, Frank E (1997) Identifying an abnormal electroencephalographic sleep profile to characterize major depressive disorder. *Biol Psychiatry* 41:964-973.

Trivedi MH, Rush AJ, Wisniewski SR, Nierenberg AA, Warden D, Ritz L, Norquist G, Howland RH, Lebowitz B, McGrath PJ, Shores-Wilson K, Biggs MM, Balasubramani GK, Fava M; STAR*D Study Team (2006) Evaluation of outcomes with citalopram for depression using measurement-based care in STAR*D: implications for clinical practice. *Am J Psychiatry* 163:28-40.

Udupa K, Sathyaprabha TN, Thirthalli J, Kishore KR, Lavekar GS, Raju TR, Gangadhar BN (2007) Alteration of cardiac autonomic functions in patients with major depression: a study using heart rate variability measures. *J Affect Disord* 100:137-141.

Uguz F, Akman C, Kucuksarac S, Tufekci O (2009) Anti-tumor necrosis factor-alpha therapy is associated with less frequent mood and anxiety disorders in patients with rheumatoid arthritis. *Psychiatry Clin Neurosci* 63:50-55.

van den Berg JF, Tulen JH, Neven AK, Hofman A, Miedema HM, Witteman JC, Tiemeier H (2007) Sleep duration and hypertension are not associated in the elderly. *Hypertension* 50:585-589.

Walden J, Grunze H, Bingmann D, Liu Z, Düsing R (1992) Calcium antagonistic effects of carbamazepine as a mechanism of action in neuropsychiatric disorders: studies in calcium dependent model epilepsies. *Eur Neuropsychopharmacol* 2:455-62.

Walker AF, De Souza MC, Vickers MF, Abeyasekera S, Collins ML, Trinca LA (1998) Magnesium supplementation alleviates premenstrual symptoms of fluid retention. *J Womens Health* 7:1157-65.

Walker AF, Marakis G, Christie S, Byng M (2003) Mg citrate found more bioavailable than other Mg preparations in a randomised double-blind study. *Magnes Res* 16:183-91.

Walton RG, Hudak R, Green-Waite RJ (1993) Adverse reactions to aspartame: double-blind challenge in patients from a vulnerable population. *Biol Psychiatry* 34:13-7.

Weston PG (1921-22) Magnesium as a sedative. Am J Psychiatry 1:637-8. (http://george-eby-research.com/html/weston.html - accessed august 15, 2010)

Whyte KF, Addis GJ, Whitesmith R, Reid JL (1987) Adrenergic control of plasma magnesium in man. *Clin Sci (Lond)* 72:135-8.

Widmer J, Bovier P, Karege F, Raffin Y, Hilleret H, Gaillard JM, Tissot R (1992) Evolution of blood magnesium, sodium and potassium in depressed patients followed for three months. *Neuropsychobiology* 26:173-9.

Widmer J, Henrotte JG, Raffin Y, Bovier P, Hilleret H, Gaillard JM (1995) Relationship between erythrocyte magnesium plasma electrolytes and cortisol and intensity of symptoms in major depressed patients. *J Affect Disord* 34:201-9.

World Health Report 2004: *Changing History Annex Table 3: Burden of disease in DALYs by cause, sex and mortality stratum in WHO regions estimates for 2002.* Geneva, The World Health Organization.

Xiong ZG, Raouf R, Lu WY, Wang LY, Orser BA, Dudek EM, Browning MD, MacDonald JF (1998) Regulation of N-methyl-D-aspartate receptor function by constitutively active protein kinase C. *Mol Pharmacol* 54:1055-63.

Young LT, Robb JC, Levitt AJ, Cooke RG, Joffe RT (1996) Serum Mg^{2+} and Ca^{2+}/Mg^{2+} ratio in major depressive disorder. *Neuropsychobiology* 34:26-8.

Zofkova I, Kancheva RL (1995) The relationship between magnesium and calciotropic hormones. *Magnes Res* 8:77-84.

Zofková I, Lamberg-Allardt C, Kancheva RL, Stárka L (1993) Effect of hypermagnesemia on the adenohypophyseal-gonadal function, parathyroid hormone secretion and some other hormonal indicators. *Horm Metab Res.* 25:29-33.

Zorrilla EP, Luborsky L, McKay JR, Rosenthal R, Houldin A, Tax A, McCorkle R, Seligman DA, Schmidt K (2001) The relationship of depression and stressors to immunological assays: a meta-analytic review. *Brain Behavior immunity* 15:199-226.

Magnesium in drug abuse and addiction

Mihai Nechifor ✉

Department of Pharmacology, "Gr. T. Popa" University of Medicine and Pharmacy, Iasi, Romania.
✉ mnechif@yahoo.com

Abstract

Addiction to different substances is considered to be a psychiatric disorder. Magnesium reduces the intensity of addiction to opiates and psychostimulants (cocaine, amphetamine, nicotine, cocaine and others). It also decreases the auto-administration of cocaine and the relapse into cocaine and amphetamine intake, as well as reducing the experimental addiction to morphine, cocaine and other substances in animals. In heroin addicts, alcohol consumers and other drug abusers, the plasma and intracellular magnesium concentration is lower compared to healthy subjects. We consider that one of the mechanisms by which magnesium reduces the consumption of some highly addictive substances is its moderate effect of stimulating the reward system. However, other main mechanisms involved in magnesium's action are the reduction of dopamine and glutamate release at presynaptic terminals in the brain, the decrease of NO synthase activity, the stimulation of GABAergic system activity, the reduction of postsynaptic NMDA receptor activity, and the reduction of some neuromediators released by Ca^{2+} and acting at calcium channels. Apart from the action of magnesium ions during emerging addiction, administration of this cation after the appearance of withdrawal syndrome reduces the intensity of the clinical symptoms. There are data that show that stress increases the vulnerability of people to develop addiction to different substances, and also reduces drug-free time and increases the incidence of relapse in heroin addicts. Stress increases catecholamine release and stimulates magnesium release from the body. This decrease in magnesium concentration is one of the important factors that hastens relapse.

Introduction

Drug dependence is today considered a chronic medical illness (Kosten, 1998) producing significant changes in the biochemistry and function of the brain (McLellan *et al,* 2000). Koob and Le Moal (2001) presented the neurobiology of addiction from the perspective of allostasis, whereby addiction is considered a cycle of progressively increasing dysregulation of reward systems, producing compulsive use of drugs with the loss of control over drug-taking.

There is a large group of substances that result in more or less intense addiction, which is characterized by three major features: compulsive use (intake), craving, and withdrawal syndrome (when the administration is stopped). The number of substances for which a more or less intense dependence was signaled is relatively high and is growing continuously. These include the opiates (morphine, heroin, etc.), the psychodysleptics (LSD), alcohol, cannabinoids and psycho-stimulants.

The main brain structures involved in development of drug dependence are the nucleus accumbens, ventral tegmentum, the periductal grey substance, the mesolimbic system, and the nucleus coeruleus. Dysfunction in the mesolimbic system, nucleus accumbens, prefrontal cortex, and ventral tegmental area are considered involved in the mechanism of drug abuse disorders (Miguel- Hidalgo, 2009).

The molecular mechanisms involved in addiction are complicated but the main chemical neuro-mediators involved are dopamine, glutamate, serotonin, endogenous opioid peptides, nitric oxide (NO) and others. The glutamatergic, dopaminergic and opioid mechanisms are considered the most involved (Grass and Olive, 2007). These mechanisms involve not only the neurons but also the neuroglia. There are many factors that can influence the intensity of addiction or withdrawal syndrome symptoms. Amongst them are magnesium and other bivalent cations (Ruiz Martinez *et al*, 1990).

Opiates

Opiates are the cause of one of the most powerful and frequent addictions, with heroin intake especially resulting in unique medical and social problems. There are data that show that magnesium decreases the intensity of opioid addiction, with administration of Mg acetate (0.5mEq/Kg/day) reducing the experimental physical dependence (Nechifor *et al,* 2004b). The intensity of symptoms in naloxone-induced withdrawal syndrome reduced, even when magnesium administration was stopped during the period of withdrawal syndrome. Administration of Mg aspartate (732 mg mg/day) for 12 weeks in heroin-addictive patients was also beneficial (Daini *et al,* 2006; Karakiewicz *et al,* 2007). Magnesium can potentially reduce the intensity of addiction through a number of mechanisms (Figure 1), including:

- decreasing dopamine synthesis and pre-synaptic release in brain;
- decreasing the activity of glutamate NMDA receptors;
- decreasing the activity of brain NOS and NO synthesis;
- modulating the opioid coupling at brain μ receptors;
- increasing glutamate metabolism (as the main excitatory amino acid involved in addiction) by enhancing glutamate decarboxylase activity;
- increasing GABAergic activity in some brain areas by increasing the vesicular GABA transporter synthesis (Gerstein *et al*, 2005).

Magnesium also potentiates the function of $GABA_A$ receptors suggesting a putative Mg^{2+} binding site on the $GABA_A$ receptor protein (Möykkynen *et al*, 2001).

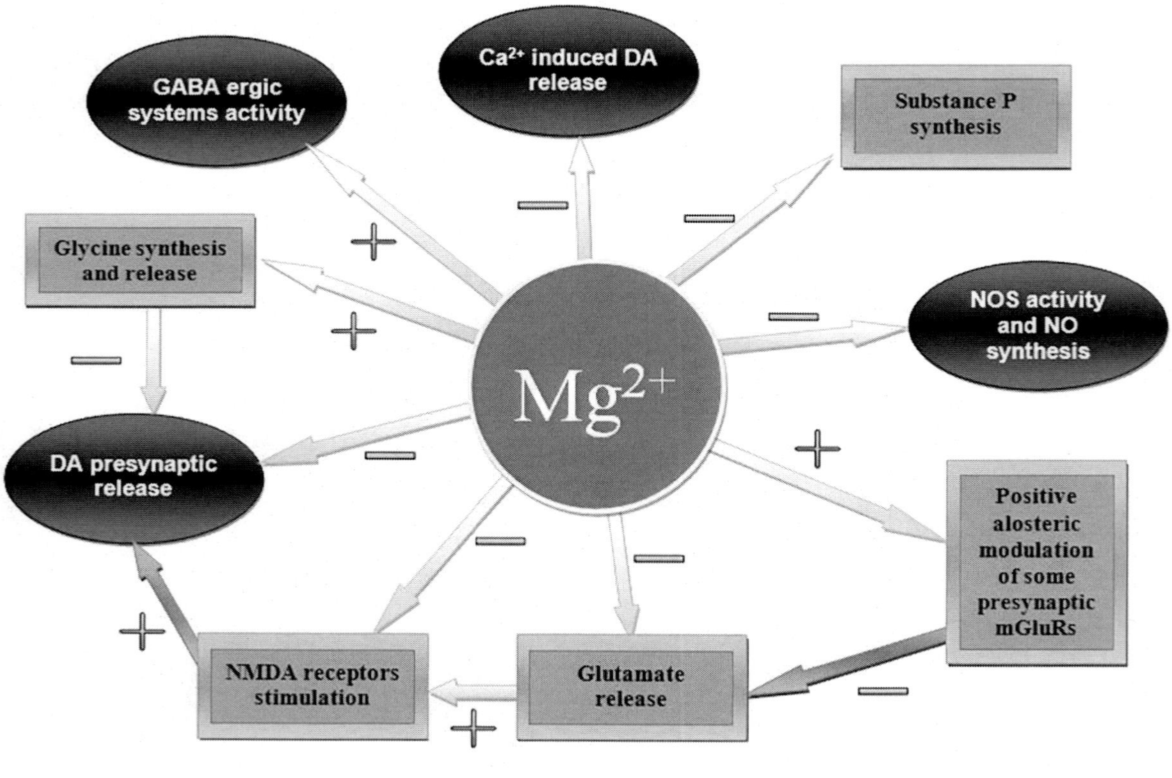

Figure 1. Mechanisms by which magnesium reduces the intensity of opiate addiction. – = inhibition; + = stimulation; DA = dopamine; NOS = nitric oxide synthase.

Dopamine is considered the most important molecule in development of pharmacodependence. Indeed, substances that result in pharmaco-dependence strongly increase the level of dopamine in midbrain. As an example, morphine produces a dose-dependent increase in dopamine-containing neurons in the substantia nigra and ventral tegmentum in rat brain (Trulson and Arasteh, 1985). Magnesium can reduce dopamine release in some brain structures through direct presynaptic action at the level of some dopaminergic synapses, by inhibiting calcium induced brain dopamine release, and by decreasing the stimulatory action of glutamate upon dopamine release. Brain dopamine level in mice is significantly increased following icv administration of $CaCl_2$. Magnesium, an antagonist to calcium, inhibits the dopamine release (Sutoo and Akiyama, 2000).

There are NMDA receptors at the level of some dopaminergic nerve endings whose stimulation also increases dopamine release. The reduction in NMDA receptor stimulation by magnesium can reduce dopamine release induced by the addictive substance (Chéramy *et al*, 1994). Extracellular Mg^{2+} blocks NMDA ion channels in a voltage dependent manner and increases the receptor affinity for glycine (Paoletti *et al*, 1995). Glycine inhibits the glutamate-evoked release of norepinephrine, and possibly other catecholamines (Johnson *et al*, 1994). In this way, the facilitating effect of magnesium on glycine linkage at its binding sites could reduce the glutamate stimulating effect of presynaptic catecholamine release (dopamine release being an essential step of addiction development). A selective inhibitor of the glycine transporter (Gly T1) significantly increased dopamine release (Bennett and Gronier, 2005). This fact indicates that glycine reduces dopamine release, in this way decreasing the intensity of addictive processes. Notably, magnesium increases both glycine synthesis and release.

Vaupel et al (1995) showed that nitric oxide synthase (NOS) inhibitors (L-nitroarginine, L-nitroarginine methyl ester) reduce several signs of opiate withdrawal (Kimes *et al,* 1993). This fact supports the involvement of nitric oxide in the pathogenic signs of the withdrawal syndrome. Mg^{2+} also inhibits NOS and we consider that in this way, it also reduces the intensity of symptoms from the withdrawal syndrome.

Chronic morphine administration decreases the NMDA receptor sensibility to Mg binding. The glutamatergic systems provide important regulation of dopamine function, while the GABA system can modulate basal levels and stimulate dopamine and glutamate release. The idea of a major role of the glutamatergic system in morphine addiction has also been proposed (Sekiya *et al*, 2004) on the basis that icv administration of DLBOA (a potent glutamate transporter inhibitor) to morphine dependent rats significantly facilitates the expression of naloxone-precipitated withdrawal. Mg^{2+} action is mainly due to its effects on neuronal activity, but also impacts upon neuroglial activity. Glial cells from CNS play an important role in regulation of glutamatergic transmission. Some substances that give rise to addiction alter the functions of astrocytes while others affect glial cell functions (Miguel-Hidalgo, 2009). Astrocyte involvement in the control of glutamate uptake and release is important for the development of addiction.

Substance P and its NK1 receptors also play a role in opiate addiction and in stress (Commons *et al,* 2010). This neuropeptide modulates NMDA receptor responses to glutamate stimulation (Parker *et al*, 1998). Magnesium reduces the synthesis and action of substance P and we believe that in this way, it can decrease the intensity of addiction. Stress induces magnesium depletion and increases the vulnerability to development of addiction or of relapse. We consider that low magnesium levels play an important role in this vulnerability.

Psychostimulants

Psychostimulants are a group of substances with various chemical structures and different mechanisms of actions, partly common, partly different, which results in a strong activation of some CNS processes. All psychostimulants induce a certain degree of addiction, but its intensity is very different. The most utilized psycho-stimulants are cocaine and its derivatives, amphetamines, caffeine and nicotine.

Cocaine

In cocaine abusers, magnesium reduced the craving for this substance (Margolin *et al*, 1992). Cocaine craving scores were 78% lower in those taking magnesium than in patients taking placebo. Mg^{2+} also reduced cocaine self-administration in patients and cocaine consumption in rats (Kantak *et al*, 1998). In cocaine addicts, the plasma level of Mg^{2+} is higher than in heroin addicts (Tonioni *et al*, 2009). NMDA receptors are essential for cocaine action in brain. NMDA antagonists and some NMDA-coupled ion channel blockers (like magnesium) may modify the cocaine effects (Kantak *et al*, 1998).

Our data shows that magnesium never determines dependence. Mg^{2+} has a moderate effect of stimulating the brain reward system. $MgC1_2$ results in an increase in time spent in the conditioning compartment in the case of conditioned place preference (CPP)(Nechifor *et al*, 2010). We consider that, apart from other mechanisms, the small stimulation on the brain reward system is important in realizing magnesium's effect of reducing cocaine consumption.

There are also data showing that genes are important for the behavior of drug abusers who have a strong genetic determination. The allelic variations related to the dopamine transporter showed a relationship with the paranoia of cocaine-dependent people (Gellertnet *et al*, 1999). We consider that genetic deficiencies in magnesium transport at the level of the neuronal membrane may be involved in the speed of addiction development and in the severity of the withdrawal syndrome.

Caffeine

Caffeine is one of the most consumed psychoactive substances, although the existence of caffeine dependence is controversial (Huges *et al*, 1992; Daly and Fredholm, 1998). There are data suggesting that caffeine results in a clinical dependence syndrome very similar to that produced by other psychoactive substances, as well as from the point of view of the caffeine-induced craving (Ogawa and Ueki, 2007). Caffeine has only week reinforcing proprieties, but the withdrawal syndrome is a reality and is similar to that produced by other drugs of abuse. Rats chronically exposed to 1 g/L caffeine a day for 20 days developed caffeine withdrawal syndrome (Dingle *et al*, 2008).

Caffeine blocks both A_I and A_2 adenosine receptors. Chronic administration of xanthines (caffeine, theophylline) causes a significant increase in the number of adenosine, nicotine and serotoninergic receptors in the brain. It also increases the number of L-type calcium channels in the neuronal membrane. The blockade of both A_1 and A_2 receptors is necessary for the full spectrum of caffeine pharmacologic effects.

The Ca^{2+} ions from the endoplasmic reticulum are very important for normal cell function. Any change in intracellular calcium concentration can have an impact on neuronal activity. Caffeine enhances the intracellular Ca^{2+} peak. This effect is higher in young animals and is altered with aging (Alshuaib *et al*, 2006). Caffeine releasable calcium ions may stimulate glutamate synthesis and release, which increases NMDA receptor activity. Wang (2007) showed that caffeine-mediated glutamate release is produced by activation of protein-kinase C pathways and involves an interaction between caffeine and presynaptic adenosine A1 receptors. The importance of caffeine action on adenosine receptors also comes out of the fact that these receptors act as regulators of neurotransmitter release in the brain (Sebastiao and Ribeiro, 2009). Adenosine stimulates all types of adenosine receptors. The omnipresence of A1, A2 and A3 receptors in CNS neurons and neuroglia reflect the major role of adenosine in modulating synaptic activity in many brain regions, including those involved in dependence.

Blockade of adenosine A_{1A} and A_{2A} receptors is involved in the development of caffeine addiction. Burgalassi et al (2009) showed that a substantial number from heavy caffeine drinkers satisfy the research criteria for dependence. Adenosine A_I and A_2 receptors have a greater involvement in addiction processes well as development of withdrawal syndrome rather than in development of caffeine dependence.

Adenosine and adenosine receptors are also involved in morphine dependence and opioid withdrawal. Adenosine is able to reduce the dose-dependent, naloxone-precipitated withdrawal in guinea pigs exposed to morphine. Caffeine significantly increases naloxone-precipitated withdrawal (Capasso, 2000). Research on guinea pig isolated ileum exposed to morphine showed that the contraction induced by naloxone was increased by caffeine (P1 antagonist) in a concentration dependent manner (Capasso and Loizzo, 2001). The caffeine effect is amplified by low Mg^{2+} concentration.

A1 receptor antagonists such as caffeine increase the presynaptic release of dopamine and glutamate. This is thought to be the main mechanism for caffeine dependence. A1 receptors are located in presynaptic areas of glutamatergic neurons and Mg can reduce caffeine dependence by blocking NMDA coupled Ca channel activity, reducing the capacity of A_1 receptor antagonists (such as caffeine) to stimulate the glutamate and dopamine release, or by reducing the glutamate stimulation of dopamine presynaptic release. It is not very clear if caffeine enhances magnesium elimination from the human body.

Amphetamine

Amphetamine is a very potent sympathomimetic agent in stimulating the CNS. The main mechanism of action is by release of biogenic amines from their storage sites in presynaptic parts of central synapses. The dependence and stereotypical behavior associated with amphetamine is induced by stimulation of dopamine release. Disturbance of perception and psychotic behavior may be due to release of serotonin and dopamine in the mesolimbic system (Hoffman, 2001). There is also a small stimulating effect of amphetamine on some serotonin receptors. Increased intraneuronal Mg^{2+} concentration is thought to reduce the intensity of psychostimulant addiction. Evidence in favor is the fact that Li^+ (which increases intracellular magnesium concentration) has an antagonistic effect with amphetamine at the level of the nucleus accumbens. Li^+ also decreased dopaminergic transmission stimulated by amphetamine (Gray *et al,* 1997). After administration of 1 mg/kg amphetamine, dopamine levels increases by 427% versus the basal level. This dopamine release is calcium potentiated. The replacement of calcium by magnesium reduces the response to amphetamine administration (Warburton *et al,* 1996). It was also remarked that structural brain abnormalities are associated with amphetamine abuse. These differences included lower cortical gray matter quantity and higher striatal volume than in normal subjects (Berman *et al*, 2008). We do not know how magnesium influences these modifications.

Nicotine

Existing data shows that nicotine addiction develops in chronic smokers with over 10-20 cigarettes/day. Chronic smoking decreases the level of serum magnesium (Niemela *et al* 1997; Nechifor *et al*, 2004a), while magnesium administration decreases the number of smoked cigarettes as well as nicotine addiction. Specifically, 2 ampoules/day Magne-B6 administration for four weeks significantly decreased the number of cigarettes smoked by heavy smokers (smokers with over 20 cigarettes/day) (Nechifor *et al*, 2004a). The Fagerstrom score was significantly reduced in the smoker group that received magnesium, from 7.93 ± 0.17 before magnesium to 6.78 ± 0.18 after magnesium ($p<0.05$). Mg^{2+} can potentially reduce nicotine addiction by:

- acting as a partial antagonist of calcium entry into neurons, thereby decreasing glutamate release and glutamatergic transmission which is stimulated by nicotine;
- decreasing nicotine-induced pre-synaptic release of dopamine and other catecholamines;
- increasing magnesium concentration in the neuron producing a decrease in sodium concentration. This decreases the stimulant effect of nicotine on nicotine receptors.
- decreasing the nicotine addictive effect by diminishing the nicotine effect on GABA synthesis. Nicotine diminishes GABA synthesis and release in some brain areas by stimulation of nicotine presynaptic receptors;
- enhancing some of the GABA effects and diminishing some effects of the excitatory amino acids in drug dependence. GABA antagonizes some of the glutamate-induced stimulatory effects of NMDA receptors.

Like nicotine, synaptically released acetylcholine stimulates nicotinic receptors and in this way enhances glutamatergic activity (Guo *et al*, 2005).

The release of DA from the nucleus accumbens and substantia nigra was stimulated by glutamate, and nicotine enhanced this release (Marien *et al,* 1983). Such DA secretion induced by glutamate and nicotine is Ca^{2+} dependent and was inhibited by Mg^{2+}. We think that this is an essential mechanism for magnesium action to reduce the nicotine dependence.

Ethanol dependence

Alcohol induced dependence is one of the most widespread dependencies. Abuse and addiction depend, at least partially, on the activation of mesolimbic dopaminergic systems. The activation of these systems is achieved directly by ethanol, but also by acetaldehyde, which results from ethanol metabolism. Acetaldehyde increases dopaminergic neuronal activity in the nucleus accumbens, ventral tegmental area and in other parts of the CNS (Foddai *et al*, 2004; Diana *et al*, 2008). Alcohol-dehydrogenase drastically inhibits the effects of ethanol on dopaminergic neurons of the ventral tegmental area (VTA). We consider that magnesium could reduce the stimulating effect of ethanol on dopaminergic systems by directly reducing the presynaptic release of dopamine, but also by decreasing acetaldehyde production.

There is important evidence implicating the endogenous opioids in the processes of reward and reinforcement (Gianoulakis, 2009). Endogenous opioids, like morphine, induce an increase of dopamine concentration in the nucleus accumbens, which is considered the most important structure for drug addiction. This is considered a common effect for many drugs involved in abuse. Ethanol increases beta endorphin release. The stimulation of opioid receptors (especially of μ receptors) seems to be important for ethanol addiction, with low morphine doses increasing ethanol consumption (Hertz, 1997). Magnesium reduces receptor binding of morphine and other μ receptor agonists (Mendez *et al*, 2001; Rodriguez *et al*, 1992). This way, magnesium could reduce the stimulation of dopamine synthesis produced by large quantities of opioid peptides, which themselves are induced by ethanol in the nucleus accumbens and VTA. We therefore consider that Mg^{2+} could decrease ethanol addiction and hypomagnesemia could increase alcohol consumption. Mendez et al (2001) showed that the reinforcing properties of ethanol may be partially mediated by ethanol regulation of μ receptors in dopaminergic neurons from mesolimbic systems. A modulation of μ receptors from the frontal and prefrontal cortex is also possible.

There are also findings that suggest that mGluR5 receptors modulate ethanol self-administration in rats (Schroeder *et al,* 2005). Dopamine is the most important neurotransmitter involved in the reward mechanism and it influences the development of alcohol dependence and relapse. Two polymorphisms of the D2 dopamine receptors seem to suffer 2.5 times more risk to develop ethanol dependence (Prasad *et al*, 2010). Embry and Lippman (1987) considered that magnesium deficiency plays an important role in the alcohol-withdrawal system. There are data that show that magnesium administration decreases the intensity of symptoms from the withdrawal syndrome. The alcohol induces hypomagnesemia and increases urinary magnesium loss. Low concentrations of ethanol deplete free intracellular magnesium (Babu *et al*, 1999). Consistent with Shane and Flink (1992), we believe that magnesium deficiency is involved not only in the intensity of the alcohol withdrawal, but also in the development of alcohol dependence.

The NMDA receptors from the nucleus accumbens and the mesolimbic structures are involved in drug reward and reinforcement. Ethanol sensitivity of NMDA receptors from the nucleus accumbens is important for ethanol induced neuroadaptation of the reward system. Chronic alcohol administration results in an increased glutamate binding to the NMDA receptors (Hu and Ticku, 1995). This highlights the importance of glutamate action in development of alcohol addiction. The activation of NMDA receptors in rats increases during the alcohol withdrawal syndrome (Sanna *et al* 1993). Electrolyte abnormalities are common in chronic alcoholics and during alcohol withdrawal syndrome (Stasinkyniene, 2002). Alcohol consumption is one of the major causes for hypomagnesemia, which is one of the most important cation imbalances in alcoholic patients and during withdrawal (Carl and Halzbach, 1994). In alcoholic patients urinary magnesium loss increases 2-3 fold (Romain, 2008) and brain intracellular Mg^{2+} level are reduced (Li *et al*, 2001; Pasternak, 1999). Low ethanol concentrations deplete type 2 astrocytes of intracellular free magnesium (Babu *et al*, 1999). The Mg^{2+} dependent decay off-rate of NMDA miniature synaptic currents (mEPSes) was also significantly reduced by ethanol (Zhang *et al*, 2005), suggesting that ethanol not only contributes to increase the release of magnesium from the body, but also to increase magnesium's effect at the NMDA receptor level.

Mg^{2+} ions modulate neuronal excitability and are involved in alcohol-related behaviors. Uusi-Oukari et al (2001) found that the putative Mg^{2+} binding sites differ between alcohol insensitive (AT) and alcohol sensitive (ANT) rats lines. In the presence of GABA, the effect of low Mg^{2+} concentration was higher in cerebral cortex and in the caudate-putamen of AT rats than in the ANT animals. Alcohol sensitive rats have alterations of the alpha 6 subunit – containing GABA A receptors. It is possible that these receptors might be involved in the sensitivity of different lines of rats to alcohol and also in the different sensibility of animals to sedative drugs (Uusi-Oukari M *et al*, 2001). Magnesium administration only during the withdrawal syndrome of ethanol addicts reduced the clinical symptoms.

Hallucinogens (psychedelic substances)

Hallucinogens are substances that induce hallucinations, disorders of thinking and delusions. The most potent hallucinogen is LSD (lysergic acid diethylamide) that produces a significant hallucinogen effect at a dose of as little as 25-50 ug. Other psychedelic drugs are derivatives with indolaminic structure (psylocibine, DMT and others) and substances with phenethylaminic structure (mescaline, MDMA, and DOM). The precise mechanism of action of these substances is not yet known, but a positive correlation between the relative affinity of hallucinogens for serotonin 5-HT2 receptors and their potency to induce hallucination has been observed (Titeler *et al*, 1988).

The hallucinogens (LSD, phencyclidine, psilocybin, mescaline, DMT and others) give a strong psychic dependence, but the concept of addiction is controversial. The presence of withdrawal from hallucinogens has not been clearly established because these drugs don't seem to induce physical dependence. The most utilized hallucinogen is LSD.

There are data that favor the idea that all phencyclidine receptors in the brain are associated with NMDA receptors. Notably, there is an interaction of L-glutamate and magnesium with the phencyclidine recognition site in the brain (Loo *et al*, 1987). The agonists of NMDA receptors induce a high affinity state in the phencyclidine receptors. This is another possibility by which Mg^{2+} can influence phencyclidine action. Mg^{2+} inhibits MK-801 (a ligand for the NMDA ion channel phencyclidine site) binding in the cortex (Chahal *et al*, 1998). It is possible for magnesium to also decrease phencyclidine action this way. However, Rothman et al (1989) demonstrated the existence of a high-affinity phencyclidine binding site associated with the dopamine reuptake carrier. The hallucinogen could therefore influence synaptic dopamine concentration. It is still unknown how Mg^{2+} influences dopamine reuptake.

Regarding other hallucinogens such as psilocin (from Psilocybe mushrooms) and phenylethyl-amine, subchronic experimental intoxication in rats disturbs magnesium concentrations (Majdanik *et al*, 2007). Low magnesium concentration also resulted from chronic mescaline and LSD administration. Hypomagnesemia is associated with an increased intracellular entrance of Ca^{2+} in these conditions. In cerebral vasospasm, which appears in chronic hallucinogen intoxication, both magnesium and the calcium antagonist verapamil block this effect (Altura and Altura, 1983). The NMDA receptor is coupled with an ion channel and has regulatory sites for phencyclidine, glycine, and also for magnesium and zinc. In this way, it might be possible for an interaction between magnesium and phencyclidine to exist with respect to the activity of NMDA receptors.

Lerma et al (1991) suggest that interactions between Mg^{2+} and phencyclidine at the level of the NMDA channels are competitive. Indeed, 0.5 mM Mg caused a four-fold decrease in phencyclidine potency. In vitro incubation of phencyclidine stimulated brain slides with 1.2 mM $MgC1_2$ shows that Na efflux produced by the NMDA receptor stimulation is decreased.

Benzodiazepines

Magnesium aspartate decreases benzodiazepine addiction (lorazepam, alprazolam, or bromazepam) (Hantouche *et al*, 1998). The decrease in addiction intensity was manifested as prolonged delay in benzodiazepine reintake, reduction of withdrawal intensity, and reduction of anxiety during benzodiazepine discontinuation. In benzodiazepine withdrawal syndrome, strong anxiety is present. This phenomenon is associated with a potentiation of AMPA receptor activity and AMPA receptor currents in hippocampal pyramidal neurons. Calcium/ Calmodulin–dependent protein kinase II has a contribution by enhancing the glutamatergic synaptic activity during benzodiazepine withdrawal (Shen *et al*, 2010). In some patients that received Mg L-aspartate, cessation of benzodiazepines was obtained without onset of withdrawal syndrome. It is possible that magnesium ions acting at the level of AMPA receptors influence the calcium/calmodulin dependent PK II to reduce the anxiety and other clinical symptoms present in benzodiazepine withdrawal syndrome.

Cannabinoids

Delta 9-tetrahydrocannabinol is the principal psychoactive compound in marijuana, although it is widely used in a number of forms. It induces an important psychic dependence, but only a modest physical dependence. Bac and Germain Fattal (2006) showed that magnesium deficiency increased the neurotoxicity of THC at low doses in rats. Hyperagressiveness and THC induced muricidal behavior in rats was also increased by magnesium deficiency. Otherwise, there is very little data regarding the influence of magnesium and other bivalent cations in cannabinoid addiction.

Conclusion

Regarding the involvement of magnesium in addiction, we consider that is important not only at the neuronal level, but also at neuroglial level. According to data that shows that the glial cells are involved in addictive behavior mainly through the regulation of glutamate transport and activity, we believe that magnesium acts at the neuroglial level by reducing the action of glutamate. There are NMDA receptors at the glial level (in oligodendrocytes, microglia and astrocytes) (Verkhratsky and Kirchhoff, 2007), and at both these receptors and the neuronal NMDA receptor level, there is a calcium channel that can be influenced by magnesium.

We consider that the ability of magnesium to reduce addiction to different substances and reduce the intensity of addiction to different substances is essentially related to the association of two different factors:

- its ability to produce a moderate stimulation of the brain reward system (Nechifor *et al*, 2010);
- its capacity to reduce the activity of glutamatergic substances, importantly involved in compulsive use disorders.

Compulsive drug-taking behavior is an important characteristic element in addiction. The existence of a strong reinforcement activity is a determining factor for drug addiction (Koob and Bloom, 1988). Reducing the intensity of dependence on different compounds involves reducing their reinforcing proprieties. Response-reinforcement learning is dependent on NMDA receptor activation (Kelley *et al*, 1997). We consider that magnesium reduces reinforcing proprieties of different compounds by action on these NMDA receptors.

References

Alshuaib WB, Cherian SP, Hasan MY, Fahim MA (2006) Modulation of neuronal [Ca2+]i by caffeine is altered with aging. *Int J Dev Neurosci* 24:389-94.

Altura BM, Altura BT (1983) Pharmacologic inhibition of cerebral vasospasm in ischemia, hallucinogen ingestion, and hypomagnesemia: barbiturates, calcium antagonists, and magnesium. *Am J Emerg Med* 1:180-90.

Babu AN, Cheng TP, Zhang A, Altura BT, Altura BM (1999) Low concentrations of ethanol deplete type-2 astrocyte of intracellular free magnesium. *Brain Res Bull* 50: 59-62.

Bac P, German-Fattal M (2006), Potentiation of Delta9-tetrahydrocannabinol (THC) effects by magnesium deficiency in the rat. *Ann Pharm Fr* 64:207-13.

Bennet S., Gronier B (2005), Modulation of striatal dopamine release in vitro by agonists of the glycine B site of NMDA receptors.Interactions with antypsychotics. *Eur J Pharmacol* 527:52-9.

Berman S, O'Neill J, Fears S, Bartzokis G, London ED (2008) Abuse of amphetamines and structural abnormalities in the brain. Ann NY Acad Sci 1141:195-220.

Burgalassi A, Ramacciotti CE, Bianchi M, Coli E, Polese L, Bondi E, Massimetti G, Dell'osso L (2009) Caffeine consumption among eating disorder patients: epidemiology, motivations, and potential of abuse. *Eat Weight Disord* 14:212-18.

Carl G, Holzbach E (1994) Reversible hypokalemia and hypomagnesemia during alcohol withdrawal syndrome. *Nervenarzt* 6 :206-11.

Capasso A (2000) Adenosine receptors are involved in the control of acute naloxone-precipitated withdrawal: in vitro evidence. *Life Sci* 66:873-83.

Capasso A, Loizzo A (2001) Purinoreceptors are involved in the control of acute morphine withdrawal. *Life Sci* 69:2179-88.

Chahal H, D'Souza SW, Barson AJ, Slater P (1998) Modulation by magnesium of N-methyl-D-aspartate receptors in developing human brain. *Arch Dis Child Fetal Neonatal Ed* 78:F116-20.

Cheramy A, L'Hirondel M, Godehen G, Artaud F, Glowinsky J (1998) Direct and indirect presynaptic control of dopamine release by excitatory amino acids. *Amino Acids* 14: 63-9.

Commons KG (2010) Neuronal pathways linking substance P to drug addiction and stress. *Brain Res* 1314:175-82.

Daini S, Tonioni F, Barra A, Lai C, Lacerenza R, Sgambato A, Bria P, Cittadini A (2006) Serum magnesium profile in heroin addicts –according to psychiatric comorbidity. *Magnes Res* 19:162-6.

Daly JW, Fredholm BB (1998) Caffeine- an atypical drug of dependence. *Drug Alcohol Depend* 51:199-206.

Diana M, Peana AT, Sirca D, Lintas A, Melis M, Enrico P (2008) Crucial role of acetaldehyde in alcohol activation of the mesolimbic dopamine system. *Ann N Y Acad Sci* 1139:307-17.

Dingle RN, Dreumont-Boudreau SE, Lolordo VM (2008) Caffeine dependence in rats: effects of exposure duration and concentration. *Physiol Behav* 95:252-57.

Embry CK, Lippmann S (1987) Use of magnesium sulfate in alcohol withdrawal. *Am Fam Physician* 35:167-70.

Foddai M, Dosia G, Spiga S, Diana M (2004) Acetaldehyde increases dopaminergic neuronal activity in the VTA. *Neuropsychopharmacology* 29:530-6.

Gass JT, Olive MF (2008) Glutamatergic substrates of drug addiction and alcoholism. *Biochem Pharmacol* 75:218-265.

Gerstein M, Huleihel M, Mane R, Stilman M, Kashtuzki I, Hallak M, Golan H (2005) Remodeling of hippocampal GABAergic system in adult offspring after maternal hypoxia and magnesium sulphate load: immunohistochemical study. *Exp Neurol* 196:18-29.

Gelernter J, Cubells JF, Kidd JR, Pakstis AJ, Kidd KK (1999) Population studies of polymorphisms of the serotonin transporter protein gene. *Am J Med Genet* 88:61-6.

Gianoulakis C (2009) Endogenous opioids and addiction to alcohol and other drugs of abuse. *Curr Top Med Chem* 9:999-101.

Gray JA, Moran PM, Grigoryan G, Peters SL, Young AM, Joseph MH (1997) Latent inhibition: the nucleus accumbens connection revisited. *Behav Brain Res* 88:27-34.

Guo JZ, Liu Y, Sorenson EM, Chiappinelli VA (2005) Synaptically released and exogenous ACh activates different nicotinic receptors to enhance evoked glutamatergic transmission in the lateral geniculate nucleus. *J Neurophysiol* 94:2549-60.

Hantouche EG, Guelfi JD, Comet D (1998) Alpha-betha L-aspartate magnesium in treatment of chronic benzodiazepine abuse: controlled and double blind study versus placebo. *Encephale* 24:469-79.

Hernandes MS, De Magaihaes L, Troncone LRP (2005) Glycine stimulates the release of labeled acethylcholine but not dopamine nor glutamate from superfused rat striatal tissue. *Brain Res Bull* 26:418-30.

Herz A (1997) Endogenous opioid systems and alcohol addiction. *Psychopharmacology (Berl)* 129:99-111.

Hoffman BB (2001) Cathecolamines, sympathomimetic drugs, and adrenergic receptor antagonists, In: *Goodman & Gilman's The Pharmacological Basis of Therapeutics* (Hardman JG, Limbird LE, eds.) Tenth International Edition, Mc Graw Hill, New York, 215-68.

Hu X, Ticku MK (1995) Chronic ethanol treatment upregulates the NMDA receptor function and binding in mammalian cortical neurons. *Mol Brain Research* 30:347-56.

Hughes JR, Oliveto AH, Helzer JE, Higgins ST, Bickel WK (1992) Should caffeine abuse, dependence, or withdrawal be added to DSM-IV and ICD-10? *Am J Psychiatry* 149:33-40.

Kantak KM, Edwards MA, O'Connor TP (1998) Modulation of the discriminative stimulus and rate-altering effects of cocaine by competitive and non-competitive N-methyl-D-aspartate antagonists. *Pharmacol Biochem Behav* 59(1):159-69.

Karakiewicz B, Kozielec T, Brodowski ., Chlubek D, Noceri I, Starczewski A, Brodowska A, Laszczylnska M (2007) Serum magnesium concentration in drug addicted patients. *Magnes Res* 20:55-7.

Kelley AE, Smith-Roe SL, Holahan MR (1997) Response-reinforcement learning is dependent on N-methyl-D-aspartate receptor activation in the nucleus accumbens core. *Proc Natl Acad Sci U S A* 94:12174-9.

Kimes AS, Vaupel DB, London ED (1993) Atenuation of some signs of opioid withdrawal by inhibitors of nitric oxide synthase. *Psychopharmacology* 112:521-24.

Koob GF, Bloom FE (1988) Cellular and molecular mechanisms of drug dependence. *Science* 242:715-23.

Koob GF, Le Moal M (2001) Drug addiction, dysregulation of reward, and allostasis. *Neuropsychopharmacology* 24:97-129.

Kosten TR (1998) Addiction as a brain disease. *Am J Psychiatry* 155:711-13.

Lerman J, Zukin RS, Bennett MV (1991) Interaction of Mg2+ and phencyclidine in use-dependent block of NMDA channels. *Neurosci Lett* 123:187-91.

Li W, Zheng T, Babu A., Altura BT, Gupta RK, Altura BM (2001) Importance of magnesium ions in development of tolerance to ethanol: studies on cultured cerebral vascular smooth muscle cells, type 2 astrocytes and intact rat brain. *Brain Res Bull* 56: 153-58.

Li-Smerin Y, Johnson JW (1996) Effects of intracellular Mg2+ on channel gating and steady-state responses of the NMDA receptor in cultured rat neurons. *J Physiol* 491:137-50.

Loo PS, Braunwalder AF, Lehmann J, Williams M, Sills MA (1987) Interaction of L-glutamate and magnesium with phencyclidine recognition sites in rat brain: evidence for multiple affinity states of the phencyclidine/N-methyl-D-aspartate receptor complex. *Mol Pharmacol* 32:820-30.

Majdanik S, Borowiak K, Brzezńska M, Machoy-Mokrzyńska A (2007) Concentration of selected microelements in blood serum of rats exposed to the action of psilocin and phenylethylamine. *Ann Acad Med Stetin* 53:153-8.

Marien M, Brien J, Jhamandas K (1983) Regional release of 3H dopamine from rat brain in vitro effects of opioids on release induced by potassium, nicotine and l-glutamic acid. *Can J Physiol Pharmacol* 61: 43-60.

Margolin A, Kantak K, Copenhaver M, Avant SSK (2003) A preliminary controlled investigation of magnesium L-aspartate hydrochloride for illicit cocaine and opiate use in methadone-maintained patients. *J Addict Dis* 22: 49-61.

McLellan AT, Lewis DC, O'Brien CP, Kleber HD (2000) Drug dependence, a chronic medical illness. *JAMA* 284:1689-95.

Méndez M, Leriche M, Calva JC (2001) Acute ethanol administration differentially modulates mu opioid receptors in the rat meso-accumbens and mesocortical pathways. *Brain Res Mol Brain Res* 94:148-56.

Miguel-Hidalgo JJ (2009) The role of glial cells in drug abuse. *Curr Drug Abuse Rev* 2:72-82.

Moykkyen T, Uusi-Oukari M, Heikkila J, Lovinger DM, Luddens H, Korpi ER(2001) Magnesium potentiation of the function of native and recombinant GABA A receptors. *Neuroreport* 12:2175-9.

Nechifor M, Chelarescu D, Mândreci I, Cartas N (2004) Magnesium influence on nicotine pharmaco-dependence and smoking. *Magnes Res* 17:176-81.

Nechifor M, Chelarescu D, Miftode M (2004) Magnesium influence on morphine-induced pharmacodependence in rats. *Magnes Res* 17:7-13

Nechifor M, Chelarescu D, Ciubotariu D (2010) The influence of magnesium-induced stimulation of the reward system. *Magnesium Res* 23:41-7.

Niemela JE, Cecco SA, Rehak NN, Elin RJ (1997) The effect of smoking on the serum ionized magnesium concentration is method-dependent. *Arch Pathol Lab Med* 121:1087-92.

Ogawa N, Ueki H (2007) Clinical importance of caffeine dependence and abuse. *Psychiatry Clin Neurosci* 61:263-68.

Paoletti P, Neyton J, Ascher P (1995) Glycine-independent and subunit-specific potentiation of NMDA response by extra cellular Mg^{2+}. *Neuron* 15 :1109-20.

Parker D, Zhang W, Grillner S (1998) Substance P modulates NMDA responses and causes long-term protein synthesis –dependent modulation of the lamprey locomotor network. *J Neurosci* 18:4800-13.

Pasternak K (1999) Tissue concentrations of magnesium in rats receiving various dosages of ethano. *Magnes Res* 12:167-70.

Prasad P, Ambekar A, Vaswani M (2010) Dopamine D2 receptor polymorphisms and susceptibility to alcohol dependence in Indian males: a preliminary study. *BMC Med Genet* 11:24.

Rodriguez FD, Bardaji E, Trayno Jr R (1992) Differential effects of Mg^{2+} and other divalent cation on the binding of tritiated opioid ligands. *J Neurochem* 591:467-72.

Romani AM (2008) Magnesium homeostasis and alcohol consumption. *Magnes Res* 21:197-204.

Rothman RB, Reid AA, Monn JA, Jacobson AE, Rice KC (1989) The psychotomimetic drug phencyclidine labels two high affinity binding sites in guinea pig brain: evidence for N-methyl-D-aspartate-coupled and dopamine reuptake carrier-associated phencyclidine binding sites. *Mol Pharmacol* 36:887-96.

Ruiz Martinez M, Gil Extremera B, Maldonaldo MD, Cantero-Hinojosa J, Moreno-Abadia V (1990) *Klin Wochenschr* 68:507-511.

Sanna E, Serra M, Cossu A, Colombo G, Follesa P, Cuccheddu T, Concas A, Biegio G (1993) Chronic ethanol intoxication induces differential effects in GABA A and NMDA receptor function in the rat brain. *Alcoholism: Clin Exp Research* 17:115-23.

Schroeder JP, Overstreet DH, Hodge CW (2005) The mGluR5 antagonist MPEP decreases operant ethanol self-administration during maintenance and after repeated alcohol-deprivations in alcohol-preferring (P) rats. *Psychopharmacology* 179:262-7.

Sebastião AM, Ribeiro JA (2009) Tuning and fine-tuning of synapses with adenosine. *Curr Neuropharmacol* 7:180-94.

Sekiya Y, Nakagawa T, Ozawa T, Minami M, Satoh M (2004) Facilitation of morphine withdrawal symptoms and morphine-induced conditioned place preference by a glutamate transporter inhibitor DL-threo-beta-benzyloxyaspartate in rats. *Eur J Pharmacol* 485:201-10.

Shane SR, Flink EB (1991-1992) Magnesium deficiency in alcohol addiction and withdrawal. *Magnes Trace Elem* 10:263-8.

Shen G, Van Sickle BJ, Tietz EI (2010) Calcium /calmodulin-dependent protein kinase II mediates hippocampal glutamatergic plasticity during benzodiazepine withdrawal. *Neuropsychopharmacology* 35:1890-9.

Stasiukyniene V (2002) Blood plasma potassium, sodium and magnesium level in chronic alcoholism during alcohol withdrawal. *Medicina (Kannas)* 38:892-5.

Rosenzweig-Haugbol S, Ebert B, Ulrichsen J (2005) Upregulation of glutamate receptor subtypes during alcohol withdrawal in rats. *Alcohol Alcoholism* 40(2):89-95.

Sutoo D, Akiyama K (2000) Effect of magnesium on calcium-dependent brain function that prolongs ethanol-induced sleeping time in mice. *Neurosci Lett* 204:5-8.

Titeler M, Lyon RA, Glennon RA (1988) Radioligand binding evidence implicates the brain 5-HT2 receptors as a site of action for LSD and phenylisopropyl-amine hallucinogens. *Psychopharmacology* 94:213-6.

Tonioni F, Martinotti G, Barra A, Martinelli D, Autullo G, Rinaldi C, Tedeschi C, Janiri L, Bria P (2009) Cocaine use disorders and serum magnesium profile, *Neuropsychobiology* 53:159-64.

Trulson ME, Arasteh K (1985) Morphine increases the activity of midbrain dopamine neurons in vitro. *Eur J Pharmacol* 114:105-9.

Uusi-Oukari M, Makela R, Soini S, Korpi ER (2001) Cation modulation of GABA A receptors in brain section of AT and ANT rats. *Alcohol* 25:69-75.

Vaupel DB, Kimes AS, London ED (1995) Nitric oxide synthase inhibitors.Preclinical studies of potential use for the treatment of opioid withdrawal. *Neuropsychopharmacology* 13 :315-322

Verkhratsky A, Kirchhoff F (2007) NMDA Receptors in glia. *Neuroscientist* 13:28-37.

Wang SJ (2007) Caffeine facilitation of glutamate release from rat cerebral cortex nerve terminals (synaptosomes) through activation protein kinase C pathway: an interaction with presynaptic adenosine A1 receptors. *Synapse* 61:401-11.

Warburton EC, Mitchell SN, Joseph MH (1996) Calcium dependence of sensitised dopamine release in rat nucleus accumbens following amphetamine challenge: implications for the disruption of latent inhibition. *Behav Pharmacol* 7:119-29.

West O, Roderique-Davies G (2008) Development and initial validation of a caffeine craving questionnaire. *J Psychopharmacol* 22:80-91.

Xing H, Azimi-Zonooz A, Shuttleworth CW, Connor JA (2004) Caffeine releasable stores of Ca^{2+} show depletion prior to the final steps in delayed CA1 neuronal death. *J Neurophysiol* 92:2960-7.

Zhang TA, Hendricson AW, Morrisett RA (2005) Dual synaptic sites of D1-dopaminergic regulation of ethanol sensitivity of NMDA receptors in nucleus accumbens. *Synapse* 58:30-44.

Made in United States
North Haven, CT
10 November 2026

22065386R00193